Psychiatric Clinical Skills

Psychiatric Clinical Skills

David S. Goldbloom, MD, FRCPC
Professor of Psychiatry,
University of Toronto;
Senior Medical Advisor,
Education and Public Affairs,
Centre for Addiction and Mental Health,
Toronto, Canada

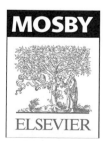

MOSBY

ELSEVIER

ELSEVIER
MOSBY

1600 John F. Kennedy Blvd.
Ste 1800
Philadelphia, PA 19103-2899

PSYCHIATRIC CLINICAL SKILLS

ISBN 13: 978-0-323-03123-3
ISBN 10: 0-323-03123-4

Notice

Knowledge and best practice in this field are constantly changing. As new research and experience broaden our knowledge, changes in practice, treatment and drug therapy may become necessary or appropriate. Readers are advised to check the most current information provided (i) on procedures featured or (ii) by the manufacturer of each product to be administered, to verify the recommended dose or formula, the method and duration of administration, and contraindications. It is the responsibility of the practitioner, relying on their own experience and knowledge of the patient, to make diagnoses, to determine dosages and the best treatment for each individual patient, and to take all appropriate safety precautions. To the fullest extent of the law, neither the Publisher nor the Editors assume any liability for any injury and/or damage to persons or property arising out or related to any use of the material contained in this book.

Library of Congress Cataloging-in-Publication Data

Psychiatric clinical skills / [edited by] David S. Goldbloom.
    p. ; cm.
    Includes index.
  ISBN 0-323-03123-4
  1. Psychiatry. 2. Clinical competence. I. Goldbloom, David S.
  [DNLM: 1. Mental Disorders–diagnosis. 2. Mental Disorders–therapy. 3. Psychology, Clinical–methods. WM 141 P9733 2006]
RC454.4.P759 2006
616.89–dc22   2005052276

Editor: *Susan F. Pioli*
Editorial Assistant: *Joan Ryan*
Project Manager: *David Saltzberg*

Printed in the United States of America.

Last digit is the print number: 9 8 7 6 5 4 3 2 1

For Will, Daniel, and Nancy

Contents

Contributing Authors

SUSAN E. ABBEY, MD, FRCPC
Associate Professor of Psychiatry, University of Toronto;
Director of Program in Medical Psychiatry, University
Health Network, Toronto, Canada

LISA FRANCESCA ANDERMANN, MPHIL, MDCM, FRCPC
Assistant Professor of Psychiatry, Culture, Community and
Health Studies, University of Toronto; Staff Psychiatrist,
Mount Sinai Hospital, Toronto, Canada

PAUL D. ARNOLD, MD, FRCPC
Fellow in Psychiatry, University of Toronto; Staff
Psychiatrist, Child, Youth, and Family Program, Centre for
Addiction and Mental Health, Toronto, Canada

R. MICHAEL BAGBY, PHD, CPSYCH
Professor of Psychiatry, University of Toronto; Director of
Clinical Research, Centre for Addiction and Mental
Health, Toronto, Canada

JOSEPH H. BEITCHMAN, MD
Professor and Head of the Division of Child and
Adolescent Psychiatry, University of Toronto; Clinical
Director of Child, Youth, and Family Program, Centre for
Addiction and Mental Health; TD Bank Financial Group
Chair in Child and Adolescent Psychiatry, The Hospital for
Sick Children, Toronto, Canada

ASH BENDER, MD, FRCPC
Lecturer, Department of Psychiatry, University of
Toronto; Medical Director, Psychological Trauma
Program, Centre for Addiction and Mental Health,
Toronto, Canada

ELSPETH A. BRADLEY, BSc, PHD, MBBS, FRCPC, FRCPSYCH
Associate Professor of Psychiatry, University of Toronto;
Psychiatrist-in-Chief, Biomedical Services and Research
Division, Surrey Place Center, Toronto, Canada; Staff,
Department of Psychiatry, Hamilton Health Sciences,
Hamilton, Canada; Consultant Psychiatrist in Learning
Disabilities, Learning Disabilities Service, West Resource
Centre, Cornwall Partnership Trust, Cornwall, United
Kingdom

PIER BRYDEN, MD, MPHIL, FRCPC
Assistant Professor of Psychiatry, University of Toronto;
Staff Psychiatrist, Child and Adolescent Psychiatry,
The Hospital for Sick Children, Toronto, Canada

CORINE E. CARLISLE, MD, FRCPC
Clinical Fellow in Child and Adolescent Psychiatry,
University of Toronto; The Hospital for Sick Children,
Toronto, Canada

BARBARA J. DORIAN, MD, FRCPC
Assistant Professor of Psychiatry, University of Toronto;
Staff Psychiatrist, Mood and Anxiety Program, Centre for
Addiction and Mental Health, Toronto, Canada

NATHAN B. EPSTEIN, MD, FRCPC
Professor Emeritus of Psychiatry, Brown University
School of Medicine, Providence, Rhode Island;
Psychiatrist-in-Chief Emeritus, St. Luke's Hospital,
New Bedford, Massachusetts

ANTHONY FEINSTEIN, MPHIL, PHD, FRCPC
Professor of Psychiatry, University of Toronto; Staff
Psychiatrist, Sunnybrook and Women's College Health
Sciences Centre, Toronto, Canada

DAVID S. GOLDBLOOM, MD, FRCPC
Professor of Psychiatry, University of Toronto;
Senior Medical Advisor, Education and Public Affairs,
Centre for Addiction and Mental Health, Toronto, Canada

BENJAMIN I. GOLDSTEIN, MD, PhD
Resident, Department of Psychiatry, University of
Toronto; Sunnybrook and Women's College Health
Sciences Centre, Toronto, Canada

CURTIS HANDFORD, BSc, MD, CCFP
Staff Physician, Nicotine Dependence Clinic, Centre for
Addiction and Mental Health; Staff Physician,
Department of Family and Community Medicine, Inner
City Health Program, St. Michael's Hospital, Toronto,
Canada

SHEILA HOLLINS, MBBS, FRCPsych, FRCPCH
Professor of Psychiatry of Intellectual Disability,
University of London; Consultant Psychiatrist, Joan
Bicknell Centre, South West London and St. George's
Mental Health NHS Trust; President, Royal College of
Psychiatrists, London, United Kingdom

ALLAN S. KAPLAN, MD, FRCPC
Director of Postgraduate Education and Professor of
Psychiatry, University of Toronto; Loretta Anne Rogers
Chair in Eating Disorders and Head of Program for Eating
Disorders, University Health Network/Toronto General
Hospital, Toronto, Canada

MARK R. KATZ, MD, FRCPC
Assistant Professor of Psychiatry, University of Toronto;
Staff Consultant-Liaison Psychiatrist, Toronto General
Hospital, University Health Network; Coordinator of
Psychiatric Services, Psychosocial Oncology and Palliative
Care, Princess Margaret Hospital, University Health
Network, Toronto, Canada

GABOR I. KEITNER, MD, FRCPC
Professor of Psychiatry, Brown University School of
Medicine; Director of Adult Psychiatry and Mood
Disorders Program, Rhode Island Hospital, Providence,
Rhode Island

PHILIP KLASSEN, MD, FRCPC
Assistant Professor, Departments of Psychiatry and
Medicine, University of Toronto; Deputy Clinical
Director, Law and Mental Health Program, Centre for
Addiction and Mental Health, Toronto, Canada

ANDREA J. LEVINSON, MD, FRCPC
Clinical and Research Fellow in Psychiatry, University of
Toronto; Mood and Anxiety Program, Centre for
Addiction and Mental Health, Toronto, Canada

ANTHONY J. LEVITT, MD, FRCPC
Professor of Psychiatry, University of Toronto;
Psychiatrist-in-Chief, Sunnybrook and Women's College
Health Centre, Toronto, Canada

PAUL S. LINKS, MD, FRCPC
Arthur Sommer Rotenberg Chair in Suicide Studies,
Department of Psychiatry, University of Toronto; Deputy
Chief of Mental Health Services, St. Michael's Hospital,
Toronto, Canada

HUNG-TAT (TED) LO, MBBS, MRCPsych, FRCPC
Assistant Professor of Psychiatry, University of Toronto;
Staff Psychiatrist, Culture, Community, and Health
Studies, Centre for Addiction and Mental Health; Mt. Sinai
Hospital, Toronto, Canada

JODI LOFCHY, MD, FRCPC
Associate Professor of Psychiatry and Director of
Undergraduate Medical Education, University of Toronto;
Director of Emergency Services, Department of
Psychiatry, University Health Network, Toronto, Canada

NATASJA MENEZES, MDCM, FRCPC
Clinical Research Fellow in Psychiatry, University of
Toronto; Staff Psychiatrist, Schizophrenia Program,
Centre for Addiction and Mental Health, Toronto, Canada

JARRET D. MORROW, MD
Resident in Psychiatry, University of Alberta, Edmonton,
Canada

JULIA NUNES
Journalist and Author, Toronto, Canada

LARA J. OSTOLOSKY, MD, FRCPC
Staff Psychiatrist, Eating Disorders Program, University of
Alberta Hospital; Department of Psychiatry, University of
Alberta, Edmonton, Canada

NEIL A. RECTOR, PhD, CPsych
Associate Professor of Psychiatry, University of Toronto;
Psychologist and Head of Anxiety Disorders Clinic, Centre
for Addiction and Mental Health, Toronto, Canada

GARY RODIN, MD, FRCPC
Professor of Psychiatry, University of Toronto;
Department Head and Joint University of
Toronto/University Health Network Harold and Shirley
Lederman Chair in Psychosocial Oncology and Palliative
Care, Princess Margaret Hospital, University Health
Network, Toronto, Canada

CHRISTINE E. RYAN, PhD
Assistant Professor of Psychiatry and Human Behavior, Brown University School of Medicine; Director of Family Research Program, Department of Psychiatry; Assistant Director of Mood Disorders Program, Rhode Island Hospital, Providence, Rhode Island

ISAAC SAKINOFSKY, MD, FRCPC, FRCPsych
Professor Emeritus of Psychiatry and Public Health Sciences, University of Toronto; High Risk Consultation Clinic, Centre for Addiction and Mental Health, Toronto, Canada

MARK SANFORD, MBChB, FRCPC
Associate Professor of Psychiatry (Division of Child Psychiatry), University of Toronto; Head of Child Mood Disorders Service, Child, Youth, and Family Program, Centre for Addiction and Mental Health, Toronto, Canada

FIONA S. M. SCHULTE, MA
Department of Public Health Science, University of Toronto; Clinical Research, Centre for Addiction and Mental Health, Toronto, Canada

PETER SELBY, MBBS, CCFP, MHSc, ASAM
Assistant Professor, Family and Community Medicine, Psychiatry, and Public Health Sciences, University of Toronto; Clinical Director, Addictions Program, Head, Nicotine Dependence Clinic, and Principal Investigator, Ontario Tobacco Research Unit, Centre for Addiction and Mental Health, Toronto, Canada

KENNETH I. SHULMAN, MD, SM, FRCPC
Professor of Psychiatry, University of Toronto; Staff Psychiatrist, Sunnybrook and Women's College Health Sciences Centre, Toronto, Canada

IVAN L. SILVER, MD, MEd, FRCPC
Professor of Psychiatry and Associate Dean of Continuing Education, University of Toronto; Director, Centre for Faculty Development, St. Michael's Hospital, Toronto, Canada

SCOTT SIMMIE
Journalist and Author, Toronto, Canada

PERCY WRIGHT, PhD, CPsych
Psychologist, Forensic Assessment Program, Mental Health Centre Penetanguishene, Penetanguishene, Canada

L. TREVOR YOUNG, MD, PhD, FRCPC
Professor and Cameron Wilson Chair in Depression Studies, University of Toronto; Physician-in-Chief, Centre for Addiction and Mental Health, Toronto, Canada

ROBERT ZIPURSKY, MD, FRCPC
Professor of Psychiatry and Tapscott Chair in Schizophrenia Studies, University of Toronto; Clinical Director, Schizophrenia Program, Centre for Addiction and Mental Health, Toronto, Canada

Preface

"Go interview that new patient." This instruction from a clinical teacher or supervisor may be the immediate prelude to a first clinical encounter in a clinic, an inpatient unit, an emergency room, or a home visit. For the student in any of the mental health professions—psychiatry, psychology, social work, nursing, and counseling—there may be a sense of dread related to not knowing what to ask or how to ask it. Lectures and readings on the theoretical causes of psychiatric disorders, memorized mnemonics of diagnostic criteria, and laminated cards of algorithmic treatment approaches provide little help for that ultimately human encounter of two individuals.

Psychiatric assessment and engagement are not entirely separable concepts. The art of asking the right questions in the right way leads to a sense in the person being interviewed that the interviewer knows what he or she is doing and understands the problem at hand. This combination of expertise and empathy can result in the provision of hope and trust, which serve as foundations for engagement.

Psychiatry is virtually alone in medicine in lacking any diagnostic laboratory or imaging tests. The absence of such external markers of validity that make both the patient and the mental health professional know that the problem is "real" dramatically heightens the need for clinical skills of assessment and engagement. Understanding the problem helps confer legitimacy to the associated distress; understanding the person helps cement the therapeutic alliance necessary for trust and hope to be buttressed by help.

Psychiatry is all about the reconciliation of the unique nature of human experience and individuality with the highly reproducible patterns of human behavior and psychiatric illness across centuries and cultures. Pattern recognition is the foundation of all expertise in medical diagnosis, and no less so in psychiatry, but the reduction of assessment to diagnostic checklists robs the field of its richness as a human encounter and deprives people with mental illness of the hope that can emerge from a sense of connection with a professional who knows and understands.

Through the contributions of numerous senior academic clinicians, this book provides a guide to psychiatric assessment and engagement across a number of clinical problems and settings. While this book is targeted toward students in the mental health professions, all of us benefit from the clinical pearls of our colleagues, whose years of dedication and experience are reflected in these pages.

David S. Goldbloom

Acknowledgments

This book was unabashedly inspired by the work of my father, Richard Goldbloom, whose similarly conceptualized textbook *Pediatric Clinical Skills* (Saunders, 2003) is now in its 3rd successful edition. He continues to emphasize the importance of clinical interviewing as the most sophisticated form of diagnostic technology in his field. At the same time, my father-in-law, Nathan Epstein (one of the contributors to this book), has profoundly shaped my own views of the primacy of clinical skills in psychiatry.

The planning for and production of this book was made immeasurably easier by the friendly support and wise counsel of Susan Pioli, Editor, and Joan Ryan, Senior Editorial Assistant, at Elsevier. The commitment and enthusiasm of the contributors, largely from the University of Toronto, as well as the response from students to early drafts, reassured us that the project was worthwhile. Finally, all the authors are grateful to the patients, families, students, and colleagues who helped us to hone our psychiatric clinical skills and to share them with our readers.

David S. Goldbloom

1

General Principles of Interviewing

David S. Goldbloom

INTRODUCTION

Your initial encounter with a patient—whether it is a brief meeting in a hallway or an extended interview in an office—represents an opportunity to begin to understand the patient's difficulties and to begin to establish a therapeutic relationship. These processes are simultaneous and interdependent rather than sequential and autonomous.

In the chapters that follow, you will learn about some of the specific contexts of diagnostic interviewing and how they affect the types of questions you will ask and the ways you will try to engage the patient. However, they also appropriately reflect some current commonalties of approach in psychiatry where diagnostic methodologies are largely limited to listening, asking, and talking.

THE PRELIMINARIES

Setting the Stage

You should consider in advance where you are going to conduct an interview. Is there a room that affords comfort and privacy? Emergency room waiting areas and shared inpatient accommodations are among the least conducive settings—and yet by default preliminary assessments are often carried out there. Is there a room somewhere nearby where you can interview the patient in private? It's worth the extra time to locate one—and patients appreciate the fact that you have made the extra effort to do so; in other words, one brick for the foundation of a therapeutic alliance has already been laid, and you haven't even started talking yet.

The room should be a setting where both you and the patient feel safe (see Chapter 14, Emergency Assessment) and comfortable, free from distracting noises (e.g., your cell phone, pager, or the jackhammer used in the ongoing renovation of the adjacent room). Given that many patients will be in some sort of distress, a box of facial tissues available at the outset is a thoughtful gesture, and it is preferable to a frantic look by both of you around the room at an emotional moment for something other than a sleeve to absorb the tears.

Are the chairs at roughly the same height, or are you towering over the patient? Are you sitting behind a desk? Why? For some patients, the desk will be a symbolic barrier between them and you.

As a general rule, never stand during an interview when the patient is either sitting or lying on a bed. Meet patients at their level in terms of eye contact. Patients who are in bed should remain there for an interview **only** if they are too debilitated (or are restrained) to sit up. Even then, cranking up the head of the bed if tolerated and then sitting adjacent to the bed will assist in normalizing the encounter. Assisting a patient out of bed and into a chair is a physical act of helping that underscores your role nonverbally.

One of the commodities you offer is your time. Does the interview environment you have selected allow you to know what time it is without checking your wristwatch repeatedly? Many mental health professionals have strategically located clocks in various regions of their offices to allow tracking of time more subtly. They don't need to be hidden; patients also like to know what time it is.

The Greeting

Introducing yourself clearly and formally to a patient on first meeting sets a tone. Formality need not imply a lack of friendliness. Do you find it irritating when people you don't know call you by your first name? Does it feel falsely friendly? I prefer to begin with *"Mr. or Ms._____"* in addressing the patient while introducing myself as Dr. Goldbloom. Some patients may say, "Call me Bob" (particularly so if that is their first name). However, there may be an expectation of reciprocity that they should be able to address you by your first name. Although some mental health professionals will go along with that informality, it can create a false level of mutual intimacy and disclosure. You will (and should) know far more about your patients' lives than they know about yours.

Shaking hands in many but not all cultures is a physical and normative form of greeting. Many patients have told me that the memory of a firm handshake on first meeting was a tangible form of support at a time they were feeling overwhelmed and alone. Think of the possible meanings for patients already feeling marginalized by their experiences if you do not offer your hand in greeting. In my experience, only extremely paranoid, angry, or obsessional patients have refused to offer theirs in return. It is the only sanctioned "laying on of hands" within mental health that has been such a comfort to patients in the rest of medicine.

To Write or Not To Write?

All too often, I have witnessed students and psychiatry residents taking notes furiously during interviews. Let's consider the advantages and disadvantages. The only advantage is the immediate availability of an almost-literal transcript of the encounter. The following are disadvantages:

1. The cognitive preoccupation that writing requires: It's a multi-tasking challenge to write down great quotes from patients while simultaneously processing what they say and thinking about how to explore it further.
2. The lack of eye contact that writing demands: Unless you are blessed with an ability to write without looking at what you are writing (I would veer eventually onto my pant leg if I tried that), time looking at your penmanship is time lost with the patient.
3. The fantasies that writing engenders: As patients watch you write (they do exactly this), they may wonder why you write down only certain parts of what they say—and what that means. They may wonder who else is going to read your notes and what happens to those notes after you are done. Patients don't have to be paranoid to be morbidly curious.

The more you build a structure into your interview and the more you use the interview to test out hypotheses about the person and the diagnosis, the less you will need to take notes. Some dates of events or doses of medication may require jotting down, but often these in-the-moment notes are far too inclusive and defeat the task of synthesizing and filtering information.

As an exercise, you should try interviewing a patient for whom someone else has already done and documented an assessment that you haven't seen. Don't take any notes while you conduct a diagnostic interview. Then sit down immediately afterward and write it up. You will be surprised, particularly if you take a semistructured approach, at how much relevant detail you recall. Compare it to the previously documented assessment and you may begin to understand what, if anything, you left out—and why. It will make you a better interviewer.

Explaining the Interview

There are two extremes in approach to explaining the interview; one style assumes that the purpose is obvious—after all, you're a mental health professional—and any explanation is redundant. The other generates a 10-minute explanation that starts to sound like a term life insurance policy.

Don't assume that the patient knows who you are, why this interview is happening, how long it will take, or what it will lead to. Remember that when people are feeling anxious, they often have difficulty listening to long and elaborate explanations.

Have you ever had the experience, most commonly at a party, when someone tells you his name and as he says it you forget it instantly? The same experience can happen in a clinical encounter. After meeting a patient in a public area and introducing myself, I usually repeat my name once we are seated for an interview and acknowledge that it is not an easy name to remember (rather than putting the possible blame for forgetting on an already anxious patient).

As for explaining the purpose of the interview, I describe a process that has three goals.

1. To find out who you are
2. To find out what kind of problems you're having
3. To find out how I can help

This is a plain-language statement that reflects multiple tasks. First, it acknowledges that I am speaking with a unique individual about whom I know little but need to learn; second, it states that there will be a diagnostic focus to the encounter; and third, it makes it clear that I am there to help. This message of help, which may seem incredibly obvious to you by virtue of your mere presence, benefits from overt statement and repetition.

Once this overview has been provided, I then explain the process, which may include the following: *"I'm going to be asking you lots of questions over the next hour, and I may need to interrupt you from time to time so I can understand things better, but at the end I'll give you my sense of what is going on and how I can help. You'll have a chance to ask me some questions as well."*

THE MAIN EVENT

Every interview has a structure—even those that seem on the surface quite disjointed. Having a template in your mind will assist you in progressing through the interview and does not require a rigid or formulaic approach. However, many novice interviewers display their template overtly by the questions they ask, such as "Now I'd like to ask you about your past personal and developmental history." What you actually want to know is about patients' experiences growing up. Why not say so in plain language rather than using the actual section headings of your write-up?

As an exercise, write down the stock phrases you use in introducing various sections of the interview. Try to imagine how they sound to a patient. Get together with some colleagues and compare notes on this task.

Identifying Data

The advantage of beginning the interview with this section is that, for most patients, it is less threatening and easier to answer than questions related to their problems. It also begins what you have already described as the first task of the interview—finding out who they are. And yet, far too many interviewers race through it as a pit stop en route to the diagnostic finish line. Components include the following:

- Age
- Occupation
- Relationship status
- Living arrangements
- Ethnocultural and racial heritage

In asking about occupation, remember that it is generally no longer acceptable or accurate to ask homemakers (usually women), "Do you work or are you at home?" Rather, *"Do you work outside the home?"* conveys an appreciation of the role within it. If someone is unemployed, you should find out how financial support occurs. Is the person receiving public assistance? How much? What does he pay in rent? How much does that leave him to live on? This line of questioning helps for several reasons:

1. It gives you a picture of the financial realities the patient faces and puts his problems in that context.

2. It conveys your interest in the day-to-day realities he faces.
3. It helps you put solutions for him in a context of feasibility.
4. It helps you gauge his financial competency.

For someone who is unemployed, you should find out when he last worked and what he did. Again, this helps establish the identity of the person at the outset, rather than simply regarding the patient as someone who is currently receiving public assistance or lives on the streets.

Asking whether someone is *"single, married, or in a relationship"* covers most of the ground. If the person is currently single, then it is reasonable to ask, *"What about in the past?"* Asking this way doesn't presume sexual orientation, and its openness may allow disclosure early in the interview.

Remember that single people have children. All too often, I see students forget to ask this of people who are not currently in a relationship or who are currently living alone. Similarly, single people may be living in nonintimate relationships with a variety of friends and relatives.

Finally, in our multicultural and multiracial universe, it's worth asking up front about the patient's background. A name, an appearance, or an accent may all trigger your curiosity, and the question is an opportunity at the outset of the interview for the patient to teach you something about himself and his community.

The Chief Complaint

It's somewhat archaic that this section heading persists in medicine. Who likes a complainer? But the various meanings of the word "complaint" include dissatisfaction, resentment, a bodily disorder or disease, and an expression of pain. It is that last category that probably comes closest to capturing what you are looking for. What is bothering this person? What does he identify as a problem for which he is seeking help? The stock question of "What brought you here today?" commonly evokes the concrete response of "a taxi." *"What sort of problem or difficulty have you been having?"* makes the question clearer.

Unless your patient has recently read a textbook of psychiatry, he will answer with words that reflect his vocabulary, perspective, and priority. The labels he has come up with can serve as a common language and reference point for further elaboration of the history. For instance, "My head's messed up" may be the anchor for your subsequent questions about chronology and other symptoms, such as *"Since your head's been messed up, have you noticed any change in your sleeping?"* Some patients will talk about having had a "breakdown." This is not the time to point out to them that this term does not exist in the diagnostic nomenclature. Rather, while using the word, you can find out what they mean by it.

History of the Present Illness

Before you have asked a single question, this history-taking has begun. Whether it is the information you received about the patient beforehand, her appearance in the waiting room, the way she spoke with you, or all of the above, you have already begun generating hypotheses about the nature of her problem.

An exercise I gave to medical students working with me in a psychiatric inpatient unit involved their meeting with patients for 1 minute and speaking with them casually about anything **except** their psychiatric difficulties or treatment; the students then had to tell me what possible psychiatric illnesses the patients had. To their amazement, without asking any of the symptom checklist questions, they had generated hypotheses worthy of testing—based on everything from appearance to affect to thought form to interaction.

One way (and there are many) to conceptualize the history is to think of it in a two-paragraph model; this may also help you when it comes to writing up your findings. In this model, the first paragraph is for the patient to elaborate what he thinks is wrong, based on his chief complaint. If you can restrain yourself from interrupting him (health professionals usually allow about 15 to 20 seconds to elapse before doing so when a patient describes a problem), this first paragraph may serve multiple functions:

1. It reveals the patient's priorities.
2. It reveals the patient's understanding of the problem, including commonly the mention of those factors the patient views as causal.
3. It sends a clear message that you are interested in how the patient views things.

For some patients, this first paragraph may be brief but still informative, as in the following:

- "Nothing's wrong." When something clearly is wrong, this answer may help you understand the patient's limited awareness.
- "Beats me. You're the doctor." This answer may be the harbinger of anger and resentment that you will experience repeatedly through the interview and that the patient has also likely expressed repeatedly before the interview.
- "Where should I start? It was a cold Tuesday in February, 1957, when I first became aware . . ." This response may induce a sinking feeling that you and the patient are going to grow old gracefully together before you reach a tenta-

tive diagnosis. It is also a signal that you are going to have to play an active and directive role in keeping the patient on track throughout the interview.

The second paragraph is for you; it allows you to follow up on all the leads obtained thus far to probe for symptoms, stressors, sequelae, and risk factors associated with particular diagnoses. Many of the subsequent chapters in this book will address the specific symptoms you need to ask about and how to ask about them. However, the following general rules still apply:

1. Do not ask about a group of symptoms at once, such as, "Have you noticed any problems with your sleep, energy, appetite, concentration, memory, libido, or interests?" The message conveyed is one of expectation of a negative response; the task of recalling this laundry list is significant and potentially embarrassing for the patient, who may opt to simply say no.
2. Do not ask about a specific symptom in a way that telegraphs your desired answer, such as, "You're not thinking about killing yourself, are you?"
3. In the face of chronic symptoms, be sure to ask whether things have changed or gotten worse. Be clear in your questions. Patients have very sensitive antennae and will quickly detect your discomfort. The two areas that evoke the most discomfort in interviewers and result in the greatest number of verbal approximations are, of course, sex and death. It is no accident that there are many approaches to these sensitive areas.

Interviewers often "forget" to ask about sexual issues, even though it represents a fundamental aspect of human behavior. The first rule is to remember that people who are single and alone, older and younger than you, have sexual lives—even the person who reminds you intensely of your grandmother. The caricature of the squirming health professional, asking reluctantly, "So . . . how are things . . . down there?" often evokes a laugh because it reflects a common discomfort. You can ask in a direct, matter-of-fact way about both sexual desire and sexual activity. Both psychiatric disease and psychiatric treatment can affect these core features of human pleasure adversely, and you can ask about it without appearing obsessed by it.

In terms of questions about suicidality, I favor a direct approach of asking plainly, for example, *"Have you been thinking of killing yourself?"* Other interviewers may prefer a graduated approach but the risk is that this conveys your discomfort with being direct. I have never seen a patient who was offended by the direct question or (as some students fear) inspired by it, for example, "No, I hadn't but that would really address my problems." Rather, people who have been suicidal are typically relieved that an interviewer has raised the issue in a straightforward, nontimid, nonjudgmental way and appears to understand the severity of their distress. Sometimes interviewers will ask, "Do you feel like harming yourself?" As an exercise, you should ask patients who have been suicidal whether this turn of phrase actually captures their subjective experience at that worst moment.

With regard to stressors and potential precipitants, it's important to remember that all of us try to make sense of nonsensical experiences by causal attribution; we look for something to blame. While these may be related to current suffering, they also may not—and other stressors may have been rendered completely unconscious. That being said, across the three principal domains of love, work, and play, you should conduct a scan for recent events of note. And do not settle for the event itself. The impact and meaning of the event for the individual are important. The most common response to verifiable trauma is resilience, not adversity.

Related to this is the search for risk factors that, like stressors, are used to provide a model of understanding for why this person is ill now. These may range from previous episodes of the same or related illnesses to a family history of psychiatric illness, temperamental traits such as introversion or perfectionism, or experiences such as repeated abuse and deprivation.

You should also know by the end of the second paragraph what the impact of the symptoms has been; this is not simply to satisfy the diagnostic requirements of the DSM-IV-TR but rather to contextualize the illness within the fabric of a person's life and to gauge its severity.

Past Psychiatric History

Elements of the past psychiatric history may blend well into the second paragraph of your history. It is important to remember that there is both an informal and a formal element to this part of the patient's experience. Asking, "When was the first time you saw a mental health professional?" skips over potentially significant information. Many episodes of illness remit spontaneously without professional intervention, and many people cannot access help even if they want it.

Sadly, many types of psychiatric illness and interpersonal difficulties are recurrent. Asking, *"When was the first time you felt this way?"* may reveal previous episodes; asking, *"When was the worst time you felt this way?"* helps gauge relative severity for that individual and may reveal more clearly diagnostic previous episodes.

For the previous formal encounters with mental health professionals, you need to know who, when, where, why, what (assessment and treatment), and how (it turned out).

Specific treatments and their benefits and toxicities, previous hospitalizations and their durations, etc. are all useful. However, for some patients who have experienced years and decades of illness and treatment, this prospect of information gathering can be daunting. You may need to get the patient to help you in a synthetic way, for example, you might ask questions such as these:

- *"What's the usual reason for which you get admitted to hospital?"*
- *"Of all the antidepressants you have taken, which one was the best, and which one was the worst? Why?"*
- *"You've been in therapy with several different therapists. In general, what's the reason that therapy usually comes to an end for you? What do you usually find helpful about being in therapy?"*

Some of the details you need for this section, in terms of reliable information, may come from old records rather than the vagaries of memory for your patient.

Given the frequent interplay between psychiatric symptoms and substance use, it is worth documenting substance use and misuse in this section of the interview if it has not already formed part of the second paragraph of your history. See Chapter 10 for some of the approaches you can use to elicit this information.

Family Psychiatric History

Just as past episodes may predict the present one for an individual, so to a lesser degree may a family history of psychiatric illness, even if it is not exactly the same illness as your patient is experiencing. Psychiatric illness is common. But so is the fear of being judged. Sometimes the question, "Does anyone else in your family have any psychiatric illness or emotional problems?" may generate less response than the more permissive *"Who else in your family . . ."* The same rules about formal versus informal history apply to family members.

Often, people will take "family" to mean immediate nuclear family. It is worth asking, *"What about your aunts, uncles, cousins, and grandparents?"* This covers virtually all blood relatives and may trigger recollection of an alcoholic uncle or a cousin who killed himself.

Medical History

This section, which is commonly brief unless the patient is being seen in hospital as part of a psychiatric consultation service, should focus on those current medical problems that might influence either diagnostic understanding or treatment. However, there are certain elements to keep in mind:

1. Like traumatic events, physical illnesses may display their relevance to your assessment through their impact and meaning, which could include anything from body image disturbance to functional limitation. For example, the body image disturbance in adolescents with diabetes mellitus may influence mood and behavior. What are the implications of physical illnesses or injuries for your patient?

2. For females, have they ever been pregnant? Although pregnancy is far from a disease state, it is a significant and medicalized body change, and it can be associated with a variety of outcomes, both medical and psychiatric. A childless woman may divulge to you a spontaneous or therapeutic abortion, and you need to know how this person weathered that experience.

Medications

"I take a blue oblong pill in the morning and a green capsule at night." This can be a discouraging but not uncommon answer to interviewers about medications. Sometimes the name and phone number of their pharmacy will lead to a more reliable recounting of pharmacotherapy—but some people are particularly conscientious regarding their medications (and may be more current than you on their side effects, thanks to the Internet).

You should remember that:

1. For some women, oral contraceptives are not viewed as medications and may not be mentioned at first. Be sure to ask any girl or woman of reproductive age whether she is using any form of birth control. The answers may trigger further inquiry about her reproductive status.

2. For many people, over-the-counter medications and alternative/complementary medicines are not considered "medication" in the traditional sense. You need to ask about these separately.

Personal/Developmental History

For many interviewers, the personal and developmental history can be the most daunting element of the entire interview. Under time pressure, it is the most likely session to be truncated, resulting in the idea that in 5 to 7 minutes you can trace out the trajectory of someone's life. This inevitably leads to the race past familiar nodal landmarks of developmental psychopathology—an absent father, school refusal, death of a relative, etc.—in a whirlwind effort to fit into a model of how the past explains the present.

Do you think someone could understand the course of your life, its richness and significance, in the matter of 10 or 15 minutes? An hour? Probably not. So you need to ask yourself what realistic goals are achievable during your tour of a person's growing up. One view (mine) is that you are looking for two things:

1. Recurring patterns of behavior and experience in relationships, in jobs, etc.

2. An evolving sense of personal identity across the nonvegetative spheres of human behavior—namely, love, work, and play

Using this as an underlying theme, traversing the path of someone's life may become more focused.

Learning about a patient's family of origin is a good place to start. You should find out who the key players were and are. How old are her parents? If they are dead, what did they die of and when? What was the impact on the patient? What do/did they do for a living? What were they like? This latter question can often trigger, if asked exactly in this way, a simple response such as "Nice." A more fruitful approach may be to ask, *"How would you describe your father to someone who never met him?"* This places an expectation of activity, reflection, and synthesis on the patient. Are there siblings? Is she close to any particular sibling? Why?

Do you know your own developmental milestones? Most students I teach have no idea when they actually walked and talked. And yet they relentlessly ask these questions of patients. It is worth remembering that:

1. There is a significant range of "normal" with regard to milestones.

2. No one remembers her own milestones unless someone else told her.

3. The relevance of these milestones is only present when they are dramatically delayed.

If you ask, *"As far as you have been told, did you walk and talk at the usual ages?"* you will usually hear, "I think so" or "I have no idea." If, however, you are told, "I didn't speak until I was 5 years old," this is a more ominous delay that requires further corroboration.

For most of us, the first intimate relationships are with our own families. Although these do not produce an unalterable template for all future relationships, it is helpful to know what they were like in understanding the person's trajectory. Chapter 22, Family Assessment, provides techniques for assessing relationships and family functioning in the present tense. Asking someone to reconstruct relationships from 30 years earlier is inevitably colored by intervening events and perceptions, as well as the unreliable nature of memory.

Nevertheless, research on personality suggests that major traits are about 50% genetically determined and 50% shaped by the environment. However, that latter determinant is almost entirely the "non-shared" environment, that is, not the general environment affecting a whole family but the unique individual relationships between the person and the environment.

Getting a sense of the person as a young child is challenging. People don't recall their early childhood with great detail and accuracy—but they have often been told what they were like. Asking in a way such as,*"What have you been told you were like as a young child?"* may produce more information as well as family mythology and expectation. Did he make friends easily? Did he have a best friend? Was he outgoing or shy? These are all early markers in the journey toward relationships. The major work task of children is going to school. Did he have trouble leaving home at the beginning to go to school? If so, why? The reasons could be as varied as bullying at school to worry about an ill parent. Don't assume that the reason for school refusal is automatically psychopathology in the child. How did he do in school? What was he good at? What did he struggle with? This may help identify strengths and competencies at a time when interviewers are focused on isolating difficulties. With regard to the third life task of play, what did he do outside of school for fun? Many interests, like sports or music, take root in these early years.

In adolescence, the journey related to these life tasks takes a different shape and so should your questions. First, there are physical pubertal changes that bring new psychological challenges and rewards. Did she undergo these changes at the same time as her peers? What was the impact? For some adolescents, this can result in significant body image preoccupation, weight concern, and disordered eating.

Commonly, adolescents begin their first intimate relationships (both sexual and nonsexual), which may be fleeting or enduring. You need to know what these were like. You can ask, *"Did you have any kind of intimate relationships with boys or girls as a teenager?"* This leaves the door open for exploration of both heterosexual and homosexual experience in an accepting way. You may also need to define what you mean by *intimate*, remembering that some sexual experiences may be lacking in a broader sense of intimacy.

If there have been relationships in adolescence, how many were there? How long did they last? How and why did they end? Who ended them? Generally, I never accept the "We agreed to break up" response. I believe there is always a "dumper" and a "dumpee" if you dig hard enough! In the case of multiple relationships, you need the person to help you synthesize them rather than laboriously review each one. You can ask, *"What's the typical reason for which relationships end for you?"* or *"What generally attracts you to people in relationships?"* People are remarkably adept at assisting you in this task.

With regard to work and play in adolescence, school again remains the major yardstick for measuring the former; evolving and enduring extracurricular interests represent the latter. People often start to think about adult roles to which they aspire in adolescence, and this is often reflected in the mentors they choose or the people they admire.

The duration of adolescence seems to be extending at both edges, dipping into prepubertal life and traversing much of people's early 20s. People are marrying and entering the workforce at an older age than several generations ago. As a result, a sense of professional and personal identity may not gel until the end of the third decade of life. However, the patterns of behavior in relationships, work, and play will be evident before then.

All too often, students conclude the personal history section of the interview with no sense of the person's competencies, strengths, and interests. This reflects a pathology-focused interview seeking to justify a current diagnosis based on the past. While you are looking for antecedents and precursors, you are also trying to know this person better. If you cannot answer the question, "What is this person good at?" at the end of the interview, then imagine how the patient feels about the journey just taken.

Mental Status Examination

Students sometimes introduce this section with an apology: "Now I have to ask you some questions that I have to ask everyone. They may seem stupid or silly, and I'm sorry but I need to ask you . . ." If you have to apologize in advance for doing something, why are you doing it? Does a cardiologist, before applying a cold stethoscope or inflating a tight blood pressure cuff, apologize for what she is about to do? An explanation is different than an apology.

Every chapter that follows in this book will repeat that the mental status examination begins the moment you first have contact with the person. The appearance, motor activity, speech, affect, thought process, and interaction are all evident to you early on in the encounter, long before you arrive at point in the sequence (typically packed into the last 60 seconds of an interview) where the mental status examination is supposed to occur.

As an exercise, if you are observing someone else conduct an interview, try predicting and writing down the mental status exam 5 minutes after the interview has started. You may be surprised by your predictive accuracy as well as the amount of informal evidence garnered early in the encounter.

The most relevant aspects of the mental status exam will have occurred during a well-conducted history. If a person is depressed, you will know by the end of the history about the quality of his mood, his degree of suicidality, or any psychomotor abnormalities. His memory and concentration difficulties will have already exposed themselves. Similarly, for someone who is psychotic, you will have asked about relevant hallucinations and delusions early on.

However, there are some subtle disturbances, often in cognitive capacity, less evident initially, which formal testing may reveal. If a patient shows up on his own at the right time and location for a scheduled appointment, do you need to assess his orientation to time, place, and person? However, someone who is accompanied because he is too depressed to organize himself or is showing signs of confusion requires more careful evaluation of orientation. Cognitive tasks can be introduced simply and truthfully with the statement, *"I'm going to ask some questions now that will help me check your memory and concentration."* No apology is needed.

In testing memory and concentration (it can be difficult to separate them at times), several routine tests are used. One is a test of immediate recall in repeating a series of numbers forward and backward. Your first challenge will be to remember the numbers yourself! Some of us have had the humbling experience of not recalling them as soon as we have given them to the patient. Generally, you will never give the patient a forward sequence longer than seven numbers. Since this happens to be the same number of digits as a telephone number, you have to avoid giving the numbers the same rhythmic vocal cadence as you would a telephone number. As an exercise, try saying your phone number aloud; you will hear the irregular rhythm, with a pause after the first three numbers and the usual downshift in vocal tone that signals the end of the sequence. For memory testing, try to say the numbers evenly in rhythm and tone so that the patient does not plug them into a telephone sequence.

In testing recent recall, you will often give the patient three things to remember and tell her you will ask her to recall the three things in 5 minutes. I have sometimes had patients say to me as they left an interview, "By the way, Dr. Goldbloom, those three things you meant to ask me for again were . . ." In other words, when it hasn't been clinically important to test their recall, I have forgotten to complete my evaluation of it! If you are testing it, try to select three words that don't automatically flow together—such as *long, book,* and *chapter*! I sometimes use *table, purple,* and *New York* to reflect an object, a visual perception, and a place. More detail on cognitive assessment can be found in the chapters on geriatric assessment (Chapter 21) and assessment in people with neurological disorders (Chapter 16).

Insight and judgment are important components of the mental status examination and are excellent transition points toward the end of an initial interview. Two of the simplest questions that will explore these areas are *"What do you think is going on with you now?"* and *"What do you think would be helpful?"* These are, after all, the exact same questions you have been asking yourself throughout this interview. Since there is no blood test for insight and judgment, your evaluation is in part a measure of the congruence between the patient's views and your own.

You need to factor in individual and cultural variables in the gauging of insight (see chapters on assessment of people with intellectual disabilities [Chapter 17] and cultural competence in psychiatric assessment [Chapter 4]). The vocabulary of distress and its origins need not match the committee consensus-based language of the DSM-IV-TR. You are trying to find a common ground of understanding that will allow you to move forward and engage in treatment. "My nerves are shot . . . that's what's making me act this way, I guess" is more likely than "I suspect that underactivity in serotonergic projections from the dorsal raphe nuclei accounts for a variety of these vegetative disturbances"! It is likely that the insight formally gauged at the end of an interview will mirror the insight displayed in the first paragraph of the history.

As for judgment, I have never asked a patient what he would do with a stamped addressed envelope found lying in the street. Severely mentally ill people refusing life-saving treatment still know to put that letter in the mailbox, and the question is entirely irrelevant to why they are seeking or needing help. However, you need to guard against viewing judgment as impaired whenever a patient disagrees with you about what needs to be done. It is important to make questions about judgment as specific and contextual to the individual as possible, and often that relates to decisions about treatment. When asking about judgment in the context of treatment, it is important to ask about anticipated consequences of both receiving and not receiving treatment. Our therapeutic zeal drives us to recommend all kinds of treatment, and patients' reluctance may be based on a variety of sources, including previous experience, personal and cultural values, and their own sources of information such as the Internet. Refusing treatment is not always a sign of impaired judgment and needs to be understood for its context and determinants.

CLOSING THE CURTAIN

In student examination situations, observed interviews often end abruptly with a terrified look by the candidate at the clock and a quick, "We're out of time. Thanks very much for speaking with me."

You need to allow a couple of minutes to end an interview. This is your opportunity to turn the tables on the process of the interview and provide a couple of key messages.

1. Explanation
2. Hope

You should provide the patient with a brief and integrative verbal summary of what you've heard. This demonstrates that you have been listening and thinking while the patient has been talking. It allows you to display the wizardry of pattern recognition in integrating the information into a cohesive model of understanding, thus providing hope through the demonstration of expertise. It gives the patient a chance to correct any major errors in how you have heard the history. And it sets the stage for the diagnostic impression you are about to deliver and the treatment you may recommend.

You should thank patients for speaking with you, acknowledging that it isn't always easy to speak about personal things with someone they haven't met before. You may want to ask whether there is anything important for you to know that has not been covered, acknowledging the time constraints. This may result in the surfacing of a key detail that the patient previously felt uncomfortable disclosing. Alternatively, the patient may say no and express surprise at how much you have covered together.

The suffering associated with mental illness is often isolating and associated with fears of permanency and hopelessness. Consistent with your provisional diagnosis, your explanation at the end should convey the following:

1. Why you think she has this problem
2. How common this problem is
3. How frequently people get better
4. How treatment makes a difference

If you achieve this, you have conducted a diagnostic and a therapeutic interview. That being said, the above represents just one of multiple approaches to interviewing. How do you find the way that works best for you? Here are some suggestions:

1. Observe as many different interviewers as you can. Your style will ultimately reflect an amalgam of multiple styles.
2. Do as many interviews as you can. After each interview, take a moment to write down what went really well and what you had difficulty with.
3. Videotape yourself interviewing, and watch the videotape with a teacher. You will appreciate the disparity between what you say and think you do and what you actually do.

Interviewing is an art and a skill. It is also the primary tool of mental health professionals. It takes time and experience to hone it—but every interview will teach you how to do it better the next time.

RECOMMENDED READINGS

Carlat D: *The psychiatric interview,* ed 2, Philadelphia, 2005, Lippincott Williams & Wilkins.

Cruz M, Pincus HA: Research on the influence that communication in psychiatric encounters has on treatment, *Psychiatr Serv* 53:1253–1265, 2002.

Shea S: *Psychiatric interviewing: the art of understanding,* ed 2, Philadelphia, 1998, Saunders.

2

The Use of Standardized Rating Scales in Clinical Practice

R. MICHAEL BAGBY, DAVID S. GOLDBLOOM,
AND FIONA S. M. SCHULTE

INTRODUCTION

This chapter introduces standardized rating scales, instruments that can be applied in clinical practice to aid in the assessment process. A central tenet is that standardized rating scales afford a systematic, quantifiable, and reliable approach to diagnosis, especially when compared with the alternative—clinical judgment. In addition, rating scales provide a consistent means by which to monitor illness and reliably track change in illness severity. This can be accomplished as a result of the overarching objective of these scales—to provide a consistent and objective means to evaluate illness. This chapter, therefore, attempts to describe in detail the value of such instruments as compared with subjective impression formation. We begin with a comprehensive outline of what standardized rating scales are and try to justify the benefits of their use; this is followed by a review of the conventional guidelines for selecting rating scales. Finally, we describe the clinical use of rating scales and provide examples of some commonly used scales. Although we acknowledge the limitations of standardized rating scales, we hope that at the conclusion of this chapter the advantages of using such instruments in lieu of relying solely on clinical judgment should be clear. We also want to be clear that clinical interviews and standardized rating scales should not be considered to be mutually exclusive; they can complement one another, and taken together, can enhance an understanding of the patient.

STANDARDIZED RATING SCALES

Standardized rating scales provide a way to evaluate symptoms of psychopathology and illness and are often used to assist the clinician in making a particular diagnostic evaluation of a patient, as well as to assess severity of illness or to track illness change. Typically administered in an interview or self-report format, rating scales most often require a person to quantify the degree to which a particular quality or behavior is present or absent by indicating where it lies along a continuum for a series of related items. For example, a question might ask whether a patient feels anxious "not at all," "some of the time," "most of the time," or "always." Rating scales are usually interpreted by summing a sequence of individual rating scores that, when aggregated, are understood to relate to a particular construct (such as anxiety). This total score is then compared with empirically generated standards or norms to ascertain where a particular individual might rank in comparison to others.

Standardized rating scales allow clinicians to assess an individual in relation to a particular predefined standard. *Standardized* means that individual test scores obtained from the test are interpreted with regard to test scores acquired from a normative sample. In other words, before being introduced as an official clinical measure, the scale is administered to a large sample from the population in an attempt to obtain the most reliable set of statistical data—means, standard deviations, standardized scores, and percentiles. It should be noted, however, that norms can be derived from any group selected as a sample, and thus no one population can be considered the ultimate normative group.

Standardized scale users can expect a reliable and consistent approach to assessment. For example, using a standardized scale ensures uniformity in the questions that are asked and consistency in the way responses are scored and interpreted. The degree to which an instrument has been standardized can extend as far as to include the seating pattern for the test and the lighting conditions required. Obviously, the degree of standardization fluctuates with each measure, and some tests, such as self-report measures, allow for a greater degree of control than others, such as interviews.

Within the arena of mood disorders, the Hamilton Rating Scale for Depression (Ham-D),[1] typically administered in interview format, serves as a concrete example of a standardized rating scale. The Ham-D originated as a means to evaluate the severity of depressive illness, and a score is assigned to a variety of documented depressive symptoms to determine depression severity. The scale consists of 17 symptoms, which are ranked on a scale of 0 to 4 or 0 to 2, depending on their degree of quantifiable severity. The total score for this instrument can range from 0 to 50, with greater than 23 indicating very severe depression; 19 to 22, severe; 14 to 18, moderate; 8 to 13, mild; and 7 or less, normal.[2] The Beck Depression Inventory (BDI)[3] provides another example of a standardized rating scale designed to assess depression severity. This instrument uses a self-report format. The scale consists of 21 items related to depressive symptoms; respondents are asked to report their severity for each of the 21 items based on a scale of 0 (absent or mild) to 3 (severe). The total score is typically interpreted according to the following severity distinctions: severe, 30 to 63; moderate, 17 to 29; mild, 10 to 16; and minimal, 0 to 9.

Standardized rating scales similarly exist for other clinical domains, such as anxiety, attention deficit disorder, and personality disorders, to name just a few.

Improvement in Accuracy of Diagnosis

Accuracy of diagnosis is integral to the clinical process in optimizing efficacy of treatment and ultimately the well-being of the patient. Despite the significance of this step in the clinical process, however, clinicians have been found to form their diagnostic decisions and evaluations of illness for their patients from very early on in the assessment process. Pressured by time limitations characteristic of day-to-day practice, clinicians are often compelled to make diagnostic decisions as quickly and as easily as possible. Moreover, as clinicians advance in their careers and gain experience and confidence with the diagnostic process,

using rating scales often takes lower priority in the assessment. In fact, standardized rating scales are often considered a "second level" of assessment.[4] Inherent in the course of making a clinical judgment, however, are the potential impediments of human judgment errors. Biases, as an example, are cognitive processes that have the ability to taint the way in which you might arrive at a decision about a patient. Two of the more common errors are the "confirmatory bias" and the "hindsight bias."

Clinical Judgment Biases and Heuristic Errors

The confirmatory bias is the tendency of clinicians to search for information to confirm existing beliefs or hypotheses that have been formed. Once a diagnostic decision has been made, therefore, you engage in confirmatory hypothesis testing. As such, subsequent probing throughout the assessment and the resulting information provided by the patient tend to be carefully assimilated in ways that only seek to confirm the initial impression. For example, if you have concluded that a patient is suffering from anxiety, the confirmatory bias posits that you will formulate your pattern of questioning to elicit responses in accordance with your hypothesis, while simultaneously construing the client's responses to align with this hypothesis. Clearly, some measure of this is absolutely necessary in the fleshing out of a clinical history from a patient based on presenting complaints and clinical hypotheses; however, the risks of this approach on its own should be evident to you as well.

Another bias that has been recognized to influence clinical judgment is the hindsight bias, which refers to the way in which impression or perception can be changed after learning the actual outcome of an event.[5] In other words, it is the tendency for people with outcome knowledge to believe falsely that they would have predicted the reported outcome of an event. In clinical practice, the hindsight bias can interfere when a patient has been referred to you with a speculated diagnosis prereported. Clinicians exaggerate the extent to which they had foreseen the likelihood of its occurrence. For example, learning that an outcome has occurred, such as the attempted suicide of a patient, might lead you to perceive your initial formulation, perhaps of suicidal thoughts, as being correct.[5]

Heuristics, or rules that guide cognitive processing to help make judgments more quickly, introduce another source of error in human judgment. In that clinicians are often pressured by time constraints in everyday practice, it is not unusual to expect that heuristics be employed to help make decisions; indeed, you would be completely lost clinically without heuristics. However, while providing ease in assessment, heuristics often sacrifice accuracy of judgment for speed. For example, the availability heuristic is the tendency for decisions to be influenced by the facility with which objects and events can be remembered. When applied to clinical practice, the availability heuristic would posit that you might be more likely to make a diagnosis of depression as opposed to anxiety if you can more readily recall patients diagnosed with depression. Coinciding with the availability heuristic is the tendency for people to be influenced by more graphic or dramatic events, rather than real-life probabilities, otherwise known as the "base-rate fallacy." Thus, disorders that receive considerable attention from the media tend to be perceived as occurring more often than they actually do. This can be especially problematic when it is recognized that the media tend to be fascinated by the more rare disorders, thereby implanting a view that these disorders occur with a greater frequency than is actually true.[6]

The representative heuristic occurs when a decision is made based on whether a person is representative of a particular category. In other words, when making a decision as to whether a patient might be diagnosed with borderline personality disorder, you may compare this patient's behavior and experiences to what has been understood as the typology of a borderline patient to determine whether the situations can be considered similar.

It is clear that there are many factors that might influence your perception on any given day. Error in human judgment is inevitable, regardless of the amount of training or the years of expertise a clinician has obtained. Standardized rating scales, therefore, are a means by which to reduce the threat of error inevitable in human decision-making.

Actuarial Approach to Diagnosis

The documented threat of biases and heuristics to human judgment can be circumvented by using standardized rating scales, which instead provide an actuarial approach to diagnosis and illness monitoring. In other words, by way of statistical models, a more formal method of assessment is available that does not allow for the influence of human judgment error. This is not an argument for giving up on clinical assessment by interview but rather is a way to systematically validate it.

Systematic and Comprehensive Evaluation

Assess Objectively the Severity of the Clinical Condition

Actuarial approaches to diagnosis allow for a more objective evaluation of patients. As already mentioned, rating scales allow clinical decisions to be made while reducing the risk of judgment biases or heuristics. In addition, there is considerable benefit to the use of a measure that has been standardized against a large, normative population as opposed to relying on a small sample derived from personal

case examples. The severity of each individual case can then instead be compared systematically to a reliable sampling of a particular population. These standards allow illness severity to be accurately quantified. Finally, the objective assessment of condition severity can also be derived from the consistency of questions asked and the uniformity with which a patient's responses are rated and interpreted.

Track Change in Illness Profile Reliably

It follows that through the uniformity afforded by standardized rating scales, it is possible to reliably track illness over time. In other words, rating scales provide you with a consistent way to evaluate the progress of a patient's illness throughout the course of treatment. With the ability to ask the same questions at each testing and to record responses in a systematic way, you can objectively evaluate your patient's improvement. The first administration of the instrument provides a baseline against which subsequent administrations of the measure may be compared. For example, you may administer the BDI upon the first presentation of a patient and conclude that the patient's depression severity lies within a particular range. After beginning treatment, a period of time may pass after which you may administer the same measure again and determine how illness severity has changed over time.

Clinical Versus Actuarial Assessment

Given the aforementioned qualities of the standardized rating scale and the depicted unreliability of clinical judgment, you may wonder why the former is not the universally designated approach to assessment. There continues to be debate, however, over clinical versus actuarial assessment. Not surprisingly, as a means to resolve this controversy, researchers have attempted to determine empirically which approach can be considered more accurate.

Throughout the 1950s and 1960s, the late and eminent psychologist Paul E. Meehl played an integral role in reviewing the available literature that evaluated the accuracy of clinical versus actuarial assessment.[7] From these reviews, he was able to conclude that statistical procedures could be considered at least as accurate, and in most cases, more accurate than judgments made by trained professionals. Despite these fairly robust findings, however, the debate continues between both these approaches to assessment. For many clinicians, the resources for detailed standardized assessment are simply unavailable. Simple scales for common disorders, however, are readily accessible and have been compiled in various compendiums (see Recommended Readings). Ultimately, assessment should incorporate components of both clinical observation and standardized assessment tools.

SELECTING A RATING SCALE

Psychometric Standards

To enjoy the precision that a standardized rating scale affords, certain standards need to be set in place and followed to ensure optimal efficacy of the instrument. This involves not only evaluating the validity and reliability of a test, but also understanding the theoretical orientation, practical considerations, and appropriateness of the standardization sample for each scale administered. These details are often offered by a test manual designed specifically to outline the administration procedures of the instrument (e.g., how to administer the test), as well as to detail the standardization sample (e.g., mean age of standardization sample) and the reliability and validity of the test. A more comprehensive discussion of validity and reliability follows.

Validity

The *validity* of a rating scale refers to the degree to which a test accurately measures what it is designed to measure. There are a number of ways to evaluate the validity of a measure, including face validity, content validity, criterion validity, predictive validity, and construct validity, each of which will be outlined below.

Face Validity

Face validity refers to how a measure or procedure appears and whether it is considered, at the surface, to represent the construct it is supposed to be measuring. The assessment of face validity calls on the subjective judgment of individuals to identify whether the measure being implemented is appropriate for the clinical question at hand. Simply put, does the scale "look" and "read" like the construct it is intended to measure? For example, a scale assessing depression would include items such as sad mood, feelings of worthlessness, low energy, etc.

Content Validity

Content validity expands on the notion of face validity and assesses the "operationalization" of a concept against the "relative content domain." For example, if you were assessing for the presence of major depression in a patient according to current diagnostic criteria in the *Diagnostic and Statistical Manual*, Fourth Edition, Text Revision (DSM-IV-TR, 2000), the scale you would use to assess this must include the seven diagnostic criteria (i.e., the "content domain") for this disorder; if it includes all these criteria, the scale would be considered to have "content validity."

Criterion Validity

The evaluation of criterion validity involves comparing scores on one test with another test considered to be assessing independently the same variable. Assuming that both measures are theoretically related, performance on one test should parallel the performance on another. For example, the BDI and the Ham-D should be highly correlated because they both measure depression and depressive severity.

Predictive Validity

The goal of predictive validity is to assess the instrument's ability to predict something it should theoretically be able to predict. For example, is a person's score on a social anxiety scale predictive of how that individual behaves in anxiety-provoking situations? Similar to criterion validity, however, one of the limitations of predictive validity is the ambiguity surrounding the determination of what a construct should theoretically be able to predict.

Construct Validity

Construct validity is interested in determining whether scores obtained from a particular test actually provide an accurate measure of a specific construct. This is perhaps the most rigorous of validity evaluations and entails a more objective and empirical approach to analysis. For example, if a scale measures the construct of depression, then the items on that scale should empirically "map onto" the diagnostic criteria that compose the depression construct. Nowadays, complicated statistical procedures such as confirmatory factor analysis are used to establish construct validity. Involved in the analysis of construct validity is also the determination of the specificity and sensitivity of the test. *Specificity* refers to the percentage of true negatives that a measure has identified, whereas *sensitivity* refers to the percentage of true positives. Put differently, and continuing with the depression motif, a test is said to have a good "hit rate" if it demonstrates sensitivity (accurately detects depression in those who have depression) and specificity (accurately detects "non-depression" in those who do not have depression).

Reliability

Whereas the validity of an instrument addresses the issue of whether a rating scale measures what it is designed to measure, *reliability* refers to the accuracy and consistency of a scale. As with validity, there is a variety of ways by which reliability can be assessed, including internal consistency, retest reliability, inter-rater reliability, and alternative form reliability. Typically, reliability is interpreted by way of a reliability coefficient, a statistic that indicates the degree to which there is agreement among scores.

Internal Consistency

The internal consistency of a rating scale is a measure of agreement among the individual components of a measure. It assesses the degree to which individual items of a scale measure the same construct or syndrome. This is usually assessed using a "split-half" method in which the items composing a scale are divided in half and the responses for the two halves are then correlated to obtain a reliability coefficient. Typically, coefficients greater than 0.70 are thought to display adequate internal reliability.

Retest Reliability

Retest reliability refers to the degree to which multiple administrations of an instrument by the same rater yield the same result. This assessment of reliability is especially important when a measure is intended to track illness over time so that changes in test score can actually be ascribed to change in the status of the illness and not, instead, to the unreliability of the test. Retest reliability is assessed by administering a particular rating scale at various points in time and determining whether, upon retesting, the scale has the ability to obtain the same results. The scores obtained from each testing are then correlated to determine the reliability coefficient. Again, a coefficient of 0.70 is considered to demonstrate adequate reliability. It should be noted, however, that the nature of administering the same measure at different points of time introduces certain threats to the evaluation of reliability. More specifically, you should be wary of practice effects or the influence of memory on your patients. Someone completing a self-report rating scale for the fifth time may fill it in mechanically, anticipating the sequence of questions.

Inter-rater Reliability

The inter-rater reliability of an instrument is specific to tests that must be scored by an examiner and refers to the degree to which the judgment of one scorer is similar to the judgment of another. In other words, to what degree can multiple raters obtain the same results from an instrument? In a clinical context, it is not unusual that patients will be seen by different clinicians over the course of their treatment. Using scales where inter-rater reliability has been established enhances the communication between clinicians about the status of the patient. Correlating the scores obtained by the two independent raters generates the inter-rater reliability coefficient. Different statistical methods exist for assessing inter-rater agreement, including the intra-class coefficient (for continuous ratings) and the kappa coefficient (for dichotomous ratings). The magnitude of these coefficients to signify statistical significance varies depending on the number of raters and subjects, but usually coefficients ranging from 0.60 to 0.70 represent good agreement.

Alternative Form Reliability

The alternative form method of assessing reliability entails administering a series of scales assumed to be equivalent with regard to content, response process, and statistical characteristics and subsequently determining their ability to achieve the same results. Using this method allows the reliability of a measure to be assessed through two or more different, but parallel, scales. For example, based on the two examples provided at the beginning of this chapter, administering both the Ham-D and the BDI to one person, as a way to gauge depression severity, would allow for the reliability of these scales to be determined. Although it eliminates the threat of practice effects or the influence of memory as discussed in the context of retest reliability, the alternative form method does introduce disadvantages such as expense and the need to be confident in the content of the various scales being used.

Clinical Utility

In addition to requiring that certain psychometric standards be met, there are particular practical issues that must be taken into consideration when selecting a standardized rating scale. For example, you must take into account the ease with which the test can be administered, the degree of expertise required, and finally, the brevity of the instrument. Think about the time implications from the patient's perspective.

Ease of Administration

Crucial to the test administrator, but also relevant to the test taker, is the ease with which the test can be administered. Complicated assessment procedures will contribute to a frustrating evaluation for the patient and likely limit compliance, in turn affecting validity and reliability. Moreover, the greater the number of steps involved as part of the test administration, the more room there is for errors to be made. Thus, when determining which tests to employ, you must consider the ease with which each test can be administered.

Expertise Required

Coupled with the need to take ease of administration into account, you must also consider the training that may be required to administer each test. Some tests may require additional training so that the procedure involved with test administration can be adequately understood. In addition, you may need training to ensure the accurate interpretation of the test results once it has been completed. Some of you will be working in settings where colleagues with psychometric expertise are able to provide consultation and assessment with these instruments. Also related to this issue is the degree of expertise required by the test taker.

More specifically, you must keep in mind the level of education and reading ability of the test takers, as well as the influence of culture and language differences.

Brevity

Also of importance to both the test examiner and examinee is the length of the test being administered. If the examination is too long or contains too many items, the test taker may become tired, frustrated, and unable to concentrate. Clearly, this can influence the validity of the test and must be taken into consideration. Several rating scales now offer a short form of their instrument; but in the same way that the reliability and validity must be carefully assessed for the original version, so too must it be evaluated for any shortened version, as there are consequences of an examination that is too short.

USING A RATING SCALE

The details surrounding the use of a rating scale are typically specific to each individual scale, and such particulars are usually included in the manual that accompanies each test. There are, however, some general guidelines that you should follow when considering how to use a rating scale.

When to Administer

Standardized rating scales are administered in a variety of clinical settings. As already mentioned, they can be used when you are making a diagnosis. In addition, they might be used as means to determine the severity of a patient's illness. These instruments, then, should be administered in situations when you are looking to understand the characteristics of a patient's illness. They can also play an important role in monitoring the impact of your treatment and to provide a concrete statement of that progress for both you and your patient.

How to Administer

Standardized rating scales should be administered in accordance with the manual that accompanies each test. It is important to note that the nature of standardized rating scales does not allow for subjective interpretations to be made by the test administrator. Testing instructions must be followed closely.

What to Administer

You should maintain an up-to-date repertoire of rating scales that meet all of the aforementioned criteria. This way, when a patient reports symptoms of anxiety, you are able to administer the appropriate measure that corresponds with the reported symptoms. The test to administer to a patient, therefore, should be dictated by the description of symptoms offered by the patient.

Multiple Administrations and Tracking Change

Standardized rating scales are also often used to track change in the patient and subsequently to gauge the effectiveness of particular treatments. In this case, you might decide to administer the test at different periods of time to evaluate how the illness and its treatment are progressing. The point at which the test is first administered serves as a baseline, and each subsequent administration is often compared to this initial score.

EXAMPLES OF POTENTIAL USES

Some Existing Scales

Both the Ham-D and the BDI have been presented as examples of existing standardized rating scales. Other examples of such scales include the General Assessment of Functioning scale (GAF),[8] the Childhood Behavior Checklist (CBCL),[9] the Personality Diagnostic Questionnaire – 4 (PDQ4),[10] the Symptom Checklist-90-Revised (SCL-90-R),[11] the Yale-Brown Obsessive Compulsive Scale (Y-BOCS),[12] and the Structured Clinical Interview for DSM-IV Axis 1 Disorders (SCID-1).[13] Compendiums that offer an exhaustive listing of tests and measures can be found in the Recommended Readings at the end of this chapter. These sources will help the clinician identify and locate standardized tests for a wide range of different uses.

LIMITATIONS AND CONCLUSION

Several limitations to the actuarial approach to assessment must be highlighted. First and foremost, this method assumes the world is stable and static, which it is not. Second, even if one assumes an unchanging environment, standardized rating scales do not take into account events that may be particular to one individual. Moreover, this approach does not consider events that may occur rarely but still have an effect on the patient. Third, despite efforts at construct validity, there is no diagnostic blood test or radiological way of confirming the existence of a psychiatric illness. Psychiatric assessment remains a method of trying to make sense of the moods, thoughts, and behaviors of another person through pattern recognition. Rating scales and standardized assessment assist in that task, enhance communication between clinicians, and provide an important yardstick for evaluation and engagement. They compel patients to reflect on their experience and, to some extent, to order it. In that regard, they may assist patients in making sense of the nonsensical and in seeing the tangible impact of getting help.

REFERENCES

1. Hamilton M: A rating scale for depression, *J Neurol Neurosurg Psychiatry* 23:56–62, 1960.
2. Kearns, NP, Cruickshank, CA, McGuigan, KJ, Riley, SA, Shaw, SP, Snaith, RP: A comparison of depression rating scales. *The British Journal of Psychiatry* 141: 45–49, 1982.
3. Beck AT, Ward CH, Mendelson M et al: An inventory of measuring depression, *Arch Gen Psychiatry* 4:53–63, 1961.
4. Murphy KR, Davidshofer CO: *Psychological testing: principles and applications*, ed 5, Upper Saddle River, NJ, 2001, Prentice Hall.
5. Garb HN: *Studying the clinician: judgment research and psychological assessment*. Washington, DC, 1998, American Psychological Association.
6. Elstein, AS, Schwarz, A:. Evidence base of clinical diagnosis: Clinical problem solving and diagnostic decision making: selective review of the cognitive literature. *British Medical Journal*, 324:729–732, 2002.
7. Meehl PE: *Clinical versus statistical prediction: a theoretical analysis and a review of the evidence*, Minneapolis, MN, 1954, University of Minnesota Press.
8. Hall RC: Global assessment of functioning: a modified scale, *Psychosomatics* 36:267–275, 1995.
9. Achenbach DM: *Manual for the child behaviour checklist 4–18 and 1991 profile*. Burlington, VT, 1991, University of Vermont.
10. Hyler SE: *Personality diagnostic questionnaire–4*, New York, 1994, New York State Psychiatric Institute.
11. Derogatis LR: *SCL-90-R, brief symptom inventory, and matching clinical rating scales in psychological testing, treatment planning, and outcome assessment*. Hillsdale, NJ, 1994, Lawrence Erlbaum Associates, Inc.
12. Goodman WK et al: The Yale-Brown Obsessive Compulsive Scale, I: development, use, and reliability, *Arch Gen Psychiatry* 46:1006–1011, 1989.
13. First MB et al: *Structured clinical interview for DSM-IV (SCID-1) (user's guide and interview)*, New York, 1996, New York Psychiatric Institute.

RECOMMENDED READINGS

American Psychiatric Association: *Handbook of psychiatric measures*, Washington, DC, 2000, American Psychiatric Association.

Anatasi A, Urbina S: *Psychological testing*, ed 7, New York, 1997, Prentice Hall.

Corcoran K, Fischer J: *Measures for clinical practice*, New York, 2000, The Free Press.

Lam RW, Michalak EE, Swinson RP: *Assessment scales in depression, mania, and anxiety*, Boca Raton, 2005, Taylor & Francis.

McDowell I, Newell C: *Measuring health: a guide to rating scales and questionnaires*, Oxford, England, 1996, Oxford University Press.

3

Documentation

DAVID S. GOLDBLOOM

INTRODUCTION

This chapter, like effective documentation, will be short. The 17th century mathematician Blaise Pascal once apologized for writing a long letter, saying that he didn't have time to write a shorter one. It takes more thought and effort to write a brief, synthetic note than to provide a literal transcript of a patient encounter. How do you decide what to write?

PURPOSE

The first answer to this question is another question: What is the purpose of the documentation? Most documentation serves multiple purposes.

1. To provide a record of the encounter itself (as a response to the medicolegal maxim that "if it isn't documented, it never happened")
2. To summarize the evidence for both diagnostic impressions and treatment plans
3. To communicate with another person

LENGTH

You should summon up your empathic skills in documentation, but this time your empathy should be directed to the reader of your note rather than your patient. What would the reader of your note want to know? What will the reader of your note actually have the time to read? Think about detailed reports you have received and read. How often have you turned quickly to the final page of a detailed consultation report to seek answers to the questions, "What did he think was going on? What did he recommend?" The information a cardiac surgeon needs about the psychiatric status of her patient is different than that desired by a psychotherapist requesting a second opinion from a colleague. Of course, the ultimate in brevity would be a couple of sentences that convey a diagnosis and recommended treatment. However, that would be incompatible with standards of professional practice and terse even for a surgeon! Surgeons, in my experience, are always grateful for a report that can fit onto a single page. Readership plummets as length increases.

STRUCTURE

Most readers appreciate a road map to a report, reflected by discrete subject headings that guide them toward (or away from) particular areas. In addition, the subject headings (as reflected in Chapter 1, with additional sections for diagnosis and treatment recommendations or plans) also provide insurance that those areas that are expected by professional practice standards are covered. This is preferable to a meandering narrative letter. Indeed, in recognition of the time exigencies and priorities of some medical and surgical colleagues, many psychiatric consultants will even begin their documentation with the diagnosis and treatment recommendations, knowing that a certain number of their readers will stop after those points. Numerous textbooks provide examples of the structures of write-ups as well as samples; an excellent source is Appendix IIIB of Shea's classic textbook.[1]

LEGIBILITY

Poor penmanship plagued health care long before the rise of computers, and word processing has been a boon to those with incurable bad handwriting. Documentation serves multiple purposes, but illegibility undermines all of them. There is no communication when your writing cannot be deciphered. I have even witnessed health professionals struggling to read their own handwriting, let alone someone else's. Consider dictating or typing your report if you have bad handwriting. Brief verbal or handwritten communication can meet some immediate needs, but a full note should follow.

CONTENT

You are given an extraordinary privilege in knowing intimate details of someone's personal life and mental health. As fascinating and helpful as these details may be, a person's right to privacy is also important. Balancing that right with the importance of communicating clinical information requires thought. Again, you should think about what the reader of your documentation needs to know to justify the diagnosis and assist in treatment. Key symptoms may support both those aspects. You also need to consider the information whose presence or absence is most relevant to the context of the patient's problems.

The specific content should reflect the kind of material that is described in the following chapters that are relevant to specific problems and people.

DIAGNOSES AND TREATMENT PLANS OR RECOMMENDATIONS

Diagnoses and treatment plans comprise the one area on which readers are most likely to focus. You should exercise both rigor as a mental health professional and specificity as a helpful colleague. You should use the DSM-IV-TR multiaxial classification system (until it is replaced by something better) for diagnostic coding. It provides a common language of understanding among clinicians, even when people do not fit neatly into its somewhat arbitrary categories.

It provides important information related to treatment, such as whether a major depressive episode is a single episode or a recurrence, or whether a condition includes psychotic features. It may even stimulate the reader to find out more about a specific diagnosis.

Treatment plans or recommendations should be as specific as possible to be as helpful as possible. Telling a primary care physician that a patient you have seen "should be treated with an antipsychotic" is far less useful than specifying a recommended agent, dose (initial, titration schedule, dose range), duration, and potential benefits and side effects. Stating that the patient "would benefit from a course of psychotherapy" is less helpful than a more precise opinion on a specific type of psychotherapeutic intervention and/or psychotherapist that realistically reflects what is possible, acceptable, and available.

CONVERSATION AS AN ADJUNCT TO DOCUMENTATION—OR VICE VERSA?

In our busy professional careers, documentation all too often serves as the only form of communication between clinicians about patients. This was the subject of a lament written by my father 30 years ago.[2] However, a phone call or a hallway chat can reveal much that documentation never reflects. It can rapidly unearth the real reason for a referral for psychiatric evaluation beyond the standard "please assess" request. It can help focus the evaluation in relation to this real agenda. Similarly, direct verbal communication afterward may provide significant relief, reassurance, or redirection for the referring clinician. These conversations typically require only a few minutes, but their benefits are palpable. From a patient's perspective, imagine the difference between *"I am going to speak with your doctor personally"* and "I am going to send your doctor a letter." Which one builds more hope regarding this admittedly transient collaboration among clinicians? The documentation provides a permanent record; the conversation provides the true dialogue.

REFERENCES

1. Shea S: *Psychiatric interviewing: the art of understanding*, ed 2, Philadelphia, 1998, Saunders.
2. Goldbloom RB: The lost art of consultation: A plea for the return of striped trousers, *Pediatrics* 56:347–348, 1975.

4

Cultural Competence in Psychiatric Assessment

Lisa Francesca Andermann and Hung-Tat (Ted) Lo

INTRODUCTION

The request to "go and see that new patient" takes on a new twist when you are asked to "go and see that new Tamil-speaking (or Chinese-speaking or Hungarian-speaking) patient." You may look out into the waiting room and see the patient surrounded by a large extended family taking up most of the seats. Or you may see a woman wearing a full head covering, making any facial expression beyond eye contact difficult to assess. A common first reaction is to think, "Oh, no," and to experience a sinking feeling when you have to see either a unilingual patient whose one language is different than yours or someone from a different cultural background.

The place to start is with your own reactions. Recent imaging studies have shown that different reactions occur in the brain when working cross-culturally. Using functional magnetic resonance imaging, Richeson and colleagues[1] found increased frontal lobe activities in people identified by questionnaire to have racial biases and prejudices, suggesting that much more effort has to be exerted to control emotions and thoughts. They also found that racial bias was linked with poor cognitive performance on a test of thinking ability, perhaps because people with implicit racial biases find it more mentally exhausting to interact with others from different backgrounds, or they are trying to suppress certain feelings.[1] In terms of clinical work, cross-cultural work may be taxing. On the other hand, this work can also be more interesting and rewarding, offering a wider vista for clinicians. The message is that learning and adapting to these situations is not only possible, but also can be fruitful. However, this may take a bit

more time and effort and some new skills, which will be described in this chapter.

In this age of political correctness, many of us have been taught to treat all others in the same manner. To do so, however, is to deny our differences. In cross-cultural psychiatry, there is much to be learned from differences as well as similarities, and avoiding discussions of difference can lead us to miss potentially important information for a full understanding of the person, which is necessary for making a correct diagnosis, formulation, and treatment plan.

Cultural competence is one of the routes to good clinical practice. In some ways, every encounter can be viewed as a cross-cultural encounter if we take into account differences in life experience, education, and beliefs. This chapter is recommended as part of the development of basic assessment skills. Do not refer to this chapter only when you see someone from a visible minority waiting for you in the emergency room—this is basic knowledge for everyone!

CULTURAL COMPETENCE

Cultural competence is the term used to describe a set of attributes that allow us to work successfully across cultures.[2,3] It can also be divided into generic and specific competencies. For example, having specific knowledge of a certain language or ethnic community may give you an advantage in working with members of that group. However, with so many diverse ethnic groups in a large multicultural society, it is impossible to become familiar with every single one in depth. This is where generic cultural competence skills come in. These skills include approaches to interviewing, beginning from a position of curiosity, and not being afraid to ask questions about the person's background and beliefs. The interviewer must be able to tolerate a certain degree of ambivalence and ambiguity, allowing the person to express himself and not jumping too soon to closed-ended questions and answers, or worse, making assumptions without checking with the patient. Clarification is a process that continues throughout the clinical encounter. Do not worry at first about not knowing the intricacies of every group you see. Starting with generic competence can go a long way. Specific information can then be sought from consultants from the particular ethnic group of relevance.

During an assessment, one can keep in mind a model suggested by a quote from anthropologists Kluckholn and Murray[4]: "Every man is in certain respects like all other men, like some other men, and like no other man." This is represented by a triangle divided into three layers (Figure 4-1). The bottom layer, which is the widest, represents the universal, "all other men." This includes issues around life and death, rites of passage, and the full range of human emotions. The top part of the triangle, the smallest area, represents the individual, or "no other man." Here one looks at the personal significance of life events and their meaning for one individual. The middle layer of the triangle, "like some other men," is where the social and cultural identity is located, and this is what is often left out of standard psychiatric assessments.

WORKING WITH INTERPRETERS AND CULTURAL CONSULTANTS

Case Example 1

Mrs. Horvath, a 43-year-old Hungarian Roma (Gypsy) woman, recently arrived in Canada and told her family doctor of some problems she had been having with anxiety and difficulty sleeping for the past few months. She was referred for a psychiatric assessment. Even though Mrs. Horvath spoke enough English to make an appointment over the phone, a Hungarian-speaking interpreter was arranged for the interview.

What We Learned: Although Mrs. Horvath spoke only Hungarian at first, as she was able to trust us more in the presence of the interpreter, she then was able to feel more confident using her limited English. As the interview progressed, we were able to gain a better idea of her level of functioning and degree of acculturation. The direct communication also enhanced our rapport.

Learning Point: Recognize partial language barriers—it might seem like the patient can speak enough basic English to communicate, but she may not be able to express inner thoughts. The use of an interpreter can help.

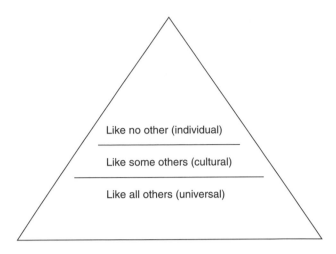

FIGURE 4-1 *Kluckholn and Murray's assessment model. (Adapted from Kluckholn C, Murray HA, editors: Personality in nature, society and culture, New York, 1953, Knopf.)*

Case Example 2

Mr. Li, a 35-year-old Chinese man with a wife and two children who recently emigrated from Beijing, was referred for a psychiatric assessment. He was frustrated by difficulties in finding a job at the same level he had before coming to Canada. He spoke English very well, and he had actually taught English in China.

What We Learned: With the suggestion of a cultural consultant, someone familiar with cultural issues in this population, we focused on the family dynamics. With the collateral history from his wife, we learned that there were more than job issues involved, and that Mr. Li was actually very stressed by family concerns, particularly the relationship of his wife to his mother. To complicate matters, his parents were about to come to Canada for a long visit—6 months. His wife was not pleased with these plans. As the oldest son, this placed Mr. Li in the center of a conflict because he was responsible to care for and to honor his parents. The home atmosphere had deteriorated considerably, with frequent arguments and concerns about physical violence. Mr. Li had made no mention of this as a problem in our first meeting.

Learning Point: For minority patients who are fluent in English, cultural issues may not be obvious at first, and a cultural consultant can help.

With changing populations, performing psychiatric assessments with the help of interpreters is happening more and more frequently. However, clinicians do not have much training in this area and are often uncomfortable with this situation. There is a lack of trained mental health interpreters, so volunteers, hospital workers, or worse still, family members are used in this position. There are a few guidelines to follow that can make this work easier. If at all possible, avoid using family members as interpreters because patients may be reluctant to reveal certain details in front of their relatives. It does take longer to do an assessment with an interpreter, so make sure you book enough time. Brief the interpreter before the interview and debrief afterward. It is important to recognize that the interpreter is not a "black box," taking in information at one end with output in another language at the other.[5] Find out who your interpreters are. This includes where they are from, their background, whether they are from a similar or different group than the patient, where they learned the language, and what, if any, dialects they are familiar with. Be aware of any reasons why it might not be suitable to match them with your patient (e.g., having been on opposite sides of a political conflict).

Seating arrangements in the interview should be in an equilateral triangle. With the clinician and the translator close together, the patient may feel intimidated. With patient and translator close together, especially when they are deeply involved in a discussion in their own language, the clinician may feel left out.[5] Westermeyer favors this triangular arrangement over the black box model but stresses that it is more complex because it involves three relationships—patient to interpreter, patient to clinician, and interpreter to clinician. However, the triangle can yield much more valuable data in an interview. Look directly at the patient, and speak directly using his or her name, rather than speaking only to the interpreter.

Indicate whether you want the interpreter to give you a verbatim account of whatever the patient says or a summary of the patient's responses. For mental status examination, the verbatim approach is advisable. You may ask for some clarification at certain points in the interview, for example, *"Did the patient's thought processes seem coherent?"* or *"Did the patient say anything that seemed unusual to you?"* Be careful not to take any interpretations completely at face value; the interpreter may be inserting his or her own issues or explanations.

In certain situations, an interpreter can sometimes act as a cultural consultant, providing important information about cultural context and historical background. Often, a request for a specific cultural consultant from an ethnic community may be necessary to integrate these details into one big picture. A cultural consultant is someone familiar with the patient's ethnocultural background who can act as a cultural interpreter, making sense of certain behaviors, ideas, and beliefs by placing them in cultural context. A cultural interpreter may also be familiar with community resources, which may become components of the treatment plan. In working with interpreters and cultural consultants, your responsibility is to get a complete picture in order to arrive at a clinical judgment, integrating different sources of information into a coherent whole.

If an interpreter is not available in a more urgent situation, AT&T Language Line Services can offer assistance across North America in 150 languages over the telephone at 1-800-752-6096. There is a fee for this service. For more details, see www.languageline.com.

Even when language difficulties do occur, recording, pronouncing, and using names properly, and being able to say hello or a few words in another language can go a long way toward indicating respect and an open attitude toward difference.[6]

USING THE CULTURAL FORMULATION

One of the useful tools for cross-cultural assessment is a cultural formulation, as described in Appendix I of the *Diagnostic and Statistical Manual*, Fourth Edition, Text Revision (DSM-IV-TR).[7] Cultural formulation consists of five sections that help to guide the interview and information-gathering process and suggest questions that will be helpful for formulation and treatment planning. The clinical assessment process is very well described by Lu et al,[8] along with one of the first research studies on evaluation of cultural consultation by Kirmayer and colleagues.[9]

Cultural Explanations of the Patient's Illness

The assessment begins with a basic question: why is the patient here? You should focus on the patient's understanding of illness (also known as the *explanatory model*) by asking open-ended questions such as, *"What do you think is wrong?"* and *"Do you think you have an illness?"* Although this is listed as the second part of the DSM-IV-TR cultural formulation, in some ways these questions are asked more naturally at the very start of the assessment. You should clarify what kind of problem the patient thinks it might be and ask what kinds of treatment expectations the patient has. During this introductory discussion, it is also important to explain your role and to let the patient know what to expect during the visit because it may likely be a first contact with psychiatry.

Focusing on cultural explanations of illness allows us to challenge any stereotypes we might have using our own preexisting cultural knowledge. For example, a Jamaican woman being treated for depression came to an appointment describing a "bad feeling" in her stomach. The psychiatrist assumed this was a somatic symptom of depression, a way of expressing distress using a physical, rather than a psychological, description, which is common in many parts of the world. In fact, the bad feeling turned out to be nausea, a side effect from antidepressant medication started the previous week. This highlights the importance of checking with the patient before making any assumptions.

Somatization, the presentation of a psychological problem within a physical symptom, is an important form of illness behavior around the world.[8] Many people believe that they can only approach a physician with a physical problem, and that this is their "ticket of entry" to be medically assessed. Others may feel there is a greater stigma in presenting with a psychological rather than a physical complaint. Still others may be unaware of the psychological aspects of their condition altogether. In any of these situations, it is important to start with a physical examination and a medical approach by a physician to rule out organic problems. No matter how sure you may be that a physical complaint is stress related or psychological in origin, for the safety of the patient you need to be reasonably sure. In addition, this helps you gain medical credibility. For a meaningful therapeutic interaction to occur, it is important not to devalue somatization as a lesser form of expression than psychologization.[10] Because of training that may overvalue psychological expression, clinicians often have difficulty relating to somatizing patients. When symptoms are given due respect, it is easier to then try to connect them to other problems in the patient's life.

Cultural Identity

Exploring cultural identity includes questions about culture, race and ethnicity, country of origin, and languages spoken. Questions about immigration history and degree of acculturation to the host country would also be included here, as would a discussion of age and gender roles as well as sexual orientation.[8] You should note the differences between an immigrant, a person who chooses to leave a home country for better opportunities elsewhere, and a refugee, who is forced to leave home and seek refuge because of violence or other life-threatening situations. Traumatic experiences, both physical and psychological, may be part of this journey. There may also be many losses involved along the way and ongoing concerns about relatives and friends who remain behind.

In-depth inquiry about cultural identity will address many issues pertaining to the social and personal history in a standard psychiatric assessment. This is also a chance to reflect on the cultural identity of the physician, who is not a "blank slate." These issues will be addressed further in later discussion.

Cultural Factors Related to the Psychosocial Environment

This part of the cultural formulation deals with social stressors and supports, and adds further information to the personal and social history. It is important to explore the role of family, which may be more extended than the typical North American nuclear family, including surrogate families developed by many refugees. Involvement with the ethnic community needs to be addressed. This can be a source of both support and stress at various times, especially if the immigrant community is a small one and there are or issues of stigma and shame or internal strife. It is also useful to make sure that the patient's level of functioning is appropriate within his or her cultural setting. For example, an Italian male in his 30s who is unmarried and living at home may be quite within cultural expectations, so you cannot jump to conclusions about dependent personality traits without having some basis for comparison with others of the same age, ethnocultural group, and social situation.

Impact of Culture on the Clinician-Patient Relationship

This section of the formulation deals with the equivalent of transference and counter-transference (feelings the patient has for the therapist and vice versa), but also takes into account particular cultural issues. The concept of ethnic match is important here. Ethnic match, the pairing of patients and clinicians from similar backgrounds, has been found to be helpful, particularly where language barriers exist. However, it is not a guarantee of success. There can be certain pairings that do not work well. This can be for political or other reasons. For example, one has to be very careful in pairing certain clinicians and patients from North and South Vietnam, Yugoslavia, or Rwanda. In smaller ethnocultural communities, patients may actually try to avoid contact with any treatment providers from their own group because of stigma or concerns about confidentiality. Furthermore, patients bring their own prejudices and stereotypes to the encounter in terms of who is a good clinician—and that may well not be someone from their own ethnocultural group.

Different pairings may include minority with minority or minority with majority. Before making assumptions that an ethnic minority patient would like to see a therapist from the same group, ask some questions such as, *"What sort of person would be helpful as a therapist?"* or *"Would I be the right person to see you?"* Comas-Diaz and Jacobsen[11] have studied these interactions in depth, looking at the ways that cultural factors influence therapeutic relationships. They describe four basic groupings: intraethnic transference and counter-transference (within one ethnic group), and interethnic transference and counter-transference (with clinician and patient from different groups). For example, they caution about the risks of "assumption of sameness," when therapists believe they know what a patient from a similar background may be experiencing without checking their beliefs. Being from the same background as patients may also lead to distancing, guilt, or anger in therapists if issues arise that remind them too much of their own lives. However, there are positive and negative factors attached to any possible dyad. Minority patients may be inspired by the success of a minority therapist.

It is also important to remember that while you are assessing the person, you are being assessed as well—in terms of your age, gender, appearance, and ability to relate. You may need to clarify your role as well as the patient's expectations and impressions.

Overall Cultural Assessment for Diagnosis and Care

This final piece of the cultural formulation brings together all the elements described and relates how this newly acquired cultural knowledge may affect diagnosis, formulation, and treatment plans.

Using the familiar biopsychosocial model, modified to include the spiritual, you should create a table with predisposing, precipitating, perpetuating, and protective factors (Figure 4-2). For each box, consider possible cultural contributions. For example, biological precipitating factors may include the use of traditional herbal medications leading to depressive or psychotic symptoms. Cultures that emphasize honor and shame may predispose their members to develop psychological symptoms when personal weakness is revealed. Spiritual practices in many cultures may have an ameliorating or protective effect.

The journal *Culture, Medicine and Psychiatry* has published a case series of cultural formulations that follow this format and provide excellent models for formulation of various disorders, including psychotic disorders, anxiety disorders, and other diagnoses within in a cultural context. Lim and Lin's[12] formulation of psychosis in a Chinese immigrant after his use of a traditional Chinese healing practice is one such example.

	Predisposing	Precipitating	Perpetuating	Protective
Biological				
Psychological				
Social				
Spiritual				

FIGURE 4-2 *Biopsychosocial-spiritual formulation.*

ELABORATION OF METHODS: MENTAL STATUS EXAMINATION

The mental status examination begins with observation, and your assessment starts as soon as you enter the room, before a word is spoken. Ideally, it is woven into the fabric of the interview rather than being done as a checklist. General appearance, including age, gender, mode of dress and grooming, and behaviors, including posture or formal greetings such as bowing, provide valuable data for your assessment.

Observations of nonverbal communication are an important part of the mental status. In many countries, including Ethiopia and parts of Asia, avoiding direct eye contact is a sign of respect and should not be mistaken for shyness or withdrawal. People may use different gestures to indicate yes or no, and shaking one's head from side to side to indicate disapproval is not a universal sign.

With regard to verbal communication, some languages are spoken faster and some much slower. The technique of mirroring, following the person's rate of speed or gestures, can be used to achieve rapport more quickly but may also have the unintended result of making the person uncomfortable if he or she does not expect you to behave in this manner.

The use of silence in some cultures is well known. For example, many Aboriginal patients, especially among the older generation, tend towards silence and will not initiate conversation with a clinician. Clinicians need to learn to respect silence instead of filling it with words.

The examination of psychopathology can be a challenge when performing a mental status examination across cultures. In some ways, it can be most difficult to accurately gauge mood and affect. Nonverbal expression of emotion can vary across cultures and may be difficult for a clinician of a different background to recognize accurately. With regard to verbal communication, certain cultures may not share our psychological vocabulary or the categories of emotion needed to differentiate between subtle feeling states. In these cases, it is important to compare with community norms and to ask the cultural consultant about normal ranges of emotional expression within that culture.[8]

The same principles apply to the assessment of delusional beliefs, which can sometimes be difficult to distinguish from nonpathological, culturally normative beliefs when one is unfamiliar with the background of the patient. Learning more about the religious and political beliefs of others, which are often common themes for delusions, can be valuable. Community norms are particularly relevant here. You should obtain a collateral history and look for any changes in the person, with regard to social and occupational functioning, over time. For example, a Tamil refugee from Sri Lanka escaping a situation of political oppression may have ongoing suspicion of police, even after reaching safety in another country, which may continue long after resettlement. Without knowing that this is a very common reaction among refugees and understanding the person's background and previous experience, one might jump too quickly to a conclusion about paranoia or delusional beliefs. If unsure, you might ask a family or community member or a cultural consultant to verify the situation. If others do not substantiate the circumstances described, then you would need to look more closely for pathology.

Although we may always have some unanswered questions when doing a cross-cultural assessment, what we do know is that the major categories of mental illness, including psychotic, anxiety, and affective disorders, are universal, and therefore we can expect there to be more similarities than differences when dealing with major axis I diagnoses. Using schizophrenia as an example of a universal mental disorder that is found around the world, the processes of thought disorder, delusions, and hallucinations are observed to be similar across cultures, although the content of the thoughts or delusions may be very different. For example, an Ethiopian man from a Muslim background described particular beliefs about having the special power to see good and evil in the world. Asking questions such as, *"Is it common for people at your mosque to share these beliefs, or are you the only one?"* may help to elucidate between culturally acceptable religious beliefs and a delusional process.

RATING SCALES

There are some cross-culturally validated rating scales for psychiatric symptoms. However, these are normally used for research purposes rather than for regular clinical practice. Care needs to be taken in the translation process to ensure reliability. The process of "back-translation," wherein the questionnaire is translated from English to another language and then back to English again by a different translator, can be used to reduce errors or misunderstandings. Often, it is the concept that is difficult to translate, not simply the words. This can lead to issues with validity: is the questionnaire measuring what it says it does? For example, many cultures do not identify depression as an illness category or associate behaviors such as crying with depression, so a question such as, "Have you felt sad or blue?" or "How many times have you cried in the last 2 weeks?" may not be answered in the same way.

ENGAGEMENT AND ONGOING CARE

Once you have completed the interview, assessment, and formulation, the real work begins. The most skillfully written report will not benefit anyone if it lies untouched in the filing cabinet. Some form of follow-up, either with a psychiatrist or other health care or social agency staff, is generally part of the treatment plan. Ensuring that this follow-up will take place is one of the most important parts of the assessment process. Many studies have documented that ethnic minorities do not access health care resources, particularly mental health care resources, with the same frequency as mainstream populations.[3] Therefore, careful attention to follow-up is especially needed. The success of this process begins with the level of engagement during the assessment. To create a situation of enhanced engagement with the patient, several conditions must be met. The patient must feel listened to and understood. Avoiding the tendency to go down a list of questions when dealing with people with language difficulties will go a long way in this regard. Patients need to feel that something was accomplished within the interview, and that they are not just being asked to leave because their time is up. Checking in with patients at intervals throughout the interview about how they are feeling, with regard to anxiety level as well as comfort about sharing their feelings, and especially how they feel at the end of the interview compared to the beginning, will provide a sense of whether a clinical encounter has been therapeutic for them.

Another aspect in developing the treatment plan involves a discussion and negotiation with the patient around your diagnostic impressions and proposed course of action. When different health beliefs intersect, this becomes particularly important. Katon and Kleinman[13] describe ways to work with different explanatory models to arrive at a common understanding and agreement. This is an ongoing process, to be adjusted as the patient proceeds through different stages of the therapy. For example, let's say you have just diagnosed a 30-year-old Chinese woman with schizophrenia and propose a course of antipsychotics. Your explanatory model is one of a biological illness based on neurotransmitter function and neuroanatomy. In contrast, the patient believes that her nerves are weak, and she would like an herbal tonic to treat neurasthenia, as recommended by her family members. After eliciting her explanatory model, you may then negotiate a compromise, which could include a low dose of antipsychotic medication in addition to Chinese traditional medicine from an herbalist. Of course, you would need to be cautious about medication interactions. However, an outright rejection of the patient's model, and her ideal treatment, would almost certainly lead to noncompliance with medication, and of more concern, the possibility of her leaving treatment altogether.

Finally, make sure that the patient leaves the consultation room with a "gift," represented by greater understanding, reassurance, or symptom relief, or something tangible, like a prescription or appointment card.[2]

CONCLUSION

Acquiring cultural knowledge alone is not sufficient. As with the development of any skill, cultural competence in assessments requires practice. With some experience, any feelings of frustration will decrease, and this work will become more enjoyable. Being able to work with patients of different cultures over time, rather than in a single assessment, increases your opportunities to deepen your knowledge and also reaffirms your increasing cultural competence.

MYTHS

1. *I need to act the same way as my patient to be accepted.* Just be respectful and professional. Your patient knows very well whether you are from his culture.

2. *I could never ask that question.* Don't avoid certain areas because of ideas you have about a cultural group—any topic can be approached tactfully and respectfully. Use a preamble to explain why you are asking certain questions.

3. *I have to know that culture very well before I can be helpful.* You don't have to pretend to know everything beforehand. Acknowledge your limitations and ask questions.

4. *If I speak louder, maybe they'll understand.* Volume is not correlated with increased understanding of English. Try to speak clearly and slowly, and ask one question at a time—don't use compound questions.

5. *An interpreter is only there to translate.* An interpreter is not a "black box." She needs to be treated as part of the treatment team, with briefings and debriefings before and after the interview. She might also provide some valuable cultural context.

Key Points:

1. If a patient's first language is not English, make sure to get an interpreter, at least for part of the assessment process, even if the patient speaks some English. An accurate psychiatric assessment and mental status exam depends on good communication

2. Obtain collateral history—this is especially important if you are dealing with unusual symptoms or a possible psychosis.

3. Don't jump too quickly to diagnose delusions; you need to rule out culturally accepted beliefs or religious ideas first.

4. Working with the family is very important—family dynamics carry more weight in the social structure of many cultures than in western society, where the focus is more on the individual. Regardless of background, involving family members is important for the outcome of the treatment.

5. Don't assume that patients want to have an ethnic match with a clinician; clarify preferences and degree of comfort.

---

6. During an illness episode, patients may often seem more regressed (especially in a foreign setting like a hospital) and less adjusted or acculturated than they might be when they are feeling well. Therefore, it is important to assess people in a familiar environment, such as home or a community center, if possible.

7. Gender, age, and social status are issues that may affect communication during the clinical encounter.

8. Be aware that somatic presentations (e.g., headaches, backaches, stomachaches) may mask a psychiatric problem.

9. Get to know the "real reason" why the patient has come to see you. The patient may have different expectations of the clinical encounter, which can then be understood and negotiated.

10. Look for strengths: resilience and resourcefulness.

REFERENCES

1. Richeson JA, Baird AA, Gordon HL, Heatherton TF, Wyland CL, Trawalter S, Shelton JN: An fMRI examination of the impact of interracial contact on executive function, *Nat Neurosci* 6:1323–1328, 2003.

2. Lo HT, Fung KP: Culturally competent psychotherapy, *Can J Psychiatry* 48:161–170, 2003.

3. U.S. Department of Health and Human Services. *Mental health: culture, race and ethnicity—a supplement to mental health: a report of the Surgeon General—executive summary,* Rockville, MD, 2001, Public Health Service, Office of the Surgeon General. Available online at www.surgeon-general. gov/library.

4. Kluckholn C, Murray HA, editors: *Personality in nature, society and culture,* New York, 1953, Knopf.

5. Westermeyer J: Working with an interpreter in psychiatric assessment and treatment, *J Nerv Ment Dis* 178(12):745–749, 1990.

6. Goldbloom RB: Skills for culturally sensitive pediatric care. In Goldbloom RB, editor: *Pediatric clinical skills,* New York, 2003, WB Saunders.

7. American Psychiatric Association: *Diagnostic and Statistical Manual,* ed 4, text revision, Washington, DC, 2000, APA Publishing.

8. Lu FG, Lim RF, Mezzich JE: Issues in the assessment and diagnosis of culturally diverse individuals. In Oldham J and Riba M, editors: *American Psychiatric Press annual review of psychiatry,* Washington, DC, 1995, APA Press, pp 477–510.

9. Kirmayer LJ, Groleau D, Guzder J, Blake C, Jarvis E: Cultural consultation: a model of mental health service for multicultural societies, *Can J Psychiatry* 48:145–153, 2003.

10. Kirmayer LJ, Groleau D, Looper KJ, Dominice Dao M: Explaining medically unexplained symptoms, *Can J Psychiatry* 49:663–672, 2004.

11. Comas-Diaz L, Jacobsen FA: Ethnocultural transference and countertransference in the therapeutic dyad, *Am J Orthopsychiatry* 61(3):392–402, 1991.

12. Lim RF, Lin K-M: Cultural formulation of a psychiatric diagnosis: psychosis following Qi-Gong in a Chinese immigrant, *Culture, Medicine and Psychiatry* 20:369–378, 1996.

13. Katon W, Kleinman A: Doctor-patient negotiation and other social science strategies in patient care. In Eisenberg L, Kleinman A, editors: *The relevance of social science to medicine*, Dordrecht, The Netherlands 1981, Reidel.

RECOMMENDED READINGS

Barrett RJ: Cultural formulation of a psychiatric diagnosis: death on a horse's back, *Culture, Medicine and Psychiatry* 21:481–496, 1997.

Fadiman A: *The spirit catches you and you fall down: a Hmong child, her American doctors and the collision of two cultures*, New York, 1997, Farrar, Straus and Giroux.

Kleinman A: *The illness narratives: suffering, healing and the human condition*, New York, 1988, Basic Books.

Lee E: Overview: the assessment and treatment of Asian American families. In Lee E, editor: *Working with Asian Americans: a guide for clinicians*, New York, 1997, The Guilford Press, pp 3–36.

Linde P: *Of spirits and madness: an American psychiatrist in Africa*, New York, 2002, McGraw Hill.

Kirmayer L, Minas H: The future of cultural psychiatry: an international perspective, *Can J Psychiatry* 45(5):438–446, 2000.

Manson SM: The wounded spirit: a cultural formulation of post-traumatic stress disorder, *Culture, Medicine and Psychiatry* 20:489–498, 1996.

Mezzich J, Kleinman A, Fabrega H, Parron D, editors: *Culture and psychiatric diagnosis: a DSM-IV perspective*, Washington, DC, 1996, American Psychiatric Press.

Sue DW, Sue D: *Counseling the culturally different: theory and practice*, New York, 1990, Wiley.

Tseng W-S: *Clinician's guide to cultural psychiatry*, San Diego, CA, 2003, APA Press.

5

Assessment of Patients with Psychosis

Natasja Menezes and Robert Zipursky

INTRODUCTION

The more experience we gain in the mental health professions, the more many of us realize the privilege we have of getting to know our patients personally—of knowing them not just as functions of their symptoms, but as functioning beings themselves. The "art of medicine"—that is what it is about. But what is the true art? In psychiatry, many would say that it is knowing *how* to ask *which* question and *when*. How you phrase a question—and at what point in the interview you pose it—can make a significant difference to both your information yield and your therapeutic relationship. It's an intimidating fact! This is not at all minimized by the fact that we have no diagnostic laboratory tests and few physical signs in psychiatry, and we must rely on our clinical and interpersonal skills to work with our patients.

This can be all the more challenging when the questioning revolves around psychosis. Many a student has prefaced a psychosis screen by saying, "These may seem like weird questions, but I ask everybody this." This usually reflects their own discomfort with the content, rather than the patient's. Anybody can ask a checklist of diagnostic criteria, but not everybody can actually elicit an accurate history of psychosis symptoms from the patient.

Being comfortable with what you have to know is key to developing skills in the art of medicine. This chapter aims to help you do just that. By the end of the chapter, the questions should not feel weird, and you should be able to ask them in the most efficient, high-yield way that fosters a relationship with your patient.

Case Example 1

John first met Dr. Yates when he was 17. He had gone through a gradual change in functioning and personality over the last 2 years, involving a slow withdrawal from his friends and family, an increased use of marijuana, and a decline in his self-care, culminating in his dropping out of school. He had become very interested in religious matters and developed a philosophical way of thinking and expressing himself. Despite his parents' concerns, he had refused to seek help. He finally ended up in contact with Dr. Yates when psychiatric treatment was mandated by the court as part of his probation term. He had broken the window of the neighbor's car because he felt that a camera had been placed in the body of the car to spy on his bedroom window. He never acknowledged this to Dr. Yates, although he had previously explained his behavior to his parents. For the first 7 months of follow-up, he denied any symptoms or distress and came only by obligation of the court. His mother administered his medication, so he was grudgingly compliant. After the first 7 months, he started to admit regrets at the losses he had gone through with school and friends but continued to deny any psychotic symptoms. He became depressed, increased his marijuana consumption, and became floridly psychotic and agitated, requiring a 3-week in-patient admission. After this admission, he began to question what had led to his behavior and admission, and he started to work with his case manager to understand the persecutory ideation he had been living with. He attempted a return to school but had to drop out because of concentration difficulties. He succeeded in holding a part-time job in a real estate agency. He felt so well that he stopped taking his medications. Since things were back to normal, he started hanging out with some new friends from work, started a romantic relationship, and did well for several months, never reporting that he had quit his medications. Gradually, he started to reuse marijuana and to withdraw, finally being fired from his job for poor attendance. He agreed to restart medications at the urging of his girlfriend and has been stable now for 2 years.

What are the issues involved in working with such a patient? This chapter can help clinicians to elicit these issues and work with them by using the following questions:

- What diagnosis accounts for the change in personality and functioning?
- What differential diagnosis needs to be considered?
- How do you engage such a patient so that he may receive treatment and follow-up earlier on?
- What are the phases of illness that patients go through?
- What risk factors affect the course of illness, and how do we elicit them?

The American Psychiatric Association's *Diagnostic and Statistical Manual of Mental Disorders*, edition 4, text revision (DSM-IV-TR),[1] notes, "The term *psychotic* has historically received a number of different definitions, none of which has achieved universal acceptance. The narrowest definition of *psychotic* is restricted to delusions or prominent hallucinations, with the hallucinations occurring in the absence of insight into their pathological nature . . . Broader still is a definition that also includes other positive symptoms of schizophrenia (i.e., disorganized speech, grossly disorganized or catatonic behavior)". In the DSM-IV-TR, the term *psychotic* refers to different combinations of delusions, hallucinations, negative symptoms, disorganized speech or behavior, cognitive deficits, and catatonia, varying according to diagnosis (Box 5-1). We view psychosis as a syndrome with different causes (Box 5-2), much as a headache can be caused by a hangover, the flu, a migraine, caffeine withdrawal, a long day, or a long book chapter!

In this chapter, we use our own clinical experience (positive and negative) to provide a starting place for addressing some of the clinical issues involved in working with people with psychosis, with an emphasis on the schizophrenia-spectrum disorders. The chapter aims to elaborate on the clinical interview of a patient with psychosis, addressing the components and challenges of the interview, the techniques to optimize engagement and information-gathering, and the knowledge base to be acquired. By the end of this chapter, you should be able to answer the following questions:

1. What techniques can I use to sufficiently engage patients with psychosis so that they stay and answer the questions in a meaningful way?

Box 5-1. The Categories of Psychotic Symptoms

POSITIVE SYMPTOMS

Delusions
Hallucinations

NEGATIVE SYMPTOMS

Affective flattening
Alogia: impoverished thinking reflected in poverty of speech
Avolition: inability to initiate and sustain goal-directed
    activities
Anhedonia: loss of interest or pleasure

DISORGANIZATION SYMPTOMS

Thought disorder
    Loose associations
    Tangentiality
    Word salad
Behavior

COGNITIVE SYMPTOMS

Attentional deficits
Memory impairment
Information-processing deficits

CATATONIC SYMPTOMS

Stupor: decreased awareness of the environment
Rigidity: rigid posture
Negativism: active resistance to instructions or attempts to be
    moved
Posturing: inappropriate or bizarre postures
Excitement: purposeless and unstimulated excessive motor
    activity

Box 5-2. The Etiologies of Psychosis

PRIMARY PSYCHOTIC DISORDERS

Schizophrenia
Schizophreniform disorder
Schizoaffective disorder
Delusional disorder
Brief psychotic disorder
Shared psychotic disorder
Psychotic disorder NOS

Secondary to . . .

General medical condition (e.g., dementia, delirium, temporal
    lobe epilepsy)
Substance-induced (e.g., illicit drugs or medication-induced)
Mood disorder

---

2. What are the goals of my interview with a patient with psychosis?
3. What differential diagnoses do I have to keep in mind, and how do I evaluate for these?

4. How do I phrase questions so they do not seem odd, but nevertheless efficiently elicit the symptoms?
5. What should I observe?
6. What additional tools can I use?
7. What challenges should I be ready for, and how can I get around them?
8. Where else can I get information?
9. What do I need to elicit from a patient seen in follow-up?

THE GOAL OF THE INTERVIEW

For the purposes of this chapter, we will consider the goals of the interview to be:

1. To engage the patient;
2. To elicit a history (symptoms, etc.) leading to provisional and differential diagnoses;
3. To determine the needs of the patient and the appropriate management;
4. To make the contact a positive enough experience that the patient will consider coming back.

Key Point:

We should strive to make every interaction with a patient a therapeutic one in which he takes something away from the contact. This applies to first-time consultations, follow-up appointments, and even brief hallway encounters.

Getting Started

Before even meeting the patient, it is important to ensure that your setting is adequate and that you are thinking about how to make both yourself and the patient feel most comfortable in the upcoming interaction. Special consideration should be paid to the following.

Comfort
- Is the setting too warm/cold?
- Does the patient have any basic needs (bathroom, food/water, etc.) to be met prior to the interview?
- Is the patient suffering any psychological/physical symptoms that could interfere with the process (e.g., anxiety, side effects such as motor restlessness or extreme sedation)?
- Does the patient require any medication prior to the interview?
- If there are observers present, are the chairs angled such that the patient does not feel stared at or ganged up on?

Key Point:

Ensuring a comfortable and safe setting before starting the interview will increase the probability that the patient will stay long enough to complete the assessment without distraction or interruption.

Safety
- From what you know about the patient (ambulance or police notes, triage assessment), do you require another person to be present?
- Is there an alternate escape route for the interviewer and/or the patient?
- Is there sufficient space that the patient won't feel threatened or crowded?
- Have you secured any loose objects that might be used to throw or strike someone?

Key Point:

It is essential that both the interviewer and the patient feel safe. If the interviewer is anxious, it will be difficult for the patient to feel comfortable in the interview setting.

Engagement

Engagement can encompass many different concepts and is applicable to any interview setting. See Chapter 1 for further general discussion on engagement.

How do you "engage" a patient with psychosis? It is an ongoing process that can be started by considering the following:

- Does the patient understand why he is here? What are the patient's goals/expectations for the encounter?
  - The purpose of the interview should be explained beforehand, setting the ground for what is to come.
  - You can address these issues in the following ways:
    - *"Perhaps you can start with telling me your understanding of the reason for our meeting today."*
    - *"Dr. X has asked me to meet with you today to clarify . . ."* or *". . . to determine whether . . ."*
    - *"I've asked you to come back for a follow-up today so that I can have some extra time to explain . . ."* or *". . . so that I can get an idea of how you are doing and whether there are any problems you would like me to know about."*
    - *"Tell me what you would like to get out of today's meeting,"* or *"How I can help you?"* or *"What do you need help with?"*

- Does the patient know what will be involved in the interaction? This should include the duration and break-down of the interview.
  - This is helpful in preventing potential stalls in the interview, such as when the suspicious patient says, "I don't see why you need to know that," or "You can get that from the chart," or "I didn't know this was going to take so long; my parking meter was up 20 minutes ago."
  - You can address this with the following tactics:
    - *"In order to make recommendations, I would like to be able to understand what has led to your coming here and what you have been experiencing."*
    - *"I understand you saw Dr. X in consultation 2 weeks ago. The questions I ask you today may repeat some of those. I find it helpful to hear about people's experiences in their own words."*
- Does the patient understand that the discussion is confidential?
  - This is particularly important for patients who are guarded or frankly paranoid.
  - You can address this with the following statements:
    - *"We may discuss some personal issues today. I would like to reassure you that all you tell me is confidential and will only be written in a report to your family doctor who referred you here. No one else can have access to that information without your permission."*
- Does the patient feel safe? Ask the following questions:
  - *"Is there anything making you uncomfortable right now?"*
  - *"I noticed that you keep looking at the door. Is there something in particular you are looking for?"*
- Are you aware of cues that the patient gives, for example, of questions she does not understand or of uncomfortable topics?
- Are you adapting your questioning style to the patient's capacity to understand or her level of education?

Key Point:

A key long-term goal is to keep a patient with psychosis in treatment, given the frequent chronicity of some psychotic illnesses. The early contacts can lay the positive foundation for an ongoing therapeutic relationship and low dropout rate.

Key Point:

It is important to realize that many patients with psychosis have elements of disorganization and deficits in attention. In this context, it is helpful to make questions brief and straightforward, sometimes using examples to clarify. Keep in mind not to use leading questions.

- Once the interview is underway, do you attempt to give a context for (i.e., normalize) questions that may seem to be of a prying/odd/judgmental nature?
  - Do not feel compelled to preface such questions by labeling them (e.g., "Now I am going to ask you some questions that may seem strange"). This ends up putting the patient on guard and reduces the probability that he will feel comfortable enough to respond honestly. It is best to personalize it to the patient.
    - *"You mentioned before that you have been under a lot of stress lately and haven't been feeling yourself. In those situations, sometimes people can have new experiences such as . . . I wonder if this has happened to you?"*
    - *"I noticed you hesitated when I asked you about X. I ask you that because in working with people who have had similar experiences, we have noticed that they often report X, and I was wondering—has that been the case for you?"*
    - *"It is important for me to have a clear idea of the amount of drugs you have been using because we know that they can sometimes have a role in X."*

COLLECTING INFORMATION FROM THE PATIENT

After your initial contact and introduction, you are finally underway with the interview. Depending on the situation, the chief complaint (*not* the whole story, but a brief introduction to the problem in the patient's own words) is a reasonable way to get started, while giving you and the patient a focus on the goal of the interview. For those patients who are not comfortable starting with an elaboration of their difficulties, and who may need a more neutral lead-in, nonthreatening data-gathering can also be an acceptable place to start, while giving you a larger contextual view of the patient (e.g., name, age, living situation).

Key Point:

It may be helpful to start with the chief complaint because it permits the patient a few minutes to talk freely, in the absence of structuring or directive questions. This allows you to observe thought form, reliability, processing capacity, etc. It gives you a sense of how organized the patient is and how open-ended your interview should be. This also permits you to develop a targeted structure for the remainder of the interview, driven by your hypotheses about the primary diagnosis and its differential.

The History of Present Illness

The history of the present illness (HPI) is the foundation of your database, the big picture overlying the details of what has led this patient to you. A properly conducted HPI should be directed by your hypotheses about the diagnosis and its differential. These hypotheses evolve from the time you first see the patient (e.g., Is she euphorically singing in the hallway while waiting for the interview? Is she stooped over with poor eye contact?) and should also be directed by the patient's cues. It is important to feel comfortable enough with what you need to know by the *end* of the interview and to ensure that you are not formulaic *during* the interview. It is helpful to be flexible with the order in which you elicit information.

Case Example 2

Sara is a 21-year-old waitress who was brought in to the psychiatry emergency department by police. She was found in the street, stripped to the waist, singing in the snow with no shoes on, claiming that if she stopped singing, the devil would take her in punishment for her sins. In the emergency department, she refused to talk for the first 2 hours, appearing to be asleep. Her vital signs were stable; she refused to comply with any blood or urine tests, and there were no signs of intoxication. She had no identification on her, and there was no source of collateral information. On waking, she was irritable and suspicious, demanding to leave. She agreed to a 10-minute interview with the psychiatry resident and swore that she would stop talking after that time.

The issues:

- How do you collect information from an uncooperative patient?
- What type of details should be prioritized in information collection?
- What emergency issues need to be considered?
- What other sources of information can be used?

In evaluating psychosis, there are several key features that must be clear by the end of the interview (they do not necessarily have to be elicited in this order, although a good start is to get an idea of the cross-section of the psychosis and its qualities and then to use this information to drive the questioning of the differential diagnosis and evolution of symptoms):

- Why now? What was the trigger for consultation being solicited at this time?
  - *"I understand that things have been different for you recently. I wonder what led you to seek help right now?"*

- What are the actual symptoms of psychosis? Remember that you want to phrase the screening questions in such a way as to elicit more than just "yes" or "no." Or, if that's what you get, you should follow up with something such as "Tell me more about that," or "Can you give me an example?" (Table 5-1).

Key Point:

Accurate data-gathering implies exploration of what patients say, and not just taking all they say at face value.

- It is important to keep in mind that most patients will have some difficulty freely expressing psychotic symptoms. It can be helpful either to normalize the question or to personalize it to this particular patient's context. You should at least start with broad conceptual questions and then hone in on the actual delusional content.
  - *"You mentioned earlier that when you smoke a joint, you get paranoid. Can you tell me a little bit more about that?" (In other words, ensure that the patient is using the word "paranoid" in the same way you understand it.) "Does that ever occur unrelated to pot?"*
  - *"Often when people have gone through a period of difficulty sleeping, they may start to feel that their thinking is different. Has that ever happened to you? Can you tell me about that? Or, you don't think it has? Perhaps if I give you an example that I often see, it might help. Patients report that when they haven't been sleeping well, they start to question things or have thoughts that run in circles, like 'I'm being followed' or 'Is it safe here?' Have you ever experienced something similar?"*

- You must be cautious and ask initial questions as broadly as possible so as to not lead the patient toward your anticipated answer (Box 5-3). Patients can often be passive, and their simple answer of "yes" may not reveal much information and may in fact be misleading.

- As mentioned earlier, in the context of attention and processing deficits intrinsic to psychosis, it is also important to *not* ask single questions that cluster multiple experiences (e.g., *"Have you ever felt your life was in danger or that people were following you or meaning you harm?"* The questions are difficult to follow for a patient with psychosis, and the answer will rarely be reflective of the true experience.

Table 5-1. Questioning Psychotic Symptoms

Symptoms	Examples	Questions
Delusions		*"Do you ever get the feeling that:*
	Persecutory	*. . . others mean to harm you/your life is in danger?"*
	Control	*. . . some outside force is controlling your actions/thoughts?"*
	Mind reading	*. . . others know what you think/you can read others' minds?"*
	Grandiosity	*. . . you have some special skills/have been selected for some special mission?"*
	Reference	*. . . things seem to happen because of you?"*
		. . . people are talking about you?"
	Thought insertion	*. . . you think something and it just didn't come from you?"*
	Thought broadcasting	*. . . your thoughts were being broadcast, on television or radio for example?"*
	Thought withdrawal	*. . . your thoughts are taken out of your head by some outside force?"*
	Somatization	*. . . something has changed in your body recently?"*
Hallucinations	Auditory	*"Do you ever hear things (whispers, sounds, voices) that others don't hear, or that you wonder if they are real?"*
	Quality	*"Do they come from inside/outside your head? Do you hear them like my voice now? Do you ever turn to see who spoke? Do they ever answer back?"*
	Number of voices	*"Are there one or more voices? Are they recognizable?"*
	Running commentary	*"Are the voices are doing a play-by-play on your actions, like in a hockey game?"*
	Command	*"Are the voices telling you what to do?"*
	Visual	*"Do you see things other people don't see and wonder if they are really there?"*
	Other (e.g., tactile, olfactory, gustatory)	*"Do you notice any strange smells, tastes, or sensations on your skin?"*
Negative	Affective flattening	*"Have others commented that your facial expression is different (e.g., that you don't smile as much)?"*
	Poverty of speech or content	*"Do you ever find that you don't have much to say?"*
	Apathy (self-care)	*"Has there been any change in your motivation to do things, or do you just not feel like it (e.g., showering, going to movies)?"*
	Anhedonia	
	Asociality	
	Interpersonal	*"Do you still see your friends? Who initiates this?"*
	Recreational	*"What did you enjoy doing 5 years ago? Has there been any change in the level of enjoyment of those things?"*
	Attention	
	Cognitive inattention	*"Has there been any change in your concentration/memory or distractibility? Can you read a book?"*

(*Note:* Examples are not exhaustive.)

■ The conviction of a belief must be evaluated to confirm that it meets criteria for a delusion (i.e., a firmly held, fixed belief that is discordant with cultural norms). If the conviction is not there, it may suggest an idiosyncratic overvalued belief, or a prodromal symptom.

　□ *"You spoke about being followed everywhere you go. Have there been times when you questioned whether this could really be true? Or times when you thought you were being followed and then you told yourself, 'But that's impossible, it doesn't make sense'? Have you talked yourself out of believing it? What have you done about it?"*

　□ *"When you have such a thought, how much do you believe it, with 100% being that it is the truth and you are convinced, and 0% being you don't believe it at all?"*

　□ *"Do you think that X is happening to you only, or does it happen to others as well? Why would you be selected more than anyone else? What is your understanding of what is happening?"*

■ It can be diagnostically helpful to evaluate the quality (i.e., content) of the psychotic symptoms. This can help to drive the rest of your questioning in clarifying the differential diagnosis. For example:

　□ A mood-congruent delusion can be suggestive of a mood disorder (e.g., a grandiose delusion in mania, a nihilistic delusion in depression).

　□ Schneiderian symptoms (e.g., audible thoughts, voices arguing or discussing, voices commenting, thought influencing or withdrawal or broadcasting, delusions) can be suggestive of schizophrenia. Although they may occur in other illnesses with psychosis, such as mania, these bizarre symptoms are weighted more heavily in the DSM-IV-TR criteria for schizophrenia.

▫ Catatonia is more often due to a mood disorder than to a medical disorder or schizophrenia.

■ Explore the evolution of the psychosis phase.

▫ Was the onset gradual or abrupt? When did it start? The duration of symptoms is important for establishing a diagnosis.

▫ Are there any triggering factors or precipitants? Acute stressors?

▫ How did it evolve until now?

▫ When was the first contact for help, and what was done?

▫ What is the current status? Are symptoms/functioning better than before? Worse? The same?

■ What has been the evolution of events and symptoms predating the onset of psychosis?

▫ It can be diagnostically helpful to have a clear timeline of functioning, symptoms, and changes in these domains, given their characterization of schizophrenia.[2] The chronology can be elicited for the following phases (some components of the early premorbid personality can be elicited in the personal/developmental history section of Chapter 1).

• **Premorbid.** It is helpful to have an idea of the personality at baseline, with a focus on capacity for interpersonal relations, odd features of personality (e.g., with respect to interests), behavioral difficulties, etc. A history suggestive of schizoid or schizotypal personality may be present before the onset of full psychosis.

• **Prodrome.** This refers to the period when some changes in functioning and mild symptoms have begun. In this period, patients may have some psychotic symptoms, but they are of a transient nature or attenuated intensity (e.g., ideas, not delusions, of reference). Patients may have new interests (e.g., philosophy, religion), a change in their thinking style (e.g., more abstract), perceptual changes, and bizarre ideas with abnormal affect. Prodrome is differentiated from full-blown psychosis by its attenuated symptoms. These can be explored with the following questions:

○ *"When did you first notice that things seemed different or not right?"*

○ *"You suggested earlier that you just weren't doing well; can you tell me a little bit about what that means?"*

○ *"You mentioned you were having a tough time with things; can you tell me what impact this had on your schooling? On your friends? Your family? How did you deal with that?"*

○ *"Patients have often told me that when they were feeling stressed, similar to what you have described, they might start to question things a lot, for example, whether people were looking at them differently. Has that been the case for you? Or, they might start to notice a lot of coincidences or connections between things; for example, it seems like whenever they cross the street, the light turns red because of them. Has something similar happened to you?"*

■ What is the current level of functioning, and how is this a change?

▫ *"Has there been any change in your sleep/ appetite/energy? What was it like before?"*

▫ *"What is an average day like for you these days? What do you do? How does this compare to 2 years ago?"*

▫ *"If I had met you 5 years ago, what would you have been like compared to today? What would have been similar/different?"* (This can be a high-yield question for eliciting symptoms and changes in personality, functioning, interpersonal capacity, etc.)

■ Are there cognitive difficulties?

▫ Impairments in concentration, memory, processing, and executive functioning are common in schizophrenia and important for management. They can also be more predictive of outcome and functioning than positive symptoms alone, and thus are important to evaluate from the patient's perspective:

• *"Have you noticed a change in your ability to remember things? Do you forget names? Misplace objects?"*

• *"How is your concentration lately? Do you have difficulty doing two things at once, for example, watching TV and having a conversation?"*

■ Are there safety/risk issues?

▫ Self-care

• *"How many times do you shower in a week? Is this a change?"*

• *"Is there anything that has affected how often you eat? Has there been a change? Do you ever go for a few days without eating because you are X? Has there been any problem with your food?"*

▫ Activities of daily living (This can also give you an idea of the patient's capacity for self-care and his executive functioning.)

• *"How often do you forget to pay the rent? How do you keep track? Have you had any problems with your landlord lately?"*

- *"Where do you get your groceries? Are there ever times where you don't have food for a few days?"*
- *"How do you keep track of your medications? What do you do if you forget?"*
  □ Dangerousness
    - *"It sounds like you've been going through tough times lately . . .*
      ○ *". . . have you ever felt like giving up?"*
      ○ *". . . have you ever wanted to escape it all by dying?"*
      ○ *". . . have you made a plan to escape by killing yourself?"*
      ○ *". . . have you tried to hurt/kill yourself?"*
      ○ *". . . have you taken any steps to prepare (e.g., buying a gun or rope)?"*
    - *"You've spoken a lot about being followed and feeling your life is in danger. What steps have you taken to protect yourself? What weapons do you have access to?"*
    - *"What would you do if you ever found out the identity of the people responsible for spreading these rumors? Have you made any attempt to contact them? To hurt them? Have you had thoughts or fantasies of killing them?"*

Key Point:

Note that in clinical interviewing, it is often more efficient to start with an assumption, for example, "What steps have you taken to protect yourself?" versus "Have you taken steps . . . ?" the latter of which permits them to answer "no" easily. This is important in other sensitive areas of questioning, such as substance use. It is best to start with an assumption that they **do** use.

Box 5-3. Steps for Questioning

- Start broad →"*You mentioned earlier you have been having trouble getting along with others. Can you tell me more about that?*" Or, if the patient has not endorsed this, you can simply start by asking, "*How have you been getting along with others lately? Any conflicts with work/friends/landlord?*"
- Use the patient's example and get more specific → "*Sometimes when people experience difficulty getting along with others, trust becomes an issue. Has that ever been the case for you?*"
- Question in a more detailed way → "*For example, you might start to feel that your friends do not have your best intentions at heart, and that they are out to get you. Have you felt like that?*" Or, "*When you walk in a hallway, you may feel that people are talking about you behind your back, making a plan to hurt you. Has that ever crossed your mind?*"

You have now set the ground to question different elements of a persecutory delusion, having eased the patient into it.

- Are there any comorbid conditions?
  □ Part of evaluation and management is evaluating what other diagnostic entities may contribute to the current state.
  □ Patients with schizophrenia have a high rate of comorbidity with certain illnesses such as depression (which can be concurrent or secondary) and anxiety disorders (including social phobia and obsessive-compulsive disorder, which have had comorbid prevalence rates as high as 46% reported).[3] A screening of these disorders should be done. In fact, in examining the criteria for major depression, you can see that they cover crucial components (sleep, energy, appetite, concentration, suicidality, etc.) and should always be questioned, irrespective of the diagnosis.

The Differential Diagnosis of Psychosis

The goal of collecting detailed information is to confirm the presence of psychosis and to arrive at a provisional diagnosis with a differential. Based on the criteria for each diagnosis (refer to the DSM-IV for the diagnostic criteria and to Chapters 6 and 7 on mood disorders), the following specific items and questions can help differentiate certain diagnoses.

Schizophrenia

It is helpful to note that, whereas two or more psychotic symptoms are required during the majority of 1 month to make a diagnosis, only one criterion is required if the delusions are bizarre or the hallucinations are Schneiderian-like (i.e., running commentary or more than two voices conversing with each other).

Schizophreniform Disorder

This disorder is differentiated from schizophrenia only by its duration criterion; an episode lasts between 1 and 6 months, including the prodromal, active, and residual phase.

Bipolar Disorder, Severe, with Psychotic Features

- You should be aware that a number of studies have suggested that adolescent boys with a first episode of mania tend to have prominent psychotic symptoms. These, combined with symptoms of psychomotor agitation, grandiosity, disorganization, and decreased sleep, are also seen in schizophrenia and can thus obscure the diagnostic picture.
- It is important to evaluate the *quality* of the psychotic symptoms. A mood-congruent delusion of grandiosity (particularly in the absence of any other psychotic symptoms) may lend more support to a diagnosis of mania.

- The decreased *need* for sleep is very suggestive of mania and differentiates it from the decrease in sleep (due to agitation or paranoia) and the day/night reversal more commonly seen in the schizophrenia-spectrum disorders.

Major Depressive Disorder, Severe, with Psychotic Features

- Many symptoms of depression overlap with schizophrenia, and thus the details must be carefully evaluated (e.g., it can be high yield for you to clarify whether "not sleeping" actually means day/night reversal with pacing at night, which is more suggestive of schizophrenia, or initial insomnia with early-morning awakening, which is more suggestive of depression).
- Again, the quality of the psychotic symptoms can be contributory, with mood-congruent nihilistic, somatic, and guilty delusions lending support to a diagnosis of depression.

Schizoaffective Disorder

- Schizoaffective disorder is not simply the coexistence of separate disorders of psychosis and mood. If you examine the criteria carefully:
  - The patient must meet criteria for active symptoms of schizophrenia, and for some concurrent substantial period he must meet criteria for a mood episode.
  - In the same period of illness, the patient must have had at least 2 weeks of psychotic symptoms *without* mood symptoms (so, if psychotic symptoms occur only in the context of mood episodes, the diagnosis is likely a mood disorder with psychotic features).
- You may find a collateral source of history invaluable in sorting out the temporal relationship between mood and psychotic symptoms.

Delusional Disorder

- The diagnosis of delusional disorder has some criteria that can be helpful in differentiating it from schizophrenia (the criteria of which must have never been met).
  - The delusions are non-bizarre (i.e., involving situations that can occur in real life, such as being followed, infected, poisoned, loved by another, or having an unfaithful partner).
  - Functioning and behavior are intact (and non-bizarre) except for the direct impact of the delusion.
  - Hallucinations, if present, are *not* prominent.

Brief Psychotic Disorder

- The criteria differentiating brief psychotic disorder from schizophrenia include the following:
  - Only one active symptom is necessary.
  - Symptoms last between 1 day and 1 month, with a full return to premorbid level of functioning.

Substance-Induced Psychotic Disorder

- Many patients presenting to psychiatry personnel for evaluation have concurrent substance use disorders complicating the presentation and diagnostic process. Some helpful hints for raising your suspicions of a substance-induced psychotic disorder follow:
  - It tends to have an acute onset (within hours of use), with rapid resolution upon substance discontinuation. The symptoms must exceed those expected of an intoxication or withdrawal phase.
  - Note that drug-intoxication symptoms usually resolve within 1 to 3 days, but this may depend on the substance consumed. For example, amphetamines, cocaine, phencyclidine (PCP), and cannabis (THC) can cause prolonged psychotic states for weeks, despite discontinuation of the substance. This can depend on the abuse history and the amount ingested, among other factors.
- To meet criteria for a primary psychotic disorder, the symptoms must persist beyond 1 month after substance discontinuation (the reality of being able to observe a patient who has been truly substance-free for 1 month is a whole other story!).
- Keep in mind that diagnosing substance-induced psychotic disorders is rarely an *either/or* situation. Sometimes, an underlying psychotic disorder may be precipitated or triggered by drug use.
- If there is ongoing substance use, symptoms sometimes fluctuate with the amount used.
- The use history and the amount and type of substance consumed can all have an effect on the vulnerability of a particular patient to a substance-induced psychosis.
- Psychosis can be due to medications (e.g., steroids, anesthetics, anticholinergics) and toxins (e.g., insecticide, carbon monoxide).

Key Point:

In the context of the high rate of comorbidity between substance use disorders and schizophrenia, remember that a psychotic state may be influenced by a consumed substance, even if not entirely causal. It is important to establish the patient's symptoms with drug use, her temporal association, the symptom severity related to drug consumption, and her degree of symptoms in periods of abstinence.

Key Point:

Consideration must be given to the *type* of substance consumed. Some classes of drugs (e.g., stimulants, hallucinogens) are more acutely psychotogenic than others (e.g., opiates, alcohol). Some cause positive symptoms (e.g., stimulants), whereas others may cause positive and negative symptoms suggestive of schizophrenia (e.g., PCP).

Key Point:

Although THC may be a less potent inducer of psychosis than stimulants or hallucinogens, it may be a more common precipitant of psychosis by virtue of the higher prevalence of use in the general population. There is substantial evidence to suggest that THC use may increase the risk of developing schizophrenia and result in a poor prognosis for those with an established vulnerability to psychosis.4

Psychotic Disorder Due to a General Medical Condition

- The index of suspicion can be raised by atypical features:
  - □ Acute onset and change in personality
  - □ Atypical age of onset
  - □ Physical symptoms (e.g., gait change, new-onset headache, incontinence, change in neurological function, symptoms suggestive of seizures)
  - □ Visual or olfactory hallucinations
  - □ Fluctuating course

Key Point:

There is an extensive and expanding list of medical conditions that can cause psychosis (Box 5-4). It is important to keep in mind that medical etiologies of psychosis are rare; thus, it is hardly necessary to memorize lists of such causes of psychosis. However, organicity should be considered a remote possibility, particularly in the case of atypical features as above. Other factors that should increase the index of suspicion for an organic cause are the setting (e.g., first onset of psychosis in an internal medicine ward) and risk factors for medical illness versus psychiatric illness (e.g., older age, multiple medications).

Obsessive Compulsive Disorder

- In some persons, obsessions can reach a delusional intensity when reality testing is lost. The presence of psychotic features does merit an additional diagnosis of delusional disorder or psychotic disorder not otherwise specified (NOS).

Box 5-4. Examples of General Medical Conditions Causing Psychosis

Alzheimer's dementia
Autoimmune disorders (e.g., systemic lupus erythematosus)
Central nervous system infection (e.g., acquired immune deficiency syndrome, Jakob Creutzfeldt disease, neurosyphilis, herpes encephalitis)
Cerebrovascular disease (e.g., stroke, brain trauma)
Endocrine/metabolic disorders (e.g., hypothyroidism, hyperthyroidism, acute intermittent porphyria, Cushing's disease, homocystinuria)
Epilepsy (particularly, temporal lobe epilepsy)
Huntington's disease
Multiple sclerosis
Neoplasm (primary or metastatic brain tumors)
Normal pressure hydrocephalus
Pellagra
Toxic poisoning (e.g., heavy metals, carbon monoxide)
Vitamin B_{12} deficiency
Wernicke-Korsakoff syndrome
Wilson's disease

- Given that the degree of reality testing can be on a continuum and difficult to accurately elicit, it is not uncommon for there to be some difficulty in differentiating obsessions from psychosis, particularly since the DSM-IV-TR does have a "with poor insight" specifier for obsessive compulsive disorder, often applied to patients whose symptoms are on the boundary between an obsession and a delusion.
- An additional factor differentiating from a delusion is that the patient should recognize that the obsession comes from within himself and is not imposed externally.

Delirium

- There are key features that differentiate delirium from a psychotic disorder:
  - □ Fluctuating course of symptoms
  - □ Fluctuating level of consciousness (this does *not* occur with schizophrenia)
  - □ Presence of a causal medical etiology

Dementia

- Again, as in delirium, there are important features that should raise your index of suspicion:
  - □ A later age of onset
  - □ Delusion often (but not always) of a personal and persecutory nature (e.g., someone stealing her possessions)
  - □ Prominent cognitive (memory, attention) deficits (although these may sometimes arise later in the course of illness, after the presence of psychotic symptoms)

> **Key Point:**
>
> Remember that even people with established diagnoses of psychotic disorders can have medical problems or other psychiatric illnesses (keeping in mind the high rates of comorbidity). The above differential should be kept in mind when evaluating a symptom relapse in patients known to have schizophrenia.

Borderline Personality Disorder

- The psychotic symptoms tend to be:
  - Transient (less than 2 days)
  - Often stress related
  - Circumscribed (i.e., encapsulated and focused)
  - Of fluctuating conviction
  - Interpersonally and environmentally reactive
- Qualitatively, these "quasi-psychotic" symptoms are often described as the following:
  - "Paranoid ideation": often of a personal nature, but not of a delusional intensity
  - "Auditory hallucinations": often described as their own self-deprecating voice/thoughts
  - Dissociative symptoms: depersonalization and derealization are much more common in borderline personality disorders than in schizophrenia
- Patients usually have significant affective lability and a long-standing history of functional and interpersonal instability

Schizotypal/Schizoid/Paranoid Personality Disorder

- These patients do not have full symptoms of psychosis, although they have some shared features with schizophrenia (e.g., poor social functioning, vague and abstract style of speech, paranoid ideation, magical thinking).
- Attenuated symptoms tend to be more longitudinal in presence, not episodic (i.e., a trait, and not a state).

Pervasive Developmental Disorder

- Symptoms are usually present from early childhood and involve prominent disturbances in language, affect, and interpersonal functioning.
- These symptoms are common with schizophrenia but usually occur in the absence of prominent delusions or hallucinations.

Factitious Disorder with Psychological Symptoms, Malingering

- Look for inconsistencies in the presentation and history.
- Evaluate for secondary gain (e.g., outstanding legal charges).

Completing the Information Gathering with the Patient

The detective work of a clinical interview involves more than just the history of present illness. Many other pieces must be gathered and brought together. The reader is referred to Chapter 1, General Principles of Interviewing, for the components of a thorough clinical interview. In this chapter, we would like to draw your attention to certain parts of the interview that are crucial and should be thoroughly evaluated in a first assessment for psychosis, as well as during follow-up (in a targeted fashion). By the end of your patient encounter, you should have a clear understanding of the following.

Substance Use (see Chapter 10)

- Be nonjudgmental. Asking a patient, *"Do you have a problem with drugs or alcohol?"* is not likely to get you an honest answer.
- Start with the assumption that the patient does use substances.
  - *"How much alcohol/drugs do you use in a week?"* (*Not* "Do you drink?" *or* "Have you ever had a problem with drinking?")
- Get a clear idea of the use history.
  - *"When did you last use?"*
  - *"How much in 1 week?"*
  - *"What effect does it have on you? Positive? Negative?"* You should specifically screen for emerging psychotic symptoms, or worsening of existing symptoms as well as improvement of those symptoms (this is helpful in understanding the patient's propensity and vulnerability to developing psychosis).
  - *"What has been your longest time without drugs? What was the impact of withdrawal? What was the state of psychotic symptoms then?"*

Legal History

- It is important to understand both premorbid history in regard to legal history as well as the current impact of psychosis on behavior.
- If you can place the question in a context personal to the patient, all the better.
  - *"It sounds like your neighbors have really been getting on your back. Have you called the police to complain? Have they ever called the police about you?"*
  - *"What contact have you ever had with the police?"*
  - *"Have you ever pressed charges against someone? Have charges ever been pressed against you?"*
  - *"Have you ever spent time in jail?"*
  - *"Have you ever done anything that you could have ended up in jail for, but weren't caught doing?"*

Medical History (Past and Present)

- You must explore any risk factors and nonpsychiatric differential diagnoses associated with psychosis, particularly as governed by the evolution and quality of each patient's psychosis:
  - Medical illnesses: for example, hyperthyroidism, systemic lupus erythematosus, acute intermittent porphyria
  - Neurological illnesses: for example, epilepsy, head injury, loss of consciousness, new headaches, unexplained nausea and vomiting, visual changes, or other focal neurological signs
  - Other risks: pregnancy complications, developmental abnormalities or delay
- Keep your ears open for any information suggestive of atypical symptoms/history that may be linked to an organic etiology, particularly of a neurological, endocrine, autoimmune, infectious, or neoplastic cause.

Past Psychiatric History

- Previous diagnoses, treatments (biological and psychological), untreated episodes related to psychosis, and its differential diagnosis must be elicited.
- This should include past dangerous behavior, in and out of psychosis.

Medication History

- What is currently being taken?
  - For how long, and prescribed by whom?
  - What positive effects has the patient experienced?
  - What side effects have been experienced? (You should specifically ask about sexual side effects, since many patients do not make the association or are uncomfortable spontaneously discussing it.)
  - What has the patient's compliance been? (*"How many times do you forget in 1 week?"*)
- Is the patient taking any over-the-counter, herbal, or natural products?
- Has the patient taken any medications known to be associated with psychosis (e.g., steroids)?

Family Psychiatric History

- It is important to start with lay terminology in eliciting family history, in addition to symptoms and specific diagnoses. The stigma of mental illness means that it is often not discussed or acknowledged within families, and it is thus helpful to normalize it as much as possible.
  - *"Has anyone in your family (siblings, parents, aunts/uncles, or cousins) had difficulties similar to you?"*
  - *"Has anyone ever had any nerve problems? Difficulties with mood/thinking?"*
  - *"Has anyone had a nervous breakdown?"*
  - *"Has anyone needed help for psychological problems?"*
  - *"Is there anyone that the family thought was 'weird'?"*
  - *"Has anyone ever tried to kill himself or herself?"*
  - *"Has anyone ever had any difficulties with alcohol or drugs? With violence or aggression?"*
  - *"Has anyone lost touch with reality? Maybe talking to themselves, or lost in their own world?"*
  - *"Has anyone ever received a diagnosis, such as depression, schizophrenia, etc.?"* (Remember to not ask multiple aspects in a single question. Ask one at a time and leave time for an answer).

Targeted Background

- In addition to the other issues discussed in Chapter 2, specific to psychosis, it is important to elicit the following:
  - Developmental history (this may be better sought from the parents)
    - Premorbid personality
    - Milestones and motor coordination (e.g., sports, clumsiness)
  - Functioning
    - School
    - Work
    - Interpersonal/social
- This is important in creating a longitudinal picture of the patient, that is, past and current functioning with a focus on what was different or problematic in childhood and what has changed and how.
- This can point to a history suggestive of a vulnerable brain, such as learning disabilities, attention deficit hyperactivity disorder, pervasive developmental disorders, mental retardation, or even mild neurological abnormalities (e.g., many children who later develop schizophrenia have motor coordination and school difficulties in childhood).
- This can also clarify any character traits that can be premorbid to the onset of schizophrenia, such as in schizotypal or schizoid personality disorder.

The Mental Status Examination

The mental status examination (MSE) is not just formal questioning. It starts from the first time you see the patient, even if you cross paths in the hallway. It involves your observations. Active questioning is actually a smaller part of the MSE.

Case Example 3

Ali was a 19-year-old man coming for a first assessment of psychosis. When Dr. Simon went to the chart room to get Ali's file, he noticed Ali peering into the men's washroom, and on return to his office, Ali was knocking on the wall behind his chair. However, once in the office, Ali did not get up from his chair. However, he often rocked back and forth or bounced his legs, all the while shooting darting glances to the corners of the room behind him and above him.

Your Observations

You should be watching and examining the patient from the beginning. Your observations will permit you to direct your interview toward developing a particular differential diagnosis, to optimize the patient's comfort and safety, to pick up on cues that show that you are listening and in tune with the patient's needs, and to decide where to go from here. Aspects you should be looking for include the following:

- Hygiene/self-care, general appearance (e.g., Is the patient overweight from medications or underweight from poor nutrition?)
- Appropriate dress for the weather (a function of organization or impoverishment)
- Patient's comfort level (e.g., Is he looking around everywhere, as if anxious or paranoid?)
- Physical aspects (you should do some physical examination for this)
  - Signs of intoxication
    - Pupils (dilated or restricted), tremulousness, sweating. You can check blood pressure and pulse if indicated.
  - Signs of medication side effects
    - Akathisia: Is the patient fidgety, unable to remain sitting?
    - Extrapyramidal side effects: Check for tremor, rigidity, decreased arm swing, slowing, choreiform or dyskinetic movement.
    - Anticholinergic: dry mucosa
  - Signs of motor abnormalities associated with psychosis
    - Tics
    - Dyskinesias
    - Mannerisms
    - Posturing
- Other observations you should note
  - Affect and demeanor
    - Level of cooperation, eye contact, range of affect (e.g., blunted affect)
  - Speech and psychomotor
    - Slowing, intonation (speech may be more monotonous in schizophrenia, fast and labile in mania)
  - Level of consciousness: This should not be altered in schizophrenia or other primary psychoses. If it is, delirium should be considered.
- You should also be listening carefully to elicit the following:
  - Thought form and content
  - Level of mental organization and concentration capacities
  - Insight and judgment

Active Questioning for the MSE

For the most part, you will be able to compose an MSE from your observations of the patient during the interview. Specific questioning may be needed for the following components (emphasis on psychosis):

- Mood: *"How are you feeling today?"*
- Thought content
  - Psychosis screen discussed in the above section should be applied for "currently" as well, if indicated
  - Suicidal and aggressive/homicidal ideation *today*
- Perceptual changes: hallucinations today
- Cognitive screen
  - Orientation
  - Current events: *"Can you tell me what has been going on in the news recently?"*
  - Concentration and memory: This is observed throughout the history (e.g., Does she recall dates? Is she able to focus on your questions and answer appropriately?) and then can be tested through serial 7s, saying the months of the year or days of the week backward, immediate and delayed recall of four words (e.g., honesty, tulip, eyedropper, brown), etc.
  - Abstraction: Proverbs are often not culturally universal, and so word pairs (similarities/differences) may be preferable.
- Insight: *"Is there anything you think you need help with? Why are your parents concerned? Why do you take this medication? Do you plan on continuing to take it?"*

Key Point:

As in a medical interview, information must be obtained for three stages: remote, recent, and current. In a medical interview, a patient with a fever of unknown origin should be asked about ever having had serious febrile illnesses or unexplained fevers, about recent fever (in the last few weeks), and should have his temperature taken now as part of the physical examination. The psychiatric interview parallels this for many issues, for example, suicide, mood, psychosis, aggression. For all these, you should clearly understand whether it has been ever, recently, or is currently an issue.

Key Point:

The MSE is not a conglomeration of the three time points. It is the equivalent of a physical examination, the patient's signs and symptoms today. It is the body temperature you measure now, not the recent or past history of fever.

COLLECTING INFORMATION FROM OTHER SOURCES

Issues Related to Using Other Sources of Information

The observations of a third party who knows the patient can be invaluable. This is particularly so for issues that patients themselves may have difficulty describing, or may not be aware of, such as type of onset, evolution over time, what actual changes have occurred (e.g., in personality and functioning), self-care issues, or fluctuations in state. However, getting information from a third party is not always a clear process. Consideration must be given to the following:

- Confidentiality: It is important to have as transparent a process as possible. It is helpful to let the patient know from the beginning that you will need additional information, but to reassure him that you cannot *give* information without his consent. Ways to communicate this include the following:
  □ *"It's a bit like writing a school project . . . you collect information from as many sources as possible—textbooks, internet, lectures—so that you can form a representative picture of what is really going on."*
  □ *"You should know that although I may ask your mother some questions on how things have been going at home, I will not give her information or answer her questions without your permission. In fact, I prefer to meet her with you in the room."*
- Seeing the patient alone versus with the collateral source: People are different when they are alone versus with others (particularly family members). It can be helpful to see the patient alone to cover sensitive issues.
  □ Current substance use
  □ Current risk assessment
  □ Current symptomatology
  □ Current interpersonal functioning
  □ Sexual functioning and adverse effects
- Seeing collateral sources alone versus with the patient: This will depend on the patient and what he agrees to. Many family members feel more comfortable not speaking in front of the patient. Again, explicit permission must be obtained from the patient to meet with the family. If the patient has a very different story from the family, it can sometimes be therapeutically helpful to ask him to give his version of explanations for the family's concerns.

Other Sources of History

- What to ask: This can depend on the source. Remember to focus on *change*:
  □ Family

- Change in functioning and personality
- Premorbid history
- Risk issues (e.g., self-care, threats)
- Fluctuations
- Signs of organicity
- Objective signs of psychosis (e.g., talking to self, acting on delusions)
- Change in sleep/appetite/mood
  □ Group home caregiver
- Aggressive outbursts
- Getting along with co-tenants
- Sleep/appetite/hygiene issues
- Changes in behavior
- Signs of psychosis
  □ School
- Behavior
- Aggression
- Academic functioning
- Change in personality/coping style

LABORATORY TESTS/PHYSICAL WORKUP

A thorough medical history and physical examination are key to dictating the extent of the further workup to be done. All patients should ideally have a family physician who conducts a physical exam every 1 to 2 years. In addition, if there is anything atypical about the psychosis, special attention should be given to evaluating for possible organicity, both on history and physical exam. *Then* consider what workup is indicated based on the information already obtained. Whether in an initial assessment or in follow-up, lab tests are done for two purposes:

1. To ensure that there is no organic contribution (e.g., thyroid function and toxicology screen are often done at baseline, but other tests to be considered if indicated include renal and liver function, glucose, B12, HIV, tuberculosis, ceruloplasmin [Wilson's disease], autoimmune workup [systemic lupus erythematosus], cortisol [Cushing's disease], electroencephalography, neuroimaging, etc.)

2. At baseline, ideally before starting antipsychotic medications (given their side effects): complete blood count and basic biochemistry, liver and renal function tests, prolactin, fasting cholesterol/triglyceride and glucose, weight, electrocardiography (if the patient has a cardiac history or is older than 45 years), and then for monitoring of medication effects

---

Key Point:

The differential diagnosis has to be clearly explored on history, given its importance in determining which tests are indicated.

Key Point:

The setting is also important in determining the extent of testing indicated. An emergency department physician seeing a patient with psychosis will have a much broader differential diagnosis to investigate, and thus more laboratory tests to order, compared with a tertiary care specialty clinic that only sees first-episode psychosis patients who have usually been through multiple assessments before their current one.

Key Point:

Even if patients have a family physician, a crucial part of the mental health care team's follow-up is to monitor for risk factors and adverse effects of antipsychotic medications. This means regularly checking for extrapyramidal symptoms, tardive dyskinesia, weight, and blood pressure; metabolic/endocrine laboratory tests; and electrocardiogram monitoring for corrected Q-T (QTc) interval prolongation.

Key Point:

It is not uncommon for a neurological condition to initially present with psychiatric manifestations that trigger help-seeking. Thus, a thorough history is crucial to identifying atypical features.

RATING SCALES

Rating scales can be administered at baseline and on an ongoing basis. These are helpful for having structured, replicable questions that can be administered at different times or by different people. They may be used for three different purposes:

1. Diagnosis: the Structured Clinical Interview for DSM-IV (for the primary diagnosis and that of concurrent disorders)

2. Symptom monitoring: the Brief Psychiatric Rating Scale, the Positive and Negative Symptom Scale, the Calgary Depression Scale, etc.

3. Antipsychotic side effects: the Abnormal Involuntary Movement Scale, the Barnes Akathisia scale, the Simpson-Angus Scale, etc.

AGE-SPECIFIC ISSUES

The differential diagnosis may vary according to the age of the patient you are seeing. For example, whereas you should always have an ear for atypical features suggesting an organic cause, this would be much more prevalent in the geriatric population in whom delirium and dementia are often the etiology of psychosis. Some of the issues to consider according to age categories are:

Children/Adolescents

- Schizophrenia is rare in children (approximate incidence of 1/10,000).[2]
- Generally, the collateral information is very important for the history and diagnosis. This should include the primary caregivers and the school.
- Specific interests include premorbid personality and functioning, school functioning, interpersonal capacity, drug use, and family history.
- Increased consideration should be given to certain diagnoses in the general differential:
  □ Developmental phase (e.g., having an imaginary friend can be normal in young children; in adolescents, the struggle for independence may make them appear withdrawn from family, when in fact they are functioning in their social group and school)
  □ Pervasive developmental disorder
  □ Attention deficit hyperactivity disorder
  □ Anxiety disorder
  □ Prodrome phase of a psychotic illness
  □ Substance-induced psychosis
  □ Schizophrenia

Adults

- Sex: the peak age of onset of schizophrenia is later in women than in men. Thus, a woman in her late 30s or early 40s with a first presentation of psychosis is not as unusual as a man in this age group with his first presentation.
- Extra consideration should be given to these diagnoses in the differential of a later-onset psychosis:
  □ Delusional disorder
  □ Mood disorder
  □ General medical condition

Geriatric Population

- Collateral information can also be important in the geriatric population, particularly if the patient is not a reliable historian. The history can come from staff at the residence of a patient, family, or partners. An additional resource may be a family physician who knows the patient well and can comment on changes over the years.
- It is important to evaluate the descriptive quality of the psychosis because there can be trends suggestive of diagnosis (e.g., persecutory delusions of a personal possession nature often occur in dementia).

- Particular attention must be paid to the possibility of the following diagnoses:
  - □ Dementia
  - □ Delirium
  - □ General medical condition
  - □ Medication interaction as a contributory factor

OTHER CONTRIBUTING VARIABLES

In addition to age, there are other variables that must be considered when interviewing a patient for psychosis. These variables may set the context for understanding the etiology, management, and functioning in a psychosis. They may dictate the resources available and the attitudes of patients and their families.

Geography

Where in the world are you working? This can be an important consideration with respect to:

- Prevalence and type of infection: Are you interviewing a patient in a country where an illness, such as tuberculosis, malaria, or parasitic infections, is endemic or highly prevalent?
- Prevalence and type of substance use: Is the consumption of hallucinogens highly prevalent and socially sanctioned?
- Cultural attitudes: Are symptoms considered negative and psychotic by Western standards actually revered and considered a sign of spiritual power in this culture? In such a situation, will people be willing to be treated with medications, or are they given a special protected role in the community?
- Treatment availability and accessibility: Is there a supply of medications? Are patients able to pay for them? Is taking medications culturally sanctioned?
- Standards of patient management and care

Setting

The setting in which you see the patient will also have an effect on what you are likely to see, how you will conduct your interview, and the goals of your interview.

Emergency Department

Emergency department (ER) interviews tend to be brief and more directive. Priority should be allocated to:

- Risk issues
- Clinical state: Is the patient psychotic or not?
  - □ If psychotic, is the etiology psychiatric, substance-induced, or organic?
  - □ The further specifics of the diagnosis do not always need to be resolved in the ER.

- Management
  - □ Does the patient need to be kept in the ER or discharged home with follow-up?
  - □ Should the admission be voluntary or involuntary?
  - □ What medications are indicated?
  - □ What emergency workup is necessary?

Outpatient Clinic Follow-up

- Acute phase (as discussed earlier, in the assessment phase)
- Chronic phase
  - □ Ongoing engagement: Your goals are to get to know your patient, get an update on her life and what is important for her.
    - *"How are you doing these days?"*
    - *"What is an average day like for you? How do you structure it? What do you like to do?"*
    - *"The last time we met, you were planning to apply for a job; how did that turn out?"*
  - □ Clinical state: Is the patient better, worse, or the same? Evaluate symptoms and functioning, including a risk assessment.
    - *"How have things been since the last time I saw you?"*
    - *"The last time we met, you were having some difficulty feeling comfortable with the people at work. How is that going?"*
    - *"How is your school/work/social life going?"*
  - □ Evaluate medication compliance, adverse effects, and positive effects (remember to start with a nonjudgmental assumption, such as, *"Everyone forgets a dose of medication once in a while."*).
    - *"How many times in a week do you forget a dose of medication?"*
    - *"What tricks do you have for remembering your medication?"*
    - *"Have you had any problems with the medications?"*
    - *"Have you noticed any positive things about the medication?"*
  - □ If there seems to have been a relapse, evaluate for a possible cause.
    - Noncompliance
    - Substance use
    - Life stressor
    - Medical condition
    - Medication interaction

Key Point:

Keep in mind that even people with well-established diagnoses of schizophrenia or other psychotic illnesses can have medical conditions such as delirium. A relapse of psychotic symptoms does not always mean there is a psychiatric issue. Look for atypical features.

Inpatient

- Longitudinal picture: What has the patient's progress been like? How is she now compared with before?
- Diagnostic clarification through observation of functioning, interpersonal capacity, activities of daily living, and regular activities (e.g., eating, sleeping, hygiene)

THE CHALLENGING INTERVIEW

Psychiatry relies on case history and human relationship, tools we carry with us everywhere. But we must ask the right questions in the most high-yield manner. So what happens when we do, but the yield is low? How do we handle the interviews where we don't get any information, where the patient shuts down or wants to leave? No matter what the setting or situation, there are a few basic rules that you should always apply:

Safety First. Your safety and your patient's safety must be priorities. If the patient is escalating in terms of agitation, you must not feel obliged to continue with a 45-minute assessment.

Multiple Sources of Information. The patient is not your only informant. Often, the collateral source is able to give details about the course and evolution of the patient's condition that are essential for making a diagnosis. If you are not able to interview the patient now, move on and come back. Also, your observations of the patient's state and responses can be crucial in clarifying the diagnosis and its differential.

Prevention. It is better to avoid problems than to have to deal with them once they occur. Be prepared. If you have information on the patient beforehand, familiarize yourself with it. Before starting the interview, lay it out for the patient, including the goals, duration, and structure. Minimize surprises for the patient. When things are slowing down, emphasize and search for the patient's strengths and interests.

There are different scenarios of challenging interviews. It is essential to be prepared and flexible while keeping cool. The following cases are common enough, particularly when interviewing for psychosis.

Case Example 4

The Paranoid (or Guarded and Evasive) Patient. Joe is a 23-year-old man coming in for his follow-up appointment. He is accompanied by his elderly mother, who tells you beforehand that he has been locking himself in his room for the last 2 weeks and drilling holes in the walls to check for wires and cameras. He comes into your office and starts tapping on the walls, checking behind the doors, and looking out the window. When you ask him how things are going, he replies, "Why would you want to know, so you can tell my mother and then she can report it to them?"

- Reassurance is important but should not be trivial or overdone.
- Confidentiality of the information discussed should be clearly mentioned.
- It is important to remain detached from the delusion (i.e., not to reinforce or play into it).
- It is rarely therapeutic to challenge the delusion, particularly early in the relationship.
- Questioning symptoms in different ways can help elicit information and can draw attention to inconsistencies, while presenting different scenarios that the patient may hopefully connect with.
- It can be helpful to ally with the patient's fear and anxiety (not the delusion itself) or whatever distress point he has:
  - *"I understand you have been feeling harassed. Is there anything I can do to make you feel more comfortable here?"*
  - *"You've mentioned a few times that you have been the most bothered by your poor sleep. Can we try to help you with that?"*
  - *"In the past when I have worked with people who also felt that they were being followed or were in danger, I observed that it was a very stressful and tiring time. They often said that coming to the hospital was a bit like coming to a safe place, given there is staff around all the time. We would like you to be able to rest. What are your thoughts about that?"*

Case Example 5

The Patient with No Insight (denying any problem, not endorsing any symptoms). Jill is a 28-year-old university student who has failed courses in the last year and has been asked to leave her program in the last month. She is coming in for a first assessment following her family's observation that she has withdrawn socially, won't eat in public places, and when with family, checks her food and will not eat it unless someone else tries it first. They have also observed her speaking to herself. When you interview her, she denies any psychotic symptoms, saying that her family has misinterpreted her actions, and that she has always sung songs to herself.

- It can be helpful in this situation to start with nonthreatening material (i.e., stay away from symptoms):
  - *"How have things been going for you?"*
  - *"What is going well for you? What are your strengths? What are you satisfied with right now?"*
  - *"What are you interested in? What are your passions?"*

- □ *"What is an average day like for you?"*
- Psychosis questioning should be broad-based, starting with the following:
  - □ *"Have you been dealing with any challenges lately?"*
  - □ *"How are you getting along with your classmates/neighbors/coworkers? Has anyone been getting on your nerves?"*
  - □ *"Has anything felt different lately? Have you noticed anything out of place or strange/off/weird lately?"*
- Try to place things in a context that is personal to this person.
  - □ *"You mentioned you've been under a lot of stress with your school difficulties lately. Sometimes in those situations, people can get a different perspective, and they start to question things in a new way. Have you ever noticed that about yourself?"*
  - □ *"You mentioned you haven't been eating much lately. People often don't eat for many different reasons. They may feel sick, or they may be worried about gaining weight, or they may worry that the food is not good for them. Which of these apply to you?"*
- Search for and go with the patient's area of distress.
  - □ *"Is there anything that has been bugging you lately?"*
  - □ *"Are you happy with how things are going? If I asked you to make a problem list with three items on it, what would you list?"*
  - □ *"Is there anything we can help you with?"*
- You can try bringing up what you know and asking for her version or explanation.
  - □ *"I understand that some people have observed you doing X. Tell me about that in your own words."*
- If nothing works and the patient continues to deny having any symptoms or problems, sometimes you just have to agree to disagree, and try to engage her for a trial period.
  - □ *"It sounds like your parents have some concerns, but you don't agree with what they are saying. I can't say that anyone is right or wrong. What do you think of coming back a few more times to make sure things are on track, and if there is nothing more we can do, then it will be your choice to continue with follow-up?"*

Key Point:

Remember that even though the patient's family is saying something is wrong, and you think something is wrong, you cannot force a patient to submit to evaluation and treatment unless there is a risk issue. Unfortunately, sometimes a patient must get sicker before she will accept treatment or before it can be given to her.

- When the patient is agitated/violent, remember the following:
  - □ Safety first.
  - □ Consider giving the patient some medication to calm down before the interview.
  - □ If a brief attempt at verbal negotiation does not work, consider giving the patient a break or calling for assistance—whichever the situation dictates.
- When the patient is thought-disordered, remember the following:
  - □ Patients are not always aware that their thought form has changed or that others are having difficulty understanding them.
  - □ As mentioned earlier, information processing and attention deficits are common in schizophrenia. It is helpful to ask short questions and to give examples if a patient does not seem to grasp an open question.
  - □ You may need to adapt a more direct/closed-ended style of questioning if the open-ended approach is low yield.
    - *"Sometimes when people have been having difficulty concentrating like you have, they experience a change in their thinking. Have you noticed any change?"*
    - *"Has anyone commented that your way of expressing yourself has changed?"*
    - *"I'm going to change my style of questioning now. I'll give you some scenarios and you can just answer 'yes' or 'no' as it applies, and then I will ask you more details about it as needed."*
- When the patient refuses to give information, remember:
  - □ Again, a nonthreatening approach can be helpful. Start with innocuous themes.
  - □ Try to go with the patient's agenda: What does *she* want to talk about; what is not working for *her*?
- When the patient is on the brink of leaving, consider the following:
  - □ Evaluate the reasons. Is there anything you can fix or explain?
  - □ Can reassurance buy a few more minutes?
  - □ If you have collateral sources of information, there are few things that absolutely have to come directly from the patient. The most important information that you should obtain from the patient is as follows:
    - Risk assessment: current suicidal and homicidal ideation
    - Mental status exam
    - Substance use: current
    - Her problem list
    - Psychosis screen (if you can get it; otherwise, family can often give sufficient information to point to psychosis)

CLOSING THE INTERVIEW

The closing of an interview, whether a first assessment or a follow-up, can have a crucial impact on the patient's impression of the interaction. Similar to a good dessert turning around a bad meal, so can the last few minutes of a session place a seal on whether the patient returns and whether the patient trusts you.

Addressing the Diagnosis

"So what is it, doctor?" Families and patients want to know why they are here and why they have to see you. There has been a traditional approach of shying away from the diagnosis of schizophrenia. However, we cannot ignore the enormous wealth of information available from the Internet, and the fact that many people arrive with their own impressions and information, correct and incorrect. It is part of our duty as mental health professionals to be aware of what they know or believe, to ensure that they have the correct information, and to explain our theories and impressions.

You do the patient a service if you do the following:

- Tell the patient the provisional diagnosis *if* you have sufficient information to back it up.
- Emphasize that the diagnosis will be reevaluated over time.
- *Don't* just tell the patient a diagnosis and leave it at that.
  - □ Explain what the diagnosis means and how you arrived at that diagnosis.
  - □ Elaborate that it is not set in stone, and that diagnoses should be confirmed over time.
  - □ Explain a brief version of the differential diagnosis.
  - □ Explain the different possible outcomes of a diagnosis.
  - □ Explain the treatment approaches available for this diagnosis.
  - □ Answer questions about etiology, risk factors, and prevention.

On the other hand, you render the patient and his family a *disservice* if you do the following:
  - □ Don't tell them a diagnosis when there is one.
  - □ Don't discuss the various outcome scenarios (given many people are not aware that some people with psychotic illness can go on to resume functioning, they automatically associate the diagnosis of schizophrenia with the end of life as they know it).
  - □ Don't relay clearly that this is a medical illness that requires treatment.
  - □ Don't discuss ways to optimize recovery, for example, taking medications, avoiding illicit substances, and stress management.

Key Point:

Remember that these are guidelines, and in clinical practice, what and how much you tell a patient and his family must be judged on a case-by-case basis. This must take into consideration the setting in which you are seeing the patient, how well you know that patient and family, how aware you are of their value system, how insightful the patient is into his illness, how agitated the patient is, and many other factors. The information is sometimes revealed in an ongoing process because it is too overwhelming to do entirely in the first encounter. It is crucial to pay attention to the family's cues about how much they want to know, instead of making assumptions about their needs.

Laying the Grounds for New and Ongoing Treatment

In both the initial and ongoing phases, the manner with which you convey the importance of pharmacotherapy and psychosocial rehabilitation can have a significant impact on future compliance and the therapeutic relationship.

Key Point:

Remember that patients are dealing with having an illness, with the stigma of it being a mental illness, with self-esteem issues, with family's expectations, with misconceptions and preconceived notions, and in general, with having to follow treatment for an extended period of time. A significant task of any mental health professional is to ensure that all of the above are addressed openly, and that the patient walks away with a clear understanding:
- *Why* treatment is necessary (including target symptoms)
- *How* progress is monitored (i.e., What is the goal of treatment, and how will you know it is working?)
- *What* the treatment is (recommended and alternatives)
- *How* it works (you should address the misconceptions about medications, for example, that you get addicted, or that it changes your personality)
- *What* the benefits and risks are (including a clear discussion of the adverse effects and long-term risks of medications)
- *What* the expected duration of treatment is

The *why* is perhaps the most important foundation of facilitating compliance. How many people in the general public have difficulty being compliant with a 10-day course of antibiotics taken three times per day, especially once the acute discomfort of infection resolves? How many women occasionally forget their daily oral contraceptives?

> **Key Point:**
>
> It is important to remember that medication compliance is an issue of human nature, and not only of mental illness. People do not like to take pills, especially if they are not in acute distress themselves. The onus is on you, the professional, to convince them of the need for the treatment, preferably within the structure of a partnership and collaboration.

There are different approaches to explaining the usefulness of pharmacotherapy (few patients resist other psychosocial modalities of treatment; thus for this purpose, we will address only medication therapy).

- The "tell it like it is" approach
  - Few patients will respond solely to being told that they have psychosis and thus need antipsychotic treatment. However, some patients will accept this, particularly those who work in the health field, or who have had previous experience of the illness (e.g., through family members).
- The "tap into their distress point" approach
  - This approach is particularly useful when patients do not admit psychosis symptoms but are able to acknowledge some other symptom, for example, that they are having difficulty sleeping, or their thoughts have been racing/confused lately.
    - *"You mentioned that you have been very disturbed by the poor sleep lately. The medication I am recommending can help with that as well."* (*Note:* You should not mislead patients and tell them that you are simply giving them a sleeping or nerve pill or a "tranquilizer.") *"In addition to helping to give you clearer thinking, it may take that anxious edge off enough for you to be able to sleep"* or *"one of its side effects is sleepiness, which may be helpful for you."*
- The "give an analogous paradigm for the patient's psychosis symptoms" approach
  - This can also help normalize her experiences and provides another context for perceiving her symptoms.
    - *"Try to think of your brain as a radar in an airplane. Both serve to alert you of things in the environment. In an airplane, the radar is meant to pick up on potentially dangerous objects for collision, like an airplane. Sometimes, however, the radar malfunctions, and it becomes too sensitive. It goes off because there is a cloud or another airplane that is very far away. Neither poses a significant problem. But the captain trusts his radar and changes his course.*
    "Sometimes, the brain is like that oversensitive radar. It is too sensitive, and picks up on things in the environment that you don't need to know about, such as people walking around you, or people looking at each other in passing while on the subway. Your brain alerts you, you interpret that there is a problem, and you act. So you are not imagining things, but your brain is working overtime.
    "The point of an antipsychotic medication is to get your brain back to working at a usual pace rather than overtime. We want it to pick up what it is supposed to from the environment, so that you don't have to make sense of things that may not be important to you."

Giving Hope

Both professionals and the public shy away from the diagnoses of schizophrenia and other psychotic illnesses because of the poor prognosis and hopelessness they may associate with them. This is often the reason that there is great hesitation to diagnose someone with schizophrenia, even when it is the working diagnosis.

Professionals have a duty to themselves and to their patients to do the following:

- Be truthful
- Be realistic
- Be optimistic, but not deceiving

We must temper our global expectations and apply them case by case. Some people *do* get well. Some people *do* improve. Some people *do* stay the same. And some people *do* get worse.[2] But, at this point in time, we cannot accurately predict who will fall into which category, and so we must relay all these possibilities to the patients and families we work with, along with a sense that we are willing to work toward the more optimistic outcomes. If we, the professionals, have a fatalistic dread about giving a diagnosis of schizophrenia to a patient, we cannot give hope and educate otherwise.

We must change our own misconceptions and work with that optimism. It is up to us to relay this optimism to our patients and their families.

It comes full circle in the task of trying to engage a patient while arriving at a correct diagnosis. Perhaps in the end, the most crucial component in completing these tasks and having the patient return to see you is giving hope.

REFERENCES

1. American Psychiatric Association: *Diagnostic and statistical manual of mental disorders*, ed 4, text revision, Washington,

DC, 2000, American Psychiatric Association, pp 297–343, 345–398.

2. Zipursky RB, Schulz SC, editors: *The early stages of schizophrenia,* Washington, DC, 2002, American Psychiatric Publishing Inc.

3. Poyurovsky M, Fuchs C, Weizman A: Obsessive-compulsive disorder in patients with first-episode schizophrenia, *Am J Psychiatry* 12:1998–2000, 1999.

4. van Os J, Bak M, Hanssen M, et al: Cannabis use and psychosis: a longitudinal population-based study, *Am J Epidemiol* 156:319–327, 2002.

RECOMMENDED READINGS

Hamilton M: *Fish's schizophrenia,* ed 3, Boston, 1984, John Wright and Sons Ltd.

Lieberman JA, Murray RM, editors: *Comprehensive care of schizophrenia: a textbook of clinical management,* London, 2001, Martin Dunitz Ltd.

6

Assessment of Patients with Bipolar Disorder

Andrea J. Levinson and L. Trevor Young

INTRODUCTION

"When you're high, it's tremendous. The ideas and feelings are fast and frequent like shooting stars, and you follow them until you find better and brighter ones. Shyness goes, the right words and gestures are suddenly there, and the power to seduce and captivate others is a felt certainty. There are interests found in uninteresting people. Sensuality is pervasive and the desire to seduce and be seduced irresistible. Feelings of ease, intensity, power, well-being, financial omnipotence, and euphoria now pervade one's marrow.

But somehow this changes: the fast ideas are far too fast, and there are far too many; overwhelming confusion replaces clarity. Memory goes. You are irritable, angry, frightened, uncontrollable, and enmeshed totally in the blackest caves of the mind."[1]

Bipolar disorder is a common disorder that affects approximately 1.5% of the population and is generally considered the most severe form of mood disorder; relapse and recurrence occur frequently, psychosis is common, and a significant proportion of patients develop a chronic, refractory course.

In this chapter, we focus on the clinical skills that are most useful in assessing patients with bipolar disorder. We have tried to include the essential content areas of the assessment of the patients. In addition, we describe many aspects of the interview process; that is, how to interact with the patient and obtain the information you need. We have used three case vignettes to make the content of the chapter more applicable to real-life clinical contexts. We begin with a brief overview of diagnostic criteria, although this is not the emphasis of the chapter. The bulk of the

chapter describes the various components of the psychiatric interview and how they pertain to patients with bipolar disorder. Finally, we discuss the assessment of a patient with bipolar disorder who is in longitudinal ongoing care. The process of working with and treating patients with bipolar disorder is highly rewarding. Manic patients can be among the most disheveled and psychotic you will ever see. Remarkably, in short order they can become completely euthymic and remain that way for prolonged periods of time. The contrast between the high-functioning well periods and those of utter disorganization and despair, and seeing how your intervention and treatments can influence the transition, is one of the most remarkable aspects of all medical practice.

DEFINITION AND DIAGNOSIS OF BIPOLAR DISORDER

All people experience variations in their mood: feeling happy, sad, angry, and irritable are normal mood changes. Bipolar disorder, or manic-depressive illness, is a mood disorder that is accompanied by extreme mood "swings" that differ significantly from normal mood variation. Bipolar disorder typically consists of three states: (1) a high state, called "mania"; (2) a low state, called "depression"; and (3) a well state, during which many people feel normal and function well. The manias and depressions may be "pure" episodes (containing only typical manic or depressive symptoms) or they may be "mixed" episodes (containing a mixture of manic and depressive symptoms at the same time). The presence of manic or hypomanic episodes

---

Box 6-1. Subtypes of Bipolar Disorder

Bipolar disorder type I: mania, with or without depression
Bipolar disorder type II: hypomania with major depression
Cyclothymia: hypomanic symptoms plus subthreshold
depressive symptoms for 2 years

Box 6-2. Neurovegetative Symptoms of Depression*

S–Sleep: *Sleep is decreased or increased, nearly every day.*
I–Interest: *Interest in all or almost all activities is lost nearly every day.*
G–Guilt: *One feels excessively guilty about things one has done or not done, nearly every day, or has feelings of worthlessness.*
E–Energy: *Marked loss of energy is noted nearly every day.*
C–Concentration: *Concentration is decreased.*
A–Appetite: *Appetite is either decreased or increased, nearly every day.*
P–Psychomotor Changes: *Psychomotor retardation represents moving or thinking more slowly than usual, and psychomotor agitation represents physical restlessness.*
S–Suicide: *Suicidal ideation may be present.*

---

*All these criteria contain a severity aspect, which means that they are not brief or transient.

---

defines a bipolar disorder; that is, the *sine qua non* of the diagnosis of bipolar disorder in the nosology of the current *Diagnostic and Statistical Manual of Mental Disorders*, edition 4, text revision (DSM-IV-TR) is the presence of manic symptoms.

The DSM-IV-TR includes two primary subtypes of bipolar disorder (Box 6-1). *Bipolar I disorder* is characterized by at least one manic episode with or without major depression. Only one single spontaneous manic or hypomanic episode ever is required to diagnose bipolar disorder. A person could have had many previous depressive episodes, but the onus is on the clinician to rule out a single manic/hypomanic episode.

In *bipolar II disorder*, a single manic episode is never identified, one or more hypomanic episodes occur, and at least one major depressive episode is identified. In *cyclothymia*, major depressive symptoms do not reach the severity threshold for diagnosis of a major depressive episode, and mood elevation symptoms, although present, do not reach the severity threshold for diagnosis of a manic episode.

To diagnose a major depressive episode, a patient must have depressed mood ("sad, down, blue") most of the day, nearly every day, for at least 2 weeks continuously, along with four of eight other symptoms as described in DSM-IV-TR. Alternatively, a patient may have anhedonia (complete loss of interest in all or almost all of one's activities) most of the day, nearly every day, for at least 2 weeks continuously, along with four of the seven depressive symptoms. One can have a major depressive episode without having a depressed mood. The neurovegetative symptoms of depression can be remembered with the mnemonic "SIGECAPS" derived by Carey Gross, MD, at Massachusetts General Hospital[2] (Box 6-2).

A manic episode involves elevated mood incorporating euphoria, irritability, or both, accompanied by a sufficient number of cardinal symptoms of mania. It is important to note that a manic episode does not require one to have euphoric mood. Many people report "high" or "extremely happy" mood, while others may only have "irritable" mood. Either type is still described as pure mania. Depressed mood can also co-occur with manic symptoms, which, with other depressive neurovegetative symptoms, can meet criteria for a mixed episode. Mixed manic episodes are as common as pure manic episodes.

For diagnosis of a manic episode to be made, the patient must experience an irritable or euphoric mood with three (if euphoric) or four (if irritable) of the seven cardinal symptoms of mania (Box 6-3) for 1 week. The cardinal symptoms of mania can be remembered using the mnemonic "DIGFAST" developed by William Falk, MD, at Massachusetts General Hospital.

Key Point:

The key difference between mania and hypomania is that mania is associated with significant social or occupational dysfunction (often spending sprees, sexual indiscretions, reckless driving, and impulsive traveling) whereas hypomania is not.

Case Example 1

Jack. It is mid-winter. A 28-year-old man, Jack, disheveled, barefoot, and dirty, wearing a torn shirt and khaki pants with no sweater or jacket, is brought to the emergency department of a local hospital by the police. His mother had contacted the police after he had been missing for 2 days. She had become increasingly concerned about his behavior over the past few weeks and had noticed that he was extremely irritable. In addition, he had only been sleeping 2 to 3 hours each night and appeared to have more energy than usual. She found his speech to be more pressured and intense, and he had expressed some unusual ideas. He had repeatedly stated that he had "superior abilities" and believed that he "controls the entire city." The police reportedly found him attempting to destroy a monument in the city.

Box 6-3. Cardinal Symptoms of Mania

D–Distractibility: *It represents being unable to focus on tasks for an extended duration of time.*

I–Insomnia: *This means decreased need for sleep, unlike depressive insomnia, which means decreased sleep. The best way to differentiate the two is to ask the patient about energy level. In manic insomnia, despite decreased sleep the energy level is average or high. In depressive insomnia, it is low.*

G–Grandiosity: *This reflects inflated self-esteem.*

F–Flight of Ideas: *Racing thoughts represent rapid progression in one's thought process.*

A–Activities: *This represents increased goal-directed activities, which are functional and often appear useful. They fall into four categories: social (increased socializing, going out more than usual), sexual (increased libido or hypersexuality), work (increased productivity), and school (producing more projects, studying more than usual). In all cases, usual levels of activity need to be based on the euthymic state.*

S–Speech: *Patients have pressured speech or increased talkativeness.*

T–Thoughtlessness: *This involves pleasure-seeking activities that do not display usual judgment and therefore, unlike increased goal-directed activities, are dysfunctional. There are four common types: sexual indiscretions, reckless driving, spending sprees, and sudden traveling.*

In addition to the above criteria, there must also be significant social or occupational dysfunction arising from the previously mentioned symptoms. If there is no social or occupational dysfunction, then the diagnosis is a hypomanic episode. For a diagnosis of a manic episode, the symptoms must last at least 1 week (or lead to hospitalization). The minimum duration for hypomania according to the DSM-IV-TR is 4 days.

Case Example 2

Laura. A 38-year-old married woman and mother of three young children, Laura presents to your office for an appointment. She describes a 2-month history of "feeling overwhelmed, teary, and sad." She is having difficulty playing with her children and is experiencing poor sleep, decreased appetite, and ongoing fatigue throughout the day. She has thoughts about wanting to end her life, but states she could never do this to her children. During the assessment, you establish that she has experienced two previous depressive episodes in the past. In addition, she had a period of elevated mood when attending university in her early 20s, where she felt euphoric and "sped-up" for a week, slept less, talked more, and felt more confident in her abilities.

Case Example 3

Victoria. You assess a 43-year-old lawyer, Victoria, who states, "I feel wound up, agitated, like I want to jump out of my skin." She describes this feeling lasting for the past month with other symptoms of increased energy, rapid thoughts, and increased spending. She regrets having charged $2000 to her credit card over the past week. She adds that she wishes she felt good, but she feels teary and depressed on most days. In addition, she cannot concentrate on simple tasks, feels continually hopeless about the future, and has thought about suicide as an option.

CONDUCTING THE ASSESSMENT

Setting and Stage

In Case Example 1, Jack is agitated, and you should attempt to provide as safe an environment as possible; an empty room is preferable. Simple furniture, for example a chair or side table, can easily be thrown or used in an impulsive manner by the patient in a manic state. Often, the emergency department can provide a safe environment for such an assessment. You should approach the interview of an acutely manic patient with the potential for violence in mind. You should always set up the interview area so that you can exit the room immediately if things become unsafe.

In Case Examples 2 and 3, which would most likely occur in an outpatient setting, you should try to assess the patient alone first. Family members or significant others may accompany the person to an interview to provide additional history. Any collateral history you can obtain, including previous hospital notes or clinical notes, is often very helpful. In the outpatient setting, the patient needs to consent to family members providing additional history.

In Case Example 1, the acutely manic patient will likely not tolerate a long interview. In these cases, you may be able to do only a mental status examination and rely on collateral information to piece together the story. While assessing the acutely manic patient, you may feel as if it is extremely difficult to interrupt the patient or to ask necessary questions to establish safety and take an adequate history. The acutely manic patient will often speak very rapidly, in a pressured and intense manner. You will need to determine when it is appropriate to contain the interview, and interrupt where necessary, without disregarding the patient or seeming disrespectful. Most importantly, when you are interviewing an acutely manic patient, you need to maintain a *flexible* approach because a controlled, ordered, sequential assessment is highly unlikely to flow, given the patient's own disorganized thought form and behavior.

In Case Examples 2 and 3, which occur in outpatient settings, it is important for you to allow the patient to tell her story. If you do not allow this to happen, the patient will not perceive you to have really listened and may leave feeling unheard and disregarded.

> **Key Point:**
>
> When you are interviewing an acutely manic patient, you need to maintain a flexible approach. A controlled, ordered, sequential assessment is highly unlikely to flow, due to the patient's own disorganized thought form and behavior.

> **Key Point:**
>
> The patient should never feel hurried and should always feel as if you are really listening to her story.

Explanation of the Interview Process

Always introduce the people present in the room (sometimes there will be more than one interviewer or observer). Make sure the patient is comfortable. Inform the patient of the approximate length of the interview and what to expect in terms of the format. For example, if there are two interviewers in the room (e.g., a staff person and student), it is useful to identify each person by name and indicate why they are there. Also, explain to the patient that after the interview, you will ask the patient to step outside in order for the two interviewers to discuss the interview, and then the patient will be asked to return for feedback.

It often helps to put the patient at ease to state, *"Please feel free to ask any questions at any time."* The assessment should feel like a conversation and not an interrogation. By putting the patient at ease and developing therapeutic alliance early on, you have a greater chance to gain the information you need to assess the patient.

In Case Example 1, Jack may be too disorganized to provide a reliable history, and collateral information from people who have been in close contact with him may be essential in understanding his condition. Acutely manic patients will often have little insight into their behavior and how it may be affecting their lives or the lives of those around them.

> **Key Point:**
>
> It is essential to gain as much collateral information as possible when interviewing the acutely manic patient. It is sometimes useful to gain collateral information before interviewing the patient, particularly in emergency assessments.

Identifying Data

Gathering identifying data is an important beginning to the interview because it sets the stage for the rest of the interview. From the start, you should try to put the patient at ease and establish an alliance. In the case of a patient with bipolar disorder, certain aspects of the identifying data may give you clues as to the impact and consequence of the illness, for example:

- Marital status: Regardless of whether the patient is single, married, separated, divorced, or living with a common law partner, it is worthwhile asking for how long this has been the case. The patient may volunteer that a long-term relationship has ended or has changed as a result of the illness.
- Living situation: This may have changed precipitously due to recent mania or depression.
- Employment: If the patient is unemployed, you should ask when he last worked and what he was doing. This provides you with a context for how the patient is coping on a functional level and gives you an early window into the possible impact of the illness.
- Source of income: Previous manic episodes may have caused financial havoc on the patient with bipolar disorder. Additionally, this line of questioning provides context for the assessment of spending behavior and financial competency, both of which can be dysregulated by a manic episode.
- City and country of origin: You should establish whether the patient has always lived in this city or has recently moved from another city or country of origin. Patients with bipolar disorder are vulnerable to traveling and leave their home dwelling impulsively during a manic episode.

Method of Referral

In outpatient assessments, it is important to obtain from patients what *their* understandings are of the method of referral, even if you have this information at hand. It is helpful for you to understand who initiated the referral. If, for example, the patient's family doctor or a family member suggested it, this may be a clue to the patient's indifference to any problem. Alternatively, if the patient states that he requested a consultation or an assessment, it already tells you that this patient is probably motivated to seek help. This is unlikely to be the case in an interview with an acutely manic patient. Insight appears to be state dependent; that is, insight is characteristically lacking in the manic state.[3] This would prevent someone who is acutely manic from seeking help in the traditional manner due to this distinctive lack of insight when the person is in a manic episode. Therefore, the person who is manic would not view his mood, behavior, and overall experience as in need of any assessment or medical attention.

Chief Complaint

The chief complaint is the patient's subjective complaint and should include the duration it has been a problem. Try to elicit this in the patient's own words because this will most accurately capture subjective experience and personal priorities. We find that using open-ended questions allows the patient's story to flow and reflects the level of awareness of the illness and its impact, for example, *"Who initiated this referral? Why is your family doctor/mother so concerned about you? What would you like to address during today's assessment?"* In the outpatient setting, it is often difficult to establish a time frame, as in a patient with long-standing bipolar illness; the "chief complaint" may be years in duration. Try to establish early on in the interview what is *most* disturbing/bothersome to the person. Ask, for example, *"What is/are the major problems for you?"*

History of Presenting Illness

The history of presenting illness (HPI) is the core section of the interview in which the chief complaint is explored more extensively. That is, you discover what the patient has been experiencing *recently*. You and the patient determine where the history of presenting illness begins, as it will vary depending on the individual. In all three vignettes, the start of the history of presenting illness is clearly defined. In Case Example 1, it would most likely be a few weeks' duration, when his mother first noticed he was "acting strangely." However, it may start prior to this point, and you need to remain flexible in your approach. In Case Example 2, you would need to quantify how long the patient has been feeling depressed, and she would tell you approximately 2 months. Some patients find it hard to pinpoint the start of their presenting illness, but with gentle questioning you can elicit this information. Other patients, particularly those with recurrent mood episodes, will know and recognize the heralding signs of a relapse—be it a change in the perception of color or a sleep disturbance. It is worth exploring and documenting this very carefully with the patient so that the next episode can be recognized and treated quickly. For example, if in Case Example 2, you asked, *"How were you at Christmas time?"* the patient may respond, "Fine, I was feeling like my normal self." Then you would have a time index from which to work. In general, people typically underestimate the duration of their episodes, and careful retrospective review and information from others close to the patient may give a more precise sense of when an episode began.

The manic patient may be too agitated and disorganized to provide you with a clear history of presenting illness. In these cases, reliable collateral history will be essential to help appraise the recent events leading up to this assessment. It can be difficult to communicate with an acutely manic patient, so try to keep your questions clear using simple, emphatic speech to which the patient can give isolated suitable replies. Patients with mania are often extremely distractible and stimulus bound, and by using clear questions and simple language that require short answers, you help contain the already overladen environmental stimulation the patient may be experiencing. Furthermore, you may easily find yourself wanting to break into laughter while interviewing a euphoric and disinhibited manic patient. Often, the patient's euphoria and grandiosity are "infectious"; however, you must try to remain calm, clear, and objective during the assessment. However, it is important to take note that you feel like giggling during the assessment because this is another clue that the patient may be manic. While resisting the urge to laugh, you can use your sense of humor appropriately to engage the patient if it is a natural skill of yours. If it doesn't come naturally to you, we recommend against it; it will feel forced to the patient and will likely not be funny or engaging. The manic patient often tests interpersonal boundaries, and it may be difficult to maintain your composure during the assessment. The patient may inquire about you and aspects pertaining to your personal life. For example, questions such as "Do have any children?" or "Do you find me attractive?" need to be reflected back to the patient. An appropriate answer would be: *"I understand you're curious to know more about me, but I don't think that it's relevant to today's meeting."* In certain situations, you might answer briefly around demographic questions, for example, *"Yes, I have children,"* but you would not want to engage in questions of a more intimate nature. Alternatively, you could choose to move on to a different topic, but this may be interpreted as not having heard their question. In addition, some manic patients will have sensitive antennae to your discomfort and will readily exploit it! They may also be subtly or overtly seductive with clinicians—a type of libidinous incontinence that can be another clue to the underlying illness.

Key Point:

Do not engage in conversation of a personal nature, as it relates to you, with the manic patient. Calmly redirect the conversation back to the pertinent history of the patient.

> **Key Point:**
> _____
>
> You will need to remain flexible in your interviewing style
> when trying to establish the history of presenting illness with
> an acutely manic patient.

Before trying to elicit lists of symptoms, try to explore
what the patient has been experiencing in the recent past.
Once you do start to obtain specific symptoms, for example, depressive symptoms in Case Example 2, you need to
place these symptoms in the individual context of the person's life. It may help to imagine you are constructing a narrative of her recent circumstances. If you try to do this, you
will gain the richness of detail and the context in which to
place her mood symptoms. Remember that each person's
symptoms, despite her characteristic patterns and clusters,
manifest in a uniquely individual and interesting way,
according to the person's individual life circumstances.
Focus on the story, instead of simply obtaining a symptom
or diagnostic criteria list.

> **Key Point:**
> _____
>
> Try to create a narrative of the person's history of presenting
> illness. Remain flexible and contextualize the symptoms to
> the individual.

Eliciting Mood Symptoms

Once you have elicited the patient's story of the recent
period of "unwellness" or "feeling markedly different
than usual" (this value-free description may be more
palatable to a euphoric manic patient), and you understand the context for these difficulties, you need to flesh
out the specific mood symptoms the patient has experienced recently.

Inquiring About Depressive Symptoms

In Case Example 2, Laura describes her mood recently
as "bleak and flat." Try to elicit the patient's recent mood
state by capturing her experience in her own words. Try to
avoid asking leading questions, such as, "Have you been
feeling depressed recently?" If the patient is having difficulty with the more open-ended questions, then you can
provide options such as sad, depressed, or calm.
Remember that patients may not describe their mood as
"depressed" but may indeed be depressed.

In Case Example 2, you inquire further and find out that
Laura enjoys very little in her day, including her time spent
with her children, which before she started feeling
depressed would have given her much pleasure. When

exploring a patient's interest in activities in her world, you
need to understand her "outside world"; don't ask a question about interest in daily activities without understanding
the person at baseline. Appropriate open-ended questions
may be: *"What do you usually enjoy doing? What do you
do for fun in your week? What activities do you look forward to?"* In Case Example 2, for example, Laura can tell
you that normally she loves to be with her young children,
and now that has significantly changed.

> **Key Point:**
> _____
>
> When exploring a patient's interest in daily activities, you
> need to understand her "outside world"; that is, don't ask a
> question about her interest in daily activities without
> understanding her at baseline. Only then can you interpret
> whether her mood is affecting her baseline level of
> functioning.

In depressed states sleep is often disturbed, and it is also
important to explore in detail how sleep is affected. We ask
the patient, *"How many hours do you sleep each night? Do
you have difficulty falling asleep, staying asleep, or waking
up in the morning? Is your sleep restful, or has it changed
in quality?"* In depressive episodes, increased need for
sleep is a characteristic of a depression with atypical features and is more common in bipolar illness. This detailed
qualifying and quantifying of sleep disturbance has implications for treatment because different medications are
shown to be more effective in patients with atypical depression. In addition, a depressed patient with melancholic
features will often endorse early morning awakening, and
this, too, will help characterize the nature of the patient's
depressive symptoms.

Always establish whether there has been a significant
change in a person's appetite in either direction. A patient
may endorse eating three good meals each day but describe
a lack of enjoyment while eating, with little interest in food.
You should also remember to inquire about fluctuations in
body weight.

In Case Example 2, Laura endorses significant cognitive
changes, including difficulty concentrating, feeling confused, ruminating about her life with an inability to focus
on her children's needs, and feeling inadequate and useless
each day. Overall, she feels slowed down both mentally and
physically and constantly feels guilty for her "inadequacy"
as a wife and mother.

Inquiring About Manic/Hypomanic Symptoms

Manic or hypomanic symptoms fall into three major
groups: (1) mood, (2) behavior changes, and (3) cognition
and perception.

Mood

Here, one should inquire in an open-ended manner about how the patient is feeling during the assessment; that is, *"How would you describe your mood today and over the past few weeks?"* Try to limit the patient to how he has been feeling *recently*, in order to ascertain his *current* mood status. Patients will not usually volunteer that they feel "manic" or "hypomanic" because these are technical terms. In fact, these terms should be avoided during the assessment because they can be misleading. It is important to elicit the patient's subjective feeling of elevated mood without leading the patient in a directive manner. For example, in Case Example 1, if one had asked Jack a few weeks before his presentation in the emergency department about how he was feeling and how he would describe his mood, he may have spontaneously described a feeling of "self-confidence" or "euphoria," "feeling exalted" or "the best I've ever felt." These descriptions would give you an individualized sense that his mood is elevated. Interviewers often equate elevated mood with mania or hypomania, but one must remember that one needs to demonstrate additional disturbance of behavior and cognition/perception to be considered manic/hypomanic. During the interview with Jack in the emergency department, he may describe his mood as "great," but you would observe his striking irritability in his interactions with you during the interview. It is important to be attuned to the underlying irritability, which is common in manic patients. The mood elevation that is expressed is often fluctuating and volatile. If one persists in interviewing a manic patient for more than a few minutes, it is likely that the irritability, anger, and fear will be revealed. Patients who are manic will often demonstrate extreme lability of mood, with rapid shifts from unrestrained euphoria to weeping and irritability.

Behavior

A decreased need for sleep is a hallmark feature of mania and can often help distinguish manic or hypomanic symptoms from "simply having a good time." In addition, a "decreased need for sleep" is probably the most useful and reliable criterion for mania. You have to persist with questions about sleep and not accept a quantification of "enough." Sometimes manic patients will either overestimate their sleep or provide a socially desirable normative response like, "Oh, about 6 or 7 hours." You should then ask, *"What's the* least *amount of sleep you've gotten away with in the last 2 weeks? How have you felt the next day? Have you had any nights where you haven't slept at all?"* This may help unmask previously covert manic sleeplessness and elevated energy. In Case Example 1, Jack had been sleeping 2 to 3 hours each night over a period of more than a week. This lack of sleep, in conjunction with his behavioral agitation, increased energy, and other symptoms of mania, helps establish a diagnosis of an acute manic episode. Patients often endorse feeling "really happy, and more outgoing and confident" for a period of days to weeks. It is important to establish whether there was sleep disturbance as well as the other symptoms of mania/hypomania concurrently, as this will help distinguish mania from a normal elevation in mood state. There is a low sensitivity for eliciting previous hypomanic episodes from the patient, and, subsequently, they are often missed in clinical interviews.

Patients with mania are very often impulsive and disinhibited in their behavior. The challenge is to elicit the information from the patient in a way that does not seem artificial or judgmental. An opening question to *avoid* using would be: "Have you noticed that you are more impulsive or behaving differently than usual?" Manic patients have little insight into the recent change in their behavior, and it is often through interviews of family and friends that the full extent of behavioral change becomes clear. In Case Example 1, Jack was brought into the emergency department by police who observed his behavioral disinhibition. He reportedly tried to destroy a public monument. It would be important to explore with Jack the reasons for this act and to try and understand whether there was an impulsive aspect to this behavior. Increased impulsivity is a hallmark feature of behavioral change in manic patients. Collateral information is often vital in determining the severity of recent bizarre and inappropriate behaviors. In Case Example 1, Jack is accompanied by his mother, who may be able to provide vital information regarding his potential to endanger himself or others. Jack's mother adds that he was recently found running down the street naked and that he had left a lit cigarette on the table and had almost caused a fire. In addition, when the police found him attacking the public monument, he resisted their help and began to engage in a physical fight with three policemen. These accounts of aggressive, disinhibited, and socially inappropriate behaviors provide one with essential information about the patient's safety and the risk of the patient harming himself or other people around him.

In addition to the obviously bizarre and uncontrolled behavioral change in manic patients, patients with hypomania or emerging behavioral change may present with smaller and subtler changes in behavior. It is important to try to understand the baseline or normal functioning of the patient. For example, someone who would normally be considered a cautious person may demonstrate initial changes in behavior that are subtle and small, for example, attending late parties or deciding to take a vacation without any planning. These small changes in behavior often precede more obvious, dramatic, and bizarre behavioral disturbances.

Mania is often accompanied by reported increased spending. As one patient described in an interview, "When I am high, I couldn't worry about money if I tried. So I don't. The money will come from somewhere; I am entitled and God will provide." In Case Example 3, Victoria regrets having charged $2000 to her credit card in the past week. Patients often describe the need to spend money as so great and overpowering, that the purchases occur with a great sense of urgency and importance, as if "nothing can stop it happening." One patient reported spending thousands of dollars on costume jewelry, unnecessary furniture, and four identical sweaters in a half-hour time period. She reported feeling out of control during this time. The patient's subjective feeling while spending the money is important, as the objective amount in dollars can be misleading.

Behavioral changes in manic patients often occur around changes in sexual behavior and attitude. Manic patients may first report an increased feeling of self-confidence, feeling less shy, finding that the right words and gestures seem obvious and the power to captivate others is felt to be certain. One patient reported that her sense of sensuality was pervasive, and the desire to seduce and be seduced was irresistible. Often an acutely manic patient's overt behavior during the assessment can be sexually provocative, providing one with objective evidence of heightened sexuality. However, patients may not volunteer the information, and it is important to ask about feelings of sexuality and sexual interest during an initial assessment. This can be done in a contextualized, natural manner when inquiring about recent relationships, whether the patient has a partner/spouse. In addition, collateral information from the patient's partner often provides one with this information.

Cognition/Perception

Patients in a milder hypomanic state often describe increased creativity, a profusion of ideas, and an ease and flow of their ideas, which facilitates artistic expression. Many artists who have experienced mania, including Robert Schumann and Virginia Woolf, described this heightened creativity and productivity while their thought form was still intact.[4] However, the surplus of thoughts and ideas increases as mania progresses, and as the interviewer you should be observing keenly when the person's conversation jumps from one topic to another. In a patient with disorder of thought form, incoherence predominates; patients will describe their thoughts as racing at great speed, as well as thoughts feeling disjointed and feeling overall very distractible. In addition, you should listen to the quality, speed, volume, and intensity of their speech because in mania, speech is often louder and more pressured, rapid, and urgent than normal. In an interview with a manic patient with thought disturbance, it is often difficult to direct the questions or to feel like you have any control over the interview. It is best to perform an active mental status examination, noting the patient's disordered cognition, and if possible, remembering specific examples of the patient's thought process, with rapid shifts of topic and "flight of ideas" that are pathognomonic for mania. The interviewer's questions should be kept closed ended, simple, and clear, so as to allow the disorganized patient to focus on a finite answer. Finally, in the case of the patient with mania and psychosis, thoughts and perceptions become fragmented and ultimately often psychotic and separated from reality. In Case Example 1, Jack believes that he "controls the entire city." This is a grandiose delusion that is a common delusion endorsed by manic patients. The way to uncover such a belief is not easily done through formulaic questions, for example, "Do you have any special powers?" Rather, by allowing the patient to describe his recent activities and behavior, you will be able to explore with the patient his underlying belief and understand more accurately how he views the world. For example, in Case Example 1, by exploring the recent event where Jack was found to be damaging state property, one could uncover that indeed Jack believed that he was leader of the city and that he had the authority to do this, as well as to govern the people of the city. Patients with mania and grandiose delusions often describe an inner compulsion to act (often in a dangerous manner) as a means of contributing to society. They often describe a great moral imperative that involves finding faults in society that they believe need to be corrected.

Perceptual abnormalities experienced in patients with mania are often described by the person as beginning with a mildly increased awareness of objects that ultimately leads to a chaotic disarray of the senses. Patients describe visual, auditory, tactile, and olfactory experiences that are all heightened, with "every external detail of the world becoming more etched in consciousness." In your discussion with manic patients, you should ask them about altered experiences involving the senses. Patients often describe an overall heightened sensory awareness, colors appearing brighter, words sounding like music, and the feeling that the different senses of vision, hearing, taste, and feeling are merging to form one combined experience. Furthermore, one can inquire about any religious experiences the manic patient may have had, as mania often involves mystical and pronounced religious experiences.

COMPONENTS OF THE ASSESSMENT (HPI AND PAST PSYCHIATRIC HISTORY) KEY TO INTERVIEWING PATIENTS WITH BIPOLAR DISORDER

It is important to consider the course of illness, family history, and treatment response in addition to phenomenology to aid your diagnosis and clinical assessment. In the literature there are five core features described that aid in determining a bipolar illness:

1. Features of mania or hypomania
2. Features of depression
3. Course of illness
4. Family history
5. Treatment response

Features of Mania, Hypomania, and Depression

Once you have established that the patient has had previous manic, hypomanic, and depressive episodes, you need to characterize these episodes; that is, you need to develop an accurate description of what qualities typify these episodes for your patient. Always make sure that what the patient is describing as a previous major depressive episode is indeed just that, as this makes your longitudinal history taking more accurate and useful. Patients may be telling you about a previous time they were depressed, and if you forget to ask about the duration and severity of the episode, you could be capturing milder, less specific mood symptoms that are still relevant to the history but not diagnosable manic/hypomanic/mixed or major depressive episodes.

You need to ask,

"What is a typical depressive episode like for you?" It is helpful to relate previous episodes to current functioning to give a sense of how the person is doing now compared to before. For example, if the person in Case Example 2 states, "Four years ago, my depression was much worse; I was actively suicidal, and my mood was terrible all the time. Right now, I am depressed, but not that depressed," this gives you valuable information about the severity of symptoms as they relate to the individual's past history of mood episodes.

"Tell me what happens to you when you are manic?" Patients are often reluctant or unable to volunteer information about their manic or hypomanic symptoms. First, patients often have poor insight into their behavior when they are manic, and subsequently (sometimes fortunately, with regard to humiliating behavior) have little memory for these episodes. Often, it is first the family or close friends who notice a change indicative of a manic episode in the patient. Ask, "What is worse for you— the depressions, the manias, or both?"

Longitudinal Course (Included in Past Psychiatric History)

Once you have captured the unique *quality* of the individual's characteristic manic, hypomanic, and depressive

episodes, it is equally important to *quantify* the number of depressions and manias/hypomanias (on average) the patient has experienced. It often helps to quantify the number of depressive/manic episodes each year, giving both you and the patient a way of making sense of the illness and how it has progressed over time.

Questions you need to ask include the following:

- *"How long do your depressions last? How long do your manic episodes last?"*
- *"How often do you experience the depressions? How often do you experience the manias?"*
- *"When was your last depressive episode? When was your last manic episode?"*
- *"How many times have you felt like that in the past year?"*

In Case Example 2, Laura has had relatively few previous episodes—only two previous depressions in total. However, in patients with longer histories of bipolar disorder, you need to look at episodes per year, or even episodes within time frames (e.g., before having children/after having children) to develop a description of the illness progression over time. You must make sure that you do not hurry over this section of the history. Patients need to feel that their individual narrative has been accurately captured and described. A detailed narrative of the patient's previous mood episodes would include the number of mood episodes, quality of episodes, response to medications, need for hospitalizations, and any links to significant stressors over time. We recommend taking detailed notes around when these episodes occurred, the duration of each episode, and their chronological and psychological relationships to significant life events. In addition, you should add the medications that the patient was taking during previous episodes to give you an accurate history of medication response. In an assessment with a patient with a very complex course of illness, with many previous mood episodes, it often helps to draw a picture and get the patient to help you in developing an accurate visual representation of mood episodes over time.

Figure 6-1 outlines 3 years in a patient's history of mood episodes. This provides you and the patient with a pictorial overview of the patient's mood episodes and does not capture the detail of a daily mood chart (discussed later). This is simply a tool to reflect the "larger" picture and how mood states possibly relate to medication use and significant personal stressors. If the flat line rises above baseline, for example, _____⌐‾‾‾⌐_____ this indicates an elevation of mood (i.e., hypomania or mania). For example, in 1996, this patient experienced a manic episode in May and June, and subsequently lithium was added to the antidepressant fluoxetine. When the line lowers from baseline, a depressive episode is indicated. For example, in 1997, the patient got depressed in October around the time of the death of his father:

A flat line indicates a euthymic mood state (i.e., no manic/hypomanic episodes and no depressions):

The amount of deviation from baseline is based on the severity of the episode; for example, a mild hypomanic episode may be represented as:

and a severe manic episode represented as:

Key Point:

Patients need to think that their individual narratives regarding their previous mood episodes and symptoms have been accurately captured and described.

Subsyndromal Symptoms of Mania, Hypomania, and Depression

In Case Example 2, you interview Laura at more length and continue to follow up with her on a weekly outpatient

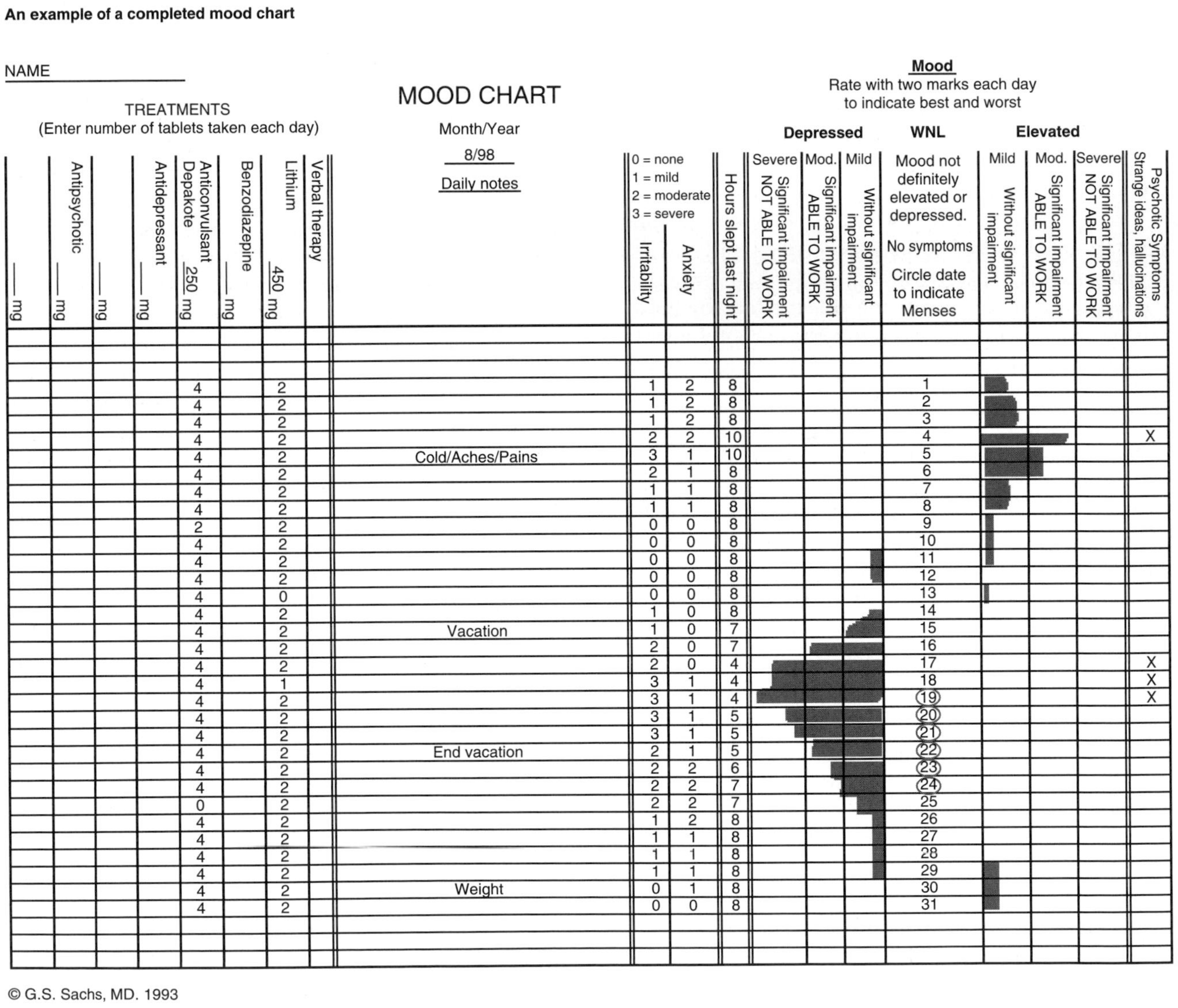

An example of a completed mood chart

MOOD CHART — Month/Year 8/98

TREATMENTS (Enter number of tablets taken each day). Columns include: Antipsychotic (mg), Antidepressant (mg), Anticonvulsant Depakote 250 mg, Benzodiazepine (mg), Lithium 450 mg, Verbal therapy.

Mood rating scale: 0 = none, 1 = mild, 2 = moderate, 3 = severe. Mood rated with two marks each day to indicate best and worst (Depressed — WNL — Elevated). Circle date to indicate Menses.

Depakote 250 mg	Lithium 450 mg	Daily notes	Irritability	Anxiety	Hours slept last night	Date	Psychotic Symptoms
4	2		1	2	8	1	
4	2		1	2	8	2	
4	2		1	2	8	3	
4	2		2	2	10	4	X
4	2	Cold/Aches/Pains	3	1	10	5	
4	2		2	1	8	6	
4	2		1	1	8	7	
4	2		1	1	8	8	
2	2		0	0	8	9	
4	2		0	0	8	10	
4	2		0	0	8	11	
4	2		0	0	8	12	
4	0		0	0	8	13	
4	2		1	0	8	14	
4	2	Vacation	1	0	7	15	
4	2		2	0	7	16	
4	2		2	0	4	17	X
4	1		3	1	4	18	X
4	2		3	1	4	(19)	X
4	2		3	1	5	(20)	
4	2		3	1	5	(21)	
4	2	End vacation	2	1	5	(22)	
4	2		2	2	6	(23)	
4	2		2	2	7	(24)	
0	2		2	2	7	25	
4	2		1	2	8	26	
4	2		1	1	8	27	
4	2		1	1	8	28	
4	2		1	1	8	29	
4	2	Weight	0	1	8	30	
4	2		0	0	8	31	

© G.S. Sachs, MD. 1993

FIGURE 6-1 *Visual representation of a patient's history of mood episodes.*

basis. You discover that even when she is not suffering from an acute episode of depression (as she was when she first presented) or hypomania (as she experienced during university), she is never symptom free. She describes having some symptoms of depression throughout most of her bipolar illness, though these are milder, less prominent symptoms that would not met criteria for a major depressive episode. Should you be concerned about this?

Most studies for patients with bipolar disorder have focused on acute episodes, namely mania or hypomania and major depression. Bipolar disorder has been conceptualized as a chronic or recurrent disorder with periods of mania or hypomania and depression, alternating with phases of euthymia. Moreover, treatment trials have primarily addressed the treatment of acute mania and acute major depression and the prevention of future manic and depressive episodes. A recent study by Judd and colleagues[5] on the long-term follow-up of a cohort of patients with bipolar I disorder concluded that, indeed, bipolar illness is a chronic disorder, but that minor and subsyndromal manic and particularly depressive symptoms are a prominent and often a predominant feature of the illness. Judd and others[5] showed that weeks with depressive symptoms predominate over manic/hypomanic symptoms in both bipolar I and II disorders, 3:1 in bipolar I and 37:1 in bipolar II. The observation that patients with bipolar disorder spend a substantial period of time with minor or subsyndromal affective symptoms has profound implications for understanding and treating the disorder and contributes greatly to the clinical presentation and morbidity of patients with this disease. In Laura's case (Case Example 2), you should take note of her ongoing milder, subsyndromal depressive symptoms and address these in your ongoing assessments and treatment plan. MacQueen and colleagues[6] conducted a study examining detailed life charting data from 138 patients with bipolar disorder. Patients were categorized into euthymic, subsyndromal, or syndromal groups according to the clinical state during their most recent year of follow-up. The three groups were then examined with respect to comorbidity, function, and treatment received. The study found that patients with subsyndromal symptoms had high rates of comorbid anxiety disorders and were more likely to have increased rates of eating disorders as well.[6] This highlights how comorbid psychiatric conditions (like anxiety disorders and eating disorders) have a significant impact on the course of bipolar disorder, and certainly, alter the person's overall functioning. Therefore, in the assessment it is crucial to explore all possible comorbid symptoms and illnesses in order to be able to assess the person's bipolar disorder fully, to engage with the patient and understand her bipolar disorder in a broader framework, and to ultimately provide treatment recommendations.

Mixed States

You assess Victoria in Case Example 3, and she presents with symptoms of mania (irritability, increased energy, rapid thoughts, and increased spending) as well as depressive symptoms, including difficulties with concentration, extreme hopelessness, appetite changes, and suicidal ideation. Mixed manic states, meeting criteria for both depression and mania, are often confusing to assess and by nature appear paradoxical, in that the person is both depressed and manic at the same time. Often in a cross-sectional assessment, you will have difficulty determining whether the patient is presenting with an agitated depression or a dysphoric mania, and this may only become clear with more longitudinal observation. When a patient appears to be in a mixed manic state, you need to think about comorbid substance abuse as a possibility because it can lead to a similar clinical presentation.

Rapid Cycling Versus Mood Lability

Many patients will endorse rapid and frequent fluctuations in their mood that occur daily or weekly. The term *rapid-cycling bipolar disorder* identifies a course of numerous mood episodes, defined as four or more episodes in a year. You need to take a careful history and obtain the necessary information to determine whether this could be a rapid-cycling variant of bipolar disorder (with distinct mood episodes) or mood lability. It is important to assess the length of these mood fluctuations as well as the severity of symptoms, that is, the degree to which they are affecting the person's functioning. In addition, the duration of mood symptoms and whether they are always triggered by environmental stressors can help distinguish true rapid cycling versus mood lability in the context of otherwise normal functioning. Certainly, "ups and downs of mood" (i.e., unstable mood regulation) has been found to be one of the strongest risk factors for bipolar disorder.[7] Therefore, the safe and cautious approach would be to have a high index of suspicion when assessing a patient with mood fluctuations, as with a more longitudinal assessment it may become clearer that these episodes are more significant episodes of mood disturbance (in duration and severity).

Bipolar Spectrum

The bipolar spectrum consists of features of bipolarity beyond the classic kind found in DSM-IV-TR criteria of bipolar I. A proposed new diagnosis, "bipolar spectrum disorder"[8] occurs in a person with major depressive disorder who does not exhibit spontaneous mania or hypomania but still manifests many signs of bipolarity. Important signs of bipolarity are a positive family history of bipolar disorder in a first-degree relative and antidepressant-induced mania/hypomania. Many, although not all, patients with antidepressant-induced mania also have a history of spontaneous manic or hypomanic episodes. If you encounter someone with antidepressant-induced mania, you should search very carefully for evidence of spontaneous episodes. Other useful signs of bipolarity include brief, recurrent, atypical, psychotic or postpartum major depressive episodes. You could view this term as a way of trying to be more specific about the DSM-IV-TR term *bipolar disorder not otherwise specified*. It is useful to conceive bipolar disorder as existing on a continuum of mood disorders, between the classic type I bipolar disorder and classic unipolar depression. Patients often do not fall neatly into discrete categories.

The course of depressive illness is also a key bipolarity factor. Depressive episodes do not recur in one third of patients with unipolar depression; they recur in almost *all* patients with bipolar disorder. Therefore, the greater the number of depressive episodes, the more characteristic this feature would be for bipolar disorder. In addition, the shorter the duration of the depressive episode, the more characteristic it is of bipolar disorder. The earlier the age of onset, the more likely the illness is bipolar in nature.[9]

Key Point:

If you encounter someone with antidepressant-induced mania, search very carefully for evidence of spontaneous episodes.

Functional History

Always establish how the person is managing on a daily basis. Start off by asking open-ended questions, for example, *"Can you describe an average day for me?"* If the patient has described significant depressive symptoms and then states that she exercises each day, attends work, attends the theater, and dines out three times a month, you should question how great an impact the depressive symptoms are having on daily functioning. This provides you with a view of possible inconsistencies in the history, and collateral history will be relevant. Bipolar illness, when active, significantly affects the person's ability to engage in relationships. Therefore, when eliciting information about mood symptoms, always ask about significant relationships. It is important to ask about intimate relationships, and specifically, to inquire about sexual intimacy and libido in a patient with bipolar disorder. Often, depressed patients will have decreased interest in sexual activity, and this is a symptom that is often overlooked. Alternatively, mania often involves increased sexual interest and activity, as well as significant sexual disinhibition. Therefore, questions

around a person's sexual life are often of high yield. However, such questions are often not asked in an initial assessment due to shyness or embarrassment on the part of the interviewer rather than the patient.

Safety

It is extremely important to inquire about recent thoughts of suicide, as well as recent suicidal intent or plan. If there has been recent suicidal thinking or an attempt, you need to explore this in detail. Bipolar disorder has considerable morbidity and mortality associated with the illness, and the suicide completion rate is the highest of all psychiatric disorders. The rate has been shown to range between 15% and 20%. The frequency of suicide attempts appears similar for the bipolar I and II subtypes. Persons with bipolar disorder repeatedly have been shown to have greater overall mortality than the general population. Known general risk factors for suicide also apply to patients with bipolar disorder. These include a history of suicide attempts, suicidal ideation, comorbid substance abuse, comorbid personality disorders, agitation, pervasive insomnia, impulsiveness, and family history of suicide.

Among the phases of bipolar disorder, depression is associated with the highest suicide risk, followed by mixed states and the presence of psychotic symptoms, with episodes of mania being least associated with suicide. Suicidal ideation during mixed states has been correlated with the severity of depressive symptoms. In Case Example 3, it would be important to establish how impairing Victoria's depressive symptoms are, as compared with her baseline, because she appears to be in a mixed manic state with suicidal ideation endorsed. In addition, you will need to collect collateral information from family members or others.

If there has been any recent dangerous behavior, this also needs to be fleshed out. In Case Example 1, the manic patient Jack may not voluntarily describe his recent impulsive behavior. However, collateral information would provide concerning information about Jack trying to destroy a monument. It is unlikely that an acutely manic patient will share with you his recent violent or impulsive acts. Therefore, it is imperative that you gain collateral history and also observe the patient very closely during the examination. In the assessment and management of potentially violent behavior, you may often need to heavily favor a reliable collateral historian and disregard a manic patient's assurances that "everything is under control." Acute mania often involves an increase in impulsive behavior, rage, and an increased risk of violence. It is also always important to inquire about any thoughts of wanting to harm another person. However, even in the absence of intent, manic agitation can be associated with high physical risk to others. You should know whether the patient drives a car and evaluate whether the mania compromises car-handling ability. Clinical experience attests to the presence of violent behavior in some patients with bipolar disorder, and violence may be an indication for hospitalization. Comorbid substance abuse and psychosis may contribute to the threat of criminal violence or aggression.

Key Point:

It is rare and unlikely that an acutely manic patient will share with you his recent violent or impulsive acts. Therefore, it is imperative that you gain collateral history and also observe the patient very closely during the examination.

Psychosis

Psychotic symptoms (e.g., delusions, hallucinations) are commonly seen during episodes of mania, mixed episodes, or depression but are more common in mania, appearing in over one half of manic episodes. In manic states, patients often experience grandiose and paranoid delusions, as well as perceptual abnormalities, resulting in visual, auditory, and olfactory experiences. These perceptual changes often start out with the patient describing a heightened awareness of the environment, which then develops into a "chaos of the senses" and finally results in frank hallucinations. A number of manic patients have described a heightened experience of sensory input, be it colors, sounds, or smells. This then becomes fused with cognitive distractibility and accelerated mental processes and even blends in with the grandiosity. More than one patient has positively endorsed a suggestion from the interviewer that they feel as if they could watch 12 television sets simultaneously, all on different channels, and follow what is going on in each show. The grandiosity found in mania often begins as simple expansiveness and a belief of superior ability. Often the prosaic and formulaic question *"Do you believe you have special powers?"* gets a quick "no" for an answer. It is useful to find out what people enjoy doing (e.g., sports, music, art) and then ask them questions like, *"If I was putting together a list of the top 10 citizens in our country in field X, would you be on that list? How long would it take you to qualify for the Olympics in your sport?"* These kinds of questions elicit more nondelusional grandiosity that might otherwise remain covert and then become delusional in its intensity.

Of course, when you assess a patient with a history of psychosis, you need to ascertain whether the psychosis was evident with manic symptoms or depressive symptoms, or if the psychosis was continuous, that is, there was evidence of psychosis in the absence of mood symptoms. This accurate longitudinal assessment will aid in diagnosis (i.e., bipolar disorder with psychotic symptoms versus schizoaffective disorder) and guide treatment decisions.

Substance Use

Bipolar disorder with a comorbid substance use disorder is a very common presentation, with bipolar disorder patients showing much higher rates of substance use than the general population. For example, the Epidemiologic Catchment Area study found rates of alcohol abuse or dependence in 46% of patients with bipolar disorder, compared with 13% for the general population.[10] Comparable drug abuse and dependence figures are 41% and 6%, respectively. Substance abuse may obscure or exacerbate endogenous mood swings. Conversely, comorbid substance use disorder may be overlooked in patients with bipolar disorder. Substance abuse may also precipitate mood episodes or be used by patients to ameliorate the symptoms of such episodes. Comorbid substance use is typically associated with fewer and slower remissions, greater rates of suicide and suicide attempts, and poorer outcome. It is very important to explore recent and past substance use very thoroughly, with detailed questioning:

- *"How often do you use _____?"*
- *"How much _____ do you use?"* Quantify the amount used for each substance on a per day/week/month basis.
- Elicit symptoms related to abuse and dependence. It is often helpful to ask patients whether they notice a difference in their mood states when not using the relevant substance. Most substances are "mood altering," and it is very helpful to explore whether they have any concerns about ongoing substance abuse/dependence. Some patients have little insight into the impact of substance use on mood stability, and this will influence ongoing alliance and treatment.
- Always ask about caffeine use (e.g., number of cups each day of tea, coffee) because caffeine affects mood and anxiety symptoms specifically.

Anxiety Symptoms

Relative to the general population, persons with bipolar disorder are at greater risk for comorbid anxiety disorders, especially panic disorder and obsessive compulsive disorder. Patients with bipolar disorder often present with comorbid symptoms of anxiety (particularly in depressed and mixed states), which are often disabling and an indicator of poor prognosis as well as inferior responsiveness to antidepressant treatment. Comorbid anxiety increases symptom severity, frequency of episodes, and suicide rates. It is important to screen for coexisting anxiety disorders (e.g., panic attacks/panic disorder, generalized anxiety disorder, obsessive compulsive disorder, social phobia, and post-traumatic stress disorder).

Past Psychiatric History

A great deal of past psychiatric history is covered in the section of the assessment related to the course of illness. In addition, you need to ask the following:

- *"When did you first see a therapist (physician, psychologist, social worker, or other counselor)?"* Inquire about the nature of the treatment (duration, number of sessions) and ask about the perceived benefits of the treatment.
- *"Have you ever been hospitalized for psychiatric illness or a suicide attempt?"* Ask about duration, dates, and treatments received.
- *"Have you thought about killing yourself before? Have you ever tried to kill yourself?"* Inquire very carefully about previous suicidal ideation, intent, plan, or attempts.

All aspects of the past psychiatric history need to be inserted into the patient's "mood map" to create a detailed, accurate history of the previous bipolar disorder over time.

Current Medications

The current medications section of the assessment should include all prescription and nonprescription medications. You should ask specifically about naturopathic remedies (e.g., St. John's wort). All medications taken should be documented with the correct name, daily doses, and duration of use; any adverse effects experienced by the patient should be noted.

Previous Medications

The section of the assessment dealing with previous medications includes all the psychotropic medications the patient has been prescribed previously. If the patient is vague about details of the medication use, it is essential that you ask the patient for permission to obtain old notes and collateral information about previous treatments. In addition to previous psychotropic medications, you should also inquire about the previous chronic use of additional medications (e.g., steroids, antihypertensive medications). Try to organize the patient's previous medications and treatments in categories, for example, groupings such as mood stabilizers, antidepressants, antipsychotics, anxiolytics, electroconvulsive therapy, and other drugs would be one way of organizing the medications. For each medication, you need to obtain the dose range, duration of use, benefits, adverse effects, mood stability while on this medication, and reason for discontinuation. This information will help you and the patient determine whether the treatment trial was adequate. Often, patients report that various previous medications they have tried simply "did not work." With careful history taking, you may establish that some or all of these trials were not adequate, that is, the patient was not administered a sufficient dose or for an adequate duration. In addition, the nonpharmacological treatments the patient has received should be reviewed thoroughly, including types of psychotherapy (e.g., cognitive-behavioral therapy, psychodynamic therapy, group therapy, light therapy, alternative therapies) to gain a complete biopsychosocial assessment of previous treatments. This will aid you in making comprehensive treatment recommendations.

Past Medical History

In this section, you should cover all current and past medical conditions. In the presence of a severe medical disorder, the disorder itself or the medications used to treat it should always be considered as possible causes of a manic episode. Neurological conditions commonly associated with secondary mania are multiple sclerosis, lesions involving right-sided subcortical structures, and lesions of cortical areas with close links to the limbic system. L-Dopa and corticosteroids are the most common medications associated with secondary mania. Furthermore, the presence of a general medical condition may also exacerbate the course or severity of bipolar disorder or complicate its treatment. For example, the course of bipolar disorder may be exacerbated by any condition that requires intermittent or regular use of steroids (e.g., asthma, inflammatory bowel disease, systemic lupus erythematosus) or that leads to abnormal thyroid functioning. In addition, treatment of patients with bipolar disorder may be complicated by conditions requiring the use of diuretics, angiotensin-converting enzyme inhibitors, nonsteroidal anti-inflammatory drugs, cyclooxygenase-2 inhibitors, or salt-restricted diets, all of which affect lithium excretion. Conditions or their treatments that are associated with abnormal cardiac conduction or rhythm or that affect renal, hepatic, or glucose function may further restrict the choice or dosage of medications. In HIV-infected patients, lower doses of medications are often indicated because of patients' greater sensitivity to adverse effects and because of the potential for drug-drug interactions.

Legal History

This should be routinely included in every assessment of bipolar patients. Often, interviewers disclose that they are shy or "embarrassed" to ask a person about previous contact with the law. However, you should have a high index of suspicion when dealing with a patient with bipolar disorder. Mood dysregulation, particularly manic episodes, often involves disinhibited and impulsive behavior, and legal contact is common. It is important to establish the nature of the charges, as well as when the last legal contact occurred. This will give you more insight into the person's current risk of violence. For example, if the person had two arrests for damage to property 10 years ago (during a manic episode) and has had no charges since that time, your level of concern should be low.

Family Psychiatric History

The family psychiatric history is an important component in an interview of any patient, but it is especially important in assessing a patient with a possible bipolar disorder because these disorders run in families. You should screen the patient for a psychiatric history in all first- and second-degree relatives, inquiring about all psychiatric disorders, including previous suicide attempts and substance abuse histories in family members. We find it useful to ask the person whether any family member received electroconvulsive therapy or was prescribed an antidepressant, mood stabilizer, or antipsychotic medication because this may give one insight into family psychiatric history and a history of treatment response that may run in the family.

Family History

The drawing of a family pedigree is an excellent way to capture the family history and structure in a visual format.

Personal History

Personal history provides you with the personal context in which to place the information you have obtained in the previous sections of the assessment. A careful and thoughtful exploration of the individual's interpersonal world at home, school, work, and play will enable you to gather a richer impression of the person in front of you. In assessments of patients who have lived with bipolar disorder for some time, you should be ready to explore their perception of how the illness has affected various aspects of their lives. If you have not explored a patient's personal history thoroughly, you will not be able to fully understand the bipolar disorder and how it affects the individual.

Mental Status Examination

In any examination, the mental status examination is key to your understanding of the patient in the here and now.

The mental status examination begins the moment patients walk through the door and you are able to observe them. When a patient is unable or unwilling to provide a history, your mental status examination becomes even more crucial.

We shall highlight some key points in the mental status examination that pertain to patients with bipolar disorder, using the first vignette from the beginning of the chapter.

In Case Example 1, Jack appears to be dressed inappropriately for the weather. This bizarre and inappropriate dress is an immediate clue that he may be manic. You notice as he enters the room that his behavior is agitated and he is unable to remain still—another nonverbal clue that he could be manic. In addition, Jack is very irritable in answering you and does not engage easily. Jack's attitude to you is very important to take note of while doing your assessment. His speech is rapid, pressured, loud, and difficult to interrupt, again making you think of mania. He describes his mood as "angry right now," but mostly "fantastic." His affect is manic and labile. His thought process is notably disorganized with tangentiality, making it necessary for you to interrupt him at times. His thought content centers around his belief that he is "superhuman" and his ideas that he is able to control the entire city (grandiose delusions, delusions of control). He denies any suicidal or homicidal ideation. The issue of safety is the most important aspect of the mental status examination. It is not sufficient to describe the person's previous history of suicidal/homicidal intent. You need to assess the person's risk of harming himself and others during the interview, and this is reported in the mental status examination. Always inquire about abnormal perceptions; these commonly occur in patients with mania and depression. Jack endorses hearing "the angels" talking to him (auditory hallucinations). Cognition is covered superficially in the mental status exam. While you are interviewing Jack, he probably would not be able to concentrate sufficiently to complete a Folstein Mini-Mental Status Examination. However, simple questions around orientation to time and place are important screening tools to assess the manic patient's organizational state. When assessing a patient in the outpatient setting, a more complete assessment of cognition is important because cognitive deficits, particularly those involving executive functioning and verbal memory, are common in patients with bipolar disorder.[11] The patient's insight and judgment are often very impaired during a manic episode, as can be clearly assessed in Jack's presentation. You ask him what he thinks is going on, and he tells you, "I am fine. Get me out of here and let me live my life." He indicates little insight into his condition, and his judgment is clearly impaired, demonstrated by his recent act of trying to destroy a city monument.

INTERVIEW SCALES

There are a number of useful interview scales that can be used in the assessment. The Hamilton Rating Scale for Depression,[12] Montgomery Asberg Depression Rating Scale,[13] Young Mania Rating Scale,[14] and the Beck Depression Inventory[15] (which is completed by the patient) are useful tools to supplement your assessment. However, these rating scales are no substitute for a thoughtful and nuanced clinical assessment.

IMPRESSION

Your impression should provide a summary of the history, with special reference to why the patient is presenting to you at this time. Your impression should review the pertinent aspects of the patient's presentation and lead logically to a DSM-IV-TR multiaxial diagnosis. It is useful to describe your understanding of the patient according to a biopsychosocial model. Always include your risk assessment of the patient in your impression. The impression section should be able to stand alone, without the preceding history, with the underlying message remaining intact and understandable. However, the entire history should provide the necessary data and support for your conclusions in the impression section. The reality of clinical practice is that many clinicians skim over the note in its entirety and focus on the impression and plan sections, so it is useful to keep this in mind when constructing your impression.

PLAN

Again, constructing your recommendations for a plan of intervention along a biopsychosocial model is a useful way to organize your thoughts. You may recommend that the patient needs to have some laboratory tests or imaging to provide you with important information, or to rule out medical causes for the clinical presentation. Common laboratory tests that are ordered in patients with bipolar disorder are thyroid indices (e.g., thyroid-stimulating hormone) because thyroid functioning influences mood regulation. In addition, lithium, a first-line mood-stabilizing treatment of bipolar disorder, can affect thyroid functioning, and so this needs to be routinely checked in patients starting or continuing to take lithium. Renal function tests (e.g., blood urea nitrogen and creatinine) are always ordered in patients treated with lithium for their bipolar disorder because lithium can affect renal function. Therapeutic levels of medications are often requested (e.g., lithium, valproate, carbamazepine levels) to ascertain whether the patient is taking the correct dose of medication.

Biological (i.e., medications and/or electroconvulsive therapy), psychotherapeutic, and social interventions should be described in your assessment documentation in a manner that makes the reader/primary physician understand the reasons behind the recommendations. The underlying thought process and logic of the recommendations should be made clear. More importantly, any recommendations you are making should be discussed extensively with the patient. The patient's reaction to the recommendations should be noted, as this will affect whether the proposed treatment will be viable and have therapeutic benefit. The patient should always be made to feel an integral part of the treatment plan, and not an "accessory" who is excluded from the treatment decisions. In the case of the first vignette, it is evident that Jack's insight into his current illness is lacking because he does not believe that there is anything wrong, and, therefore, it is unlikely that he will appreciate or concur with any treatment recommendations. The issue of his legal capacity to make treatment decisions would have to be thoroughly assessed on an ongoing basis in this case.

Key Point:

The patient's reaction to the treatment recommendations should be noted, as this will affect whether the proposed treatment will be viable and have therapeutic benefit. The patient should always be made to feel an integral part of the treatment plan, and not an "accessory" who is excluded from the treatment decisions.

ONGOING ASSESSMENT AND PSYCHIATRIC CARE OF PATIENTS WITH BIPOLAR DISORDER

Providing ongoing psychiatric care to a patient with bipolar disorder involves a broad range of clinical skills that are not referred to in an initial assessment. In ongoing longitudinal care of a patient with bipolar disorder, therapeutic alliance is critical for understanding and working collaboratively with the patient over time.

A mood chart is intended to provide patients with a simple means of generating a graphic representation of their illness over the last month (Figure 6-2). Mood charting will allow the clinician and the patient to systemically bring together important pieces of information such as medication levels, mood state, and major life events to see emerging patterns that otherwise might be difficult to discern. Mood charting is a good way to record events chronologically and may help the patient to report mood and other symptoms to you more efficiently.

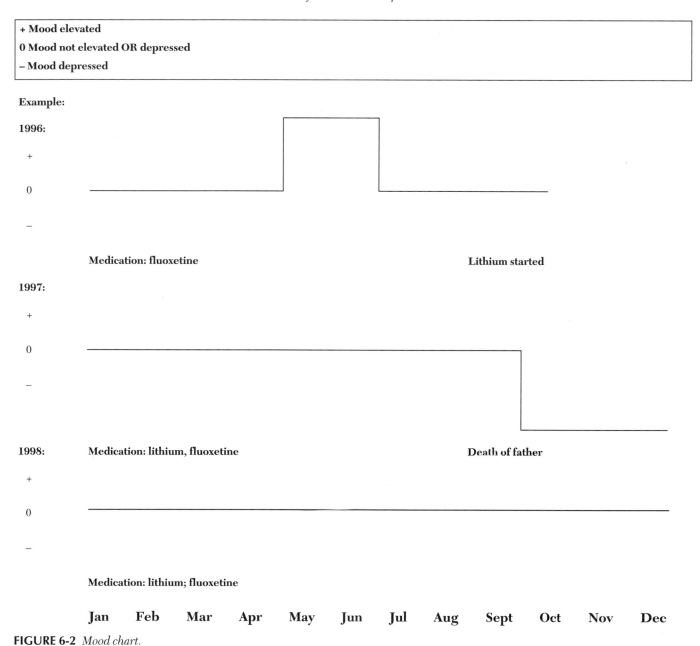

+ **Mood elevated**

0 **Mood not elevated OR depressed**

– **Mood depressed**

Example:

1996:

Medication: fluoxetine   **Lithium started**

1997:

1998:   **Medication: lithium, fluoxetine**   **Death of father**

Medication: lithium; fluoxetine

Jan   Feb   Mar   Apr   May   Jun   Jul   Aug   Sept   Oct   Nov   Dec

FIGURE 6-2 *Mood chart.*

Bipolar disorder carries significant morbidity and severity of symptoms over time, with frequent relapse and recurrence of mood symptoms. The long-term impact of the illness on the individual needs to be explored in the ongoing therapy with the patient. This involves more than prescribing maintenance medications or checking up on mood symptoms. This may involve discussions about the person's sense of loss in terms of relationships, career ambitions, or overall functioning. This could include working on the person's need to set different life goals or to look at alternative options.

As you get to know your patient well, you will learn to anticipate stressors with your patient that will aid you in identifying new episodes in a timely manner. Ongoing work with a patient with bipolar disorder involves a particular conscientious attitude, with an attention to detail and subtle changes in the patient. You should be aware that small changes in mood or behavior might herald the onset of a manic or depressive episode. Over time, the knowledge you gain about the person and his illness course allows early identification of usual prodromal symptoms and early recognition of new episodes. The patient who is manic or hypomanic often has limited insight into his or her difficulties; once again, family involvement will become important.

CONCLUSION

In this chapter, we have highlighted the important components of the interview of the patient with bipolar disorder, which pertain to both the content and the process of the psychiatric interview. The challenge of assessing these patients, which is perhaps unique to this psychiatric disorder, is due to the multiple presentations and rapidly changing clinical status. Patients' symptoms can fluctuate, ranging from severely depressed with suicidal thoughts in one instance to floridly manic and psychotic in another. In addition to these polar opposite states, there are the milder, less clear symptoms of mild depression, hypomania, and other combinations of residual mood symptoms that fall on the bipolar continuum. The patient's clinical presentation can shift along this broad continuum over time, and sometimes the shift can be very rapid and sudden. In addition, with optimal treatment and psychotherapeutic intervention, the patient with bipolar disorder can remain very stable and constant with regard to both symptomatology and functioning.

In conclusion, some of the main points covered in the chapter are as follows:

- The assessment of patients with bipolar disorder may involve working with persons in acutely agitated states because patients with bipolar disorder present as psychiatric emergencies when acutely manic. This assessment involves a flexible style of interviewing, obtaining the mental status examination as you take the history, assessing risk quickly, and relying heavily on collateral history.
- A thorough risk assessment, including assessing the patient's risks of violence and self-harm, is a vital component of the overall assessment of a patient with bipolar disorder.
- The high comorbidity of substance use and abuse in patients with bipolar disorder means that a thorough inquiry regarding recent and past substance use is extremely important.
- The active searching for hypomanic and mixed hypomanic/manic symptoms in a patient presenting with unipolar depression is very important. You need to have a high index of suspicion in dealing with patients; otherwise, these symptoms are missed in an assessment.
- In patients with antidepressant-induced manic episodes, you should probe for spontaneous manic episodes because they will have more than likely occurred in these patients.
- A longitudinal history of the patient's mood symptoms is extremely important to assess diagnosis, ongoing dysfunction, and the impact of treatment interventions. The use of a mood chart can facilitate this process and be very helpful.

Finally, the patient with bipolar disorder provides you with some of the most varied, dramatic, and memorable clinical situations you will ever face in psychiatry. The process of assessing and working with a patient with bipolar disorder on an ongoing basis is challenging and, most importantly, extremely rewarding.

REFERENCES

1. Goodwin FK, Jamieson KR: *Manic-depressive illness*, New York, 1990, Oxford University Press.
2. Ghaemi S: *Mood disorders: a practical guide*, Philadelphia, 2003, Lippincott Williams & Wilkins.
3. Ghaemi SN, Rosenquist KJ: Is insight in mania state-dependent? a meta-analysis, *J Nerv Ment Dis* 192:771–775, 2004.
4. Jamison K: *Touched with fire*, New York, 1993, Simon & Schuster.
5. Judd LL, Akiskal HS, Schettler PJ, et al: The long-term natural history of the weekly symptomatic status of bipolar I disorder, *Arch Gen Psychiatry* 59:530–537, 2002.
6. MacQueen GM, Marriott M, Begin H, et al: Subsyndromal symptoms assessed in longitudinal, prospective follow-up of a cohort of patients with bipolar disorder, *Bipolar Disord* 5:349–355, 2003.
7. Angst J, Gamma A, Endrass J: Risk factors for the bipolar and depression spectra, *Acta Psychiatr Scand Suppl* 418:15–19, 2003.
8. Akiskal HS: Validating 'hard' and 'soft' phenotypes within the bipolar spectrum: continuity or discontinuity? *J Affect Disord* 73:1–5, 2003.
9. Ernst CL, Goldberg JF: Clinical features related to age at onset in bipolar disorder, *J Affect Disord* 82:21–27, 2004.
10. Regier DA, Farmer ME, Rae DS, et al: Comorbidity of mental disorders with alcohol and other drug abuse: results from the Epidemiologic Catchment Area (ECA) Study, *JAMA* 264:2511–2518, 1990.
11. Altshuler LL, Ventura J, van Gorp WG, et al: Neurocognitive function in clinically stable men with bipolar I disorder or schizophrenia and normal control subjects, *Biol Psychiatry* 56:560–569, 2004.
12. Hamilton M: A rating scale for depression, *J Neurol Neurosurg Psychiatry* 23:56–62, 1960.
13. Montgomery SA, Asberg M: A new depression scale designed to be sensitive to change, *Br J Psychiatry* 134:382–389, 1979.

14. Young RC, Biggs JT, Ziegler VE, Meyer DA: A rating scale for mania: reliability, validity and sensitivity, *Br J Psychiatry* 133:429–435, 1978.
15. Beck A: *Beck Depression Inventory*, Philadelphia, 1961, Center for Cognitive Therapy.

RECOMMENDED READINGS

Goodwin FK, Jamieson KR: *Manic-depressive illness*, New York, 1990, Oxford University Press.
Jamison K: *An unquiet mind,* New York, 1995, Random House.

7

Assessment of Patients with Anxiety Disorders

NEIL A. RECTOR AND PAUL D. ARNOLD

INTRODUCTION

Anxiety is one of the most basic and universal human experiences and has been recognized for as long as 5,000 years. It is a negative mood state involving subjective feelings of physical tension and apprehension for the future. Few of us get through a week without experiencing anxiety or fear. But the brief and low-intensity anxiety that besets us in our lives is not comparable to the frequency, intensity, and duration of the anxiety experienced by persons with an anxiety disorder. Yet, anxiety disorders are ubiquitous with up to one in four adults suffering from an anxiety disorder sometime in their lifetime. Studies conducted in the United States demonstrate that 10% of the population suffered from an anxiety disorder in the preceding 12 months. The anxiety disorders are the most prevalent mental health problem among women and second only to substance use disorders in men. Anxiety disorders result in significant and often profound personal suffering, impairment in social functioning, and significant socioeconomic costs. For instance, it has been determined that anxiety disorders account for over one third of all costs associated with mental illness.

The fourth edition of the *Diagnostic and Statistical Manual of Mental Disorders,* text revision (DSM-IV-TR),[1] lists 12 distinct anxiety disorders, although six principal categories are proposed: phobias, panic disorder with and without agoraphobia, generalized anxiety disorder, obsessive compulsive disorder, acute stress disorder, and post-traumatic stress disorder. The anxiety disorders share many features, but each also has its own distinct elements.

Case Example 1

Brenda presents for treatment with a 2-year history of recurrent and unexpected panic attacks: "It started on a night when I was studying for my final exams. I began to feel sick to my stomach. At first I thought it was just the start of the stomach flu, but then my mind started to drift to worrying whether something's wrong. I started to shake, and it was as if electricity ran through my body. I quickly stood up, and I felt so dizzy and disoriented that I thought: I must be losing my mind. Since then, I've had dozens and dozens of these attacks, and each time I feel that I narrowly escaped losing it."

Case Example 2

Steve describes a lifelong fear of being judged in social situations: "My father taught me to never show emotion, say as little as possible, and always appear polished . . . for as long as I can remember I've worried about not living up to this standard. I'm always expecting to be judged and humiliated by others. I find it excruciating to do simple things like answer the phone, talk to strangers, or eat in restaurants. I'm sure that people think I look weird and sound stupid."

Case Example 3

Jane has struggled with contamination obsessions and compulsions since the age of 9. At the time of assessment, she provides the following overview: "I am worried that unless I am extremely careful, I am going to bump into, sit on, step on, or be poked by a blood-stained needle that is infected with HIV. I watch every step I take, I avoid sitting on chairs unless I have to, and I spend a lot of time checking my clothes before getting dressed, my bed before going to sleep, etc., in fear that I am going to get HIV from a dirty needle."

Brenda, Steve, and Jane all experience the hallmark features of an anxiety disorder: irrational and excessive fear, physical feelings of apprehension and tension, and impairment in functioning as a result of the anxiety. They differ, however, in the particular nature of their fears. While we can reliably distinguish between the different anxiety disorders, it is important to note that they are often co-occur. Depression is also highly comorbid with the anxiety disorders. In a recent study that examined rates of comorbidity in patients presenting with an anxiety or depressive disorder, 55% of these patients had at least one additional anxiety or depressive disorder at the time of the assessment. When the scope was broadened to consider lifetime comorbidity, the rates increased to 76%. This overlap between anxiety and depressive disorders becomes especially important in treatment planning, which will be addressed later in this chapter.

This chapter focuses on the clinical skills that are relevant to the assessment and formulation of the different anxiety disorders. The aim is not to provide an overview of the DSM-IV-TR anxiety disorders or to reiterate assessment procedures captured in well-developed diagnostic interviews such as the Structured Clinical Interview for DSM-IV Disorders or the Anxiety Disorders Interview Schedule. Rather, our goal is to address clinical strategies that will help you, as a clinician, to do the following:

- Readily understand the continuum of anxiety from normal to abnormal
- Distinguish between the physical, cognitive, and behavioral components of each anxiety disorder
- Establish ideal assessment conditions
- Incorporate psychometric information into the assessment formulation
- Determine patient suitability for psychological and medical treatments
- Deliver quick and effective psychoeducation

Collectively, the learning objectives are to learn the following:

1. Clinical skills to assess the phenomenology of the anxiety disorders
2. To integrate different sources of information to arrive at an idiosyncratic case conceptualization of the patient's anxiety condition
3. Strategies to assess the patient's suitability for cognitive-behavioral therapy and pharmacotherapy
4. Key points to include in the psychoeducation of the anxiety disorders

OVERVIEW OF ANXIETY DISORDERS

What is normal anxiety? Anxiety is a normal human response that alerts a person to the presence of danger or a threat and can therefore be highly adaptive when elicited in the appropriate context. This alerting signal has characteristic physical, cognitive, and behavioral features. *Fear* is another term commonly used to describe this affective response, which is considered one of the basic emotions shared by humans and other animals. Anxiety symptoms can be viewed as being on a continuum, or *spectrum*, ranging from normal behavioral traits to severe dysfunction. Normal anxiety may prompt actions that reduce threat and therefore enhance functioning. For example, a student experiencing apprehension regarding a test may study to alleviate unpleasant feelings of anxiety and avert the threat of failing a course. However, it would be cause for concern if the anxiety were so severe that it impeded performance, for example, by causing impaired concentration during the test.

When does anxiety become a clinical problem? Anxiety is deemed a clinical problem when it is persistent and the symptoms are determined to have crossed a threshold of severity on the anxiety spectrum. Determination of whether this clinical threshold has been reached is based on a number of factors including degree of distress, functional impairment, and the environmental or developmental context in which the anxiety occurs. For example, the intense "fight or flight" physiological response of a panic attack is normal and highly adaptive when faced with a direct threat to one's life or personal integrity (e.g., when being attacked by an animal). However, if this same fear response occurs spontaneously or in response to a relatively benign stimulus, it is considered excessive relative to the context in which it occurs and is more likely to be a clinical problem. The developmental context is important for anxiety triggered by separation from a caregiver, which is a normative response in infants and younger children (first seen at approximately 8 months of age) that becomes a clinical problem if it persists into later childhood or adolescence.

What anxiety disorders are commonly seen in clinical practice? When symptoms are sufficiently severe to warrant clinical attention, it is likely that the afflicted person meets the criteria for a *categorical* anxiety disorder diagnosis. Criteria for anxiety disorder diagnoses are outlined in the DSM-IV-TR (the most commonly used system in North America and the one used in this book) or the International Classification of Disorders (ICD-10; more commonly used in Europe). The following common anxiety disorders are classified based on the focus of anxiety:

- Panic disorder with/without agoraphobia (PD/A)
- Specific phobia

- Social phobia
- Obsessive compulsive disorder (OCD)
- Post-traumatic stress disorder (PTSD) (and its shorter-term variant, acute stress disorder)
- Generalized anxiety disorder (GAD)
- Separation anxiety disorder (in children)

There are some differences between the natural rates of these disorders and the extent to which people with the different disorders seek treatment. For instance, it has been suggested that between 30% and 50% of all referrals to specialized anxiety assessment and treatment clinics present with PD/A, whereas patients with GAD are less likely to seek help. Patients with social phobia may also be less able to reach out for treatment, although this appears to be changing.

What else should I be screening for? Although many patients with a chief complaint of anxiety suffer from a primary anxiety disorder, you need to be vigilant for other disorders that may present with anxiety symptoms. First, it is important to consider the possibility that general medical conditions or substance use may be involved. These disorders are classified in the DSM-IV-TR under the categories of "Anxiety Disorder Due to a General Medical Condition" and "Substance-induced Anxiety Disorder." If you suspect a contributory medical condition or substance, the underlying etiological factor should be identified through careful medical history, supplemented in some cases by physical examination or laboratory findings. As a general rule, medical and substance-related causes are more likely if the anxiety disorder has prominent physical manifestations, which is more typical of PD and GAD compared with other diagnoses.

Both panic and generalized anxiety symptoms can result from a wide variety of physical disorders, especially those originating from the endocrine (e.g., hyperthyroidism), cardiac (e.g., cardiomyopathy), respiratory (e.g., pulmonary insufficiency), or neurological (e.g., traumatic brain injury, seizure disorders) systems. Obsessive compulsive symptoms in children may occur episodically following streptococcal infections, a syndrome known as pediatric autoimmune neuropsychiatric disorders associated with streptococcal infections. Other infectious (e.g., post-viral encephalitis) and degenerative (e.g., Huntington's chorea) syndromes affecting the central nervous system may also cause obsessive compulsive symptoms, but these are relatively rare and typically associated with other prominent neurological manifestations. Substance use may also induce anxiety symptoms, either in the intoxication or withdrawal phases. The substances most characteristically associated with generalized anxiety or panic symptoms are those that activate the sympathetic nervous system (sympathomimetics). Anxiety-inducing sympathomimetic agents can be prescribed (e.g., methylphenidate), nonprescribed but available "over-the-counter" (e.g., caffeine), or illicit (e.g., cocaine). Obsessive compulsive symptoms may occur in response to treatment with atypical antipsychotic agents. Medical or substance-induced delirium may present with anxiety; however, it will also be associated with altered level of consciousness and acute cognitive changes (e.g., disorientation), which should easily distinguish it from primary anxiety disorders (in which these features should not be present).

After considering anxiety disorders due to a general medical condition, substance-induced anxiety, and delirium, the clinician should screen for other primary psychiatric disorders based on history and mental status examination. Anxiety alone is a rather nonspecific symptom that can be associated with a variety of other mental illnesses, particularly mood or psychotic syndromes. Patients with mood disorders often have comorbid anxiety features that may be a major focus of clinical attention. However, if anxiety only occurs while the patient is experiencing a major depressive, hypomanic or manic episode and not at other times, then the additional diagnosis of an anxiety disorder is usually not warranted. Patients with psychotic disorders also commonly experience heightened anxiety. However, if the anxiety only occurs while the patient is psychotic, then an anxiety disorder is usually not assigned, particularly when the anxiety seems directly related to the content of the patient's hallucinations or delusions. For example, a primary anxiety disorder is not present if the anxiety is triggered primarily by a firm, fixed belief that one is the subject of a nonexistent conspiracy, which is more consistent with a psychotic disorder.

In addition to screening for other disorders that commonly present with anxiety symptoms, you should be alert to the presence of common comorbid conditions. Symptoms of concurrent conditions may increase the level of distress experienced by the anxiety sufferer, and failure to address these symptoms may lead to poorer treatment outcomes. The most common comorbid conditions in anxiety disorder patients are other anxiety disorders. *Major depressive disorder* is also particularly common in this population. It is particularly important to recognize depression since PD patients with comorbid depression are at increased risk for suicide. *Substance abuse and dependence* are also present at elevated rates in persons with anxiety disorders compared with the general population. Patients with OCD are at increased risk for developing other conditions that share certain clinical features with OCD and are therefore often referred to as "obsessive compulsive spectrum disorders." Although not all clinicians agree on which disorders should be included in the obsessive compulsive spectrum, most would include tic disorders, body dysmorphic disorder, and trichotillomania (hair pulling).

> **Key Point:**
>
> Anxiety is a clinical problem if it is persistent, is associated with significant functional impairment, or interferes with a person's quality of life.

> **Key Point:**
>
> You should screen for medical disorders and substances that may induce anxiety symptoms. Once these are ruled out, you should also consider mood and psychotic disorders in the differential diagnosis because patients with these syndromes commonly present with anxiety symptoms.

> **Key Point:**
>
> Anxiety disorders are often comorbid with other disorders, especially other anxiety disorders, mood disorders, and substance abuse or dependence.

CONSIDERATIONS BEFORE YOU SEE THE PATIENT

Will the patient have trouble getting to and from the session? Most patients, even those with severe anxiety disorders, are typically able to get to and from sessions, but there may be circumstances where this becomes more difficult. The patient experiencing recurrent panic attacks may anticipate having a panic attack if he is required to drive or take public transit to get to the appointment. The patient with excessive checking rituals may have a history of being 3 to 4 hours late for appointments because he is compelled to return to the house to check the appliances, lights, locks, etc. Patients with agoraphobia may not be able to leave the house at all! You can help problem-solve around these potential barriers to attendance. For instance, in scheduling the first appointment, you should ask whether the patient recognizes any barriers to attending the sessions (or to being on time). The patient experiencing panic may need to be accompanied by a family member or friend; the patient with excessive checking behaviors may need a late afternoon appointment; the housebound patient may require phone contacts in the first instance or arrangements to be seen by a community worker. Likewise, it is not uncommon to hear patients report, "I don't know what I'm going to do, I'm too anxious to go back to work," or "I can't drive home feeling the way I feel," just as the session begins to wrap up. You can take the following steps to address this problem. First, anticipate this possibility prior to the session. The patient can plan to be driven home or take the day off from work. Second, save time at the end of the session to help relax the patient. This can be done through the normalizing of his symptoms (e.g., *"You're not in any danger whatsoever"*), offering reassurance, and assisting with an action plan (e.g., *"What routes could you take to get home to avoid likely panic triggers?"* or *"Whom could you call if anxiety begins to feel unmanageable?"*). Third, socialize the patient to the anxiety habituation model (e.g., *"Anxiety is very likely to decrease over the next 30 to 60 minutes"*) and plan for him to sit outside your office or in a coffee shop until he feels ready to resume his day.

Is the patient likely to request someone else to be in the session with him? This is not an infrequent request, especially for patients presenting with PD/A. Bringing in someone else to attend with the patient may serve as a safety behavior and be perceived as essential to complete the interview. There are a number of issues to be considered here:

- Will the patient consider seeing you alone with prompting?
- How much anxiety/distress will be experienced by the patient if this is not permitted?
- What is the likely success of completing the session?
- Who is actually in attendance with the patient (e.g., a friend, a parent, a partner, a child)?
- Are there special ethical issues pertaining to confidentiality that will need to be addressed?

Ordinarily, we would encourage you to try to see adult outpatients alone. Provision could be made for the person in attendance with the patient to remain seated outside the office, and the patient could be given the opportunity to take breaks, if needed. If the patient remains upset, consider starting the session with the guest present then a short time later checking to see whether the patient would accept for the guest to now sit outside.

How anxious is the patient likely to be? For many patients, just attending a clinical appointment involves significant exposure to their fears. The requirement for eye contact and personal self-disclosure can be extremely difficult for a patient with social phobia. Shaking hands, having to hang up jackets, and sitting on chairs may be the most fear-provoking triggers for the person with contamination obsessions. You should attempt to gather enough information at the time of the referral to anticipate the patient's anxiety triggers. For instance, if someone is referred for assessment and treatment of a fear of heights and your office is located on the 30th floor of a building, special arrangements to see the patient at an alternative office or perhaps at the ground floor level will be necessary. Some patients may need to engage in significant "safety behaviors" to be able to attend and remain in the session. For example, some patients with claustrophobia may require that the door be left slightly ajar, or the patient with contamination obsessions may wear gloves (and even a mask) throughout the session. You should aim to be flexible and to allow these behaviors if they are likely to make the difference between manageable versus unmanageable levels of anxiety.

It is important to remember that attentional resources become scant when we are anxious. Patients with anxiety disorders may have considerable difficulty concentrating on questions and encoding relevant information. You should therefore be extremely clear, appropriately paced, and patient with prompting to repeat questions, information, etc.

What should be done if sessions are frequently canceled due to avoidance strategies? Given that avoidance is a hallmark feature of anxiety, it is not surprising that many patients initially schedule but then do not attend sessions. This may begin as early as the first appointment or escalate in treatment as patients are requested to discuss, imagine, and write down their fears and increasingly approach situations that are likely to provoke anxiety. As before, this problem can be reduced somewhat if it is anticipated and addressed at the outset. You can ask the patient: *"Do you anticipate anything getting in the way of coming in to see me that day?"* or *"Many people that I see find it hard to attend sessions because of anxiety. Do you think that you'll be able to see me even if you're feeling anxious?"* Similarly, if there are already scheduled sessions that have been missed due to avoidance, you should attempt to address the fears that are creating barriers to attendance, normalize the experience of being anxious at the session, and communicate the important message that every time the patient allows herself to experience anxiety she is contributing to a calmer future.

What if the patient has a panic attack during the session? First, remember not to panic yourself! Since you know the patient is experiencing a nondangerous, short-lived spike in autonomic arousal as a natural consequence of fear, you can reassure the person that everything she is experiencing is "normal" and "safe." You can also attempt to draw her attention away from her somatic sensations by introducing a distraction task. For instance, try to keep the patient's attention focused on a pleasant topic of discussion, or introduce a more stringent distraction task such as counting backward by sevens or reading the labels of books on the book shelves. Some patients may resort to safety behaviors, such as breathing into a bag, lying down, or taking medication—all of which represent acceptable strategies to feel better. Other patients may request to leave or, in rare circumstances, may simply bolt from the office. You can aim to normalize this request (e.g., *"I understand completely; we all feel the need to escape when we're feeling very anxious."*) but then see whether the patient would be willing to stay to test out whether anxiety is likely to come down shortly as predicted.

If the patient persists or does get up to leave, you should leave with her. This will provide the opportunity to discuss the normal cycle of anxiety once the patient is feeling better (which is likely to be soon after leaving). It will also serve to consolidate her trust in you and the therapeutic alliance.

Case Example 4

Susan arrived at her second assessment session 20 minutes late and seemingly rushed. She had to rush away from a meeting at work to get to the appointment, and then she got stuck in traffic. She was speaking very quickly about the details of her lateness when she suddenly began to look ashen. She was visibly hyperventilating. She stopped talking and began to put her head between her knees, rocking back and forth. The clinician asked her whether she was having a panic attack, and Susan nodded in the affirmative. The clinician quickly stated, "Susan, you are perfectly safe. Even though you're feeling uncomfortable right now, you are not in any danger. You are just experiencing increased sensations of normal and natural anxiety which will stop soon. From 1 to 10, 10 being the worst, how intense are the symptoms right now?" Susan replied, "Nine." Susan next rolled onto the floor, stating that she thought she was having a seizure. The clinician responded, "It's okay to lie down; do whatever makes you most comfortable. I want you to know that you may be feeling a range of sensations that seem pretty scary, but you are not having a seizure, and you are not in any danger. Tell me more about what you're experiencing." Susan recounted that she was feeling dizzy, a rapid heart rate, and sensations like "pins and needles" through her body. The clinician clarified, "Those are all normal physical symptoms of the natural flight/flight response—they're there because you're experiencing fear." How severe are the symptoms now from 1 to 10?" Susan replied, "Eight." The clinician further attempted to introduce a distraction exercise: "Actually, I would love to hear more about the concert that you went to last night." Initially, Susan had trouble distracting herself but soon began to discuss the concert from the night before and actually ended up going into some degree of detail. The clinician checked in to see how intense the symptoms were now, and Susan indicated that they had come down to five. Next, the clinician asked whether she would be okay to stand up (slowly) and resume sitting in the chair, which she did. Susan was looking tentative but somewhat relieved. The clinician used the passing panic attack to socialize Susan further to the panic model by asking her what thoughts were going through her mind during the last 5 to 8 minutes to elicit her appraisals of danger as well as what she wanted to do (i.e., at first, leave) and then actually did (i.e., she decided to lie down as a safety behavior). The clinician was able to help Susan recognize how the three systems of anxiety (see below) interacted to create an attendant increase in anxiety.

Finally, the clinician was able to help Susan recognize the trigger for this attack (i.e., hyperventilation and early recognition of an internal trigger [dizziness]).

Key Point:

When possible, you should anticipate anxiety triggers that may create barriers to attendance and engagement in the assessment process.

Key Point:

Plan to use heightened anxiety/panic in session to begin to socialize the patient to an alternative, less threatening view of the anxiety.

Key Point:

Anticipate the clinical and ethical issues relevant to a third party being present in the assessment (and treatment). Since "helpers" are known to increase the effectiveness of exposure tasks, this situation can be framed in a positive light.

CONDUCTING THE ASSESSMENT

Semi-Structured Clinical Interviews

Your assessment should ideally begin with a semi-structured clinical interview that can aid in arriving at a reliable differential diagnosis. For the purposes of assessing the anxiety disorders, there are two gold-standard semi-structured clinical interviews: the Structured Clinical Interview for DSM-IV Axis I Disorders (SCID-I) and the Anxiety Disorder Interview Schedule (ADIS-IV). Both interviews assess the full spectrum of DSM-IV anxiety disorders (as well as other disorders). Research has demonstrated that the use of the SCID-I and ADIS-IV can significantly enhance diagnostic accuracy. Clinicians are likely to find the SCID-I to be more feasible for use in community clinical settings, as opposed to the ADIS-IV, which requires a more hefty time commitment. Table 7-1 includes questions that the clinician can ask to screen for the major DSM-IV-TR anxiety disorders.

Functional Analysis: Three Systems of Anxiety

Because the same anxiety disorder can be expressed in many different ways depending on the person, the next step after completing a differential diagnosis is to determine the specific pattern of symptoms for each individual patient. One useful classification system that captures the three major response systems of anxiety is as follows: physiological/somatic, cognitive, and behavioral. The three systems often vary in their strength across people and across contexts:

1. *Physiological aspects*: These reflect the array of symptoms activated by the flight-or-flight response and include heart palpitations or increased heart rate, shallow breathing, trembling or shaking, sweating, dizziness or lightheadedness, muscle tension, shortness of breath, nausea, and other symptoms of sympathetic nervous system arousal.

Table 7-1. Screening for the DSM-IV Anxiety Disorders

Disorder	Screening Questions
Specific phobia	*"Are there any specific things (e.g., heights, closed places, animals) that you fear or avoid? Do you think that your fear is excessive?"*
Panic disorder with/without agoraphobia	*"Have you ever suddenly felt frightened or anxious or developed intense physical symptoms?"* *"Have you ever worried that there might be something terribly wrong with you physically (i.e., heart attack, 'going crazy')?"* *"Do you avoid certain situations because of your panic attacks?"*
Social phobia	*"Are you afraid of social situations, such as speaking, eating, or writing?"* *"Do you avoid other social situations?"*
Generalized anxiety disorder	*"Do you worry excessively about minor things?"* *"Have you ever found it hard to stop worrying?"*
Obsessive compulsive disorder	*"Have you ever been bothered by intrusive thoughts that don't make any sense and just keep coming back?"* *"Have you ever had to do things over and over again that you couldn't resist doing?"*
Post-traumatic stress disorder (acute stress disorder)	*"Have you ever seen or had something happen to you that was extremely upsetting and frightening?"* *"Do you have recurrent dreams, nightmares, or flashbacks about that event?"* *"Do you get extremely upset in a situation that reminds you of a terrible event?"*

2. *Cognitive aspects:* Patients report having anxious thoughts (e.g., "I'm losing control"), anxious predictions (e.g., "I'm going to fumble my words and humiliate myself"), and anxious beliefs (e.g., "Only weak people get anxious"). Activation of the fight/flight response alerts the person to the possible existence of danger, and there is an immediate and automatic shift in attention to potential threat. This can range from mild worry to extreme terror (e.g., "I'm dying").

3. *Behavioral aspects:* As suggested, the fight/flight response prepares the body for action—to either fight or to flee from the situation. Patients report engaging in certain behaviors while refraining from others as a way of protecting themselves from perceived danger or the discomfort created by anxiety. These behaviors include *avoidance* of feared situations (e.g., driving), *avoidance* of activities that elicit sensations similar to those experienced when anxious (e.g., exercise), *subtle avoidances* or behaviors that aim to distract the person (e.g., talking more during periods of anxiety), and *safety behaviors* or habits to minimize anxiety and feel "safer" (e.g., always having a cell phone on hand to call for help).

Although the physiological, cognitive, and behavioral response systems of anxiety can be distinguished, it is important to understand their interdependency as well as their functional relationship to external and internal triggers. For instance, one patient with OCD may experience physical tension after the arrival of an intrusive sexual obsession and then attempt to neutralize the tension by engaging in neutralizing behaviors (e.g., thinking "pleasant" thoughts). Another patient with OCD may experience all of the classic symptoms of autonomic arousal when faced with having to use the public restroom, which is likely to lead to avoidance or subtle avoidance behaviors. The functional analysis thus provides the clinician with the opportunity to develop an idiosyncratic case conceptualization. Some examples of the three systems for the major DSM-IV-TR anxiety disorders can be seen in Table 7-2.

Past Psychiatric History

Previous contacts with mental health professionals should be thoroughly documented. The history must include specific and systematic exploration of both psychological and somatic therapies, including chronological details such as duration of treatment and approximate frequency of sessions or appointments. Ask the patient what was helpful about a given treatment, in addition to whether there were any negative effects.

When inquiring about previous psychotherapy, it is particularly important to ascertain whether the patient has ever received cognitive-behavioral therapy (CBT). Many patients are not aware of the therapeutic modality used by their therapists, and it is often necessary to explore this issue by asking what took place in typical sessions. For example, it is helpful to know whether the therapist assigned homework tasks in between sessions (typical of CBT) or focused on discussing recent or past life events during sessions (typical of supportive or psychodynamic therapy). Patients should also be asked about self-help books and other resources they have accessed.

A good medication history including the name, dose, and duration of medications received is critical for determining whether previous treatments were adequate. If patients are not able to freely recall the names of specific psychotropic agents, they may nevertheless be able to recognize names of previous drugs if you list commonly prescribed medications. Patients should be asked the reasons for stopping previous medications; this may reveal a history of adverse effects or potential barriers to treatment adherence, which can be addressed through psychoeducation. For example, many patients prematurely discontinue selective serotonin reuptake inhibitors (SSRIs) because they are unaware of the usual latency of several weeks for a therapeutic response and assume that the medications "aren't working."

Past Medical History

The primary purpose of a medical history is to screen for medical disorders or substance use that may influence anxiety symptoms. The presence of comorbid medical disorders may also influence choice of treatment, particularly if psychotropic drugs are likely to aggravate the physical condition or interact with other medications being used. The medical history should be tailored to the individual patient depending on contextual factors such as age. For example, relatively detailed medical questions should be asked of geriatric patients because they are more likely to be suffering from medical disorders.

A general medical history should be obtained from all patients with anxiety disorder, including current or significant past illnesses, prescribed medications, over-the-counter medications, and herbal remedies. Screening questions should be asked regarding head trauma, episodes of loss of consciousness, and seizures. If prominent physical symptoms are associated with anxiety, the medical history should include a more detailed history specific to that complaint. For example, a patient ostensibly presenting with panic attacks with prominent chest pain should be asked questions regarding chronological features of the

Table 7-2. Functional Analysis of the Anxiety Disorders: Examples of the Physical, Cognitive, and Behavioral Components

	Physical	Cognitive	Behavioral
Panic disorder with/ without agoraphobia	• Accelerated heart rate • Chest pain or discomfort • Dizziness • Paresthesias (numbness) • Trembling or shaking • Sensations of shortness of breath	"I'm having a heart attack." "I'm going crazy." "I'm having a stroke." "I'm losing control." "I'm suffocating."	**Avoidance** • Travel, malls, line-ups • Exercise, strenuous activity, sex **Safety Behaviors** • Carry a cell phone at all times • Carry medication in front pocket
Social phobia	• Blushing • Sweating • Tremors • Nausea/growling stomach • Muscle tension • Dry mouth	"I'll blush, and people with think I'm anxious." "I'll look anxious and sound stupid." "People will think I'm weird." "People will think I'm weak."	**Avoidance** • Social gatherings, parties, meetings • Public speaking **Safety Behaviors** • Use alcohol prior to social interaction • Wear clothing to hide autonomic arousal (e.g., perspiration)
General anxiety disorder	• Motor tension • Shakiness • Inability to relax • Restlessness • Fatigue	"Something's going to go wrong." "I'm going to lose everything I've got." "This worry is going to make me nuts." "I can't cope without certainty about the future."	**Avoidance** • News, newspapers **Safety Behaviors** • Excessive Internet searches for information on finance, health, world events • Body checks (e.g., checking pulse)
Obsessive compulsive disorder	• Muscle tension • Discomfort	"I'm going to get sick and infect the entire family if I touch this door handle." "If I don't check again, I'll be responsible if something bad happens." "Having a thought about an action is like performing the action."	**Compulsions** • *Behavioral*: Wash, check • *Mental*: Pray, count **Avoidance** • Doors, public washrooms • Sharp objects **Safety Behaviors** • Wear gloves • Hide objects that may cause harm
Post-traumatic stress disorder and acute stress disorder	• Sleep difficulties • Irritability or anger outbursts • Difficulty concentrating • Hypervigilance for danger • Exaggerated startle responses	"I now realize that I'm never safe." "If I hadn't acted the way I did, this would never have happened." "People aren't to be trusted." "If I keep getting anxious, I'm going to lose it."	**Avoidance** • Thoughts, feelings, conversations, activities, places, or people associated with the trauma (e.g., emergency vehicles, parking lots) • Use alcohol to block out memories of event **Safety Behaviors** • Diminished participation in significant activities

pain, aggravating and alleviating factors, previous history of heart disease, and cardiac risk factors.

Depending on your preference, you may ask about substance use either in the medical history or in the past psychiatric history. All patients should be asked about alcohol consumption, smoking habits, and street drugs (particularly psychostimulants such as cocaine and amphetamines). Caffeine intake should be ascertained specifically because excessive caffeine intake can aggravate panic or generalized anxiety symptoms. It is often revealing to ask patients how their drug or alcohol use affects their anxiety because they may be using substances to "self-medicate" their symptoms.

Family Psychiatric History

Anxiety disorders have been shown to have a strong genetic component based on family and twin studies. Family histories often reveal one or more relatives with a history of symptoms similar to the patient, which provides supportive evidence for an anxiety disorder diagnosis. The following questions should be asked to obtain a detailed family history:

- *"Does anyone else in your family suffer from anxiety? What is the nature of their difficulties with anxiety?"* Follow this up with specific questions relevant to the patient's complaint, such as asking about obsessions and compulsions in family members if the patient has OCD. For OCD, one should also ask about tic disorders because OCD and tic disorders often coaggregate in families.
- *"Has anyone in your family suffered from other emotional or behavioral difficulties, such as depression, which interfered with their functioning or caused them significant distress? Did any of your family members ever abuse alcohol or drugs?"*
- *"Did any of your relatives ever seek help from a mental health professional or receive medication to treat emotional or psychological problems? Could you describe the type of treatment they received and whether it helped them?"* These questions are particularly helpful with regard to psychotropic medications because genetic factors may influence both treatment response and the likelihood of adverse effects.

The history obtained should be recorded in the form of a genogram for easy reference. It may be necessary to specify that you are interested in *biological* relatives. Patients should be questioned specifically about children, parents, and siblings (first-degree relatives), although details about more distant relatives should be recorded if the patient volunteers them.

Personal History

The overall purpose of the personal history is to obtain information regarding the individual patient to develop a detailed biopsychosocial formulation, and much of this history is not specific to any particular diagnostic entity such as anxiety disorders. However, certain aspects of the personal history should receive particularly close attention in a patient with an anxiety disorder. The developmental history should include specific questions about whether the patient recalls experiencing anxiety at an early age. Early experiences of separation anxiety should be ascertained by asking patients whether they recall feeling highly anxious when apart from their parents, including when being left at school or in day care for the first time. Separation anxiety is relatively rare in adults, but when present in childhood may represent a developmental precursor to anxiety disorders in the mature individual (particularly PD).

A detailed *social history* will provide valuable information regarding the impact of the illness on the patient's current social and work or academic functioning. Patterns of avoidance resulting from anxiety may be particularly disabling. For example, a patient with social phobia is often socially isolated and avoidant of jobs involving interpersonal contact. This adversely affects their occupational functioning.

Mental Status Examination

No attempt will be made to provide a detailed description of the entire mental status examination in this section, which will focus on specific issues particularly pertinent to anxiety disorders.

General Description

Appearance, psychomotor behavior, and degree of eye contact may provide a variety of clues regarding the anxious patient's mental state. An example of a clue derived from general appearance is hands that appear raw or chapped, which may indicate compulsive hand washing—a common feature of OCD. Acute anxiety often produces changes in psychomotor behavior, which may range from fidgeting to more marked signs of agitation such as pacing. Sometimes these motor behaviors may be more ritualized in nature, as in the patient with OCD who crosses the threshold of your office three times to ward off bad luck. Obsessive compulsive patients with contamination concerns may also be observed to avoid touching doorknobs, shaking hands, or sitting on your office furniture. A patient who suffers from social phobia may avoid making eye contact.

Mood and Affect

It is often useful to have the patient rate her current anxiety from 1 to 10 (10 being severe). When describing a patient's *affect*, it is important to note whether the patient appears anxious at the time of the interview. Visible signs of anxiety, in addition to the psychomotor behaviors described above, may include sweating, blushing (especially characteristic of social phobia), or rapid respiration (which may indicate an impending panic attack).

Thought Process

Thought disorder is unusual in patients with anxiety disorder and should prompt suspicion of a psychotic process. However, many patients with OCD will provide excessively detailed answers to questions and at times exhibit circumstantial and overinclusive thought form. This may interfere with the process of the interview if the person insists on "finishing the story" and is difficult to redirect.

Thought Content

Careful attention to thought content will often reveal the focus of the patient's anxiety and therefore support a specific anxiety disorder diagnosis. *Worries,* defined as "apprehensive expectations," are a defining feature of generalized anxiety, particularly if the patient has difficulty controlling her worries and does not respond readily to reassurance. *Phobias* are specific, focused fears that are most characteristic of the specific phobias social phobia and agoraphobia but can also be seen in other disorders. *Obsessions* are defined as intrusive, repetitive thoughts, which are usually recognized as senseless or inappropriate by the person experiencing them and are characteristic of OCD. *Suicidal ideation* should be assessed carefully in all anxiety disorder patients. Patients experiencing both depressive symptoms and panic attacks may be at increased risk for suicide.

Perceptual Abnormalities

Although *perceptual abnormalities* are not usually present in anxiety, patients with OCD sometimes use the term *voices* to describe their obsessive thoughts. Usually, obsessions can be readily distinguished from auditory hallucinations because the patient clearly recognizes them as a product of his own mind.

Insight

The degree of insight has implications for treatment planning because it is more difficult to initiate psychotherapy in a patient with poor insight. In the adult patient with OCD, insight should have been present at some point during the illness for the diagnosis to be made, and the degree of *insight* helps to distinguish obsessions from overvalued ideas or delusions.

Collateral Information

Collateral information obtained from family members may be extremely helpful, particularly if the patient has difficulty providing a history due to embarrassment regarding his symptoms (particularly true of OCD) or disabling anxiety in the interview setting (particularly true of severe social phobia). Consultation notes from previous assessments should be sought, and direct contact should be made with current therapists or other persons actively involved in the patient's care. The patient's confidentiality must always be respected when collateral information is being sought. This includes obtaining the patient's informed, written consent to release medical records, which is a legal requirement in most jurisdictions.

Medical Investigations

A detailed medical workup is frequently unnecessary. For example, there is little to gain from ordering blood workup in a young, healthy patient with a specific phobia of snakes. However, as described in the overview, patients with panic attacks or generalized anxiety may require medical investigations to rule out physical causes for their somatic symptoms. Examples of symptoms warranting investigation include recurrent abdominal pain associated with generalized anxiety or acute chest pain that accompanies panic attacks. The workup should proceed from least to most invasive, beginning with a simple physical examination focused on the systems of interest. As noted, more careful consideration should be given to medical causes in patients who are older or who have preexisting medical conditions or risk factors. In the psychiatric setting, it is prudent to discuss any medical concerns with the patient's family physician, who can coordinate the patient's overall care and inform you of previous medical findings and investigations. If in doubt, do not hesitate to seek consultation from an appropriate specialist. The clinician should judiciously order laboratory tests to investigate specific physical symptoms rather than order a "standard battery" of investigations. The following tests may be particularly useful in the anxiety disorder setting:

- Complete blood count
- Blood glucose
- Thyroid function tests
- Vitamin B_{12} and folate levels
- Drug and alcohol screening
- Electrocardiogram

Case Example 5

Ms. A. is a 35-year-old woman who presents with a history of recurrent episodes of sudden onset intense anxiety that peaks within 10 minutes and lasts for up to an hour. Associated symptoms include diaphoresis, shortness of breath, paresthesias, dizziness, and a sensation of retrosternal "tightness." The patient was seen in the emergency department and, following a cursory physical examination, was told that her symptoms were due to "anxiety attacks" and referred for this psychiatric consultation. However, when obtaining a detailed history of present illness it becomes clear that Ms. A. has many physical symptoms, which preceded the onset of the panic attacks, including diaphoresis, tremulousness, and weight loss. The family history reveals no history of anxiety disorders, but there is a family history of thyroid illness. Laboratory investigations are normal except for a below-normal thyroid-stimulating hormone level. Ms. A. is referred to an endocrinologist and, after further investigations, is diagnosed with Graves' disease. Correction of this condition results in resolution of the panic attacks, and no further psychiatric intervention is required.

Key Point:

Past medical history is obtained to screen for other medical disorders, which may influence anxiety symptoms, and to obtain information regarding current prescribed medications, herbal remedies, and substance use.

Key Point:

Family psychiatric history should include specific inquiry regarding anxiety, mood, and other psychiatric symptoms (including substance abuse) in biological relatives.

Key Point:

A medical workup is often not necessary, but if required, should begin with a simple focused physical examination. Judicious use of laboratory investigations should be considered depending on the nature of the patient's physical symptoms and other contextual factors such as age and preexisting medical conditions.

Key Point:

Collateral history from family members, therapists, and other persons involved in the patient's care should be sought if the patient provides informed consent for the clinician to obtain this information

PSYCHOMETRIC MEASURES

The clinician can further obtain detailed and reliable information about the patient's range, frequency, intensity, and severity of anxiety symptoms by administering standardized rating instruments. This information can be used for confirming the initial diagnosis and treatment planning. It would be fair to say that there are literally hundreds of rating scales from which to choose in the assessment of anxiety and the anxiety disorders. Below is a brief listing of some of the more prominent scales for each disorder, followed a by brief description of the scales most commonly used in our clinical practice. Barlow[2] recently provided a more thorough overview of the different self-report and clinician-administered scales for each of the anxiety disorders.

General Measures

Beck Anxiety Inventory

The *Beck Anxiety Inventory (BAI)* consists of 21 self-reported items (four-point scale) used to assess the intensity of physical and cognitive anxiety symptoms during the past week. Scores may range from 0 to 63: minimal anxiety levels (0–7), mild anxiety (8–15), moderate anxiety (16–25), and severe anxiety (26–63).

Hamilton Anxiety Rating Scale

The *Hamilton Anxiety Rating Scale* is a five-point rating scale with both clinician-administered and self-report versions available, measuring 14 items pertaining to symptom severity among patients with anxiety disorders. Scores range from 0 to 24: recovered (0–4), mild (5–10), moderate (11–16), and severe (17–24).

Panic Disorder Measures

Panic Disorder Severity Scale

The *Panic Disorder Severity Scale* consists of seven items (five-point scale) and is used to assess different dimensions of PD severity in patients diagnosed with PD. The dimensions include panic attack frequency, distress during panic attack, severity of anticipatory anxiety, fear and avoidance of agoraphobic situations, fear and avoidance of panic-related sensations, and impairment in work and social functioning. The total score is the average of the scores for the individual items.

Mobility Inventory

Mobility Inventory for Agoraphobia is a self-report questionnaire consisting of 26 situations commonly avoided by a patients with agoraphobia. It measures the severity of agoraphobic avoidance (rated on a five-point scale and scored by calculating means for all items) and frequency of panic attacks (rated on a five-point scale and scored by using frequency count) during the past week.

GAD Measures

Penn State Worry Questionnaire

The *Penn State Worry Questionnaire* is a 16-item self-report questionnaire (five-point scale) measuring a person's general tendency to worry excessively. Scores can range from 16 to 80, with higher scores indicating more severe worrying.

Worry Domains Questionnaire

The *Worry Domains Questionnaire* is a 25-item self-report questionnaire (five-point Likert-type scale) that assesses the degree of worrying about five different specific domains: relationships, lack of confidence, aimless future, work, and finance. Items in each domain are added, creating the total score for a specific domain.

Social Phobia Measures

Liebowitz Social Anxiety Scale

The *Liebowitz Social Anxiety Scale* consists of 13 social and 11 performance situation items that are rated by a clinician on separate four-point scales of fear/anxiety and avoidance.

Brief Social Phobia Scale

The *Social Phobia Scale* is a 20-item scale measuring anxiety in situations involving observation by others and is rated on the five-point Likert scale. This scale is scored by summing all items.

OCD Measures

Yale-Brown Obsessive Compulsive Scale

The *Yale-Brown Obsessive Compulsive Scale* is a standardized rating scale with both clinician-administered and self-report versions available, measuring 10 items pertaining to obsessions and compulsions on a five-point Likert scale. Scores range from 0 (no symptoms) to 4 (severe symptoms), and a total score is calculated by summing items 1 to 10 and can range from 0 to 40.

Padua Inventory Revised

The *Padua Inventory Revised* consists of 41 items describing common obsessions and compulsions, which are rated on a five-point scale ranging from 0 (not at all) to 4 (very much).

PTSD Measures

Clinician-Administered PTSD Scale

The *Clinician-Administered PTSD Scale* is a semi-structured interview that measures the 17 symptoms of PTSD according to the DSM-IV. The frequency and intensity of each symptom are rated on a five-point scale. To obtain a total score, the frequency and intensity of each symptom are summed.

Impact of Event Scale

The *Impact of Event Scale* is a 15-item self-report questionnaire evaluating experiences of avoidance (numbing or responsiveness, avoidance of feelings, situations, and ideas) and intrusion (intrusive thoughts, nightmares, intrusive feelings, and imagery) in patients with PTSD. Items are rated on a four-point scale from 0 (not at all) to 5 (often).

Case Example 6

After a semi-structured clinical interview, functional assessment, detailed history interview, and relevant tests, it was determined that Mark had a primary DSM-IV-TR diagnosis of OCD. He reported a range of obsessions including contamination, harming, and sexual obsessions; overt compulsions including excessive hand washing and cleaning rituals and excessive checking behaviors including locks, doors, and household appliances; and covert rituals in response to his sexual obsessions, including counting and neutralizing with "normal" sexual images. It was decided that self-report scales should be administered to better understand the full history of past and present obsessions and compulsions, to rate the relative importance of each of his obsessions and compulsions, past and present, and to gauge the relative severity and impairment caused by each of the obsessions and compulsions. In addition, because he was being considered for CBT treatment of his OCD, it was decided that it would be helpful to know the different ways in which he cognitively appraised his intrusive thoughts, images, and impulses. He was administered the self-report and clinician versions of the Yale-Brown Obsessive Compulsive Scale (Y-BOCS) to provide a standardized assessment of obsessive compulsive frequency, intensity, and severity. He was also administered the BAI to gauge the frequency and severity of general anxiety symptoms. His score profile indicated the following: he scored in the mild range on the BAI; and in the severe range on both the self-report and clinician versions of the Y-BOCS, with the order of importance of his obsessions and compulsions being harming-checking, contamination-checking, and sexual obsessions. Collectively, these measures contributed to information about the nature and severity of his OCD as well as the identification of harming obsessions and compulsions as the most salient symptoms that would be targeted in CBT treatment.

Key Point:

Select reliable and valid self-report and/or clinician-administered assessment measures to help confirm the clinical diagnosis and aid in treatment planning.

Key Point:

Aim to include measures that assess general anxiety symptoms irrespective of diagnosis plus measures that tap aspects of patients' specific symptoms.

DETERMINING PATIENT SUITABILITY FOR TREATMENT

Patients with anxiety disorders are typically treated in outpatient settings, although there is the possibility for more intensive treatment in inpatient and day treatment programs where available. For example, the most evidence-based treatment for severe OCD is intensive inpatient exposure and response prevention therapy. There are a number of factors you should consider before embarking on treatment, irrespective of the treatment context.

What is the patient's level of anxiety sensitivity? *Anxiety sensitivity* refers to the tendency to fear anxiety symptoms as a result of perceived harmful physical, social, or psychological consequences. Patients who have high anxiety sensitivity are likely to have a low threshold for the activation of their anxiety. They are also more likely to find the symptoms of anxiety intolerable. Since treatment of the anxiety disorders typically requires exposure to the person's feared situations and symptoms, knowing a person's level of anxiety sensitivity will help you determine the likely response to early exposures and perhaps even whether the patient will stick it out in treatment. You can ask, *"To what extent would you agree with the statement that anxiety is dangerous and should be avoided as much as possible?"* or *"Have you found that you try to avoid experiencing strong emotions?"*

Another approach to determining patients' willingness to experience anxiety in treatment is to conduct a symptom induction test during the assessment phase. This could include having patients breathe through a straw for 2 minutes or run on the spot for up to 2 minutes—or any other activity that is likely to bring on physical sensations that mirror the patient's naturally occurring anxiety symptoms. Responses to open-ended questions about anxiety tolerance can be used in conjunction with the patient's response to the symptom induction test to gauge his tolerability of anxious arousal. This information can then be used, in part, to determine the particular nature, timing, and likely roadblocks in introducing exposure tasks.

Can the patient establish a treatment focus on one problem? The vast majority of patients presenting for treatment of an anxiety disorder will often present with more than one anxiety disorder in addition to other psychiatric comorbidities. An important treatment consideration is the extent to which the patient can identify and focus on a core set of problems in the interview. For instance, questions such as, *"What would you like to receive help for?"* or *"What do you think needs to change?"* will help determine the patient's treatment focality. If the patient reports a litany of problems that all appear equally important, his style is loose and rambling, and he is unresponsive to your attempts to structure the focus, then this may point to comparatively poor suitability for brief, disorder-specific treatment interventions. Patients who are able to prioritize different problems and show an ability to selectively focus on a single problem are more likely to maintain continuity across sessions and subsequently benefit from treatment.

Is the patient motivated to receive and stick with treatment? Before embarking on treatment, it is important for you to get a feel for whether the patient is really ready for the commitment that treatment will require. After all, he is going to be asked to attend regular sessions and arrive on time, face the experience of anxiety, adhere to a specific medication regimen and/or cognitive-behavioral tasks that include homework assignments between sessions, and perhaps even substantial lifestyle changes. Not all patients are ready and motivated to meet this challenge. We have found that patients who believe there is a "magical solution" to their anxiety or who believe that the therapist has all of the answers are less likely to accept the personal responsibility for change. You should ask, *"What is your understanding of the role you will play in treatment?"* or *"Do you think you will be able to put in the time and effort to get better right now?"* to better gauge this. Another factor that can adversely affect motivation to pursue treatment is the patient's level of optimism toward getting better. You can address the patient's optimism by asking: *"Do you think you can get better with treatment?"* or *"Do you think you are capable of change?"*

In addition to these general considerations, there are issues that are more relevant to determining suitability for medications and distinct issues relevant to suitability for CBT.

Considerations for Pharmacotherapy

A number of factors must be considered before initiating pharmacotherapy, including the following:

- The nature and severity of specific symptoms being targeted
- The presence of concurrent psychiatric and medical conditions
- Attitudes regarding medication

You should carefully define the nature of "target symptoms" before initiating treatment. Examples of appropriate target symptoms include hyperarousal in PTSD, panic attacks, or psychic anxiety. For this reason, medication is generally not indicated for specific phobias in the absence of comorbid conditions. Practice guidelines for anxiety disorders generally recommend medication when symptoms are more severe, whereas patients with milder symptoms are often initiated on CBT before pharmacotherapy is considered.

Patients with comorbid psychiatric disorders, such as depression, are particularly suitable for psychopharmacological intervention because the medication may potentially alleviate both conditions. This is particularly true of SSRIs, which have a high degree of efficacy in the treatment of both depression and anxiety. Concurrent medical conditions should be considered when choosing medications. There are no absolute contraindications to using SSRIs, although common adverse effects may aggravate comorbid conditions in some cases. For example, gastrointestinal side effects with SSRI use are very common and may be problematic in patients with comorbid gastrointestinal conditions. There is some evidence that SSRIs may induce gastrointestinal bleeding in some patients who are predisposed to this problem, particularly in the geriatric population. Migraine headaches may also be aggravated by SSRIs. It is extremely important to carefully document medications being used to treat medical disorders, since some of the SSRIs have significant drug interactions.

Given that SSRIs are among the most widely prescribed drugs in all of medicine and have attracted a considerable amount of media coverage, many patients will have strong beliefs and attitudes regarding these agents. Attitudes toward medication should be briefly explored in the initial interview, if this treatment option is being considered, by directly asking, *"How do you feel about taking medications to help reduce your anxiety?"* The discussion that ensues may reveal common misconceptions regarding SSRIs, for example that they are habit-forming. Other common attitudes toward psychotropic medications may be elicited in this way. For example, many patients feel that taking medications to alleviate anxiety is a sign of weakness or moral laxity. Such information regarding the patient's attitudes will be helpful when providing psychoeducation.

Considerations for Cognitive-Behavioral Therapy

In addition to the relevance of the general suitability factors outlined above, there are a number of additional questions that clinicians can ask to better determine a patient's suitability for CBT. First, because CBT highlights the role of psychological factors in the persistence of clinical anxiety, it would be useful to know what attitudes patients have toward psychological explanations of their problems. For instance, if patients strongly believe that anxiety is a disease that can only be helped with medication, they may be less interested in and therefore, not suitable for, CBT. Generally, patients who report an interest in learning more about how their thoughts and feelings contribute to their anxiety, indicate that they would be willing to face their anxiety if it were to help in the long-run, and have a history of conscientious task completion are comparatively better candidates for CBT than patients who do not endorse these elements. Patients can also be asked directly whether they would be willing to complete homework tasks between sessions, such as thought records and exposure tasks, as part of the treatment.

Case Example 7

Brenda, a 21-year-old community college student, was referred for problems pertaining to "excessive worry" and "anxiety." She had been receiving pharmacotherapy (SSRIs) for the previous 14 months but was still experiencing clinically significant distress and impairment and was seeking augmentation with CBT. After a formal assessment of her anxiety and associated psychiatric difficulties, she was assessed for CBT with a semi-structured suitability interview for the anxiety disorders.[3] Although her diagnostic profile indicated recurrent major depressive disorder (in partial remission), social phobia, and GAD, she was explicitly requesting treatment for worry.

When asked to describe a recent situation that prompted her to worry, Brenda responded, "I don't know, I was just watching TV and I began to feel real bad." Questioning about other times when she felt anxious led to similar difficulties in identifying the triggers or her appraisals of the triggers. It is not uncommon for patients to have trouble recognizing the specific triggers for their anxiety cycles, but most can do so with prompting (e.g., *"What was going through your mind when you started to feel anxious?"* or *"What did you think would happen if you weren't able to stop worrying?"*). However, Brenda had trouble recognizing the role of her thinking in the production of anxious arousal. She appeared to have a limited ability to identify and access her thoughts or to differentiate between anxious thoughts and non-anxious thoughts. She also had difficulty in differentiating between emotional states; rather, feelings related to anxiety, sadness, or frustration were lumped together under the term "bad" feelings. Brenda indicated that she was not typically bothered by feelings of anxiety although she was concerned "that worry about the worry was the worst part of her problem." She stated that she did not know much about CBT but would do whatever it took to feel better. In considering the range of her current problems, she was able to remain focused on difficulties resulting from recurring worry cycles. Finally, she indicated that she had read about CBT on the Internet before attending the session and said, "It made sense . . . I'm hopeful it can work for me too."

There were a number of factors that appeared to predict likely success for Brenda in CBT:

- She was requesting help for a specific problem and was able to remain focused on this problem in the interview.
- She had read about CBT (albeit superficially) and was willing to put the time and effort into treatment (including facing anxiety in session and doing homework).
- She communicated that she was optimistic that her condition could improve with some hard work.

However, she had considerable difficulty in identifying, distinguishing, and linking thoughts and feelings, pretherapy skills that have been found to be associated with successful outcomes in cognitive therapy. As such, it was concluded that Brenda was (moderately) suitable for CBT, although treatment would ideally focus on the behavioral aspects of treatment and limit, at least in the early going, the more complex cognitive strategies. It was also determined that early sessions should address her limitations in differentiating thoughts and feelings by teaching her foundational skills in emotion recognition. This would be achieved through in-session tasks and via homework assignments focused on understanding of the role of thoughts and feelings during periods of worry.

Key Point:

It is important to collect information regarding the patient's level of anxiety sensitivity, ability to focus on a specific problem for treatment, and level of motivation to adhere to aspects of the treatment protocol. This information can be used to identify patient strengths and weaknesses and to plan treatment so as to minimize noncompliance, early termination, or nonoptimal treatment response.

Key Point:

In assessing suitability for pharmacotherapy, it is important to explore the patient's beliefs and attitudes about medications and their use. This also serves as an opportunity to reduce misconceptions and stigma around medication use.

Key Point:

In determining whether a patient is fit for CBT, explore directly the patient's understanding of CBT, his or her readiness to "feel worse before feeling better," and his or her commitment to complete in-session exposure tasks, homework assignments, special readings, etc.

PROVIDING PSYCHOEDUCATION

Patients typically wait years before seeking help for their anxiety difficulties because of shame and embarrassment. Starting from the first visit, you should begin to provide psychoeducation to normalize the experience of anxiety and to reduce the patient's perceived stigma around having an anxiety disorder. You can aim to communicate that anxiety is

- *Normal*, and experienced by every living organism right down to the sea slug
- *Necessary* for survival and adaptation
- Although uncomfortable, *not in the least harmful or dangerous*
- Typically *short lived*
- Sometimes *useful* for performance (e.g., up to moderate levels of anxiety actually enhance performance)

However, anxiety can be expressed inappropriately at times. Therefore, the goal of treatment is reduce the inappropriate expression of anxiety.

Most patients presenting with anxiety disorders have heard the phrase *fight-or-flight response*, but most are not really sure what this means. You should aim to get across key information so that patients have a basic understanding of the physical, cognitive, and behavioral components of anxiety response:

- Anxiety is a response to danger or threat.
- The purpose of anxiety is to protect an organism.

After this introduction, you should have patients describe their particular sensations, thoughts, and behaviors when they are anxious. As the patient reports experiences, you can outline these symptoms on a whiteboard. The effect of writing down the patient's symptoms within the three-systems model has the effect of breaking down the perception of anxiety as a global, overwhelming response into an understandable and predictable reaction. It also has the effect of shifting the patient from a "victim" to an "observer" of his anxiety.

Beyond a general overview of the nature of the fight/flight response, the specifics of the three-systems model of anxiety, and an attempt to socialize the patient to the three systems model of anxiety, additional disorder-specific information can be communicated to the patient as outlined in Table 7-3.

Most patients ask why they developed this problem. You can provide information about how anxiety runs in families. You can also provide a review of factors that precipitate anxiety (disorders):

- Stressful life events
- Real or imagined loss
- Traumatic events

- Other medical or psychiatric problems
- Medications
- Use of alcohol and illicit substances

As part of psychoeducation, it is important for you to discuss the available treatment options, highlighting the role of medications and CBT. You can emphasize the very effective nature of these treatments as a means to creating hope. Finally, it is important that you provide recommended self-help readings on the nature and treatment of the patient's anxiety disorder (see suggested self-help reading list at the end of this chapter).

Table 7-3. Normalizing the Anxiety Disorders

Anxiety Disorder	Normalizing Statements
Specific phobia	• Phobia is one of the most prevalent and recognizable of human experiences. • Phobic fear is often disproportionate to the actual threat posed by the phobic cue. • Many phobias originate in childhood and are transitory and overcome through experience with the feared object. • Humans have a biological predisposition to phobias so as to learn survival-relevant associations. • Up to 11% of general population will experience specific phobia in their lifetime.
Panic disorder with/without agoraphobia	• Up to 30% of community members report experiencing (limited) panic attacks at some point within a 12-month period. • Physiological symptoms cannot lead to psychotic symptoms such as delusions, hallucinations, and disjointed thoughts and speech, which are not symptoms of general anxiety. • The fight/flight response was designed to keep an organism alert in case of danger; therefore, it cannot make an organism "lose control." • Nerves are not electrical wires, and anxiety cannot damage them. • Physiological symptoms of panic attack occur spontaneously and are unrelated to physical activity, which is not true of anginal pain. • One in 30 persons develop PD/A.
Social phobia	• Most people are slightly apprehensive (such as "butterflies" in your stomach) when approaching a situation that involves public speaking or interactions with strangers. • Studies in the community show that people's # 1 fear is speaking in front of a group. • Studies in the community show that the majority of the respondents have at least some social situations that they believe they fear more than the average person. • Up to one in eight people suffer from social phobia sometime in their lifetime.
Generalized anxiety disorder	• It is a normal feeling to show worry about multiple aspects of life. • Everyone experiences some form of anxiety on a daily basis. • Feeling anxiety during stressful times is a normal phenomenon. • Studies suggest that approximately 80% of persons in the community report continuous worrying at certain point of their lives. • It is normal and adaptive for people to be apprehensive about the future. • Up to one in 20 people have GAD.
Obsessive compulsive disorder	• Many people experience little compulsions from time to time, ranging from the desire to remember the name of a song to jumping over a crack that might "break your mother's back." • We all have a mild tendency to dwell on some thoughts. • Rachman and de Silva (1978) showed that upwards of 90% of healthy student control subjects have been found to experience intrusive thoughts that are similar in content to those reported by OCD patients.[4] • Examples of obsessive thoughts in a nonclinical sample are to hurt or harm someone, to say something nasty and damning to someone, to commit acts of violence in sex, to shout at and abuse someone, or to crash a car when driving. • Community studies show that people report increases in intrusive thoughts when exposed to stressful situations or events. • Up to one in 40 people have OCD.
Post-traumatic stress disorder and acute stress disorder	• Feelings of anxiety, a sense of helplessness, vulnerability, and feelings of grief, sadness, and anger are normal responses to traumatic events. • It is normal and universal for people to have these feelings after experiencing sudden, traumatic life events. • A traumatic experience can be considered as a new experience for which people are usually not prepared, and it has to be worked through after it happens. • Experiences of and reactions to a traumatic event are unique and vary among individuals. • Fifty-five percent of the population will experience a major traumatic event. • Approximately 7% to 10% will develop PTSD. • Five to fifteen percent of people have subclinical forms of PTSD after traumatic events.

> **Key Point:**
>
> From the initial session, try to normalize anxiety as much as possible by letting the patient know that *everyone* experiences anxiety, and it is therefore normal. And although uncomfortable, it is not dangerous. Anxiety is an "alarm" reaction to danger, and the patient can learn to stop reacting to "false alarms" to reduce distress and impairment.

> **Key Point:**
>
> Try to provide information that is current and relevant to the patient's specific anxiety problems so as to reduce self-blame and stigma and enhance feelings of universalism.

> **Key Point:**
>
> You should deliver a message of hope by reviewing the range of effective medical and psychological treatments for the patient's anxiety disorder.

SPECIAL POPULATIONS

Pediatric Anxiety

Special considerations for performing an assessment of pediatric disorders and differences from the adult assessment process are described in detail in Chapters 21 and 22, and the clinician assessing childhood anxiety should follow these general guidelines. In childhood, determination of when anxiety is pathological rather than within the normal range is complicated by developmental considerations because specific fears may be normative at certain ages. For example, fear of the dark becomes prominent in the preschool years in "normal" children and gradually dissipates between the ages of 6 and 10 years. In addition, although a child is capable of experiencing the affective and physiological components of anxiety at an early age, certain cognitive capacities may be prerequisites for the full expression of an anxiety disorder. For example, children typically develop the ability to anticipate future events by 7 to 8 years of age. This ability may be a prerequisite for experiencing the excessive worries characteristic of GAD. In contrast to worries requiring more mature forms of cognition, separation anxiety is much more likely to occur in children given the developmental importance of remaining close to caregivers during early childhood. This developmental aspect of separation anxiety is reflected in the DSM-IV-TR, in which *separation anxiety disorder* is classified as a disorder usually beginning in childhood.

In pediatric patients with obsessive compulsive symptoms, it is important to ask about recent infectious illnesses, sore throat, or upper respiratory symptoms. The rationale behind these questions is the recent identification of a syndrome known as pediatric autoimmune neuropsychiatric disorders associated with streptococcal infections (PANDAS), in which prepubertal children develop sudden onset of obsessive compulsive symptoms after experiencing a streptococcal infection, presumably as a result of an autoimmune process.

Anxiety in Elderly Patients

General geriatric assessment guidelines can be found in Chapter 23. Elderly patients with primary psychiatric disorders are more likely to present with somatic complaints rather than a chief complaint of subjective anxiety. This propensity for somatization may in part be due to increased stigmatization of mental illness in this age cohort. PD and OCD rarely begin in old age, so elderly patients with these conditions will usually have a long history of symptoms. In contrast, it is common for elderly patients to develop agoraphobia for the first time, often following a physical illness or other traumatic event.

The differentiation of primary anxiety disorders from medical or substance-induced anxiety constitutes a major diagnostic challenge in elderly patients, especially given the frequency with which prominent physical complaints are present in this population. You should maintain a high index of suspicion for medical disorders in the elderly, particularly if the anxiety symptoms have atypical features (e.g., onset of panic attacks in late life). Any suspicion of a medical cause should be investigated with a physical examination and appropriate laboratory investigations. Polypharmacy is also a common issue in elderly patients, necessitating a careful medication review to assess for possible substance-induced anxiety symptoms and for determining possible interactions with anxiolytic medications.

Cognitive disorders such as dementia and delirium are far more common in the elderly compared with younger adults and may be associated with anxiety symptoms. All elderly patients should therefore be screened for cognitive deficits using an instrument like the Mini-Mental State Examination. An altered level of consciousness may indicate delirium and should not be present in a primary anxiety disorder. Depression is commonly comorbid with anxiety in elderly patients, and a first onset of generalized anxiety symptoms in older adults is almost always due to depression rather than GAD.

TREATMENT CONSIDERATIONS

Building a Treatment Plan

Sources of information from the diagnostic assessment, detailed history, mental status examination, collateral information from family and other sources, laboratory tests, psychometric measures, and suitability considerations should provide a road map for the treatment plan. You now know the following:

1. The patient's diagnoses and the primary diagnosis for treatment
2. The developmental and contextual aspects of the problem
3. The specific symptoms of the patient's problem and the extent to which they interact
4. Some understanding of the specific triggers for his anxiety cycles
5. The patient's strengths and weaknesses in cognitive, emotional, social, and behavioral functioning
6. Any medical illnesses or disabilities that interact with the anxiety condition
7. The patient's symptom functioning in relation to standardized norms for other people with that disorder
8. The patient's readiness, motivation, and likely prognosis for first-line available treatments
9. Whether there are special issues relevant to his anxiety disorder

The next step is to consider the two evidence-based first-line interventions for the treatment of anxiety disorders: pharmacotherapy or CBT.

Starting Treatment with Medications, CBT, or a Combination

The preponderance of patients are first treated in the primary care context and are therefore likely to be taking one or more medications at the time of referral for psychiatric consultation. Presently, there are numerous medications that have been proven effective in well-conducted randomized placebo-controlled trial studies for specific disorders in the anxiety spectrum. These include fluoxetine, fluvoxamine, paroxetine, sertraline, venlafaxine, moclobemide, buspirone, imipramine, and nefazodone, among others. There are well-articulated treatment guidelines for the specific timing, dosing, and monitoring with these medications for the different anxiety disorders.

In addition to pharmacotherapy, there is considerable evidence for the effectiveness of CBT for each of the anxiety disorders. There is a consensus across different treatment guidelines and expert panels that CBT should be the first-line intervention in the treatment of the anxiety disorders. Presently, there are step-by-step patient and clinician manuals for each of the anxiety disorders (see reading lists below). Generally, unless the patient has completed a previous course of CBT and failed to significantly improve, demonstrates very limited suitability for CBT as outlined above, reports a lack of interest in trying CBT, or cannot access a well-trained CBT therapist, he should be provided this treatment modality for his difficulties.

Unfortunately, there has been very little research addressing the particular sequencing of medication and CBT treatments for the anxiety disorders. In randomized controlled trials comparing lone versus combined treatments for the anxiety disorders, there are no consistent differences between CBT, medications, and their combination in the short term. Excluded here is the treatment of simple phobias, for which CBT is the only empirically demonstrated effective treatment. There is growing empirical support, however, for better long-term outcomes and fewer relapses with CBT compared with medications. Because of our limited knowledge about the combination of treatments, the most parsimonious treatment recommendation at the present time is to follow established treatment guidelines for the provision of CBT and first-line pharmacotherapy interventions when indicated. For patients with severe anxiety disorders, the combination of CBT and pharmacotherapy is likely to be most effective. Once treatments have been initiated, they can be adjusted depending on the patient's progress. CBT sessions and medication dosages can be adjusted in intensity to reflect therapeutic progress.

Key Point:

Although there is a range of treatment options, you should aim to provide or coordinate first-line evidence-based treatments. Where possible, every patient should be considered for CBT given its short- and long-term effectiveness for each of the anxiety disorders.

ACKNOWLEDGMENTS

The authors wish to express their gratitude to Madalyn Marcus and Kate Szacun-Shimizu for their editorial assistance.

REFERENCES

1. American Psychiatric Association: *Diagnostic and statistical manual of mental disorders-TR,* ed 4, text revision, Washington, DC, 2000, American Psychiatric Association.
2. Barlow DH: *Anxiety and its disorders: the nature and treatment of anxiety and panic,* New York, 2002, The Guilford Press.
3. Rector NA, Cox BC: The development of a scale to assess suitability for cognitive behavior therapy for anxiety disorders. Paper presented at the Annual Meeting of the Association for the Advancement of Behavior Therapy. Toronto. November, 1999.
4. Rachman S, de Silva P. Abnormal and normal obsessions. *Behavior Research and Therapy* 16:233–248, 1978.

RECOMMENDED READINGS

Bourin DH, Lambert O: Pharmacotherapy of anxious disorders, *Human Psychopharmacol* 17:383–400, 2002.
Stein DJ, Hollander E: *Textbook of anxiety disorders,* Washington, DC, 2002, American Psychiatric Publishing.

WEBSITES

Anxiety Disorders Association of America: www.adaa.org
American Psychiatric Association: www.psych.org
American Psychological Association: www.apa.org
Association for Advancement of Behavior Therapy: www.aabt.org

8

Assessment of Patients with Personality Disorders

Paul S. Links

INTRODUCTION

Students at all levels of their training are going to encounter patients with personality disorders. Half of all patients in an inpatient psychiatric service and a quarter of all patients in psychiatric outpatient clinics will meet criteria for personality disorders. Patients with personality disorders are frequent service users.[1] For example, within a sample of community adults, respondents with borderline personality disorder had extremely high rates of mental health service usage, approaching those of respondents with schizophrenia.[1] Personality disorders can be diagnosed in approximately 10% to 15% of the general population. Therefore, patients with personality disorders are frequently encountered, are often in great need of care, and sometimes are the most difficult and confusing for clinicians to assess, engage in therapy, and manage.

> **Key Point:**
>
> Students at all levels of their training are going to encounter patients with personality disorders.

The overall purpose of this chapter is to give you an approach for diagnosing patients with a personality disorder and for engaging these patients in treatment. Specifically, this chapter covers the basics about personality disorders, including why it is important to recognize a personality disorder diagnosis and how to make a diagnosis of a personality disorder. I will look at ways to use your clinical interview to try to diagnose and engage personality-disordered patients. Other assessment methods to make personality disorder diagnoses will be discussed. Specific challenges related to working with patients with personality disorders will be addressed, including maintaining one's boundaries with these patients, involving family and other care providers, and the importance of taking a rehabilitative perspective. The chapter will conclude by identifying some key references for further reading.

Case Example 1

The Avoidant Jeweler. Mr. A. was a 40-year-old single man who presented for help because his anxiety was interfering with his work. For the last 4 months, Mr. A. had been avoiding customers who approached him in the jewelry store where he worked. Mr. A. described that he daily experienced a strange sense of himself leaving his body when he greeted new customers. This anxiety, when in the company of customers, prevented him from being able to focus or concentrate on the sale. The strange sensation, later labeled *depersonalization*, was now causing Mr. A. to avoid greeting any customers. Fortunately, Mr. A. was an expert jeweler and was able to spend more and more time in the back of the store. "I am better at appreciating the faults in diamonds rather than in people," he explained.

Mr. A. characterized himself as highly anxious, and he avoided most social situations; he was unable to eat in public, and he had always disliked speaking to new customers. He gave a history of occasional panic episodes, but they were much less frequent than his sense of depersonalization. Mr. A. denied being depressed, although he was concerned that his anxiety would jeopardize his work. The patient did not give a history of significant past traumatic events, obsessive or compulsive symptoms, constant worrying, or other dissociative features. Mr. A. admitted that he occasionally drank to excess to diminish his anxiety in social situations. He recognized that his drinking was dysfunctional and problematic at times.

Mr. A. had never spoken to a psychiatrist before, and he had no history of medical problems. He lived a quiet existence and still resided with his mother and an older brother. Both his mother and brother were described as shy, nervous people. Mr. A. was very motivated to deal with his difficulties at work, although he had little motivation to be more sociable outside of the context of his work. **Question: Should Mr. A. give up making sales?**

Case Example 2

Safety and Ms. Street Punk. Ms. B., a 19-year-old woman called "the Street Punk" by the emergency staff, presented herself to hospital, stating, "I'm suicidal. I don't feel safe." The staff in the emergency stressed that this patient is "trouble." They explained that she frequents the emergency department, can be loud and aggressive, and has been diagnosed as having antisocial personality disorder. However, since uttering those few words, the patient remained mute and huddled in the corner of the examination room. When I entered the room, the patient was now sitting cross-legged on the stretcher with her jacket hood covering almost all of her face. In spite of the rain jacket, scars from previous self-attacks were apparent on her wrists, ankles, and neck.

"I'm the doctor with the Crisis Team. They asked me to speak with you. You're feeling suicidal?" I began.

No response. No acknowledgment at all.

"Can you tell me your name and where you're living?"

No response.

"Have you ever been to this hospital before?"

No response.

Several questions later, I indicated, "You're obviously not feeling safe and not safe enough to speak with someone that you've never met before. Is there something I could do to make you feel safer while you're here in the hospital?"

No response, although she moved her hooded head up as if to catch a glance of my face.

"Is there someone I could talk with who knows about your problems and can help me understand why you've come to the hospital today?"

"Ryan, at Streetview, knows why I'm here," the patient abruptly responded.

"Is Ryan a counselor at Streetview?"

"Yes. He told me to get lost, so I came here."

"That sounds pretty hurtful. Can you tell me more about what happened?"

For Ms. B., identifying her hurt feelings allowed the interview to progress. The patient gave permission for me to speak with her counselor and the staff at "Streetview." However, as I left the room, the patient shouted, "Don't send me back there. I won't go back there. I need to be in hospital." **Question: What are the safety issues to consider with Ms. B.?**

Case Example 3

"I'm always thinking of suicide." "I'm always thinking of suicide," stated Mr. C. when approached by the doctor in the emergency department. This 36-year-old single man explained that he had thought of suicide every day of his life since he was 12 years old. However, Mr. C. was unable to explain his actions from the night before, when he impulsively slashed his wrists. Mr. C. cut deeply into his tendons and said he wanted to die when he made repeated cuts to both wrists. However, when he realized that his cuts were clotting; Mr. C. cleaned himself up and went to bed. The following morning, Mr. C. decided to come to the emergency department for treatment to repair the remnants of his self-injury.

Mr. C. could not explain why he acted on his thoughts the night before. He denied any particular stressful events and endorsed few symptoms of depression or anxiety. The patient described daily thoughts of suicide, and he insisted that if he owned a gun he would be dead by now. Mr. C. acknowledged that he always felt unhappy and that his life was empty. He had few close relationships and insisted that he preferred to keep people "at arm's length." He was not psychotic, although he had odd beliefs that he called his "superstitions," which made him uncomfortable with human contact. The patient admitted to drinking a half a dozen beers each day and acknowledged that he could be very impulsive. He endorsed frequent, unsafe, anonymous gay sexual encounters but did not consider himself gay. He reported bouts of gambling and episodes of dangerous driving when he had a license, but he denied that he was ever violent or assaultive. The patient did admit to drinking on the night of his suicide attempt, but he explained that he was less likely to attempt suicide when he was intoxicated. Mr. C. essentially denied any other symptoms or any history of psychiatric contacts. However, he acknowledged a difficult childhood, as his parents separated shortly after his birth. Mr. C. grew up in the unpredictable care of his alcoholic mother and indicated that his mother could be physically violent when drunk.

The patient had been reasonably successful at school and had held the same job for more than a decade. He was a troubleshooter for an internationally recognized software company. Mr. C. explained that he much preferred facing a screen than other people. "I trust machines much more than I trust people," he added.

The patient insisted he had no plans to hurt himself, but he could not ensure his safety to the doctor. Mr. C. reported that he planned to attend work tomorrow and agreed to a follow-up appointment for early next week. Given his agreement to attend a follow-up appointment, the patient was discharged from the emergency department. **Question: What are the issues to be addressed at the follow-up appointment?**

PERSONALITY DISORDER DIAGNOSIS

Personality disorders have received increasing attention within the psychiatric nomenclature since 1980, with the inclusion of a separate axis, axis II, for personality disorders in the American Psychiatric Association's *Diagnostic and Statistical Manual of Mental Disorders,* 4th edition, text revision (DSM-IV-TR). The purpose of the separate axis for personality disorders was to assist clinicians in attending to this aspect of a patient's presentation and to separate personality features from axis I disorders like depression, anxiety disorders, and schizophrenia. However, attempts to categorize or understand personality have been of interest to mankind going back to the time of Hippocrates and his four temperaments. The typologies to characterize personality disorder have varied from four temperaments to Charles Fourier's 810 character types. Personality disorder diagnoses have gone through several revisions since the first publication of axis II disorders in 1980 leading to the current classification based on DSM-IV-TR.[2] The DSM-IV-TR lists the criteria for each of the 10 personality disorders and organizes them into three clusters (see the section entitled "Interpersonal Aspects of Personality Disorder" where some of the features of each personality disorder are listed and organized by cluster). Most of the recent modifications have been made based on empirical evidence, and other changes were done to increase correspondence with the *International Classification of Diseases,* 10th edition (ICD-10).[3] The development of axis II appears to have been helpful in focusing clinicians' attention onto some aspects of personality, differentiating them from symptom disorders such as schizophrenia, mood disorders, or anxiety disorders and fostering research into personality disorders.

Personality is the synthesis of our behaviors, cognitions, and emotions, which make each of us unique. Ironically, this uniqueness is, for the purpose of personality disorder diagnosis, reflected in a predictable pattern of symptoms and behaviors. These attributes tend to be stable and enduring, allowing our family, friends, partners, and acquaintances to predict how we will respond to a given situation and permitting them to describe us to others.

Although our personalities allow others to predict and anticipate our responses to situations, a person with a healthy personality demonstrates a range of coping responses and a variety of coping styles when placed in a stressful situation. A disordered personality occurs when a person cannot display such adaptability and flexibility. The lack of adaptability and a limited repertoire of coping responses can result in distress for the individual and for those around her.

Personality disorders are generally thought to be recognized by adolescence or earlier and were first thought to continue as stable disorders throughout adulthood. There is now some evidence that personality disorders can be recognized in childhood. For example, borderline personality disorder can be diagnosed in adolescents because the symptom pattern and the level of dysfunction will be very comparable to what is found in adulthood. However, there is still some concern about whether these disorders have predictive validity—that is, whether they predict that the person will continue to have the diagnosis in adulthood. The original definition in the DSM indicated that personality disorders were deeply ingrained, inflexible, maladaptive patterns of sufficient severity to cause impairment in functioning and profound distress. However, recent research has suggested that personality disorders may be more flexible and changeable than previously considered.

The usefulness of personality disorder diagnoses for helping clinicians with the management of patients is still debated. Some have argued that the uniqueness of a person's personality, for both strengths and weaknesses, is best captured with a dimensional approach. A dimensional view is that personality exists along a continuum, whereas a categorical approach draws a line between health and pathology, allowing the diagnosis of disorder. Although there are definite advantages to characterizing personality using a dimensional approach, there still may be benefit in having diagnoses to assist in clinical management. Often, clinicians are faced with yes/no decisions, for example, deciding whether medication should be prescribed, hospitalization arranged, or involuntary assessment ordered.

Key Point:

Personality is the synthesis of our behaviors, cognitions, and emotions, which make each of us unique. Despite this uniqueness, both normal personality and personality disorder have defined patterns.

Importance of Diagnosis

The diagnosis of a personality disorder can be important to the clinician because it indicates several important facets relevant to the patient's care. For example, the diagnosis can indicate an increased risk for suicide or suicidal behavior, reflect the course and prognosis for coexisting disorders, indicate important etiological factors, inform you about the patient's course and outcome, highlight aspects of the patient's social role performance, and assist you in determining overall management parameters for the patient.

Risk of Suicide and Suicidal Behavior

Most of the research evidence on the relationship among personality disorders, suicidal behavior, and suicide focuses on antisocial and borderline personality disorder. Less literature exists on other personality disorders in relation to suicidal behavior and suicide. In discussing antisocial and borderline personality disorder, we can examine the relationship to suicide in two ways: first, we can discuss how the rates of these personalities are found in victims of suicide or those who make suicide attempts; second, we can then look at the rates of suicide and suicide attempts in samples of persons with these personality disorders. Marttunen et al.,[4] from the Comprehensive of Psychological Autopsy Study in Finland, estimated that 17% of adolescents aged 13 to 19 years who died by suicide met criteria for conduct disorder or antisocial personality disorder. When Marttunen et al.[5] studied adolescents with nonfatal suicidal behavior, approximately 45% of males and one third of females were characterized by antisocial behavior. Beautrais et al.[6] studied persons who had made medically serious suicide attempts and compared the attempters to other subjects from the same community. After controlling for the intercorrelation among mental disorders, these investigators found the risk of a suicide attempt was 3.7 times higher for individuals with antisocial personality disorder than for those without that diagnosis.

A few studies have documented the lifetime risk of suicide in samples of persons with antisocial personality disorder. Maddocks,[7] in a 5-year follow-up of a small sample of 59 persons with antisocial disorder, estimated a 5% lifetime risk of suicide. Laub and Vaillant[8] researched the causes of death of 1,000 delinquent and nondelinquent males followed up from ages 14 to 65 years. Deaths due to violent causes (i.e., accidents, suicide, or homicide) were significantly more common in delinquent compared with nondelinquent males; however, equal proportions of both groups died by suicide.

With regard to borderline personality disorder, studies of suicide completers have found that 9% to 33% of all suicide victims would have met criteria for borderline personality disorder. Crumley[9] demonstrated a high incidence of borderline personality disorder in adolescents and young adults aged 15 to 24 years who engaged in suicidal behavior. Depending on the study, the lifetime risk of suicide among subjects with borderline personality disorder has been found to range between 3% and 10%.[10] In addition, as many as 75% to 80% of persons with borderline personality disorder have a history of suicidal behavior.[11,12] Fewer studies have focused on clusters A and C; however, evidence suggests that cluster A and C personality disorders versus those without personality disorders are associated with an increased risk of suicide and suicide attempts. Nevertheless, the relationship between cluster B, particularly borderline and antisocial personality disorders, and suicide/suicide behavior has been the best documented and appears to be more robust than the relationship between suicidal behavior, suicide, and the other clusters.

The clinical assessment of borderline or antisocial patients can be complicated, particularly if they have a history of recurrent suicidal behavior. I suggest using a model that characterizes the suicide risk as either chronic or acute-on-chronic to assess and communicate the suicidal risk for patients with recurrent suicidal behavior. Typically, these patients are at a chronic elevated risk of suicide much above the general population. The risk exists on account of their history of multiple attempts, and this risk is also increased if there is a history of self-injurious behavior.[13,14] Stanley et al.[14] found that patients with self-injurious behavior were at risk for suicide attempts because of their high levels of depression, hopelessness, and impulsivity and also because they misperceive and underestimate the lethality of their suicidal behaviors. Forman et al.[15] have documented that recurrent suicidal behavior, a history of more than one attempt, may be a good marker for patients with increased risk of suicidality, high levels of psychopathology, and poor functioning. The patient's level of chronic risk can be estimated by taking a careful history of previous suicidal behavior and focusing on times when the patient may have demonstrated attempts with the greatest intent and medical lethality. By documenting the patient's most serious attempts, you could estimate the severity of the patient's ongoing chronic risk of suicide.

In patients with repeated suicide attempts such as borderline personality disorder patients, you can look for evidence of an acute-on-chronic level of risk. The acute-on-chronic risk will be present if the patient is suffering from a major depressive episode or if the patient is demonstrating high levels of depression and hopelessness. The study by Yen et al.[16] supported the need to look for an acute-on-chronic change in status; these researchers demonstrated that a worsening of depression or substance use occurred in the month preceding a suicide attempt relative to the general levels of change in these symptoms in all other months. Patients with borderline personality disorder are known to be at risk for suicide around times of stress—for example, at times of hospitalization or recent discharge. The clinical scenario of a patient presenting in crisis shortly after discharge from an inpatient setting illustrates a time when the risk assessment must be very carefully completed to ensure the proper disposition decision is made. The patient is potentially at acute-on-chronic risk, and the assessment cannot be truncated because of the recent discharge from hospital. Proximal substance abuse can increase the suicide risk in patients with borderline personality disorder. The existence of a diagnosis of substance abuse is, of course, a factor that increases a chronic risk for suicidal behavior. The risk is acutely elevated in patients who have less family support or a perceived or actual loss of important supportive relationships.

Gunderson[11] made the distinction that patients with borderline personality disorder who are attempting to manipulate their environment are at less risk than borderline patients who present in highly regressed, dissociative states. At these times, interventions frequently have to be put in place acutely to reduce the risk of suicide attempts or self-harm. Using the acute-on-chronic model can be effective for communicating decisions regarding risk assessment and management. For example, if you think a patient is at a chronic but not acute-on-chronic risk for suicide, you can document and communicate that a short-term hospitalization will have little or no impact on a chronic risk that has been present for months and years. However, an inpatient admission of a patient demonstrating acute-on-chronic risk might well be indicated. A short-term admission may allow the level of risk to return to previous levels. Managing the chronic level of suicide risk in patients with borderline personality disorder or recurrent suicidal behavior often involves strategic outpatient management such as dialectic behavior therapy, which has proved effective for reducing suicidal behavior.[13,17]

The chronic risk of suicide is often more of an issue for you as a clinician than for the patient. For many patients with severe personality disorders who persistently contemplate suicide, these thoughts are coping strategies that give them a sense of power and control over their life experiences. They often struggle against your attempts to control or modify these thoughts. You must monitor the risk regularly in such patients. Your other important task is to understand that these chronic suicidal thoughts have meaning to the patient, and therapeutic gains can sometimes be made as the patient comes to understand the meaning behind his chronic suicidal contemplation.

Coexisting Axis I Disorders

The presence of an axis I disorder and a personality disorder seems to have implications for the treatment and course of the axis I disorder. Evidence exists that the occurrence of an axis I disorder (e.g., major depression) with a personality disorder will delay the response to treatment and increase the risk of recurrence of axis I disorders. In general, these effects on treatment response and course seem to be found regardless of the type and nature of the axis I disorder and the coexisting personality disorder.[18] Mulder[19] recently challenged this conclusion, stating that the best-designed studies report the least effect of personality pathology on depression treatment outcome. Many of the studies have shortcomings, and they rarely control for other depressive characteristics, such as chronicity and severity, that may influence the outcome and be related to personality pathology. Suffice it to say that, clinically, the presence of a comorbid personality disorder or personality pathology should not be seen as an impediment to seeking a good treatment response and to aggressively treating the axis I disorder. It may be important to impart to the patient that the response to treatment may be less robust and may take longer; nevertheless, appropriate treatment is worth pursuing.

For example, I advised, *"Ms. D., I must caution you that because we are dealing with more than one clinical diagnosis, treating your depression will take a little longer, and some of the symptoms may not completely resolve. However, I do strongly recommend that we proceed with a trial of the antidepressant."*

Key Point:

The diagnosis of a personality disorder can indicate an increased risk for suicide or suicidal behavior, affect the course and prognosis for coexisting disorders, indicate important etiological factors, inform the clinician about the patient's course and outcome, highlight aspects of the patient's social role performance, and assist the clinician in determining overall management parameters for the patient.

Etiology of Personality Disorders

Diagnosing a personality disorder requires some understanding of the etiology of these disorders. Several general principles can be derived based on current evidence. About 40% to 50% of the total prototypic variance in personality functioning or characteristics is related to genetic factors, none or very little is due to shared environmental factors, and the remainder of the variance may be accounted for by nonshared environmental factors.[20]

Psychosocial adversity also appears to be related to personality pathology. Paris[21] summarized the evidence by indicating that parental psychopathology, family breakdown, and traumatic events all appear to be risk factors for personality disorders. The author felt these factors were most related to the etiology of impulsive personality disorders, although they also may be implicated in the anxious cluster disorders. The risk factors show a great heterogeneity within disorder, and there is also a significant overlap between disorders. In addition, adversity during childhood does not fully account for the development of personality disorders. Paris[21] outlined a diathesis-stress model of personality psychopathology. It is clear that traits may reflect underlying genetic vulnerability, and psychological and social factors can be crucial in determining whether these underlying trait vulnerabilities are amplified, leading to overt disorder. However, persons differ in their exposure and susceptibility to these psychological and social factors. It is clear that personality disorders are not based on single or linear cause-effect models and require the integration of biopsychosocial factors in both their understanding and their management.

Course and Outcome

Certainly, as defined in the DSM, personality disorders were said to begin by late adolescence and continue throughout much of adulthood. However, the systematic study of the course of major personality disorders is clarifying our understanding. For example, Zanarini et al.[22] examined the remission rates over a 6-year prospective follow-up study of patients with borderline personality disorder. The remission rates at 2 years were in the range of 30% to 40%, consistent with other studies in the area. In addition, there was approximately a 50% remission rate by 6 to 7 years' follow-up. The study indicated that there was a progressive pattern of remission and that very few patients showed a reexperiencing of their symptoms to the point of being rediagnosed. However, a quarter of the patients in this study were in a never-remitted group, which indicated that some patients had a very chronic disabling course. This and other evidence suggest that the course of personality disorders is more changeable than first considered. It is important to understand this possibility and share this hope for change with the patient.

Social Role Dysfunction

To make a diagnosis of a personality disorder, the features must lead to distress or impairment of social or other role functioning. More is being learned about the general aspects of social role dysfunction that accompanies personality disorders. For example, Skodol and colleagues[23] indicated that patients with personality disorders are more likely to be separated, divorced, or never married and to have had periods of unemployment, frequent job changes, and exposure to disability. However, a discrepancy exists, as often these patients tend to be more educated than their job performance would indicate. When the quality of their social functioning is studied, patients with personality disorder generally have poor social functioning with difficulties in personal relationships and poor work performance and job satisfaction. Skodol et al.[23] found empirical evidence that fit with clinical experience for a gradient of functional impairment from the less severe personality disorders to the more severe personality disorders. Patients with schizotypal and borderline personality disorder had greater and more widespread impairment of social functioning compared with patients with obsessive compulsive personality disorder or patients with major depression without comorbid personality disorders. Patients with avoidant personality disorder fell between these two extremes. Overall, the findings indicated that these patients had poor social and work functioning and that much of their difficulties with functioning were attributed to their personality disorder. You must be attuned to the fact that patients with personality disorder have significant social role impairment, and although they may have comorbid symptom disorders, much of their social role dysfunction comes from their personality disorder.

Role performance can be context-bound; for example, a patient with a paranoid personality disorder may generally be isolated and friendless but may make an excellent night watchman, enjoying the solitude but also accepting the need for vigilance during the work hours. Patients should be asked about their functioning in each of their roles including family life, intimate relationships, work, social leisure, and financial functioning. It is important to determine role functioning because it can be an important target for interventions when the management plan is being generated.

GENERAL MANAGEMENT PRINCIPLES

The diagnosis of a personality disorder should help you formulate general management plans and principles so that a patient is appropriately cared for. The progress in formulating management of personality disorders is evidenced by the recent publication of the American Psychiatric Association Practice Guidelines for Patients with Borderline Personality Disorders.[24] The publication of these guidelines implies that enough research and expert opinion have been generated to begin to formulate appropriate management guidelines. Some principles have been suggested that should direct our care of most patients with personality disorders. For example, the clinician must establish the treatment framework outlining the aspects of the treatment, indicating what she provides and what she expects from the patient. Clear boundaries around treatment relationships and tasks must be maintained. Where multiple providers are involved, early agreement must be established regarding which clinician will assume primary overall responsibility for monitoring the patient's safety and treatment response. Because of the patient's risk for crises and suicidal behavior, monitoring of safety and developing a response to a crisis are primary roles of the clinician. Plans for dealing with crises must be outlined and documented as part of the management plan. As indicated, you must attend to the diagnosis and treatment of coexisting axis I disorders. In addition, you must have a low threshold for seeking consultation because of the difficulties that are inherent in managing the clinician-patient relationship. It is understood that patients can stimulate a strong emotional reaction from the clinician, and you should be alert to this eventuality. Patients often pressure clinicians to modify or violate patient-clinician boundaries. Extra vigilance may be required, and risk management strategies must be practiced to prevent boundary violations.

RECOGNIZING A PATIENT WITH A PERSONALITY DISORDER

Diagnosing a personality disorder from a single clinical encounter is difficult. The patient may be known only from periodic visits in the outpatient department or from a cross-sectional assessment done during an emergency visit. During these encounters, try to address the following questions to assess for a personality disorder diagnosis:

1. Is this an axis I disorder or a personality disorder presentation?
2. Why is the patient seeking help?
3. How does this patient make me feel, and what do I observe on the first encounter?

Identifying Axis I Disorders

Axis I disorders such as major depression or anxiety disorders often coexist with diagnoses of personality disorders. The cognitive, affective, and behavioral symptoms of an axis I disorder and a personality disorder can overlap considerably. For example, manic patients may appear impulsive, angry, and volatile just as a borderline patient can present in the same manner.

Specific information about the onset and progression of symptoms, the repetitiveness and duration of the clinical presentation, and the way in which symptoms relate to the patient's environment and life stresses will help the clinician differentiate an axis I disorder from the traits of a personality disorder. In general, axis I disorders are of recent onset even when they represent relapses of chronic illnesses and may be assessed by taking a history of the present illness and carefully examining the mental status. However, the traits of a personality disorder usually are evident at least for the last 3 to 5 years and are uncovered during the developmental, personal, and social history. Careful attention should be paid to how patients interact, perceive, and think about their significant relationships. Personality disorder traits will tend to wax and wane over a matter of days and weeks, but historically they should characterize the pattern of interpersonal relationships and should surface repeatedly throughout adulthood.

The distinction between an axis I disorder and traits of a personality disorder is difficult to make. A common example is major depression, which can create the patient's negative view of self and others and dramatically impair interpersonal functioning. Sometimes, it is impossible to separate the impact of the axis I disorder from that of personality traits. Because of this difficulty, you may be wise to forego diagnosing a personality disorder if the patient is in the throes of a very active axis I disorder such as a major depression.

Personality disorder diagnoses in adolescent patients are a particular problem because the symptom status tends to be very changeable in adolescence over time. Borderline personality disorder has been diagnosed with acceptable validity and reliability in adolescents. Adolescents meeting criteria for borderline personality disorder will show significant psychopathology and considerable functional impairment, and they are not just going through the turmoil of normal adolescence. However, there is still some question about the predictive validity of borderline personality disorder diagnoses in adolescents. Will the disorder carry through into adulthood with reasonable stability?

The presentation of a patient with a personality disorder may be influenced by the context in which the patient is assessed. The patient with a personality disorder may appear impaired in one context, particularly when in crisis or feeling invalidated, yet appears quite normal in another context. An axis I disorder, however, is usually independent of context and will run its course over the next days and weeks. The patient being assessed for an axis I disorder versus a personality disorder should at best be assessed over a period of 1 to 2 weeks to help determine whether the course of the presentation is variable or persistent.

Determining Why a Patient Seeks Help

You must understand the reasons why the patient is seeking help. Patients may be distressed and requesting help. The patient's symptoms may be characterized as *ego-dystonic;* that is, the presentation is causing the patient distress and is leading to help-seeking. These presentations are more characteristic of the anxious cluster of personality disorders, such as avoidant and obsessive compulsive personality disorder. Other patients present for professional help because of the distress they cause to others rather than to themselves. These patients' symptoms or behaviors are characterized as *ego-syntonic.* These patients are likely to have been forced or encouraged to seek help, and if they do so willingly, they may only be doing so to protect themselves from retribution from another person. Patients with personality disorders from the so-called dramatic cluster, such as antisocial and narcissistic personality disorders, are more likely to present in this way. However, patients with borderline personality disorder are very much help-seeking.

Examining How the Patient Makes You Feel

It is important to begin your assessment as soon as you encounter the patient. Important clinical information can be garnered from your initial impressions, based on the patient's demeanor, dress, and behavior that can provide important clues about the patient's personality traits. Is the patient slow to make eye contact? Does he or she respond to cues such as an initial greeting with questions, nods, or smiles, or is the patient overly familiar at initiation of the interview? Is the patient suspicious, withdrawn, or anxious and timid?

You can learn a great deal by monitoring your own responses to patients. It is not uncommon for a clinician to feel coerced by a patient into acting in a certain way during interactions. For example, you may feel pressured to take more control if the patient presents as extremely helpless. Attempts by you to help the patient are often ineffective in resolving the patient's helplessness, and you are left feeling frustrated and angry. This type of interaction, at its worst, can lead you to transgress professional boundaries, for example, by trying to settle the patient with a soothing caress or by becoming angry and acting unprofessionally.

Patients who coerce you into taking charge but then frustrate your attempt to do so are defending themselves from the same feelings that such interactions evoke in you. Rather than acknowledge feelings of being helpless and out of control, frustrated, or angry, the patient coerces you to take on and experience these feelings. This is achieved by acting in such a way that it pressures others to respond in a certain manner. Your frustration or anger at your failed efforts accentuates the patient's attempts to fight off acknowledging these same feelings.

By looking at this type of interaction and understanding where it comes from, you can better understand the patient. You will recognize this pattern of interaction and can try to label the patient's feelings, although the patient will often deny their existence because of strong defenses. Acknowledgment by you that you feel pressure to respond in a certain way will often free the patient to discuss feelings. This type of interaction, called *projective identification,* is something that makes for difficult encounters with personality disorder patients. However, if this is experienced, it can help clarify the diagnosis because these defenses are often used by patients with borderline personality disorder. Understanding this interaction can allow you to be more in touch with the patient's inner feeling state and self-experience. However, it must be remembered that the nature of the patient's defenses are not specific to any one personality disorder, and the presence of a defense mechanism does not define a personality disorder. Nevertheless, immature defenses such as projective identification, and defenses that impair reality testing, are more typical of patients with severe personality disorders.

Although your reaction to a patient can be very enlightening and can be useful diagnostically, there are limitations to this approach. For example, patients with personality disorder, particularly borderline patients, often can be difficult and can trigger strong reactions in clinicians, but it is important to remember that not all difficult patients will end up being borderline and not all borderline patients are difficult. To avoid this pitfall, you should carefully confirm and document that the patient meets diagnostic criteria before settling on what can be a highly stigmatizing label. Although all patients with psychiatric disorders will experience some stigmatization, patients with borderline personality disorder are often stigmatized by health care professionals as being undeserving or untreatable, sometimes preventing access to appropriate care.

SPECIFIC PERSONALITY DISORDER DIAGNOSIS

Once you suspect that a patient has a personality disorder, the next step is to assess which specific personality disorder or personality traits the patient is manifesting. Diagnosing patients into categories, particularly personality disorders, is a challenge, based on one or even several clinical interviews. Many patients with personality disorders, even though they have the same diagnosis, appear quite different from one to another. Most patients with severe personality disorders also meet criteria for two or more personality disorder diagnoses. It is next to impossible for you to keep track of diagnostic criteria that are needed to make a specific diagnosis as per the DSM-IV-TR.[2] In that diagnostic system, there are at least 10 sepa-

ity. The
have g
stated t
out con
nate se
ing free
being a
borderl
but pre
instabil
and dev
on and
bility, t
threat o

Patie
terized
usually
often h
affects.
extreme
tress an
identifi
Thus, i
unwant
a way as
emotion
tial tem
Difficul
are exp
difficult
Finally,
ties that
ically th
have di
lose to
microps
patients
tion, d
intense

Bord
therapy
anger an
and vali
ing to ha
the esca
respond
Howeve
flexibili
importa

Narciss

The c
rich trac

rate categories and more than 100 criteria, in total, that would have to be assessed. Many of the criteria are complex and require considerable clinical inference to establish their presence. Many of the criteria have similar and overlapping conceptual meanings—for example, social discomfort of a patient with a schizoid personality disorder who has paranoid fears must be differentiated from the fear of embarrassment of a patient with avoidant personality disorder.

How can you make a diagnosis of a specific personality disorder? I suggest that there are four steps to be taken that will help you recognize specific personality disorders or traits:

1. Pay attention to the factors that raise your suspicion of the presence of a particular personality disorder, such as the interpersonal aspects of personality disorders that are outlined in the following section.
2. Look for the essential feature of the personality disorder as outlined in the DSM-IV-TR text.
3. Inquire for evidence of interpersonal functioning characteristic of that personality disorder in the history or evidence in the interactions during the clinical interview.
4. After the clinical interview, apply the full DSM-IV-TR criteria for the specific personality disorder to confirm the diagnosis. Or, if indicated, consider using self-report or semi-structured assessment measures to establish the diagnosis. (The use of these measures is discussed later in the chapter.)

Clinical decision making develops out of the formulation of clinical hypotheses that are then tested as further data are collected. Tentative suspicions about particular personality disorder diagnoses are common based on first encounters or first observations. Also, you should consider the setting in which the patient is being assessed. Although the prevalence of personality disorders is relatively low in the general population, the prevalence increases in certain clinical settings. For example, you would expect the lowest prevalence of personality disorders to be found in the community, slightly higher rates in outpatient settings, with again higher rates in inpatient settings, and perhaps the highest rates of some personality disorders in prisons or jail settings.

Having developed some hypotheses about what personality disorders or traits are present, review the following factors as you proceed with your clinical assessment:

- The prevalence of a particular personality disorder in a particular setting should be considered. For example, in a forensic setting, antisocial personality disorder would be more common, whereas in a medical or primary care clinic, you might expect a higher probability of anxious or dependent personality disorder diagnoses.

- How the patient has come to the clinician's attention is important. Try to differentiate whether there is an ego-dystonic or ego-syntonic pattern of distress that is explaining the presentation.
- The patient will have to be assessed for the presence of axis I disorders. Certain axis I disorders are thought to be more likely to coexist with certain personality disorders. For example, anxiety disorders may be more likely to be found in the anxious cluster personality disorders.
- A family history of psychiatric illness should be taken from the patient and available family members. You should ask about the occurrence of personality traits in family members. Disorders such as borderline personality disorder tend to run in families. Schizotypal and paranoid personality disorders are found with increased frequency in the family members of schizophrenic and paranoid psychotic patients.
- The developmental history should be reviewed, with an aim to look for specific risk factors that might be related to adult personality disturbance. For example, childhood shyness and fear of strangers in novel situations may raise the suspicion of an avoidant personality disorder. A history of childhood sexual abuse has been associated with the development of borderline personality disorder.
- A recurrent pattern of interpersonal interactions should be sought, as this pattern may point toward a specific personality disturbance.
- Assessing how severely the patient's functioning is affected is an important parameter. Personality disorders do seem to form a hierarchy based on the severity of dysfunction. As mentioned earlier, Skodol et al.[23] found empirical evidence that schizotypal and borderline personality disorder were characterized by dysfunction in essentially all realms, whereas less severe and more circumscribed dysfunction was more characteristic of obsessive compulsive personality disorder. Therefore, assessing level of functioning can lead to some understanding of the nature and severity of the personality disorder diagnosis.

INTERPERSONAL ASPECTS OF PERSONALITY DISORDERS

You should be aware that patients with personality disorders manifest their problems through cognitive, affective, interpersonal, and behavioral characteristics. *However, the key feature of all personality disorders is the pattern of interpersonal functioning that can be obtained from reviewing the patient's history of significant relationships and by observing the patient's interactions in the therapeutic*

Akhtar[33] clarified the clinical features of narcissistic personality disorder and described them in six realms. The first realm is self-concept, in which grandiosity is the central element, exemplified by a preoccupation with fantasies of outstanding success, an undue sense of uniqueness, feelings of entitlement, and a seeming self-sufficiency. This overt manifestation of grandiosity may indicate a covert feeling of inferiority. Interpersonal relationships are the second realm of this disorder. These people often demonstrate numerous shallow relationships with intense need for tribute from others. However, they typically lack empathy for others and are generally unable to participate in family life. They often have more of a relationship with their children than with their spouses. Akhtar[33] said the overt interpersonal charm hides their inability to trust others and to develop meaningful deep relationships. Persons in the third realm of social adaptation appear charming, successful, hardworking, and intensely ambitious. Underneath, however, they have a nagging aimlessness and a shallow commitment to things other than to achieve admiration. With regard to ethics, standards, and ideals, Akhtar's fourth realm, they can present with a caricatured modesty and appear moralistic, although their values will readily shift in order to gain favor. The fifth realm relates to love and sexuality. These persons are characterized with marital instability; they often have marital affairs, are promiscuous, and can be seductive without warmth or caring. They have difficulty viewing their romantic partners as separate individuals with their own interests, rights, and values. They may be unable to comprehend the incest taboo and occasionally will have sexual perversions. Lastly, the sixth realm describes cognitive style. Persons with narcissistic personality disorder in this realm can appear decisive, opinionated, knowledgeable, and articulate, with a love for language. They use language and dialogue to regulate their self-esteem and to control interactions rather than to foster intimate or meaningful dialogue.

Engaging a narcissistic person requires that you attend to his need for acknowledgment and accept, to some extent, his feelings of entitlement. For example, if you were seeing a family in which one of the spouses was narcissistic, it may require that you attend first to the narcissistic patient's needs as a means of initial engagement. By acknowledging that these needs are important and valued, often this will de-escalate the narcissistic patient's demand for recognition. Once some of the narcissistic need is acknowledged and met, often this allows for further engagement and cooperative dialogue.

Histrionic Personality Disorder

Persons with histrionic personality disorder can be charming, expressive, and dramatic. They tend to seek attention, and they can be manipulative to maintain the interest of others. They may use behavior, including seductive sexual behavior, suicide attempts, or even physical illness, to obtain your attention. Their cognitive style can be characterized by dichotomous thinking, overgeneralization, and emotional reasoning. Their typical exaggerated emotional responses are superficial but charming.

Interpersonally, these persons feel inadequate and seek the approval or attention of others, including clinicians. Horowitz[34] explained that patients with histrionic personality disorder seek attention to avoid their inner despair. However, they fear a loss of self-control when the desired attention is received. Through their demonstrations of helplessness, they provoke a rescuing response from the other person, including clinicians. Given that this response only reinforces their feelings of inadequacy, they reject the helpful response, leaving the clinician or rescuer feeling angry and helpless in return. Their personal histories will often demonstrate repeated life stories of moving from the role of victim to the aggressor and to the rescuer in their close relationships.[34] They can often play out this style of interaction with clinicians.

Engaging patients with histrionic personality disorder in therapy or clinical care can be difficult. Although they present as focusing on their emotional needs, these patients use emotions in a superficial manner, and they often need some overt behavioral response to foster a sense of trust. For example, if you are working with a histrionic patient, your adherence to a previously agreed-on plan and your demonstrating this can be very important. As one histrionic patient explained, "Talk is cheap."

Antisocial Personality Disorder

Patients with antisocial personality disorder are characterized by interpersonal difficulties that include irresponsibility, irritability, and impulsivity. However, these patients can appear slick and engaging and are quite cunning and calculating in relationships. They tend to be thrill seekers and engage in risk taking. They are impulsive and unable to delay gratification, and they lack empathy. They often show a history of criminal, aggressive, impulsive, and irresponsible behavior.

You must remember that these patients can be very engaging with a superficial charm and glibness. Such patients can pathologically lie and manipulate without experiencing guilt or remorse. Antisocial patients need to be assessed for the risk they present to other persons, particularly those who may be vulnerable when formulating management plans. Although patients with antisocial personality disorder are difficult to engage in ongoing treatment, patients with significant anxiety or depression or at a stage of readiness to tackle a substance abuse problem may benefit from appropriate treatment.

Cluster C: Anxious Cluster Personality Disorders

Obsessive Compulsive Personality Disorder

Patients with obsessive compulsive personality disorder are typically workaholics. They are concerned about productivity and order much more than emotional expression or interpersonal functioning. These persons need control more than they need interpersonal contact.

Such persons tend to be perfectionistic and dependable, although they can also be stubborn and possessive. Individuals with obsessive compulsive personality disorder are conscious of social status, obsequious to their superiors, and autocratic and demeaning to their subordinates. Their cognitive style includes concern for detail, need for certainty, and the belief that there is a correct solution for every problem. Their cognitive style is rule based, and they tend to be inflexible and unimaginative in their thinking. They have difficulty with emotional states, particularly in relation to feelings of anger and dependency. These patients demonstrate a need to control their emotions for fear of their expression. They often have difficulty with problem solving, with having appropriate empathy, and with challenges to their rigidity.

Engaging persons with obsessive compulsive personality disorder can be problematic because they are strongly defended and attempt to control or avoid therapeutic encounters. However, they can be engaged by focusing on two issues: keeping the patient in the here and now, rather than in the past or the future, and identifying with his emotional pain and distress. If you can recognize and verbalize some of the emotional distress that is defended, these patients will often feel reassured and will wish to engage. The patient may be reassured by simply having you acknowledge that he is not expected to trust the clinician after only a few sessions.

Dependent Personality Disorder

Persons with dependent personality disorder are characterized by being passive and nonassertive. Typically, they give a history of helpless behavior in their interpersonal relationships and show great indecision. They often have difficulties expressing anger directly and use passive-aggressive techniques instead. In relationships, they can appear self-sacrificing, going out of their way to be compliant and seeking the approval of others. Often they are characterized as "the nice guy." However, you may feel quite perplexed because although the patient appears to be approving, her behavior may communicate disapproval.

Dependency tends to be demonstrated in two dimensions. The first is called *attachment-related dependency,* which means that these persons show the dependency primarily in their emotional reliance on persons with whom they are involved in intimate relationships. Dependent persons tend to seek, attain, and retain a relationship with someone they see as stronger and wiser than themselves.[35] Sometimes, this attachment-related dependency can be manifest with their clinicians. The second dimension of dependency, *generalized dependency,* appears as a general lack of self-confidence and problems with assertiveness that affect all—not just intimate—relationships. These persons have more generalized relationship difficulties, and most relationships serve the purpose of eliciting assistance, guidance, and approval.[35] These persons show help-seeking behavior in most of their relationships, and they will seek out a number of people who they feel are potentially "nurturers, protectors, or caretakers."[36]

Engagement with dependent patients is not usually the difficulty. They rapidly form a dependency and initially appear as "the perfect patient." However, in the therapeutic relationship, they avoid conflict and do not openly express their needs. You have to attend to this lack of openness and expect that the patient's covert behavior could ultimately thwart the therapeutic plans.

Avoidant Personality Disorder

Patients with avoidant personality disorder are characterized by sensitivity, particularly to rejection. They desire to be accepted but keep their distance unless they have unconditional approval. They tend to be anxious, inhibited, and keep a noticeable distance, even during the interview. They lack skills to manage anxiety, to deal with social situations, and to assert themselves effectively in a relationship, including the clinician-patient relationship. They give a history of avoiding intimate or work-related relationships because they fear criticism, disapproval, or rejection.

It can be very difficult to engage patients with avoidant personality disorder. They tend to be reticent and inhibited, and you must anticipate that a true open relationship will take many months and perhaps years to develop.

CONFIRMING THE DIAGNOSIS

After a clinical interview is completed with a patient with a suspected personality disorder, you should attempt to confirm the personality disorder diagnosis by reviewing the full criteria from the DSM-IV-TR for the specific suspected diagnosis. If you can confirm the diagnosis after reviewing the criteria, then you should make a mental note of those features that first raised your suspicions for the diagnosis. Experienced clinicians can rapidly develop diagnostic hypotheses based on previous encounters with similar patients.

If you are unable to confirm the personality disorder diagnosis after reviewing the full criteria set, several steps to confirm the diagnosis should be considered. A patient with an acute axis I disorder will be difficult to assess for a personality disorder diagnosis. The personality disorder diagnosis may appropriately be deferred until the symptoms of the acute disorder have improved. During the acute state, clinicians are likely to overdiagnose personality disorders, and patients will likely overendorse personality pathology.[37] You should seek collateral information from family or friends about the patient's personality features. However, research findings indicate that agreement between the patient's report and the collateral informant is often poor,[37] and inconsistencies between the different sources of information can be difficult to reconcile. Zimmerman[37] suggested that the patient's report should be used for information about affective or cognitive aspects of personality, whereas the informant may be more reliable about the person's interpersonal or behavioral functioning.

If you are still uncertain about the personality disorder diagnosis, many assessment tools are available to confirm or refute your clinical impression. These assessment tools fall into four categories: self-report measures for personality traits rather than disorders, self-report measures for personality disorders, semi-structured interviews for personality traits, and semi-structured interviews for personality disorders. For an extensive discussion of these instruments, Clark and Harrison[38] provide an excellent overview of all the measures in each category. One example from each type of measure will be highlighted, including a discussion of how you might utilize this or other similar measures in your assessment.

Self-Report Measures for Personality Traits

The NEO Personality Inventory–Revised is a widely used instrument that assesses subjects for five domains of normal personality: neuroticism, extraversion, conscientiousness, agreeableness, and openness. The so-called Five-Factor Model of personality appears to capture the central dimensions that make up normal personality. The scale is usually administered and scored by a clinical psychologist, and the inventory contains 240 items and takes about 50 minutes to administer.[39,40]

Self-Report Measures for Personality Disorders

The Millon Clinical Multiaxial Inventory (MCMI-III) was developed to reflect its author's conceptions of the various personality disorder constructs rather than DSM personality disorders. However, this instrument has been widely used to make a range of personality disorder diagnoses for both clinical and research purposes. The test is usually administered and scored by a clinical psychologist. The test involves answering 175 true/false questions, and about 30 minutes are required to administer the test.[41,42]

Semi-Structured Interview for Personality Traits

The Psychopathy Checklist–Revised was specifically developed to assess subjects for the concept of psychopathy. The ratings are made based on information from a clinical interview and a review of collateral information; however, these ratings require considerable clinical judgment and expertise. Although psychopathy is somewhat related to antisocial personality disorder, the measure has been primarily used to predict recidivism in forensic settings.[43,44]

Semi-Structured Interview for Personality Disorders

There are five established semi-structured interview assessments for making DSM personality disorder diagnoses. One of the most widely used versions is called the Structured Clinical Interview for DSM-IV Axis II Personality Disorders. This measure requires trained interviewers and takes more than an hour to administer, sometimes several hours. The structured interviews have allowed for improved inter-rater agreement compared with that obtained from a clinical interview; however, the validity of these instruments has not been adequately demonstrated. Typically, these structured interviews are used for research purposes or in tertiary specialized clinical settings.[45-47]

SPECIFIC CHALLENGES IN WORKING WITH PATIENTS WITH PERSONALITY DISORDERS

The following is a list of some specific challenges that you might encounter in working with patients with personality disorders:

- These patients can provoke strong emotional responses in clinicians. If these patients are causing you to extend appointment times beyond their scheduled times, to have sleepless nights, or to do anything you would feel uncomfortable discussing with colleagues, a consultation regarding the patient's management is recommended.

- Patients with personality disorders often feel invalidated or dismissed by clinicians. These patients may be helped if you take the time to explain the diagnosis and validate their experience—acknowledge that there are explanations for their problems and their distress.

- Family members of a patient with a personality disorder often have no information about the patient's diagnosis and have no idea how to be of assistance to their relative. With the patient's consent, the family may be informed how to respond if a crisis arises and how to support and encourage the patient's compliance with treatment.

- Patients who have a history of repeated negative encounters with clinicians and who feel victimized by these interactions should probably not be seen alone by you or at the end of the day when no one else is in the office.

- Three fundamentals beliefs should form your attitudes when working with patients with personality disorders:
  - Self-determination: These patients should be active participants in all phases of their care and treatment. Encouraging this active involvement will reinforce the patient's feelings of empowerment and competence.
  - Focus on functioning: In assessing outcome, you should not lose sight of the improvement obtained in the patient's role functioning and quality of life. Functioning should be assessed over and above the changes in symptom status.
  - Maintaining hope: You are justified in maintaining hope rather than aggravating the sense of hopelessness. You should use a longitudinal perspective to observe and assess the person's changes.

- Patients with personality disorders may report that one clinician is all good while another clinician is all bad or even dangerous. Particularly when working with borderline patients, you must recognize that these patients are vulnerable to *splitting,* or extreme perceptions of others, and the likely reality is somewhere in between the extremes.

FOLLOW-UP ON CASES

Case Example 1

Mr. A. was thought to suffer from depersonalization disorder and avoidant personality disorder. He made significant progress with his problems at work once he was educated about depersonalization, anxiety, and avoidant behavior. He gained an understanding that anxiety was time-limited and that he could overcome his anxiety by exposing himself to stressful situations. Mr. A. found that a small dose of citalopram reduced his anxiety and

the occurrence of depersonalization. With his improvement, his doctor encouraged Mr. A. to force himself to approach customers, in spite of some remaining anxiety. The patient was rewarded with increasing sales. Mr. A. continued to avoid most other social situations and most other people, although he was more active socially with colleagues at work.

Case Example 2

Ms. B. eventually settled in the emergency department and accepted a referral to a "safe bed" with a community crisis home. Unfortunately, Ms. B. returned to the emergency department later the same weekend. As the patient's presentation was very similar at that time, she was not thought to require further intervention and certainly not an admission to hospital. When the doctor returned to the emergency cubicle to explain, rather curtly, that admission was not indicated, the patient became violent, threw her dinner tray at the unsuspecting doctor, and stormed out of the emergency department.

Case Example 3

Mr. C. was diagnosed as having a substance abuse disorder, primarily alcohol, and also met criteria for borderline and schizotypal personality disorders. He attended follow-up appointments, and his therapist was eventually able to connect his suicide attempt to the loss of an attractive coworker who had suddenly quit her job the week before. With the help of his therapist, the patient began to recognize the many negative consequences of his drinking and entered into an alcohol rehabilitation program.

Key Point:

There are four steps to be taken that will help you recognize specific personality disorders or traits:
1. Pay attention to the factors that raise your suspicion of the presence of a particular personality disorder.
2. Look for the essential feature of the personality disorder as outlined in the DSM-IV-TR.
3. Look for evidence in the history of interpersonal functioning characteristic of that personality disorder or in the interactions during the clinical interview.
4. After the clinical interview, apply the full DSM-IV-TR criteria for the specific personality disorder to confirm the diagnosis. Or, if indicated, consider using self-report or semi-structured assessment measures to establish the diagnosis.

> **Key Point:**
> _____
>
> The key feature of all personality disorders is the pattern of interpersonal functioning that can be obtained by reviewing the patient's history of significant relationships and observing the patient's interactions in the therapeutic encounter.

> **Key Point:**
> _____
>
> Patients with personality disorders can provoke strong emotional responses in clinicians. If these patients are causing you to extend appointment times beyond their scheduled times, to have sleepless nights, or to do anything you would feel uncomfortable discussing with colleagues, a consultation regarding the patient's management is recommended.

CONCLUSIONS

If you use your clinical skills to develop an understanding of what patients with personality disorders are experiencing, you will have a real opportunity to assist these patients. Understanding what a personality disorder is and what the implications of this diagnosis are and learning the skills to recognize a personality disorder will help you in your work with these patients. You must demonstrate the attitudes that foster the patients' active participation, attend to their quality of life, and maintain hope. Ultimately, you can develop the necessary skills, and you can experience what it is like to help these difficult but rewarding patients with personality disorders.

REFERENCES

1. Swartz M, Blazer D, George L, et al: Estimating the prevalence of borderline personality disorder in the community, *J Pers Disorders* 4:257–272, 1990.
2. American Psychiatric Association: *Diagnostic and statistical manual of mental disorders*, ed 4, text revision, Washington, DC, 2000, American Psychiatric Association.
3. World Health Organization: *The ICD-10 classification of mental and behavioral disorders,* Geneva, 1992, World Health Organization.
4. Marttunen MJ, Aro HM, Henriksson MM, et al: Mental disorders in adolescent suicides. DSM-III-R axes I and II diagnoses in suicides among 13- to 19-year-olds in Finland, *Arch Gen Psychiatry* 48:834–839, 1991.
5. Marttunen MJ, Aro HM, Henriksson MM, et al: Antisocial behavior in adolescent suicide, *Acta Psychiatr Scand* 89:167–173, 1994.
6. Beautrais AL, Joyce PR, Mulder RT, et al: Prevalence and comorbidity of mental disorders in persons making serious suicide attempts: a case-control study, *Am J Psychiatry* 153:1009–1014, 1996.
7. Maddocks PD: A five year follow-up of untreated psychopaths, *Br J Psychiatry* 116:511–515, 1970.
8. Laub JH, Vaillant GE: Delinquency and mortality: a 50-year follow-up study of 1,000 delinquent and nondelinquent boys, *Am J Psychiatry* 157:96–102, 2000.
9. Crumley FE: Adolescent suicide attempts, *JAMA* 241:2404–2407, 1979.
10. Paris J, Zweig-Frank H: A 27-year follow-up of patients with borderline personality disorder, *Compr Psychiatry* 42:482–487, 2001.
11. Gunderson JG: *Borderline personality disorder,* Washington, DC, 1984, American Psychiatric Press.
12. Kjellander C, Bongar B, King A: Suicidality in borderline personality disorder, *Crisis* 19:125–135, 1998.
13. Linehan M: *Cognitive behavioral treatment of borderline personality disorder,* New York, 1993, Guilford.
14. Stanley B, Gameroff MJ, Michalsen V, et al: Are suicide attempters who self-mutilate a unique population? *Am J Psychiatry* 158:427–432, 2001.
15. Forman EM, Berk MS, Henriques GR, et al: History of multiple suicide attempts as a behavioral marker of severe psychopathology, *Am J Psychiatry* 161:437–443, 2004.
16. Yen S, Shea MT, Pagano M, et al: Axis I and axis II disorders as predictors of prospective suicide attempts: findings from the Collaborative Longitudinal Personality Disorders Study, *J Abnorm Psychol* 112:375–381, 2003.
17. Koerner K, Linehan MM: Research on dialectical behavior therapy for patients with borderline personality disorder, *Psychiatr Clin North Am* 23:151–167, 2000.
18. Reich JH, Green AI: Effect of personality disorders on outcome of treatment, *J Nerv Ment Dis* 179:74–82, 1991.
19. Mulder RT: Personality pathology and treatment outcome in major depression: a review, *Am J Psychiatry* 159:359–371, 2002.
20. Jang KL, Vernon PA: Genetics. In Livesley WJ, editor: *Handbook of personality disorders: theory, research and treatment,* New York, 2001, The Guilford Press, pp 177–195.
21. Paris J: Psychosocial adversity. In Livesley WJ, editor: *Handbook of personality disorders: theory, research and treatment,* New York, 2001, The Guilford Press, pp 231–241.
22. Zanarini MC, Frankenburg FR, Hennen J, et al: The longitudinal course of borderline psychopathology: 6-year prospective follow-up of the phenomenology of borderline personality disorder, *Am J Psychiatry* 160:274–283, 2003.
23. Skodol AE, Gunderson JG, McGlashan TH, et al: Functional impairment in patients with schizotypal, borderline, avoidant, and obsessive compulsive personality disorder, *Am J Psychiatry* 159:276–283, 2002.
24. American Psychiatric Association: *Practice guidelines for the treatment of patients with borderline personality*

disorders, Washington, DC, 2001, American Psychiatric Association.

25. Sperry L: *Handbook of diagnosis and treatment of the DSM-IV personality disorders*, New York, 1995, Brunner/Mazel.

26. Paris J: *Social factors in personality disorders: a biopsychosocial approach to etiology and treatment*, Cambridge, UK, 1996, Cambridge University Press.

27. Freud S: Libidinal types (1931). In *Standard edition*. London, 1961, Hogarth Press, pp 215–220.

28. Waelder R: The psychoses, their mechanisms and accessibility to influence, *Int J Psychoanal* 6:259–281, 1925.

29. Reich W: *Character analysis (1933)*, ed 3, New York, 1972, Farrar, Strauss & Giroux (Translated by VR Carfagno).

30. Fenichel O: *The psychoanalytic theory of neurosis*, New York, 1945, Norton.

31. Kernberg OF: *Borderline conditions and pathological narcissism*, New Haven, CT, 1975, Yale University Press.

32. Kohut H: *Analysis of the self*, New York, 1971, International Universities Press.

33. Akhtar S: Narcissistic personality disorder: descriptive features and differential diagnosis, *Psychiatr Clin North Am* 12:505–529, 1989.

34. Horowitz MJ: Psychotherapy for histrionic personality disorder, *J Psychother Pract Res* 6:93–107, 1997.

35. Livesley WJ, Schroeder ML, Jackson DN: Dependent personality disorder and attachment problems, *J Pers Disorders* 4:131–140, 1990.

36. Bornstein RF: The dependent personality: developmental, social and clinical perspectives, *Psychol Bull* 112:3–23, 1992.

37. Zimmerman M: Diagnosing personality disorders: a review of issues and research methods, *Arch Gen Psychiatry* 51:225–245, 1994.

38. Clark LA, Harrison JA: Assessment instruments. In Livesley WJ, editor: *Handbook of personality disorders: theory, research and treatment*, New York, 2001, The Guilford Press, pp 277–306.

39. Costa PT, McCrae RR: Normal personality assessment in clinical practice: the NEO Personality Inventory, *Psychol Assess* 4:5–13, 1989.

40. Costa PT, McCrae RR: The five-factor model of personality and its relevance to personality disorders, *J Pers Disorders* 6:343–359, 1992.

41. Millon T, Davis RD: The MCMI-III: present and future research directions, *J Pers Assess* 68:69–85, 1997.

42. Millon T, Davis R, Millon C: *Manual for the Millon Clinical Multiaxial Inventory–III (MCMI-III)*, Minneapolis, MN, 1994, National Computer Systems.

43. Hare RD, Harpur TJ, Hakstian AR, et al: The Revised Psychopathy Checklist: descriptive statistics, reliability, and factor structure, *Psychol Assess* 2:228–259, 1990.

44. Hare RD: *The Hare psychopathy checklist–revised manual*, North Tonawanda, NY, 1991, Multi-Health Systems.

45. First M, Spitzer RL, Gibbon M, et al: The structured clinical interview for DSM-III-R personality disorders (SCID-II): part I. Description, *J Pers Disorders* 9:83–91, 1995.

46. First MB, Spitzer RL, Gibbon M, et al: The structured clinical interview for DSM-III-R personality disorders (SCID-II): part II. Multi-site test-retest reliability study, *J Pers Disorders* 9:92–104, 1995.

47. First M, Gibbon M, Spitzer RL, et al: *User's guide for the structured clinical interview for the DSM-IV axis II personality disorders*, Washington, DC, 1997, American Psychiatric Press.

RECOMMENDED READINGS

American Psychiatric Association: *Practice guidelines for the treatment of patients with borderline personality disorders*, Washington, DC, 2001, American Psychiatric Association.

Gunderson JG: *Borderline personality disorder: a clinical guide*, Washington, DC, 2001, American Psychiatric Publishing Inc.

Livesley WJ: *Handbook of personality disorders: theory, research and treatment*. New York, 2001, The Guilford Press.

Paris J: *Nature and nurture in psychiatry: a predisposition-stress model of mental disorders*, Washington, DC, 1999, American Psychiatric Press.

Sperry L: *Handbook of diagnosis and treatment of the DSM-IV personality disorders*, New York, 1995, Brunner/Mazel.

9

Assessment of Patients with Eating Disorders

ALLAN S. KAPLAN AND LARA J. OSTOLOSKY

INTRODUCTION

An eating disorder diagnosis requires the presence of both disordered eating behavior and characteristic psychological disturbance. There are two eating disorders currently recognized in the American Psychiatric Association's *Diagnostic and Statistical Manual of Mental Disorders*, Fourth Edition, Text Revision (DSM-IV-TR): anorexia nervosa (AN) and bulimia nervosa (BN). There is a third eating disorder, binge eating disorder (BED), which, although not currently officially recognized by DSM-IV-TR, has gained increasing validity as a serious clinical problem. Persons with BED are almost always overweight or obese. Obesity in the absence of disordered eating and psychological disturbance is not considered an eating disorder but rather a metabolic disturbance. Only about 30% to 40% of obese persons have an eating disorder, which is usually BED.[1] In this chapter, however, we will focus primarily on the assessment of AN and BN in adults, although the principles enunciated here are generally applicable to the assessment of children and adolescents with AN or BN and to patients with BED.

By the end of this chapter you should:

1. Know the criteria for these illnesses as defined in the DSM-IV-TR
2. Be aware of the differences in presentation of AN and BN
3. Understand the critical components in engaging patients in the interview
4. Know the basic differences between interviewing adults and children/adolescents with these illnesses
5. Understand how to fully assess a person with a potential eating disorder

6. Be aware of the medical complications.
7. Have a clear idea as to what preliminary treatment the person will need
8. Know what questions to ask collateral sources—particularly the families of persons with eating disorders
9. Have some understanding of these illnesses from the perspective of the person with the eating disorder

These eating disorders are challenging illnesses to treat; a proper comprehensive assessment is critical to the planning of appropriate treatment interventions for these disorders. Although they are most commonly seen in adolescent and young women, eating disorders also occur infrequently in young children, males, and in the elderly.

Eating disorders were once thought to only occur in white, upper-middle-class families, but the epidemiology of these disorders has changed somewhat over the past quarter century so that they now cross all ethnic and racial lines as well as all social classes. Although they are much more common in Westernized cultures, they do occur in non-Westernized societies.

The understanding of the etiology of these conditions has also changed quite dramatically over the past several decades. For many years, eating disorders were thought to be almost entirely due to environmental factors, including a society that objectified women and idealized a thin body shape, as well as due to a dysfunctional family, including family dynamics that contribute to a child being parentified and leading to fears of psychobiological maturity and arrested development in the young teenager. These factors were thought to contribute to an internal sense of a lack of control in one's life, leading to a need to control one's weight.

There have also been other hypothesized contributors to this central core feeling of ineffectiveness, including sexual abuse and characterological traits such as perfectionism.

In the last 20 years, however, interest and research into the neurobiology and genetics of these illnesses have increased. This process of elucidating important neurobiological etiological factors in eating disorders has been analogous to the process of deciphering the pathophysiology of schizophrenia, which has evolved over the past 50 years, from thinking schizophrenia was caused primarily by pathological mothering to more understanding of the neurobiological basis of this severe mental illness. It is now understood that eating disorders have biological, psychological, and sociocultural risk factors that contribute to their pathogenesis. It is important to detect the presence of an eating disorder as early as possible because these disorders generally have a better prognosis when treated earlier. In addition, they are often accompanied by serious medical and psychiatric complications, some of which can be fatal. Eating disorders may be only one aspect of the patient's psychiatric pathology, as these illnesses commonly coexist with other psychiatric and personality difficulties.[2]

Key Point:

Do not assume that all obese persons have an eating disorder; only about 30% to 40% do. An eating disorder requires two features: disordered eating behavior and characteristic psychological disturbance. Therefore, obesity in the absence of disordered eating and psychological disturbance is not considered an eating disorder but rather a metabolic disturbance or a multidetermined state involving genes and environment that does not reflect a core psychopathology.

Case Example 1

Anorexia Nervosa. **K** is a 25-year-old white woman who has two younger siblings and lives with her parents. She was attending university until she became too underweight to continue and is presently unemployed. She is 163 cm (5 ft 4 in) tall and her body mass index (BMI; kg/m^2) at presentation was 14.8 with a weight of 39.2 kg (86.4 lb). The lower end of normal BMI is 20, or a weight of 53 kg (116.8 lb) for someone of K's height. She has had two other hospitalizations for her low weight status, and she has been chronically ill for 6 years. Her highest weight before the onset of her illness was 59 kg (130 lb) at age 18. K restricts her food intake essentially to coffee during the day and overall eats less than 800 calories per day. She also walks up to 6 miles per day. She feels compelled to continue these behaviors as she becomes very anxious with the idea of any weight gain and already feels that she is fat. She

has a tearful affect, severe insomnia, and an inability to concentrate. She has numerous medical difficulties related to her AN but the most severe include bradycardia, edema, osteopenia, amenorrhea, and constipation. She also has severe social phobia, depressed mood, and compulsive grooming rituals taking hours in the morning. There is also a documented history of physical and emotional abuse toward her and her sister by her parents, but they have attempted to be supportive since she became ill.

Case Example 2

Bulimia Nervosa. **B** is a 24-year-old white woman who lives with three female roommates and works as a physical education teacher. She has a 3-year history of daily episodes of binge eating followed by self-induced vomiting. She also exercises compulsively. She has never been overweight in her life and presently weighs 53.2 kg (117.3 lb) and is 157 cm (5 ft 2 in) tall. This corresponds to a BMI of 21.2. She does have concerns that she looks fat, and the feelings of fullness after eating result in high anxiety and physical discomfort resulting in vomiting. She has also previously used diet pills and herbal weight-loss products. Her last boyfriend told her she was fat and sexually abused her. She is very sensitive to criticism and rejection, and her mood is very depressed. There is a history of alcoholism in her grandmother, depression in her sister, and bipolar disorder in her mother, who has been chronically weight and shape concerned. There are strained family relations, and B feels compelled to try to sort out the family problems. Her family is unaware of her eating disorder, and she does not feel she can tell them or rely on their support. She is quite ashamed of her disordered eating behavior, although she has found that it temporarily relieves her anxiety and depressed mood. She abuses alcohol, getting intoxicated weekly, for the same reason. Her medical complications include episodes of hematemesis, heartburn, and an irregular heartbeat.

DSM-IV-TR Diagnostic Criteria for AN

1. Refusal to maintain body weight at or above a minimally normal weight for age and height (weight loss leading to maintenance of body weight less than 85% of that expected; or failure to make expected weight gain during a period of growth, leading to a body weight of less than 85% of that expected)

2. Intense fear of gaining weight or becoming fat even though underweight

3. Disturbance in the way in which one's body weight is experienced, undue influence of body weight or shape

on self-evaluation, or denial of the seriousness of the current low body weight

4. In postmenarchal females, amenorrhea (the absence of three consecutive menstrual cycles)

Subtypes
Restricting Type
During the current episode of AN, the person has *not* regularly engaged in binge-eating or purging behavior.

Binge-Eating/Purging Type
During the current episode of AN, the person has regularly engaged in binge-eating or purging behavior.

DSM-IV-TR Diagnostic Criteria for BN

1. Recurrent episodes of binge eating. An episode of binge eating is characterized by eating, in a discrete period of time, an amount of food that is definitely larger than most people would eat during a similar period of time or under similar circumstances. It also consists of a sense of lack of control over eating during the episode (e.g., a feeling that one cannot stop eating or control how much one is eating).

2. The person engages in recurrent inappropriate compensatory behavior to prevent weight gain, such as self-induced vomiting; misuse of laxatives, diuretics, enemas or other medications; fasting; or excessive exercise.

3. The binge-eating and compensatory behavior to prevent weight gain both occur, on average, at least twice a week for 3 months.

4. Self-evaluation is unduly influenced by body weight and shape.

5. The disturbance does not occur exclusively during episodes of AN. There are two types:
   a. The purging type: During the current episode of BN, a person has regularly engaged in self-induced vomiting or the misuse of laxatives, diuretics, or enemas.
   b. The nonpurging type: The person has used other inappropriate compensatory behaviors, such as fasting or excessive exercise, but has not regularly engaged in the purging methods.

DSM-IV-TR Diagnostic Criteria for Eating Disorder Not Otherwise Specified (Including Binge Eating Disorder)

These examples do not meet the full criteria for either AN or BN:

1. All of the criteria for AN are met except the person has regular menses.

2. All of the criteria for AN are met except that, despite significant weight loss, the person's weight is in the normal range.

3. All of the criteria for BN are met except that the binge eating and the inappropriate compensatory mechanisms occur at a frequency of less than twice a week or for a duration of less than 3 months.

4. There is regular use of inappropriate compensatory behaviors by a person of normal body weight after eating small amounts of food.

5. The person repeatedly chews and spits out, but does not swallow, large amounts of food.

6. BED involves recurrent episodes of binge eating in the absence of the regular use of inappropriate compensatory behaviors characteristic of BN. BED patients are usually overweight or obese because of the regular binge eating that occurs without compensation (e.g., purging, exercise, or fasting).

Proposed Criteria for BED

1. Recurrent episodes of binge eating. An episode of binge eating is characterized by both of the following:
   - Eating, in a discrete period of time, an amount of food that is definitely larger than most people would eat in similar period of time under similar circumstances
   - A sense of lack of control over eating during the episode

2. The binge-eating episodes are associated with three (or more) of the following:
   - Eating much more rapidly than normal
   - Eating until feeling uncomfortably full
   - Eating large amounts of food when not feeling physically hungry
   - Eating alone because of being embarrassed by how much one is eating
   - Feeling disgusted with oneself, depressed, or very guilty after overeating

3. Marked distress regarding binge eating is present.

4. The binge eating occurs, on average, at least 2 days a week for 6 months.

5. The binge eating is not associated with the regular use of inappropriate compensatory behaviors and does not occur exclusively during the course of AN or BN.

Differences in the Presentation of AN and BN

There are differences in the presentation of AN compared with BN. The anorexic's symptoms are ego-syntonic; that is, the patient is not usually disturbed by her symptoms, especially her weight loss. She typically minimizes the medical complications resulting from weight loss or attributes them to other difficulties. She does not see why the people around her are concerned and secretly feels proud of her accomplishment of weight loss. If she does agree to treatment, it is often for the purposes of appeasing concerned persons or because she desires treatment for a depressed mood or similar psychiatric or medical difficulty associated with her eating disorder. Patients with AN do not usually come seeking help of their own accord; concerned people around them usually coerce them to seek care. Bulimic persons, on the other hand, are different because, although they do not wish to gain weight, they are distressed by their bingeing and purging. They are usually embarrassed that they engage in these behaviors and wish to eliminate them. It is not clearly evident to anyone else that the person with BN has any eating problems; she often appears of normal weight and tends to keep her symptoms to herself because of the shame and embarrassment associated with her binge eating and purging. The anorexic person tends to see her weight loss as an accomplishment and tends to feel proud of it and will therefore tenaciously hold on to it, whereas the bulimic wishes to be rid of her disordered eating. Many bulimic patients feel like "failed anorexics" because they would like to have the self-control to restrict their food intake, but they are unable to and end up bingeing instead. Both AN and BN patients tend to try to hide their bodies and to dress in baggy clothes, but for different reasons. Anorexic patients may try to hide their weight loss because of the obvious negative attention their emaciation brings and for fear of demands for weight increase by parents and clinicians. Bulimic patients tend to be normal or slightly overweight and to be ashamed of their bodies and their weight and shape. A significant challenge for parents and clinicians in assessing and treating these disorders is that the end goal for persons with both AN and BN—a thin body shape—is something society promotes as worthwhile and desirable. As a result, there are powerful forces that reinforce the pathological ideas and behaviors seen in patients with eating disorder. For a vulnerable person with low self-worth, little self-confidence, and a feeling of ineffectiveness, this pursuit of thinness becomes an all-consuming endeavor in the pursuit of external validation.[3]

Engaging Patients in the Interview

Assessment of eating disorders presents some challenges in engaging patients.[4] These are primarily related to their lack of trust of authority and their intense need to feel in control. Their fears can include fear of weight gain, of over-eating and bingeing, of hospitalization and confinement, and of loss of control of their lives. Their symptoms may also serve very powerful functions in their life, which can include the need to keep a family together,

attention seeking, the modulation of negative mood states, a fear of psychological and physical maturity, and a fear of sexuality.

You can facilitate the engagement process with people with eating disorders by doing the following:

- Explain that anxiety and apprehension are understandable and expected, given the nature of their problem.
- Be empathic, gentle, validating, and nonjudgmental while not colluding with their denial of illness.
- Be aware of and monitor your counter-transference; persons with eating disorders may invoke anger, frustration, and helplessness in caregivers, and these patients are very sensitive to and aware of such reactions, having evoked similar reactions in members of their own family.
- Be completely honest with patients about the need for nutritional rehabilitation and weight gain. It is best to take a matter-of-fact stance about the realities of the illnesses and not collude with the person in her denial of symptoms and the risks associated with her pathological behaviors. Persons with eating disordered will not engage with a clinician if they do not feel that the clinician is knowledgeable about eating disorders in general and if the clinician does not demonstrate specific expertise about their problems in the interview.
- Be patient and collaborative while recognizing that the person is unique.
- Ensure the interview is focused and systematic. Try to put the person at ease and take time to develop a therapeutic alliance. This is facilitated by explaining who you are and what your intention is in doing the assessment.
- Ensure that you interview the patient in a private room, setting aside adequate time to do a comprehensive assessment, which usually takes at least 1 hour. Explain from the outset what will be done, how long the assessment will take, and the potential plan after the assessment.
- Provide education about the illness, including written material.
- For a patient over the age of consent, interviewing the person alone without family members present is essential. In the absence of clear suicidal risk, for adult patients, any contact with family should occur only with the patient's consent and only in the patient's presence. For younger patients, involvement of the family in the assessment process is critical and whenever possible should occur with the patient present.

The engagement process can be *inhibited* by the following:

- Assuming the person is difficult to engage because she has an underlying personality problem that interferes with interpersonal relatedness. Patients with eating disorders may have abnormal brain chemistry, usually related to starvation, that can interfere with a patient's capacity to concentrate and that can exacerbate characterological traits.

- Using scare tactics, threats of hospitalization, and arguing with the patient.
- Trying to be too authoritative.
- Being unprepared for what you might see. Some persons may be very inhibited and shy whereas others may be outwardly hostile and threatening. Keep in mind that some persons may have been living with their eating disorder for so many years that they do not know how they would manage anxiety without the behaviors or what identity they would have without the illness. Others do not, in fact, see their behavior as abnormal and may be surprised when they are told they have a psychiatric illness.
- Using too many close-ended questions. It is important to start each section of the interview with an open-ended question and then get more specific as you hear what the patient reveals. It is also important to wait to give the patient time to answer because how she answers can give clues about the degree of resistance in revealing her symptoms and accepting treatment.

Differences Between Interviewing Adults and Children with Eating Disorders

The interview and assessment of a child or a young adolescent with an eating disorder have some unique features. There is a certain level of increased urgency involved in the assessment of children because they become medically compromised more quickly than adults do because they do not have the same energy reserves. The effects of weight loss and malnutrition are more critical because the person is in a growth and development phase, which can be permanently affected by weight and nutritional compromise. It is also much more challenging to assess for mood and anxiety in younger patients. Involvement of the family in the assessment is critical; in addition, the assessment of a child or adolescent with an eating disorder needs to involve the school and the child's primary care physician or pediatrician. After nutritional and weight stabilization, one of the primary modalities of treatment is family therapy, especially when the child is under the age of consent and still living at home.

ASSESSMENT

Five major sections will be discussed as part of the assessment process: the clinical interview, collateral information, physical examination, investigations, and differential diagnoses.[5]

Although the identification of differential diagnoses is an important part of the entire assessment process, it cannot be adequately arrived at until all other components of the assessment have been completed. The process outlined here focuses on interviewing adults rather than children.

Key Point:

The assessment needs to be very detailed, especially regarding weight, eating, and comorbid features, including medical complications. Spending the time to conduct a detailed assessment will facilitate the person in feeling you understand her distress and disorder. As well, patients may not volunteer specific information unless you ask about it. They may feel humiliated and embarrassed.

Clinical Interview

Demographics

Demographics includes age, marital status, whether there are children, the living situation, including with whom (e.g., spouse, parents, siblings, children) and where the person lives, education, employment and financial status, and religious affiliation. The person's religious or cultural background is important to inquire about because she may have food restrictions and cultural rituals around eating related to cultural or religious practice. How the patient is financially supported is important in relation to her level of practical independence.

Key Point:

Do not assume that if the person is not white that she cannot have an eating disorder. Similarly, do not assume that if a female patient is of normal weight or even overweight, she cannot have an eating disorder.

Chief Complaint

Have the person state in her own words what brought her in for an assessment. It is important to note how much insight she has into her problem; does she recognize that there is a psychological basis to her difficulties, or does she only see it only as a behavioral problem?

History of Presenting Illness
Weight History

This must be documented in the interview because it reveals the severity of illness. If the patient does not know her weight, you should weigh her without her shoes and, if possible, with her wearing a hospital gown. If the patient refuses, you should explain the importance of an accurate weight because low weights are associated with psychological, cognitive, and physical changes. Patients with eating disorders are notoriously unreliable in their self-estimation of their weight.

Possible questions to ask include the following:

- *"What do you weigh now? How tall are you?"* This allows you to calculate her corresponding BMI. A healthy BMI is between 20 and 25.
- *"What is the most you have ever weighed as a teenager? As an adult? What is the least you have ever weighed as a teenager? As an adult? When these weights occurred, for how long did you weigh that much, and what were your eating patterns like at the time?"*
- *"What weight tends to be the most stable for you without dieting?"* This may have to be elicited from family because the patient may tell you a lower weight than is realistic. This question allows the clinician to determine where the patient's weight may need to be to have the best chance of curbing eating disordered behaviors such as binge eating.
- *"At what weight did your periods become irregular or stop? At what weight did your periods stop for three months or more?"* This helps to determine a minimum goal weight associated with return of normal menstrual function.
- *"How do you feel about your weight and your sense of how your body looks?"* The importance of assessing body image cannot be overemphasized. Many persons will tell you that they have lost weight or are trying to control their weight for reasons such as health or fitness; it is important to point out to patients that typically, the more weight they lose, the more disturbed their body image becomes and the stronger their drive for thinness.
- *"What do you see as your ideal weight? Do you see certain body parts as overweight, and if so, which ones?"* These persons often see specific body parts as unrealistically large or feel that after eating their body parts are "growing." How would her life be different at her ideal weight? This may help elucidate desired and even worthwhile goals for which disordered eating is a maladaptive and largely unsuccessful mechanism.
- *"What would being at a weight that didn't require dieting mean for you in terms of how you think of yourself as a person?"*
- *"When did you first become concerned with your weight or shape? Were you ever teased about it?"*
- *"What was your weight like as a young child and as a teenager? Were you ever involved in activities such as competitive sports, ballet, gymnastics, or modeling where your weight or shape were very important?"*
- *"Do you avoid activities now that require you to expose your body, such as swimming?"*

- The patient should gently be asked about any relationship between significant life events and weight status. This can help to make her aware of the connection between emotions and feelings about weight and shape by identifying upsetting life events that contributed to dissatisfaction with weight and shape.

Eating-Disordered Behaviors History

Persons with eating disorders may engage in many typical behaviors that characterize their illness. It is important that you ask about each of these because the person may not disclose them without your asking; specific behaviors may give clues as to potential medical complications, diagnostic information, and prognosis.

An important question you should ask is regarding what methods the patient uses to control her weight. It is important to specifically ask about the nature, frequency, and duration of the following behaviors:

- Food restriction
- Self-induced vomiting
- Laxative abuse (number taken and type)
- Diuretic or diet pill use (number taken and type)
- Use of herbal weight loss products (number taken and type)
- Thyroid medication abuse or ipecac use (number taken and type)
- Manipulation of insulin, if patient is a diabetic, to lose weight
- Use of illicit substances, such as amphetamines or cocaine, to control weight
- Level of exercise

Food Restriction

Food restriction is always present in AN and BN in one form or another. Possible questions to ask include the following:

- *"How do you limit what you eat? Do you skip meals? Do you steer clear of certain food items or food groups? Do you go on fasts? Over what period of time has all this occurred?"*
- *"Do you ever hoard or hide food or try to dispose of food?"*
- *"Do you avoid eating with others?"*
- *"Do you have any 'forbidden' foods? Do you have categories of foods that are 'good' and 'bad'?"*

Exercise

Exercise, in terms of types and frequency, is important especially in the face of a compromised medical state.

Exercising in the context of an eating disorder should always be considered illness behavior. Such exercise is characteristically done alone and in a rigid, repetitive, and compulsive manner that is rarely pleasurable or has any goal other than burning calories.

Possible questions to ask include the following:

- *"Why do you exercise?"*
- *"Do you feel compelled to exercise or feel guilty if you cannot?"*
- *"Do you base the amount of exercise you do on the number of calories you eat?"* It is not uncommon to see persons who will never take an elevator or will refuse to sit down if they can stand. These can be pathological behaviors aimed at expending calories.

Food Rituals

Persons with eating disorders also may have unusual food-related rituals or patterns of eating. Possible questions to ask include the following:

- *"Do you chew and spit out food or regurgitate it?"*
- *"Do you use of a lot of caffeine or gum chewing to curb your appetite?"*
- *"Are you a vegetarian?"* In the context of an eating disorder, this is almost always driven by a fear of fat.
- *"Have you eliminated entire food groups from your diet?"*
- *"Do you have any special routines or rituals when you eat?"* Use of inappropriate utensils for eating, such as a tiny spoon, is not uncommon. A person with an eating disorder may cut her food into tiny pieces and eat very slowly. She may have to eat foods in a certain order, not have foods touching on the plate, or chew a certain number of times before swallowing.
- *"Do you cook for family members or others? If so, do you eat with them or do you eat separately?"* Persons with eating disorders often eat different food than what their family is eating.
- *"Do you feel knowledgeable about nutrition? Do you spend time reading books about nutrition and recipes?"* The nutritional knowledge of a person with an eating disorder is often distorted to justify her unhealthy eating patterns.
- *"When do you eat?"* Often such persons only eat late at night and when alone.
- *"Do you ever restrict fluids or drink fluids in order to feel full in the absence of calories?"*
- *"Do you count calories and grams of fat?"*
- *"Do you use diet products and high-fiber products?"*
- *"Do you ever use a lot of condiments on your food because you feel you are 'giving in' if you enjoy the taste of foods?"*

- *"Do you ever steal food or eat unusual items during a binge, such as uncooked or raw food?"*
- *"Do you weigh foods? Do people ever comment on the size of the portions you take for yourself?"*
- *"Do you have any food allergies or lactose intolerance?"* Patients may believe they have food intolerances or allergies that they use to justify why they cannot eat certain foods.

Checking Behaviors

A person with an eating disorder may have many checking behaviors. Possible questions to ask include the following:

- *"How often do you weigh herself? How does your actual weight affect your eating, and how you see yourself?"*
- *"Do you measure yourself with a tape or use clothes as a guide for estimating your weight?"*
- *"Do you check yourself in mirrors frequently or avoid them entirely?"*
- *"Do you repeatedly pinch areas of your body where you feel fat?"*

Binge Eating

Another area to explore is binge eating, which occurs in all patients with BN and half of patients with AN. Possible questions to ask include the following:

- *"How old were you when you started to binge eat?"*
- *"What type and amount of foods do you consume in a binge?"*
- *"How often do you binge eat?"*
- *"Can you identify triggers for binge eating, such as hunger, feeling upset, or something else?"*
- *"Are the binges planned, or are they sudden?"*
- *"What do you eat when not binge eating?"*

Pattern of Eating

Questions regarding pattern of eating can help to give a thumbnail sketch of what the patient's eating behavior is like. Possible questions to ask include the following:

- *"Do you have regular meals throughout the day? What do you eat, and how much do you eat at each meal and snack?"* This should provide an estimation of caloric intake in a typical day.
- *"What times of the day/night do you eat in addition to regular meal times?"* Nighttime eating is not uncommon in patients with eating disorders. Patients often refer to "good" or "bad" days of eating, depending on their success at caloric restriction (good day) or their loss of control and overeating (bad day). Have the person describe a "good" day of eating and then a "bad" day, noting the frequency of each in the week.

- *"Do you keep track of what you eat?"* You should suggest, as a way of more accurately assessing her food intake, that she record in writing what she eats each day for a 1-week period. At another interview, review this record with the patient. Although such dietary self-reports can be helpful, one should keep in mind that the accuracy of self-reporting of dietary intake decreases dramatically after 24 hours.

The above information should provide you with a clear sense of the presence and severity of a clinically significant eating disorder. However, it is necessary to ask about other psychiatric problems as well, such as mood changes, symptoms of anxiety, or substance use, because these are commonly found in patients with eating disorders.

Other Psychiatric Symptoms

Knowledge of psychiatric comorbidities is necessary because these should be treated concurrently with the eating disorder to optimize the chance of full recovery from the latter. Important areas to explore regarding comorbidity include the following:

- Mood, especially symptoms of depression: These include changes in sleep, eating, libido, concentration, and energy. It is important to assess risk for self-harm and suicidality, as well as any symptoms suggestive of a bipolar disorder. These would include symptoms of mania such as discrete episodes of increased energy, racing thoughts, decreased need for sleep, and poor judgment as manifested by promiscuity or excessive spending.
- Anxiety: This should include current or past non-food-related obsessive compulsive symptoms. In addition, the presence of panic attacks should be elicited as well as any phobias, including social phobia, which is not uncommon in patients with AN.
- Substance use/abuse: Patients with eating disorders have higher than expected rates of substance use for both alcohol and street drugs. Patients will specifically seek out street drugs that are associated with weight loss, such as amphetamine-containing substances. Patients will also abuse prescription drugs given for other conditions because of associated weight loss. These include methylphenidate (Ritalin) and thyroid preparations. Patients will use a variety of over-the-counter diet pills, diuretics, and natural substances such as ephedrine that are associated with weight loss.
- Personality: Persons with AN differ somewhat in terms of their personality from those with BN. Persons with AN tend to be more compulsive and overly controlled in their behavior. They are also more socially avoidant and conflict averse, more passive, and more fearful.

Persons with BN tend to be more impulsive and thrill-seeking and tend to engage in impulsive behaviors such as self-harm, stealing, and promiscuity. However, there are some similarities in terms of the psychological issues people with anorexia and bulimia face. You should inquire about the following in assessing these issues:

- A sense of ineffectiveness, perfectionism, maturity fears, and difficulties expressing emotion
- How the individual would describe her personality and then how she thinks others see her
- Feelings of guilt
- Difficulty making decisions
- Extreme sensitivity to criticism
- Tendency to sacrifice personal needs to please others
- Difficulties coping with stress
- Difficulties coping with being alone

Medical History

It is important to review the patient's medical history to rule out the other medical conditions that may be associated with weight loss or abnormal eating, as well as to be aware of ongoing medical complications associated with the eating disorder.

Eating disorders are associated with many medical complications. The effects of starvation, weight loss, vomiting, laxative and diuretic abuse, and compulsive exercising can lead to serious and potentially life-threatening medical complications. Knowledge of any preexisting medical condition associated with weight loss or abnormal eating is important to note. Not infrequently, a bout of mononucleosis in adolescence or extraction of wisdom teeth can lead to mild weight loss because the person feels unwell or cannot eat because of pain or swelling. If this is then associated with subsequent positive comments from others about the individual's change in weight and shape, increased caloric restriction can occur in pursuit of more external approval, leading to further weight loss and the eventual development of an eating disorder.

Questions in the medical assessment should include the following:

- *"Have there been any significant past medical illnesses?"*
- *"Have you had any head injuries or seizures?"*
- *"Have you had any surgery? Any plastic surgery?"*
- *"Have you had any bone pain or bone fractures?"*
- *"Are you aware of any abnormal laboratory findings that are common in people with eating disorders?"* These include abnormal levels of potassium, anemia, and/or evidence of dehydration.
- *"How old were you when you started to menstruate? How much did you weigh at that time? What are your*

periods like now? Have your periods ever stopped? For how long? Have you ever been pregnant?"

- *"Have there been any other medical diagnoses that have been given by physicians to explain your symptoms?"*

Patients with eating disorders present to their physicians with physical symptoms that often get misdiagnosed and whose treatments often exacerbate their eating disorder. Examples of this include hypoglycemia, which is common in starved persons, and irritable bowel syndrome or lactose intolerance. Cramps, diarrhea, and abdominal pain can occur in patients who abuse laxatives, and these symptoms mimic those associated with irritable bowel syndrome or lactose intolerance; this can lead to erroneous diagnoses when the laxative abuse remains covert and undisclosed. It is, however, important to note that laxative abuse in fact can often lead to a temporary state of lactose intolerance. Treatment should be aimed at ceasing laxative use rather than restricting lactose in the diet. In addition, patients often get misdiagnosed with hypothyroidism and then are given thyroid hormone, which they use to increase their metabolism and lose weight. In the face of starvation, it is common to have low normal thyroid indices, which should not be treated by thyroid replacement but by refeeding.

Key Point:

Eliciting a history of the medical complications is necessary to determine the need for further medical treatment and possible hospitalization.

Medications

Questions regarding medications should include the following:

- *"Have you used any psychiatric medications, as well as medications for gastrointestinal symptoms, vitamins, or mineral supplements?"*
- *"Are you allergic to any medications?"*

Past Psychiatric or Eating Disorder Treatment

Regarding past psychiatric or eating disorder treatment, it is important for the clinician to ask the following:

- *"Have you had any previous specialized medical or psychiatric treatment for an eating disorder? If so, were you an outpatient or were you hospitalized?"* In addition, information about the nature of the treatment

(e.g., psychotherapy, medication) and its duration and effectiveness is important.

- *"Have you received treatment for any other psychiatric disorder? If so, what was the treatment and what was the problem?"*
- *"Have you seen a dietitian? What did you learn from this experience?"*

Family History

Important questions to ask regarding the family history include the following:

- *"Has anyone else in your family had an eating disorder?"*
- *"Is there any family history of drug or alcohol problems?"*
- *"Is there any family history of a mood disorder, such as depression or manic depressive illness, anxiety disorder, such as obsessive compulsive disorder, or suicide?"*
- *"How would you describe your relationship with your parents and siblings?"*
- *"What is the weight status and eating behavior of each family member?"*

Personal History
Developmental History

Important questions regarding the patient's developmental history include the following:

- Pregnancy and birth history: *"What do you know about your feeding and growth patterns when you were a newborn? What about during infancy?"*
- Toddler period: *"What have you been told about what you were like as a toddler? Were there any delays in your developmental in terms of things like learning to walk or talk?"*
- Childhood: *"Did you experience any separation difficulties (e.g., going to school) or major stressful events? How easily did you make friends?"* You should also ask about her weight status and growth as a child in comparison with siblings and children of similar age.
- Family environment: *"Whom were you closest to, and why? How did your mother and father divide up parenting responsibilities?"*
- Eating patterns at home: "Did your family have regular sit-down meals together? As a family, was there much focus on dieting and nutrition?"

School/Occupational History

Regarding the patient's school and occupations history, it is important for the clinician to ask the following:

- School history: *"How did you do academically?"*

- Occupational history: *"How many different jobs have you had? What was the reason for ending jobs? Did any of your jobs or activities focus on weight and shape (e.g., modeling, dance, gymnastics) or food (e.g., waitressing, chef)?"*

Relationship History

Possible questions regarding the patient's relationship history include the following:

- Review both platonic and intimate relationships. This would include assessing difficulty in making friends, and comfort in relationships with others. *"How many boyfriends/girlfriends have you had? How long did your relationships last? What were the reasons for the relationships ending? Does your current partner know about your eating disorder, and if so, how does he or she try to help you?"*
- Sexual activity: *"What kind of sexual experiences have you had? At what age did you first have intercourse? Was it consensual? Did you feel pressured? What was your emotional reaction?"*
- Abuse history, including physical, sexual, or emotional: Ask in a direct but gentle way whether there ever was a time in the patient's life when she was victimized or abused. If so, *"What happened? How often did it happen? Who was the perpetrator? What was the reaction if you told family, friends, or the police?"*
- *"Did you experience any other major life events, such as significant losses, moves, etc.?"*

At the end of the interview, you should ask the patient why she thinks she has an eating disorder and how she thinks it started. You should also explore the patient's motivation for treatment. This can be done, in part, by asking the patient how she feels about her illness, how has it has affected her life, and how she sees it playing out in the future. These questions can help to uncover the patient's level of denial and can also challenge her to think about what the benefits or detriments are in recovering or staying ill. Asking the patient whether she has any questions for you is a good way to end the interview.

Mental Status Examination

The mental status examination is similar to that for other psychiatric illnesses (see Chapter 1) with a few exceptions. The core requirements include the following:

Appearance

Type of dress, grooming, cleanliness, eye contact, and cooperativeness. Does the patient look her age? What is her weight status, and how medically ill does she appear? It is also important to note characteristic visible physical

sequelae of her disordered eating and purging, which are mentioned in a section to follow.

Motor Activity

Has there been any abnormal motor activity, including excessive activity (which is used to burn calories or is a sign of anxiety)? Some patients may be fidgety due to discomfort in answering questions, or patients may even stand and pace throughout the interview to facilitate burning calories.

Mood

Ask about mood on a scale of 1 to 10, with a 1 being the worst the patient has ever felt. What is the patient's mood right at the time of the interview? The patient should be asked about suicidal and homicidal thoughts. Patients with eating disorders often become suicidal, which tends to be more pronounced at very low weights, with chaotic eating, and with approaching more normal weights with treatment. Thoughts about self-harm (e.g., overdosing, cutting, burning) are quite common in these patients and should be asked about and noted.

Key Point:

As with any psychiatric patient, persons with eating disorders do become suicidal. This should always be asked about regardless of how the person presents.

Thought Form and Content

Patients do not usually have a disorder of thought form, although the content is often near delusional regarding their body image. They should be asked directly how they feel about their bodies: *"Where do you feel fat?"* The presence of obsessions and compulsive rituals that are not food related should be explored and noted.

Perceptual Abnormalities

What do they see when they look at themselves in the mirror? Patients often see certain parts of their bodies as too big, or they may focus on a specific body part, believing it is in some way abnormal without so much of a focus on its size.

Memory and Concentration

Short- and long-term memory and concentration can be adversely affected by weight loss, dehydration, and starvation and should be assessed through standardized clinical tests.

Judgment

Assessing the patient's judgment, specifically as it relates to her medical and nutritional state, is important. In severe cases, this can be markedly impaired and may be grounds to involuntarily impose treatment if the patient's life is threatened by her illness.

Insight

Does the patient recognize that she is ill, and does she recognize the need for treatment? Patients may be extremely well informed about eating disorders in a way that can intimidate the junior interviewer but at the same time display an amazing lack of ability to appreciate their own predicament.

Key Point:

Try to understand the illness from the patient's point of view, especially in terms of what function her symptoms serve. This is a helpful way of engaging the patient.

Collateral Information

Collateral information is important to ascertain the reliability of the patient's self-report and to get an idea of how the patient is perceived by others. Interviewing significant others (e.g., spouse, family, friend) with the patient present is the ideal way to collect this information. If the patient is an adult, such an interview can only occur with the patient's consent. There is a potential risk in conducting such interviews. The interviewer needs to be careful to not be perceived as "taking sides," preserving a therapeutic alliance with the patient while also demonstrating understanding of the perspectives and needs of an often-exhausted family.

Questions to be addressed in the interview with the family and significant others include the following:

- *"When did you first notice any difficulties with your child/spouse/partner's eating or notice weight changes? What specifically do you know about her disordered eating behaviors?"*
- *"How have you been coping with her difficulties?"* You may want to explain that it would not be unusual for parents or spouses to feel very upset, sad, angry, frustrated, and helpless. *"What approaches have you tried to help her with her eating difficulties and other problems?"* It is not uncommon for parents and significant others to "police" the patient's eating behavior, which for adult patients tends to not be helpful. For children and younger adolescents, on the other hand, it may be necessary and therapeutic to do so.
- *"What behaviors have you noticed, and what is the patient's emotional state like? Have others commented on changes in her in any way?"*
- *"How is the family functioning at home? Is there a lot of stress and fighting? How is the patient's behavior affecting the family?"*
- *"How does the patient get along with her siblings, parents, etc.?"*
- *"Why do you think she developed this disorder?"*

Another major goal of an interview with family members or significant others is to provide psychoeducation about the illness and its treatment. It is important to review with the family or significant others the multidetermined nature of eating disorders and not to engage in parent bashing or blaming others. You should review in a general way what the recommended treatment for their child/spouse/partner is.

Other sources of collateral information include the family physician or pediatrician, and for younger patients, school personnel such as teachers and guidance counselors. Requests for reports from previous clinical contacts (e.g., other physicians, therapists, dietitians) can be helpful.

Physical Examination

Eating disordered behavior, whether it is starvation or any of the forms of purging, can result in physiological abnormalities that need investigation as part of the assessment. A comprehensive physical examination is an important component of the assessment of a patient with an eating disorder. This is also important because it can demonstrate to the patient the negative health effects resulting from her illness.

Many of the physical symptoms of which patients complain are the result of the downregulation of the autonomic nervous system resulting from starvation and subsequent lowering of basal metabolism. However, the physical and emotional effects are not specific to the eating disorder itself; the same effects are seen in persons who are starved but do not have an eating disorder. This was first demonstrated in a study conducted in 1944 by the U.S. military, in which conscientious objectors were voluntarily starved for several months to ascertain the effects of starvation on eating behavior.[6] The American military was mystified by the bizarre eating behavior that freed prisoners of war in Japan and survivors of the concentration camps in Europe demonstrated when they were liberated and given food to eat. Many of these persons began to binge eat, in some instances to the point of death, when they were re-fed. The subjects in this study, after 3 months of semistarvation, showed very definite changes in their eating behavior, mood, and cognitions. These subjects became apathetic, lost interest in life, and had impaired concentration. Many suffered insomnia, intense food cravings, and preoccupation with food, including hoarding of food, dreaming about food, and wanting to become chefs. They experienced episodes of binge eating when the study was stopped and they were given as much food as they wished. They reported that they had lost all sense of satiety (i.e., knowing when they were full after eating). Even when their weight was restored, they still had problems with satiety. They also complained of physical symptoms such as weakness, fatigue, dizziness, reduced libido, constipation, bloating and indigestion with eating, headaches, and cold intolerance. All these symptoms resulted from a lowering of their metabolism to conserve energy (calories), resulting in lowered blood pressure and pulse, contributing to dizziness; lowered basal body temperature resulting in feeling cold; reduced levels of testosterone, leading to reduced libido; and reduced intestinal movement, resulting in bloating and constipation. All these symptoms are common in patients with eating disorders and require nutritional rehabilitation and weight gain to reverse.

In assessing these patients, you should do the following:

- Examine their skin. Often it is pale or sallow, and they may have scars on the dorsum of the hand from friction against their front teeth while inducing vomiting (Russell's sign). Blue fingers and toes are not uncommon due to reduced peripheral blood flow to conserve heat. As a result, their skin will be cold peripherally and dry. The skin may look slightly orange due to carotenemia (excessive carotene levels in the blood). Specific signs attributable to the effects of vomiting include sores and rashes around the mouth due to irritation of skin from the acid contents of vomitus, salivary or parotid gland swelling, and periorbital petechiae from vomiting.
- Examine the mouth. Of note are dry lips and tongue (dehydration), dental erosion, caries, and mouth sores. You may be able to smell a sweet acetone smell on their breath indicative of ketosis, which occurs in starvation.
- Look for thinning scalp hair and the development of lanugo hair (a fine, downy hair that can appear on the face and chest in the context of starvation).
- Measure temperature, blood pressure (lying and standing), and pulse rate. Postural drops of blood pressure are common.
- Measure height and weight, and calculate BMI.
- Examine cardiovascular status including peripheral pulses, evidence of dependent or generalized edema, and pulse rate. Bradycardia and an irregular heart rhythm are common.
- Note the presence or absence of bowel sounds or abnormal abdominal masses or tenderness. Patients with eating disorders can develop subclinical pancreatitis and demonstrate tenderness and an abnormal mass as a result.
- Conduct a neurological examination. Patients with eating disorders can develop peripheral neuropathies and seizures. Prolonged starvation can contribute to the development of headaches, and reflexes may be diminished with electrolyte abnormalities or hyperactive with mineral deficiencies.

Investigations

There are certain tests that should always be completed to screen for imminent medical risk. These include a complete blood count and differential, electrolytes, and renal function, which include measurement of creatinine and blood urea nitrogen levels and an electrocardiogram. There are other tests that should be completed if you find other abnormalities or if the patient complains of certain physical symptoms. These include thyroid indices (i.e., thyroid-stimulating hormone, triiodothyronine, thyroxine), serum phosphate, magnesium and calcium, blood glucose, liver function tests, serum amylase, and a urinalysis. A stool examination may be necessary if gastrointestinal bleeding, abdominal complaints, and anemia are present.

Bone densitometry can be considered, but its routine usefulness is questionable other than to help the patient realize the ongoing physical damage the eating disorder is causing. It is reasonable to do this only if the person has a history of unexplained bone fractures and bone pain and has been amenorrheic for a long period of time. However, there is no known effective treatment for the osteopenia/osteoporosis that occurs in patients with AN other than the treatment of the disorder itself, which requires nutritional rehabilitation and weight gain. Exogenous hormones (i.e., oral contraceptives) should not be given, as they are ineffective for the treatment of the osteopenia/osteoporosis that occurs in AN.[7] In AN, in addition to reduced new bone formation due to decreased estrogen, there is also increased bone destruction due to the hormone changes that result from starvation that is not corrected by exogenous hormones.

Differential Diagnoses

Medical Disorders

The most common medical conditions that are associated with weight loss and therefore may be misdiagnosed as AN include thyroid disease, inflammatory bowel disease, hypothalamic tumor, or rare forms of malabsorption. However, in none of these conditions does the patient actively pursue thinness and engage in self-starvation. Medical causes of overeating are extremely rare and usually involve brain abnormalities such as rare tumors or degenerative disorders.

Other Psychiatric Disorders

The weight loss associated with AN needs to be distinguished from other psychiatric conditions associated with weight loss.[8] These include the following:

- Mood disorders, especially depression: However, in depression, the patient usually is distressed by her weight loss and attributes it to a true loss of appetite and disinterest in eating. This is completely different than the condition of a patient with AN who is obsessively preoccupied with food and is surprisingly unconcerned about weight loss.
- Anxiety disorders: These include specific food phobias not associated with caloric content. Obsessive compulsive disorder can also be accompanied by weight loss if the patient is so consumed by ritualistic behaviors that she cannot eat properly. The obsessions in obsessive compulsive disorder are not food related, but rather are related to fears of contamination or the anxiety around the need for checking or counting rituals.
- Substance abuse: Certain substances, such as amphetamines or cocaine, reduce appetite through their effects on brain function and can therefore be associated with considerable weight loss.
- Conversion disorder: Psychogenic vomiting, for example, can be accompanied by significant weight loss. In this case, the patient denies vomiting to get rid of calories but vomits because of abdominal pain or for reasons of which she is unaware.
- Schizophrenia or delusional disorder: In psychotic states such as those that occur in schizophrenia, a person can believe that her food is being poisoned and will therefore stop eating. This can lead to dramatic weight loss, the cause of which is clearly very different than in AN.

There are few other psychiatric conditions where binge eating is a prominent feature and where patients do not have weight and shape concerns. Some patients who have impulse control difficulties, like those with borderline personality disorder, may binge eat as one of many impulsive behaviors in which they engage.

Engagement for Treatment

Explanation of the Diagnosis

After you have assessed the patient, you should be able to provide a diagnosis of an eating disorder if it is present. It is important to explain the disorder without using technical language. In terms of nutrition, it is imperative that you tell the patient that treatment would include the cessation of dieting and maintaining a regular intake of an adequate number of calories. Generally, the minimum dietary intake for a young adult female is initially 1800 to 2000 calories per day and then is increased to meet the person's nutritional and energy needs. It is also helpful to explain the relationship between dieting and binge eating, as well as the dangers of purging and of the use of diuretics or diet pills. Treatment usually requires regular medical monitoring and treatment of medical complications, nutritional therapy, some form of psychotherapy, and in some cases, medication.[9] Treatment in a structured intensive specialized program is necessary in cases that are more severe, especially for AN.

Medical Signs Potentially Necessitating Admission to a Hospital

1. Electrolyte abnormalities: Symptoms associated with electrolyte abnormalities include palpitations, fatigue, muscle weakness and spasms, diminished reflexes, irritability, and convulsions. The presence of potassium under 2.5 mmol/L usually requires intravenous treatment and cardiac monitoring in a hospital.
2. Weight loss: Hospitalization may be required for weight loss that is rapid or greater than 25% loss of total body weight.
3. Cardiovascular abnormalities: These include cardiac arrhythmias on an EKG, severe bradycardia, edema, or severe hypotension.
4. Seizures and/or delirium.
5. Acute gastrointestinal conditions: These can include bowel obstruction, pancreatitis, or esophageal or gastric tears or rupture.

The highest-risk patient for serious medical complications is the purging anorexic patient with significant acute weight loss.

The primary psychiatric reason for an emergency admission to hospital is acute suicidality.

Methods of Assessment

In addition to clinical interviewing, persons with eating disorders can be assessed in many ways, including self-monitoring forms, behavioral observation, self-report measures, clinical rating scales, symptom checklists, and test meals.[10] Examples of self-report and interview-based assessment instruments include the following:

Self-Report Instruments

1. Eating Disorder Inventory (EDI): This is a standardized self-report measure assessing attitudes and thoughts about weight shape as well as characteristic psychologi-

cal domains with which persons with eating disorders struggle.[11]

2. Eating Attitudes Test (EAT): This is a standardized self-report measure of eating disorder symptoms.[12]

3. Eating Disorder Examination Questionnaire (EDE-Q): This is a self-report measure based on the EDE (see following discussion) that assesses dietary restraint, binge eating, and attitudes about shape and weight.[13]

4. Self-monitoring: This involves patients recording in a diary/journal their daily food intake, weight control behaviors, thoughts, and feelings in a systematic way. This can be a helpful way to assess 24-hour caloric intake and the degree of dietary chaos; however, it is often difficult for patients to comply with such self-monitoring.

Structured Interviews

1. Eating Disorder Examination (EDE). This is a semi-structured interview, used to assess current eating disorder symptoms, that generates DSM-IV diagnoses.

2. Yale-Brown-Cornell Eating Disorder Scale (YBC-EDS). This interview-based checklist covers rituals and preoccupations common in eating-disordered individuals.[14]

CHALLENGES IN ASSESSING AND ENGAGING PEOPLE WITH EATING DISORDERS

Some health professionals, even very experienced ones, are reluctant to see people with eating disorders. Even within the mental health professions, there may be avoidance of or frank dislike for these people. Persons with eating disorders are no less deserving of help than any other group affected by psychiatric illness—so what explains the variety of professional attitudes toward them?

Some clinicians view eating disorders as problems people have brought on themselves—as opposed to schizophrenia—and that are subject to volitional control. Although there is a volitional component to disordered eating behavior, the psychological and biological determinants and drivers of eating disorders are not under conscious control. Indeed, lack of control is a powerful and common experience among people with eating disorders, and if you haven't understood that experience, you haven't understood the patient.

Some clinicians may feel outdone by people with eating disorders—that these patients are more omniscient about their problems than most clinicians, that they can out-negotiate those people trying to help them, or that they may be frankly deceptive when it comes to compliance with therapeutic goals. This can leave clinicians feeling intimidated or angry, once again failing to connect with the distress that underlies the expressed behavior. Clinicians may also feel competitive with or jealous of the extraordinary discipline manifested by some patients with regard to weight loss or fitness, although in our experience, the more clinicians witness the suffering, the less they are weight-and-shape preoccupied themselves.

You need to be mindful of your own attitudes and prejudices, both toward your own weight and shape and toward your patients. Working with persons with eating disorders can be immensely rewarding, demanding an understanding of the complex interplay among biology, psychology, and culture; between the patient and the family; and between the patient and the clinician.

Key Point:

Monitor your reactions to the patient. Assessing and treating patients with eating disorders is difficult and requires a longitudinal view of the disorder and an understanding of its presentation, course, and outcome.

Key Point:

The assessment should be the beginning of treatment. Often patients are very ambivalent about asking for help; establishing a collaborative relationship at the first interview that engages the patient in her treatment is critical to the patient's continuing in care. The provision of information about the disorder as part of a psychoeducational approach is helpful in facilitating this process.

REFERENCES

1. Fairburn CG and Brownell KD, editors: *Eating disorders and obesity: a comprehensive handbook*, ed 2, New York, 2002, Guilford Press.

2. Kaplan AS, Garfinkel PE: General principles of outpatient treatment. In Gabbard G, editors: *Treatments of psychiatric disorders*, ed 3, Washington, 2001, American Psychiatric Press, pp. 2099 2117.

3. Vitousek K, Watson S, Wilson GT: Enhancing motivation for change in treatment resistant eating disorder patients, *Clin Psychol Rev* 18:391–420, 1998.

4. Kaplan AS, Garfinkel PE: Difficulties in treating patients with eating disorders: a review of patient and clinician variables, *Can J Psychiatr* 44(7):665–670, 1999.

5. Kaplan AS: Medical and nutritional assessment of eating disorders. In Kaplan AS, Garfinkel PG, editors: *Medical issues and the eating disorders: the interface,* New York, 1993, Brunner Mazel.

6. Keys A, Brozek J, Henschel A, et al: *The biology of human starvation,* Minneapolis, 1950, University of Minnesota Press, p. 1.

7. Klibanski A, Biller BM, Schoenfeld DA, et al: The effects of estrogen administration on trabecular bone loss in young women with anorexia nervosa, *J Clin Endocrinol Metab* 80:898–904, 1995.

8. Garfinkel PE, Garner DM, Kaplan AS, Rodin, G, Kennedy S: Differential diagnoses of emotional disorders that cause weight loss, *Can Med Assoc J* 129:939–945, 1983.

9. Garner DM, Garfinkel PE, editors: *Handbook of Treatment for Eating Disorders,* ed 2, New York, 1997, Guilford Press.

10. Fairburn CG, Wilson GT, editors: *Binge eating: nature, assessment and treatment,* New York, 1993, Guilford Press.

11. Garner DM, Olmsted MP, Polivy J, Garfinkel PE: Comparison between weight-preoccupied women and anorexia nervosa. *Psychosomatic Medicine* 46:255–266, 1984.

12. Garner DM, Garfinkel PE: The Eating Attitudes Test: an index of the symptoms of anorexia nervosa. *Psychological Medicine* 9:273–279, 1979.

13. Fairburn CG, Beglin SJ: Assessment of eating disorders: interview or self-report questionnaire? *Int. J. Eating Disorders* 16:363–370, 1994.

14. Mazure CM, Halmi KA, Sunday SR, et al. The Yale-Brown-Cornell Eating Disorder Scale: development, use, reliability and validity. *J. Psych. Res.* 28:425–445, 1994.

10

Assessment of Patients with Substance-Related Disorders

Peter Selby and Curtis Handford

INTRODUCTION

Addiction is considered a chronic, remitting, and relapsing brain disease characterized by the recurrent use of a psychoactive drug(s) and loss of control over use of the drug. This definition implies that addiction treatment needs to be chronic and biopsychosocial in nature, similar to the treatment of other chronic diseases such as hypertension, diabetes, and depression.

The goal of this chapter is to increase the confidence of medical and other mental health students, residents, and faculty in working with substance-using patients, especially those patients who also suffer from a concurrent psychiatric disorder.

To accomplish this goal, this chapter focuses on the following learning objectives:

1. Explaining the concept of addiction as a highly prevalent, chronic illness with a considerable burden of disease
2. Developing a thorough, confident approach in screening, case-finding, and diagnosing substance-use disorders in patients
3. Developing an appropriate, confident approach to managing patients with substance-use disorders

---

Case Example 1

Robert is a 39-year-old man referred by an emergency room (ER) physician for acute suicidal ideation. He had been brought to the ER 18 hours ago by his girlfriend because he threatened suicide. She reported that Robert had been more irritable and withdrawn for the previous 6 months, ever since he lost his job as a welder. He was diagnosed with depression and had been prescribed venlafaxine (75 mg/day) for the past week. Recently, he had gained 20 lb despite a loss of appetite; he reported having insomnia and complained of anhedonia, low energy, poor concentration, and feelings of guilt and worthlessness. On admission to the ER, he smelled of alcohol, was slurring his speech, and was tearful. He stated he wanted to be dead. Because of the suicide risk and Robert's unwillingness to remain in the ER, he was detained involuntarily.

When you see the patient, he is tremulous, anxious, and pacing the room. He is irritable and denies ever being suicidal. He admits to drinking 750 mL of vodka daily for the past 6 months, ever since he has been unemployed. His last drink was 18 hours ago, just before he was brought to the ER. You notice that among his laboratory results in ER, his gamma glutamyl transpeptidase (GGT) and aspartate aminotransferase (AST) levels and his mean corpuscular volume (MCV) are abnormal. He meets criteria for alcohol dependence and alcohol withdrawal. He also endorses having memory blackouts. He denies ever having withdrawal seizures. You treat his withdrawal using the Clinical Institute Withdrawal Assessment for Alcohol Revised (Appendix I) to guide the administration of diazepam.[1] He responds to a total of 80 mg of diazepam over 4 hours. He becomes more cooperative and less agitated. He no longer has tremors, and his gait is steady. He is still depressed. He consents to an admission to the general psychiatry ward.

Two days later, Robert's mood improves by 50%. He is no longer suicidal but admits to cravings for alcohol. You have him meet the hospital substance abuse counselor. He agrees to attend an alcohol treatment program as an outpatient. You prescribe him naltrexone 150 mg po bid to reduce his cravings for alcohol. In follow-up, he describes three drinking occasions over 2 months due to triggers in social situations and when he feels stressed. His plasma GGT, AST, and MCV are normal. He continues to participate in an aftercare program once per week and describes no symptoms of depression or suicidality. His depression appears to be in complete remission, and he tapers himself off the antidepressant with no ill effects.

Robert stays sober for 12 months and relapses when he breaks up with his girlfriend. He begins to drink 750 mL of vodka daily again, but this time he presents to you for care just 4 weeks after his relapse. You refer him for detoxification and readmission to a residential treatment program. He successfully completes treatment and attends aftercare. His next lapse is 4 years later but only lasts 5 days. This time, his GGT is only mildly elevated, but his MCV and AST are at normal levels. He has built sufficient social supports to maintain his sobriety, has a sponsor in Alcoholics Anonymous, and has insight into the "disease of alcoholism." Therefore, he seeks help before spiraling into a full-blown relapse. This time he meets criteria for a major depressive episode unrelated to the consumption of alcohol. He has an 80% response to venlafaxine within 6 weeks. Because of Robert's alcohol dependence history, you avoid prescribing any benzodiazepines for his insomnia. You manage his insomnia with good patient education on sleep hygiene. He is satisfied with his progress, and you taper him off venlafaxine after 6 months of full remission of his depressive symptoms. He is advised to continue with his self-management skills and attendance at Alcoholics Anonymous meetings with instructions to follow up with you should he have a relapse to alcohol dependence, depression, or both.

This case illustrates how psychiatric syndromes can be caused by underlying addictive disorders and vice versa. With appropriate engagement and multidisciplinary treatment with long-term follow-up, long-term disability can be prevented, and patients can lead relatively high-functioning lives.

Role of the Health Care Professional in Addictive Disorders

Substance-use disorders cause or co-occur concurrently with both mental health and medical disorders. Despite this fact, many health care professionals avoid, ignore, or inadequately manage their patients' substance use problems. This is partly due to the frustration clinicians feel when treating or interacting with addicted patients, who may "push our buttons" or not adhere to our recommendation to just "stop using drugs." However, with appropriate attitudes, knowledge, and skills, clinicians can be the most powerful motivators for change in the lives of these patients. Clinicians can play a role in screening, treating, referring patients to behavioral treatments, and monitoring progress.

Patient Interview

Patients usually present to clinicians with conditions that are a *consequence* of the addiction, rather than seeking help for their addiction per se. Therefore, the tasks in the clinical interview include the following:

1. Uncovering the relationship of substances of abuse to the presenting complaint(s)
2. Diagnosing specific addiction syndromes (i.e., problematic use, abuse, dependence, substance-induced disorder, concurrent disorders, intoxication, withdrawal)
3. Exploring the consequences of the patient's addiction on each of the following:
   a. Physical health (e.g., HIV, hepatitis C in injection drug users; liver disease in alcoholism)
   b. Psychological well-being (e.g., effects on mood, self-esteem, and self-worth)
   c. Social and family relationships (e.g., loss of support from friends and families)
   d. Economic and employment status (e.g., job loss, poverty, unstable or no housing)
4. Determining the level of patient motivation to change
5. Offering the appropriate intervention

Clinician-Patient Relationship

Treatment planning is a joint process, with the clinician offering a range of choices to engage the patient on a journey of recovery. It often requires multiple interactions between clinician and patient before the patient is "ready" to engage in the treatment process. This makes the clinician-patient relationship particularly important to retain the patient in treatment. Unlike most other clinician-patient relationships, relationships with actively addicted patients may not follow the rules of honesty, respect, and trust. Therefore, a fundamental task is to create a healthy relationship where the patient doesn't feel judged and feels comfortable to disclose lapses, relapses, and other confidential information such as past physical and sexual abuse. The development of this relationship is an iterative process that requires you to be consistent and honest, yet accepting (i.e., nonjudgmental) of the patient. Such an attitude is conducive to the development of a healthy relationship to effect behavior change in the patient.

SUBSTANCE-RELATED DISORDERS: A SPECTRUM

The term *addiction* is primarily a lay term. Many clinicians and patients will label people as addicted if they are physiologically dependent on a drug, use large amounts of a drug, or are unable to stop using a drug. However, current concepts of addiction focus primarily on the loss of control over drug use and continued drug use despite harmful consequences, rather than on the physiological dependence per se. In this chapter we use *addiction* and *substance-use disorder* interchangeably.

The diagnostic vocabulary of addictions requires some definition and explanation to ensure that clinicians are describing the same phenomena when they communicate with patients and with each other.

The American Psychiatric Association's *Diagnostic and Statistical Manual of Mental Disorders*, Fourth Edition, Text Revision (DSM-IV-TR) lists addictive disorders as axis I diagnoses under the broad term *substance-related disorders*. This is broadly subdivided into *substance-use disorders*[2] (substance abuse and substance dependence) and *substance-induced disorders*. Process addictions such as gambling are not included in this chapter.

Substance-Use Disorders

Substance Abuse

The presence of any one or more of the four criteria (Box 10-1) within a 12-month period determines this diagnosis.

Box 10-1. Substance Abuse*

Substance abuse is defined in DSM-IV-TR as a maladaptive pattern of substance use leading to clinically significant impairment or distress, as manifested by one (or more) of the following, occurring within a 12-month period:

1. Recurrent substance use resulting in a failure to fulfill major role obligations at work, school, or home (e.g., repeated absences or poor work performance related to substance use; substance-related absences, suspensions, or expulsions from school; neglect of children or household)
2. Recurrent substance use in situations in which it is physically hazardous (e.g., driving an automobile or operating a machine when impaired by substance use)
3. Recurrent substance-related legal problems (e.g., arrests for substance-related disorderly conduct)
4. Continued substance use despite having persistent or recurrent social or interpersonal problems caused or exacerbated by the effects of the substance (e.g., arguments with spouse about consequences of intoxication, physical fights)

*Reprinted from American Psychiatric Association: *Diagnostic and statistical manual of mental disorders*, ed 4, text revision, Washington, DC, 2000.

This reflects the tolerance of the environment to a person's substance use. This includes role obligations, the context of use, legal problems, and social problems. Note that the amount of drug consumed does not contribute to the diagnosis.

A mnemonic to remember the criteria for substance abuse is SLOP (*s*ocial, *l*egal, *o*bligations, *p*hysically hazardous).

A diagnosis of substance abuse can *never* be made if the person has *ever* met criteria for dependence on the same substance. This reflects the chronicity of substance dependence that is characterized by relapses and remission for that drug class.

Substance Dependence

This diagnosis is more reflective of a disease defined by criteria less dependent on environmental factors and more dependent on biological mechanisms.

A mnemonic to remember criteria for dependence (Box 10-2) is WET TICK (*w*ithdrawal; *e*xcess use; *t*olerance; *t*ime spent acquiring, using, or recovering from the use of the drug; *i*nterference with roles; inability to *c*ut down; continued use despite *k*nowledge of harm).

Tolerance is a physiological phenomenon characterized by the need for increasing amounts of a substance to achieve intoxication, or by the reduced psychoactive effect with continued use of the same amounts of a substance. Tolerance will result in a heroin-dependent person increasing the amount of heroin he uses to experience the euphoria associated with the drug. Tolerance does not develop at the same rate to all the effects of a drug. For example, tolerance to the constipating and respiratory-depressing effects of heroin will develop at different rates than tolerance to the euphoric effects of the drug.

Withdrawal is a syndrome that occurs when a drug is suddenly stopped or dramatically reduced in a person who is tolerant to that drug. The withdrawal syndromes differ depending on what type of drug is being abused. Some heavily dependent persons do not recognize withdrawal because they use the drug or an equivalent very regularly.

If the patient is either tolerant to a drug or experiences withdrawal upon cessation of a drug, you should specify that the patient is physiologically dependent. This provides a clue as to whether withdrawal management will be necessary for the patient. It is important to note that tolerance and withdrawal are neither necessary nor sufficient to make the diagnosis of substance dependence. This fact is particularly noteworthy when trying to diagnose dependence in a patient who is using drugs of abuse for legitimate medical reasons. For example, a patient who has been treated for years with opioids for chronic non-cancer pain of the back may experience tolerance and withdrawal to the prescribed opioid. This would indicate physiological dependence on the opioid but does not necessarily mean that the patient is addicted or psychologically dependent on opioids.

Box 10-2. Substance Dependence*

Substance dependence is defined in DSM-IV-TR as *maladaptive pattern of substance use leading to clinically significant impairment or distress* as manifested by three (or more) of the following, occurring at any time in the same 12-month period:

1. Tolerance, as defined by either of the following:
   a. A need for markedly increased amounts of the substance to achieve intoxication or desired effect.
   b. Markedly diminished effect with continued use of the same amount of the substance.
2. Withdrawal, as manifested by either of the following:
   a. The characteristic withdrawal syndrome for the substance.
   b. The same (or a closely related) substance is taken to relieve or avoid withdrawal symptoms.
3. The substance is often taken in larger amounts or over a longer period than was intended.
4. There is a persistent desire or unsuccessful efforts to cut down or control substance use.
5. A great deal of time is spent in activities necessary to obtain the substance (e.g., visiting multiple doctors or driving long distances), use the substance (e.g., chain-smoking), or recover from its effects.
6. Important social, occupational, or recreational activities are given up or reduced because of substance use.
7. The substance use is continued despite knowledge of having a persistent or recurrent physical or psychological problem that is likely to have been caused or exacerbated by the substance (e.g., current cocaine use despite recognition of cocaine-induced depression, or continued drinking despite recognition that an ulcer was made worse by alcohol consumption).

*Reprinted from American Psychiatric Association: *Diagnostic and statistical manual of mental disorders*, ed 4, text revision, Washington, DC, 2000.

Certain disease course specifiers are important to accurately specify the current status of a substance-dependent patient. For example, in the case above, when Robert lapses to drinking for 4 days, his diagnosis would still be alcohol dependence with physiological dependence, full remission. Even though he had a lapse, he failed to meet criteria for active alcohol dependence. A diagnosis of alcohol abuse in this case would be inappropriate because it is trumped by a previous diagnosis of alcohol dependence.

Differentiating Between Substance Abuse and Dependence

Substance abuse is a separate diagnostic category from dependence and most often occurs earlier in the course of a patient's substance use career (Table 10-1). Therefore, it is rare for a patient to meet criteria for dependence without having a lifetime diagnosis of abuse for that drug class, especially alcohol and cannabis use disorders. In clinical populations, abuse is as least 3–15 times more common than dependence. Exceptions include cocaine and opiates, where there is rapid progression to dependence within the same year a patient meets criteria for abuse. Criteria for substance abuse are defined by the environmental context, whereas five of seven criteria for dependence are independent of the environment.

If patients ever meet criteria for dependence for a particular drug class, they can *never* be diagnosed with current *abuse* for that drug class even if they don't currently fulfill criteria for dependence. Course specifiers for dependence (e.g., partial remission) should be used.

Categories of abuse and dependence for all substances are described except nicotine, for which dependence is the only diagnostic category, since dependence develops very rapidly for most users. The clinician should specify whether the patient has physiological dependence (i.e., displays tolerance, experiences withdrawal, or both). However, physiological dependence is *not* the *sine qua non* of "addiction." It merely indicates that the patient may experience withdrawal when stopping the substance.

Polysubstance Dependence

If a patient meets criteria for dependence and is using three or more substances (excluding caffeine and nicotine), a diagnosis of polysubstance-use disorder may be made if no single drug accounts for all the criteria. In other words, the use of a single drug is not sufficient to meet criteria but, when grouped under polysubstance use, the patient meets criteria for dependence. However, if a patient uses three different drug classes and the use of each contributes to diagnostic criteria independently, then each one should be recorded separately.

Other terms commonly used in the international substance use field include the following:

- Harmful use: Pattern of use causing damage to health.
- Hazardous use: Pattern of use that increases the risk of harmful consequences.
- Problem drinking: Drinking above low-risk guidelines (14 standard drinks per week for men and nine standard drinks per week for women, with no more than two drinks per drinking occasion) with consequences in one or more domains of the person's life. Although there is some overlap with alcohol abuse in DSM-IV-TR, there is no overlap with alcohol dependence. Compared with alcohol abuse, the consequences that define problem drinking can include health consequences such as hypertension, reversible liver disease, etc.

Table 10-1. Differentiating Substance Abuse and Dependence

	Abuse	Dependence
Clinically significant impairment/distress	Yes	Yes
Maladaptive pattern	Yes	Yes
12-month time period	Yes	Yes
Number of criteria	1 or more	3 or more of any
Criteria:		
1. Failure in role responsibility at work, school, or home	Yes	Yes
2. Using in physically hazardous situations	Yes	Yes, but not necessarily
3. Legal problems	Yes	Yes
4. Use despite repeated social or interpersonal problems	Yes	Yes
5. Tolerance	Possible	Yes
6. Withdrawal	No	Yes
7. Quantity/duration	Not necessarily excessive	Larger/longer than intended
8. Control	Intermittent	Persistent desire to cut down or inability to cut down
9. Time commitment	Moderate	Large (acquiring, using, and/or recovering from substance use)
10. Social, occupational, or recreational impairment	Yes	Yes
11. Continued use despite knowledge of harm	Yes	Yes

Course Specifications: It is important to describe the course of the diagnosis by indicating if the patient is in remission.

- No criteria are met: Note that continued use of the drug is possible without meeting diagnostic criteria for either abuse or dependence. However, that does not mean interventions to prevent progression and the development of negative consequences are unwarranted. For example, someone who continues to inject cocaine should be immunized against hepatitis B, given sterile needles, and counseled on proper needle disposal and avoidance of sharing injection paraphernalia with others.
- Early full remission: No criteria are met for at least 1 month but less than 12 months.
- Early partial remission: Fewer than 3 criteria are met for at least 1 month but less than 12 months.
- Sustained full remission: No criteria are met for 12 or more months.
- Sustained partial remission: Fewer than 3 criteria are met for 12 months or more.

- Binge drinking: Cyclical consumption of large amounts of alcohol (typically more than five or more standard drinks per occasion for men and four or more standard drinks per occasion for women). This definition is conservative and useful for public health initiatives because this pattern of drinking is associated with alcohol-related problems. However, clinicians typically define a binge as a bout of heavy drinking in excess of baseline consumption that persists for days to weeks. This pattern also has intermittent periods of sobriety or reduced consumption.

Substance-Induced Disorders

In DSM-IV-TR, these diagnoses are applied when patients meet criteria for other axis I disorders, but those disorders are better accounted for by the use or discontinuation of the substance(s). This diagnostic category includes syndromes caused by drugs of abuse, medications, and other toxins. The following are possible diagnoses associated with drugs of abuse.

Intoxication

This diagnosis is made when the patient is under the immediate influence of the drug, leading to maladaptive behaviors (e.g., slurred speech, disinhibition, belligerence, unsteady gait in patients intoxicated with alcohol). Intoxication is specific to a particular drug or class of drugs. Patients who meet criteria for intoxication do not necessarily meet criteria for substance-use disorders, but intoxication is a red flag to you to explore this further.

Intoxication delirium

This is a more severe form of intoxication accompanied by altered levels of consciousness and cognition.

Withdrawal

This diagnosis is made when the patient experiences a distinct syndrome characteristic of discontinuation of a substance. Usually, the blood levels are low to absent, and the onset is within hours to days of stopping or reducing use of the substance. Acute withdrawal usually lasts 7 to 10 days for most substances.

Withdrawal delirium

This is a more severe form of withdrawal and is typically seen in alcohol withdrawal (delirium tremens or DTs). In addition to symptoms of withdrawal, the patient is disoriented or hallucinating or experiences illusions and hallucinations, usually visual and very frightening to the patient. The onset is usually within a week of stopping or reducing alcohol. It is a medical emergency, with a 2–5% mortality and requires aggressive treatment. You will likely see such patients admitted to the hospital where the alcohol dependence and early symptoms of alcohol withdrawal have been missed. With systems in place to screen and treat withdrawal aggressively, it is possible to prevent delirium tremens.

Especially in emergency and inpatient settings, it is important to distinguish between intoxication (acute psychopharmacological effects of the drug or drugs) from withdrawal (effect of upregulated systems responding to the absolute or relative lack of drug) (Table 10-2).

Substance-induced mood disorders are characterized by the spectrum of clinically significant and impairing mood disturbances that occur within 30 days of or during intoxication or withdrawal. The mood disorder is not better explained by other causes and doesn't occur within the context of delirium.

Substance-induced anxiety disorders have similar criteria, and the clinical presentation reflects the range of anxiety disorders.

With *substance-induced psychotic disorders*, there are prominent hallucinations or delusions, but the former are not included if the patient recognizes that they have resulted from the use of a substance; the remaining criteria are similar to the substance-induced mood and anxiety disorders.

ETIOLOGY OF ADDICTION

Biological mechanisms alone do not explain the prevalence and incidence of addictive disorders. To better understand the clinical and contextual factors associated with the development of an addictive disorder, it is useful

Table 10-2. Differentiating Between Withdrawal and Intoxication

	Intoxication	Withdrawal
Depressants, Including Alcohol		
Symptoms		
Nausea, vomiting, and/or diarrhea	Often euphoric, maybe dysphoric	Usually dysphoric
Disorientation	Possible with alcohol and opiates	Possible with alcohol and opioids
Level of consciousness	Possible	Possible, but usually only in severe cases
Anxiety	Depressed, eyes may be closed, drowsy	Normal or excited, eyes often wide open
	Minimal	Pronounced
Signs		
Respiration	Depressed	Rapid or normal
Orientation	May be abnormal	May be abnormal
Gait	Staggering, unable to stand	Staggering, unable to stand
Tremors	Absent	Present
Speech	Slurred	Tremulous or normal
Autonomic hyperactivity	Absent	May be present, pronounced in opiate withdrawal
Sweating	Absent	May be present, especially with alcohol
Gooseflesh	Absent	Present in acute opioid withdrawal
Seizures	Only with alcohol and while blood levels are elevated and rising	Occurs within days of stopping, level of alcohol/drug is usually low or zero, rare in opioid withdrawal
Hallucinations	Absent	May be present in severe cases (e.g., delirium tremens)
Delusions	Rare	Absent
Levels in biological fluids (breath, urine, blood)	Elevated	Low or absent
Stimulants		
Symptoms	Agitated, restless, euphoric, garrulous	Agitated or tired, irritable, dysphoric
Nausea, vomiting, diarrhea	Rare	Rare
Disorientation	Possible	Rare
Level of consciousness	Alert/hyper-alert; unconscious if overdosed	Sleepy but easily roused
Appetite	Absent	Hungry, seeks food and water
Anxiety	Frequent	Not usually
Depression	Unlikely	Common

to broadly categorize these factors into four main categories. The interplay between these categories determines the development, consequences, maintenance, and recovery from addiction. A clinician must be aware of all these factors to develop a comprehensive clinical assessment and management plan for an addicted person.

Drug (Agent) Factors

The following are factors of various drugs related to addiction. The abuse liability of a drug (pharmacodynamics and pharmacokinetics) (Box 10-3) involves the following:

- Drug-brain receptor interaction affecting various neurotransmitters, second messengers, and brain reward pathways
- Ability to rapidly cross the blood-brain barrier (i.e., small molecular size, low plasma protein binding, unionized, high liposolubility)
- Short half-life (e.g., oxycodone is more addictive than methadone)
- Rapid onset and offset of action (e.g., crack is more addictive than MDMA)

Box 10-3. Classification of Drugs of Abuse

I. CENTRAL NERVOUS SYSTEM (CNS) DEPRESSANTS
   A. Alcohol
   B. Sedative/hypnotics and anxiolytics
      1. Benzodiazepines
      2. Barbiturates
   C. Opioids
   D. Inhalants including amyl nitrate (poppers) and Nitrous oxide
   E. Gamma hydroxybutarate (GHB)

II. CNS STIMULANTS
   A. Cocaine/crack
   B. Amphetamines
      1. Speed (d-amphetamine)
      2. Crystal/ice/meth (methamphetamine)
      3. Ecstasy (methylenedioxymethamphetamine; MDMA)
   C. Nicotine
   D. Caffeine

III. HALLUCINOGENS
   A. Lysergic acid diethylamide (LSD)
   B. Psilocybin, mescaline
   C. Cannabinoids
   D. Phencyclidine (PCP)
   E. Ketamine

IV. ANABOLIC STEROIDS

V. COMMON OVER-THE-COUNTER MEDICATIONS
   A. Antihistamines/antinauseants

- Route of administration (inhalation is the most rapid route of delivery, with the highest dose reaching the brain due to direct absorption into the systemic arterial circulation and bypass of first pass metabolism in the liver (therefore, smoked crack is more addictive than chewed cocoa leaves)
- The contaminants in the drug and/or route of administration primarily play a role in causing associated medical complications, thereby increasing the burden of disease (e.g., methanol in alcohol, starch, or anesthetics in cocaine used by injection drug users, carcinogens in cigarettes, HIV and hepatitis C virus transmission with needle use)

Host Factors

Genetic Predisposition

Genetic factors account for about 50–60% of the variance in persons who develop addictions. There is no single gene implicated in substance dependence. Moreover, treatment works despite these genetic predispositions.

Pharmacogenetics

The distribution of the type and amount of cytochrome P450 in the liver determines the metabolism of a drug of abuse. Slow metabolizers are less likely to get addicted.

Development of Tolerance

Patients who develop tolerance rapidly are also more likely to develop substance-related disorders. Therefore, those who can "hold their drinks" are more likely to develop substance dependence than those who have aversive experiences with small amounts of the drug.

Psychiatric History

The reasons for a history of psychiatric illness increasing the vulnerability to substance abuse and dependence are not obvious but include the "self-medication" hypothesis—that patients use drugs to medicate their mental health problems. However, more often than not, concurrent substance use worsens the prognosis.

Past History of Abuse

The prevalence of past trauma is especially high in substance-using populations. The history of abuse may be revealed after detoxification, when the patient has lost a pharmacological defense against these painful experiences and memories.

Personality Factors (e.g., High Risk Takers)

Patients with high novelty-seeking personality traits are more likely to get addicted.

Age

Adolescence is often a vulnerable time when substance use begins. The disease usually becomes clinically significant in young adulthood, although there are exceptions.

Sex and Gender

Men are far more likely to get addicted. However, women have a poorer prognosis in treatment.

Ethnicity

Some ethnic groups have genetic protection against dependence due to metabolic differences (e.g., Asian populations tend to have low levels of the liver enzyme alcohol dehydrogenase that leads to aversive experiences when they drink alcohol, leading to reduced consumption of alcohol).

Environmental Factors

Availability

There is a direct correlation between the availability and promotion of a drug and its use in society.

Price

The cost of the drug is inversely related to the consumption, with poor populations being most price sensitive.

Legal Status

Drugs that are legally available are used more commonly, and the onset is at a younger age.

Social and Cultural Norms

These determine the attitudes toward use, addiction, and its treatment.

Gender and Sex Roles and Expectations

Gender roles are associated with type of drug(s) used, frequency and context of use, and route of administration. Generally, male use is associated with socializing and celebration, while female use is usually a coping strategy to deal with stress. However, there is tremendous overlap, and stereotyping is not helpful.

Social Determinants of Health

Substance use is more common in those with lower education (high school or less), those living in poverty, and in those working at blue-collar jobs. However, addictions occur in all social classes and are more difficult to detect in those with higher socioeconomic backgrounds because of the stigma associated with the disease and the environmental tolerance of heavy use of some substances.

Vectors

The suppliers or dealers of drugs also play a pivotal role in addictive disorders. They often control the quality, type, and amount of drug available. Depending on the legal status of the substance, these variables are affected. However, although a legal industry, the tobacco industry has not developed or marketed a less harmful product. It is estimated that tobacco use will be responsible for over 500 million deaths worldwide in the next 50 years.

Gateway Drugs

Although most users of alcohol and tobacco do not progress to illicit drug use, there is an over-representation of smokers and drinkers in populations who use illicit drugs.

The most common progression for substances of abuse appears to be tobacco and alcohol, followed by marijuana and then other drugs of abuse, although exceptions have been noted. Thirteen percent of users of alcohol, 8% of marijuana users, and 15% of cocaine users will develop dependence on that substance within 10 years of their first use of it. Therefore, early detection of abuse and dependence, and understanding and addressing these factors, are important to induce and sustain a remission.

EPIDEMIOLOGY OF SUBSTANCE USE[7]

It is important to recognize the high prevalence of substance use in the general population, particularly among people experiencing a psychiatric disorder. Health care practitioners all too often overlook this highly prevalent condition.

General Population

The lifetime prevalence of substance-use disorders in the general population is 6.2% (7.7% males, 4.8% females). This excludes nicotine dependence, which is closer to 50%. However, in those who have *ever used* drugs recreationally, the lifetime prevalence of drug abuse or dependence is about 18%, which is triple the baseline risk.

Psychiatric Disorders

Any anxiety disorder increases the risk of an alcohol use disorder by 50%, and it increases the risk of any substance-use disorder by 70%. Patients with panic disorder and obsessive compulsive disorder are at particular risk, as are patients with post-traumatic stress disorder. Thirty-two percent of patients with any mood disorder have a comorbid addictive disorder (16.5% alcohol, 18% other, including polysubstance use). Fifty-six percent of patients with bipolar disorder have an addictive disorder, making it the axis I illness most likely to co-occur with a substance-use disorder.

> Altered level of consciousness, disorientation, thought disordered, acutely paranoid, affective disturbance, and/or abnormal behavior occur.

> Rule out other organic causes as appropriate: structural, metabolic, endocrine, medications, etc. (have a high index of suspicion for the above if the level of impairment is in excess of that expected due to withdrawal/intoxication alone or inconsistent with the expected time course).

> • Take a short history and conduct a focused physical examination to make your diagnosis.
> • Differentiate between intoxication and withdrawal and manage accordingly.
> • Complete the history once the patient is neither intoxicated nor in withdrawal.

> As a rule of thumb, intoxication with sedative hypnotics is similar to withdrawal from stimulants and vice versa. Intoxication occurs within minutes of ingestion and lasts a few hours depending on the half-life of the drug. Withdrawal occurs when the level of drug is falling, and so its onset is at least a few hours if not days after the person has stopped the drug. Over time, withdrawal tends to worsen, peak, and then gradually subside over days. Most substance users in withdrawal crave the drug to mitigate symptoms, while intoxicated individuals do not crave as much.
> Symptoms that persist after 4 weeks of last use of a drug are unlikely due to withdrawal or intoxication. However, these symptoms could still have been precipitated by drug use and persist for months and years (e.g., sleep disorders, flashbacks, and memory problems).

FIGURE 10-1 *Approach to patients presenting with potential substance-induced disorders.*

In one study, 45% of patients who presented to an early psychosis program met criteria for one or more types of substance abuse or dependence, most commonly alcohol and cannabis.[3] The use of stimulants was rare.

Alcohol and drug use disorders are also very strongly associated with antisocial, histrionic, dependent, and borderline personality disorders (57% have substance-use disorders). Therefore, routine and repeated screening for substance use is necessary for all patients you are assessing for mental health problems.

Screening for Alcohol and Drug Use Disorders

Screening is warranted in ambulatory, emergency, and inpatient settings (Figure 10-1). Many practitioners are distrustful of and cynical about patients with addictions. Therefore, many clinicians simply double the amount of substance use that a particular patient reports. This attitude is counter-therapeutic, since the patient feels mistrusted and judged. It is more useful to understand that the denial and lies are not personally directed at you as a clinician, but are rather a part of the stigma and shame associated with having an addiction.

The Approach
Screening for substance use and substance-use disorders is a part of a good clinical interview. It is important to use a straightforward, nonjudgmental approach that will allow for full disclosure by the patient. The context of screening or probing into this sensitive issue requires the establishment of trust between patient and provider. Therefore, it may take several interviews before the patient is ready to disclose the full extent of the substance use (see section on Motivational Interviewing).

A quick screen for substance use is to simply ask patients whether they ever used any substances in their lifetime. It is useful to start with the use of tobacco, alcohol, and caffeine, followed by prescribed medications, and then illegal drugs, beginning with cannabis and then reviewing the major drugs prevalent in the community (see Table 10-2).

Screening questions for problematic substance use have high sensitivity and low specificity. Therefore, positive responses indicate that a full assessment to rule in or rule out a diagnosable substance-use disorder is needed. The most popular and validated screening tool is the CAGE questionnaire[4] and its modification for other substances of abuse, the CAGE-AID.[5] These four questions are useful screening tools because they only take 2 minutes or less to conduct (Box 10-4).

More detailed screening tools can be found in reference texts (see Recommended Readings).

Detailed Alcohol/Drug Consumption History
Box 10-5 is a checklist for detailed history/examination and biological tests for substance-use disorders.

Box 10-4. Screening for Alcohol and Drug Problems

CAGE and CAGE AID

- Have you ever tried to *Cut down* on your drinking or drug use?
- Have you ever been *Annoyed* by others telling you to cut down on your drinking or drug use?
- Have you ever felt *Guilty* about your drinking or drug use?
- Have you ever needed an *"Eye opener"* in the morning or the need to use drugs in the morning?

Interpretation: Two out of four positive responses suggests a lifetime history of alcohol/drug problems, indicating the need for further exploration for substance-use disorders.

Pattern of Use

It is important to document the quantity and frequency of alcohol use at baseline for the reasons that follow.

Diagnosis

This documentation helps with diagnosis because those with alcohol dependence tend to be daily drinkers and drink more than four drinks per day.

Management

If the patient is not willing to abstain completely, reduced drinking goals and less harmful patterns of consumption need to be established and measured against baseline patterns. Drinking patterns also indicate whether withdrawal management is necessary (Box 10-6).

Prescription/OTC drug dose may be accurately assessed if the patient reveals the details of the source of the drug(s). Illicit drug dose is hard to estimate because of the variable purity of street drugs. However, in both instances, the pattern of consumption indicates whether withdrawal management may be necessary, especially with opioid and benzodiazepine users. As a rule of thumb, if a patient is unable to stop using safely for more than a week, withdrawal management is indicated.

Physical Examination

This is a vital part of the diagnosis but is often skipped. It is important to document vital signs and stigmata of substance use (e.g., track marks in injection users, nasal septal perforation in cocaine snorters, conjunctival injection in marijuana smokers, tobacco-stained fingers and teeth in smokers, odor of alcohol on the breath). Examine the patient for physical signs of withdrawal or intoxication. A thorough mental status examination will elucidate possible substance-induced disorders.

Box 10-5. Checklist for a Detailed History/Physical Examination and Biological Tests for Patients with Substance-Related Disorders

Tobacco, alcohol, and drug history: lifetime, last 30 days (quantity and frequency of consumption)
Symptoms of intoxication/overdose
Withdrawal symptoms, especially seizures
Depression/anxiety
Suicidal ideation
Consequences of drug use: school, work, home, social, legal, housing
Medical consequences: (e.g., HIV, hepatitis B and C, infective endocarditis in injection drug users; cirrhosis, pancreatitis, hypertension, insomnia, diarrhea in alcohol users)
Associated issues:
    Drinking/drug use and driving/boating/sports
    Unprotected sex
    Needle sharing
    Family violence
    Safety of children
    Birth control
Pain history and management
Physical examination to confirm above (e.g., needle track marks)
Laboratory/point-of-care testing
Complete blood cell count, serum transaminases
Breathalyzer
Urine toxicology testing

Box 10-6. Alcohol Consumption (Frequency × Quantity)

Pattern of alcohol consumption:
- Daily, weekly, monthly, sporadic
- Variations to baseline pattern if any.
- Binge pattern (≥5 standard drinks per occasion with variable periods of abstinence)

Quantity of alcohol consumed:
- Elicit specific consumption from the patient. "Social drinking" does not accurately reflect the amount or pattern of consumption.
- Convert the patient's response into standard drinks containing equivalent amounts of ethanol. A standard drink is:
    □ 341-mL (12-oz) bottle of beer (5% alcohol)
    □ or 43 mL (1.5 oz) of spirits (40% alcohol)
    □ or 142-mL (5-oz) glass of wine (11% alcohol)
    □ or 85 mL (3 oz) glass of fortified wine (e.g., sherry, port, vermouth) (18% alcohol)

Urine Toxicology

Drug/alcohol testing of biological fluids confirms the presence or absence of the drug in the body; results do not indicate the absence or presence of a substance-use disorder. Therefore, all results must be interpreted within a clinical context to guide treatment interventions.

Urine toxicology is the least invasive and most common method of detecting drugs of abuse. You must indicate to the toxicologist which drugs are of interest to choose the most appropriate methods to reduce false positives and false negatives. Table 10-3 has further details on toxicology testing. To interpret a urine toxicology result, the first step is to check the urinary creatinine concentration. If it is less than 2 mmol/L, the sample is too dilute for accurate interpretation if no drugs are detected in the sample. Of course, if the sample has 0 mmol/L of creatinine, the sample tested is not urine. The next step is to check the pH of the sample. If the pH is less than 2 or greater than 9, drugs of abuse may not be detected. This indicates that the sample has likely been tampered with to foil drug detection. If the pH is normal, the results of the drug tests are generally valid.

For example, a patient whose urine toxicology result is positive for opiates (codeine, morphine, and 6 monoacetyl-

morphine [a metabolite of heroin]) likely used heroin alone or with codeine. Another explanation is that the patient used opium or heroin made from opium rather than morphine alone. Poppy seed ingestion or prescribed codeine preparations cannot account for this result.

Laboratory markers

These tests, such as liver function tests and hematological indices, are indirect measures of alcohol consumption and health consequences because alcohol is eliminated at the rate of about one standard drink per hour. There are no specific biomarkers for other drugs of abuse.

Although laboratory markers have lower sensitivity and specificity than the CAGE questionnaire in the detection of problematic substance use, they are useful to detect use in patients who are unable to respond or communicate and to monitor response to therapy. Sometimes, they provide a reason to discuss alcohol problems with a patient who may not have revealed her true level of consumption before the blood tests were taken. The best laboratory markers currently available are the GGT and MCV. Normal values do not exclude at-risk drinking because their sensitivity is only 30% to 50% to detect consumption of four to six drinks per day. The half-life of GGT is 4 to 6 weeks and can be used as a marker of relapse. The half-life of MCV is 3 months (the life span of red blood cells). Therefore, normalization of the MCV can be used as confirmation of continuous abstinence for at least 3 months in those who had elevated levels at baseline.

The GGT, being a nonspecific marker, can be elevated by obesity, diabetes, biliary tract disease, nonalcoholic liver disease, and microsomal enzyme inducers such as phenytoin or barbiturates. The MCV can be elevated by hypothyroidism, folate or vitamin B_{12} deficiency, drugs like valproic acid, smoking, and liver disease.

The elevation of the AST levels to two to five times the normal value and double the level of alanine aminotransferase indicates alcohol-induced liver damage. And although this may be used to monitor recovery, it has very low sensitivity for diagnosing alcohol-use disorders. It normalizes within 14 days of abstinence from alcohol. AST levels may also be elevated due to cardiac muscle damage, high doses of vitamin A, herbal remedies, or muscle damage caused by strenuous exercise or an intramuscular injection.

A newer test, carbohydrate deficient transferrin, is not widely used because it provides no advantage over other cheaper tests. Moreover, it is not useful to monitor drinking in women due to high false-positive rates.

Concurrent Disorders

Certain psychiatric disorders increase a person's risk of developing a substance-use disorder. Conversely, a person

Table 10-3. Limits of Detection of Various Drugs in Urine

Drug/Drug Class	Duration of Detection
Amphetamine	1–3 days
Barbiturates	
Short-acting (secobarbital)	1–2 days
Long-acting (phenobarbital)	3+ weeks
Benzodiazepines	More likely to detect diazepam but may miss high doses of clonazepam, bromazepam, and lorazepam Up to 3+ weeks, depending on extent of diazepam use
Cannabinoids	
After cessation of short-term use	Up to 10 days
After cessation of chronic use	3+ weeks
Cocaine	1–2 days (parent drug); various metabolites may be detected and reported
Benzoylecgonine (cocaine metabolite)	3–7 days
Opiates	3–7 days
Codeine	1–2 days
Morphine	1–3 days
Meperidine (false-negative results on immunoassay)	1 day; also detects normeperidine (1–2 days)
Hydromorphone	1–2 days; insensitive to therapeutic levels
Oxycodone (false-negative results on immunoassay)	1–2 days
Methadone and methadone metabolite (EDDP)	1–4 days

with a substance-use disorder is at increased risk of being diagnosed with a primary psychiatric disorder. There are three main hypotheses to explain this association.[6] First, the self-medication hypothesis describes the concept of patients using drugs or alcohol to treat symptoms of their primary psychiatric disorder. However, the reinforcing properties of the abused substances then lead to a secondary substance-use disorder. The second hypothesis is that substance abuse induces social, psychological, and physical changes that culminate in a secondary psychiatric disorder. Finally, there may be an independent, underlying factor that predisposes a person to the development of both a primary psychiatric disorder and a substance-use disorder. Regardless of these hypotheses, it is generally not clinically useful to justify one disorder because it was "caused" by the other. "Self-medicating" should never be a reason not to treat a substance-use disorder.

Further complicating the picture is that certain substance-induced disorders can mimic common primary psychiatric disorders. Intoxication, withdrawal, substance-induced mood disorders, substance-induced anxiety disorders, and substance-induced psychotic disorders are some examples of substance-induced disorders that can be misdiagnosed as primary psychiatric disorders. Many different substances can cause these substance-induced disorders.

There are certain tools a clinician can employ to distinguish a primary psychiatric disorder from a substance-induced disorder (Figure 10-2). Arguably, the most reliable way to distinguish between the two is to observe a patient for 4 weeks of abstinence to see whether the psychiatric symptoms improve or resolve. In addition, there are historical clues that are suggestive of a primary psychiatric disorder: onset of psychiatric symptoms before the onset of substance use, persistence of psychiatric symptoms during periods of abstinence, a family history of psychiatric disorders, and severe psychiatric symptoms.

If you diagnose a substance-induced disorder (i.e., the addiction appears to be dominant), the most appropriate management is to initiate abstinence from the abused substance(s). After 4 weeks of abstinence, the patient's psychiatric symptoms can be reassessed for a possible primary psychiatric disorder. One caveat to this approach is that if the patient presents with severe psychiatric symptoms such

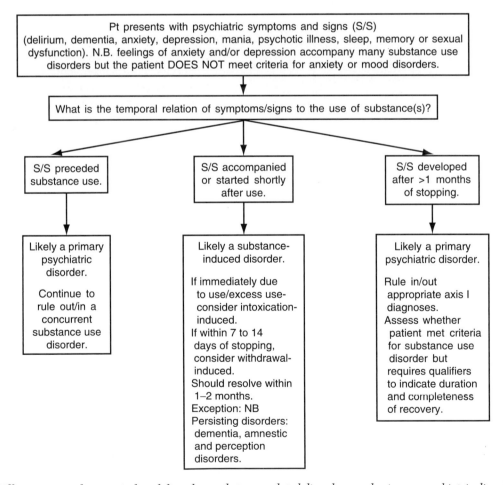

FIGURE 10-2 *Differentiating substance-induced disorders, substance-related disorders, and primary psychiatric disorders.*

as suicidal ideation (i.e., the psychiatric illness appears to be dominant), it may be prudent to treat the psychiatric symptoms immediately, even though a substance-induced disorder has not been definitively ruled out.

If a patient is diagnosed with both a substance-use disorder and a primary psychiatric disorder, then this patient has a concurrent disorder (or dual diagnosis). It is very important to treat both the psychiatric and substance-use disorder as separate but equal entities. Keep in mind that these patients are at increased risk for suicide. In addition, patients with concurrent disorders are difficult to treat and have a poorer prognosis. They require comprehensive case management and an integrated treatment approach that involves both mental health and addiction treatment. You should not treat only the psychiatric disorder and hope that the substance-use disorder will resolve itself. This validates the drug use, is not likely to work, and may in fact be dangerous due to potential drug-drug interactions.

TREATMENT OF SUBSTANCE-USE DISORDERS

Goals of Addiction Treatment

The primary goal of addiction treatment is to induce and then sustain a remission. The secondary goal is to increase the interval between relapses and to decrease the duration and severity of each relapse. Therefore, the overall goal is similar to that of other diseases: to reduce the harm caused by the disease without necessarily effecting a cure.

Despite the similarities to other chronic illnesses, there are some unique considerations with addictive disorders. Addictions are accompanied by considerable social stigma and shame for the patient and his or her family. Due to the extreme compulsive nature of addictive disorders, secondary antisocial behavior may complicate the addictive disorder. Moreover, the spiritual aspects of treatment may be more pronounced in the management of addictions than in other chronic diseases. This may make those involved uncomfortable because of religious overtones and value conflicts with patients. There are several ways to recover, and patients need to explore the risks and benefits of each modality.

Philosophy of Treatment

There are two main philosophies that exist but have served to divide the treatment community along ideological lines. The more traditional approach to addictive disorders is the abstinence-oriented approach. In this methodology, complete abstinence from all psychoactive drugs is the only acceptable goal, and failure to comply is usually met with punishment of some sort (e.g., shaming, discharge from treatment, denial of social assistance, imprisonment). The origins of this come from the temperance movement, with moralistic overtones to care. Therefore, terms with moral overtones such as *abstinent, clean, dirty,* and *in denial* have woven their way into the lexicon of addiction treatment. The underlying values may leave patients with an experience that has been provider-centric, confrontational, and disempowering. These programs tend to work for those who believe in them, accept the philosophy, and are ready to change.

Alcoholics Anonymous is a mutual-aid nonprofit organization with meetings of recovering alcoholics available on all continents at no charge. Although a common belief about Alcoholics Anonymous is that patients have to be abstinent to attend, the contrary is true. Attendees must simply have a desire to address their disease. Moreover, the structure recognizes and operationalizes the concept that recovery is a process by having 12 steps. It also recognizes relapses and has structures built into it to provide support and to recognize progress. Despite some very positive aspects to this movement, patients may be resistant due to their beliefs and experiences in mutual-aid programs.

Harm Reduction

Complete cessation of all drug use is a laudable goal and should be explored with every patient. However, most dependent patients are not ready to stop using drugs immediately, but they are certainly able to engage in behaviors that reduce the harm of their drug use. For example, an injection heroin user has the option of using sterile needles provided at a needle exchange program and/or enrolling in a methadone maintenance program. Both interventions have the potential to reduce HIV transmission and improve general health.

Harm reduction can be defined as any program or policy designed to reduce drug-related harm without requiring the cessation of drug use per se. This philosophy informs a variety of effective interventions aiming at personal or social harms in different areas of substance use (e.g., moderate drinking, methadone substitution for heroin dependence). However, modification of a single variable may lead to compensation in another domain and increased net harm. For example, snuff was promoted to smokers as a safer alternative, but it actually recruited nonsmoking youth with minimal switching by smokers. Therefore, harm reduction has to be framed within a broader understanding of the issue of total harm.

Substance Abuse

Patients with substance abuse are amenable to brief interventions by clinicians. Complete abstinence is not necessary, and reduced consumption goals are acceptable, except if there are clear contraindications to drinking due to medical, legal, or social reasons. However, patients should be advised that substance abuse is a risk factor for the later development of dependence. The use of motivational techniques (see following section), especially in brief treatment programs (four to six 1-hour sessions in either a group or individual setting), and self-help books can be very useful. Therefore, routine screening and brief advice to quit should be the standard for all patients you see, especially if you are not specialized in the treatment of addictions.

Substance Dependence

Reduced consumption in patients with substance dependence is usually not a sustainable goal in the absence of agonist/antagonist treatment. Therefore, abstinence should be recommended as the goal with the maximum benefit and best prognosis. Unfortunately, not all patients are ready and able to achieve this goal.

Withdrawal management is often the first step in the process. This can occur at home, in a nonmedical ("community") setting, or in a medically supervised setting. Medically supervised withdrawal management is generally recommended for patients who have a history of withdrawal seizures (e.g., from alcohol or benzodiazepine/barbiturate dependence), who are pregnant, or who suffer from serious medical (e.g., coronary artery disease) or psychiatric (e.g., schizophrenia, suicidal ideation) conditions.

Withdrawal management is only the first step in the process of treating substance dependence. Once detoxification is complete, the patient should be offered comprehensive addiction treatment in an inpatient treatment center or in an outpatient treatment setting.

Motivating Change in Addicted Patients

Many clinicians find it hard to treat patients with addictions because they find them manipulative, unmotivated, and unresponsive to treatment. However, rates of recovery are similar to those of other chronic conditions. Factors that influence recovery include a positive patient-clinician relationship, social supports beyond the therapeutic relationship, and the premorbid functioning of the patient. Therefore, the clinician has a very important role to play in engaging the patient in the process of change.

Understanding Motivation

Although some experts believe motivation is a trait, many others believe motivation to be a state that is determined by a combination of internal and external variables. The transtheoretical model of change has excellent face validity and states that the readiness to change exists along a continuum.[7] Patients at the various stages of change have different cognitive and affective responses to change (Figure 10-3). There are five stages of change, namely precontemplation (not ready to change in 6 months), contemplation (ready to change in 2 to 6 months), preparation (ready to change within a month), action (has changed but for less than 6 months), and maintenance (has changed for 6 or more months). Relapse occurs when the patient starts using again. Many users slip back to a previous stage and should be supported to try quitting again. This is known as "recycling." Good treatment involves planning for such lapses and preventing them from becoming full-blown relapses. Therefore, it is very important that patients should not be disengaged from treatment if they use drugs (i.e., display symptoms of the disease for which they are seeking help); they should be encouraged to stay the course.

Motivational Interviewing

This method of patient interaction is a way to operationalize nonjudgmental, client-centered yet change-oriented treatment. It promotes honesty and accountability while helping patients resolve ambivalence about changing. There are several ways to assess motivation, but the first task of the interview is to establish rapport by using reflective listening and being nonjudgmental. The latter is simply achieved by obtaining the history without using "why" questions. Explore the reasons using "how," "when," "where," "who," and "what" questions. Instead of asking, "Why do you use drugs?" you may say the following: *"Tell me how you feel/think when you use drugs,"* or *"Help me understand what happens to you when you use/don't use drugs."* The latter two questions are less likely to induce resistance to engagement in the change process. The attitude of the physician is to come "alongside" the patient rather than "at" the patient.

Examples of nonjudgmental questions include the following:

- "How many drinks do you drink every day?"
- "How many drinks does it take to make you feel high?"
- "Can you drink closer to 24 beers per day or closer to 36 per day?"
- "Can you tell me about your drug use?"
- "How many cigarettes do you smoke every day?"
- "How long can you go without having a drink or using drugs?"
- "Help me understand the good things of drug use for you."
- "Can you tell me the pattern and amount of cocaine you use?"
- "When you use heroin how does it make you feel? For how long?"
- "Where do you drink the most?"
- "How do you feel when you stop using?"
- "What helps you feel better?"
- "What is the scariest aspect of stopping drugs?"
- "What do you think you will do with your time if you stop using?"

To motivate patients to change, the mnemonic to remember is the five Rs: relevance, rewards, risks, roadblocks, and repetition.

Relevance

Patients change behavior when the change is relevant to their life experience. For example, a smoker may not be willing to change, but an abnormal cardiac stress test may motivate him to contemplate quitting or reducing smoking. Moreover, the motivating factor may not be health but other factors such as price and availability of the drug or experiencing social, legal, or other consequences of use.

To rapidly assess patients' readiness to change, you can ask the following two questions:

1. *"Given everything going on in your life right now, on a scale of 1 to 10, where 10 is the most important issue to address and 1 is the least important, how important is it for you to stop using drugs?"*
2. *"Given everything going on in your life right now, how important is it for you to change? Not at all, somewhat, very, or most important?"*

However, just because change may be important, patients may still not take action due to lack of self-efficacy or confidence. Therefore, it is necessary to ascertain patients' confidence to change.

Simply substitute "confident" for "important" in the above questions to explore this issue. Depending on the importance and confidence, you can direct the interview to boost these variables by exploring the rewards and risks.

Many substance users are ambivalent about their drug use. It has been observed that when patients are ambivalent,

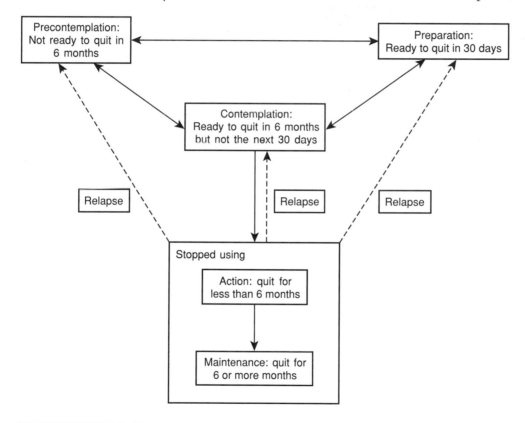

FIGURE 10-3 *The journey through the stages of change.*

they get very resistant to change if providers make arguments for change by threatening their autonomy. Therefore, the task is to create discrepancy by helping patients compare and contrast both the rewards and risks of their behaviors. When you explore this with patients and then reflect the discrepancy back to them, there is often increased readiness to change. Patients report feeling understood and are more likely to engage in the process of change.

Rewards

People use substances because of the reinforcing properties of drugs. Patients expect clinicians to be judgmental or to lecture them about using drugs. They are often ready to counter any argument about the negative aspects of drug use. To prevent arguments with them, it is best to explore the rewards of drug use for them. You may ask the following question: *"Help me understand what are the good things about using X for you."*

Once this aspect has been explored, proceed to explore the risks of ongoing use.

Risks

Explore patients' understanding of the personal negative consequences (if any) of using drugs. Explore the negative aspects on their health, as well as on the social, occupational, legal, and familial domains of their lives.

Once this task is completed, you should reflect back your understanding of the rewards and risks. An example is: *"On the one hand, using makes you forget your problems for awhile, but on the other hand your addiction is causing problems for you at work and home. I can see why you may have difficulty quitting right now. What else can we talk about today so that I can be helpful to you?"*

These statements are empathic without condoning ongoing drug use. It also allows patients the opportunity to change at a pace acceptable to them. This sets the stage for the development of a healthy therapeutic alliance in which patients feel they can trust you with the truth without being judged.

Roadblocks

To gain an appreciation of the feasibility of change in those who are ready to change, it is important to explore the roadblocks they face in making change.

Discovering Roadblocks

When a clinician is being directive and giving advice, the patient may display resistance by overtly challenging the advice. Moreover, it is subtle, and the patient will use "Yes, but. . ." statements. For example, if you state, "Why don't you just avoid going to the bar to stop drinking?" a resistant response will sound like, "Yes, I could do that, but how am I going to meet my friends? Are you telling me that I also have to give up my friends? I'd go crazy locked alone in my apartment!" This leads to an exchange in which the clinician tries to offer solutions to each added problem. However, this kind of exchange eventually leads the clinician to get frustrated with the patient who either consciously or subconsciously resists the advice. To avoid such an encounter, use positive and exploratory statements to identify roadblocks and get the patient to "brainstorm" possible solutions.

- "Which situations do you find make you want to use?"
- "I wonder, what things have worked for you to deal with these triggers?"
- "What else do you need to do to deal with these triggers?"
- "I understand that you have no one to watch your kids while you attend treatment. Who do you think you could ask to help with this? Family, friends, social services, the treatment program, or anyone else I didn't mention?"
- "It appears that you find it hard to stay off heroin despite trying repeatedly. What is your understanding of the role of methadone as a treatment?"

By the end of the session, summarize your understanding of the situation, the next steps the patient is going to take to get better, and what your role is in the treatment plan.

Goal Setting

Help patients set realistic short- and long-term goals. Explore how they are going to achieve these goals, what happens if they experience roadblocks, and how they are going to monitor progress. Some patients with low self-esteem or depression or those who have lost hope due to the severity of their illness may not be willing to set goals. It may require a few sessions to explore their past successes, current attempts at recovery, and treatment of an underlying depression, if present. The task is to elicit self-motivating statements. For example, you can ask patients how they managed to cope through the adversity of their conditions. This facilitates reflection on actual accomplishments communicated by patients.

Repetition

Follow-up visits with the patient should be spent exploring the degree of change by reassessing importance and confidence. Opening statements for the interview may include the following statements:

- "Since we last met, how have things changed?"
- "How do you feel about these changes?"
- "What has been good about these changes?"
- "What has been not so good about them?"
- "What have you done to cope with these triggers to use?"
- "What are the next steps for you?"

The remainder of the session can be spent exploring progress and next steps. In summary, motivational interviewing allows you to develop a positive therapeutic relationship without much negative counter-transference because the responsibility of recovery lies with the patient. Your role as facilitator rather than an expert empowers patients to take responsibility for their behavior. However, they still have a resource to keep up the hope and motivation to change.

CHILD PROTECTION AND DRIVING CONSIDERATIONS

Violation of doctor-patient confidentiality has been justified in several jurisdictions on the basis of greater good to individuals and society. Since substance-use disorders can affect major role obligations and are potentially physically hazardous to others, mandatory reporting of these conditions is common. These can often be reasons for disengagement from treatment and dissolution of the doctor-patient relationship. It is best to be honest with the patient at the beginning of the session as to the limits of confidentiality. If you need to break confidentiality, discuss the issue with the patient, acknowledge her feelings, and offer continued assistance. If your patient recognizes that you are simply obeying the law, she may reengage in the process once her anger passes.

Suspected Child Abuse or Neglect

Although having a lifetime diagnosis of a substance-use disorder does not preclude patients from fulfilling their role as parents, active substance use may place minors in their care at risk. Most jurisdictions have reporting requirements that must be followed and not delegated to others to file the report.

Driving While Impaired

Substance use while operating a vehicle significantly increases the chances of a motor vehicular accident. Many jurisdictions expect physicians to counsel their patients against driving while actively addicted. In inform Ontario, Canada, physicians are held liable for failing to inform the Ministry of Transportation about patients who have a condition that may impair their ability to drive. Interestingly, most drivers who are charged for driving under the influence do not meet criteria for any substance-use disorder. This means that most drivers charged with impaired driving may not have discussed their drug or alcohol use with their physicians, and their physicians will not have had a prior opportunity to intervene. As a result, public health measures such as driver education and public awareness campaigns are very effective in reducing the incidence of impaired driving in a community.

CONCLUSION

Addiction is responsible for many health-related problems, particularly in psychiatric patients. It is our responsibility as health professionals to detect addictive disorders and to offer appropriate treatment. This chapter has emphasized the need to view addiction as a chronic med-

ical illness. By understanding the impressive burden of illness associated with addiction, and by taking a nonjudgmental approach to dealing with addiction, a practitioner can turn this challenging area of medicine into many successful, rewarding encounters with patients.

REFERENCES

1. Holbrook AM, Crowther R, Lotter A, et al: Diagnosis and management of acute alcohol withdrawal, *CMAJ* 160(5):675–680, 1999.
2. American Psychiatric Association: *Diagnostic and Statistical Manual of Mental Disorders*, ed 4, text revision, Washington, DC, 2000, American Psychiatric Association.
3. Van Mastrigt S, Addington J, Addington D: Substance misuse at presentation to an early psychosis program, *Soc Psychiatry Psychiatr Epidemiol* 39(1):69–72, 2004.
4. Maisto SA, Saitz R: Alcohol use disorders: screening and diagnosis, *Am J Addict* 12(Suppl 1):S12–S25, 2003.
5. Brown RL, Rounds LA: Conjoint screening questionnaires for alcohol and other drug abuse: criterion validity in a primary care practice, *Wis Med J* 94(3):135–140, 1995.
6. Kushner MG, Abrams K, Borchardt C: The relationship between anxiety disorders and alcohol use disorders: a review of major perspectives and findings, *Clin Psychol Rev* 20(2):149–171, 2000.
7. DiClemente CC, Schlundt D, Gemmell L: Readiness and stages of change in addiction treatment, *Am J Addict* 13(2):103–119, 2004.

RECOMMENDED READINGS

Brands B, Kahan M, Selby P, Wilson L, eds: *Management of alcohol, tobacco and other drug problems: a physician's manual*, Toronto, 2000, Centre for Addiction and Mental Health.

CAMH Publications: Substance use and addiction, 2003. www2.camh.net/publications/substance_use_addiction.html

Create Canada: Medical education and training on addiction. www.addictionmedicine.ca

Gourlay D, Heit H, Caplan Y, editors: *Urine drug testing in primary care*, San Francisco, 2003, California Academy of Family Physicians. www.familydocs.org/UDT.pdf

Graham AW, Schultz TK, Mayo-Smith MF, et al, editors: *Principles of addiction medicine,* ed 3, Chevy Chase, MD, 2003, American Society of Addiction Medicine.

Health Canada: Best practices concurrent mental health and substance use disorders, 2003. www.hc-sc.gc.ca/hecs-sesc/cds/pdf/concurrentbestpractice.pdf

Kahan M, Wilson L, editors: *Managing alcohol, tobacco and other drug problems: a pocket guide for physicians and nurses,* Toronto, 2002, Centre for Addiction and Mental Health.

Rollnick S, Mason P, Butler C: *Health behavior change: a guide for practitioners*, New York, 1999, Churchill Livingstone.

World Health Organization: Neuroscience of psychoactive substance use and dependence, 2004. www.who.int/substance_abuse/publications/psychoactives/en

Appendix I: Addiction Research Foundation Clinical Institute Withdrawal Assessment for Alcohol (CIWA-Ar)

For each section, ask the prompts and/or observe behavior.

1. Time:
   24 hour clock, midnight=00:00

   __:__

2. Pulse or heart rate, taken for 1 minute

   ___ bpm

3. Blood pressure

   ___/___ mm/Hg

4. **NAUSEA AND VOMITING**
   Do you feel sick to your stomach? Have you vomited?   No nausea and no vomiting ❏0

   Mild nausea with no vomiting ❏1
   ❏2
   ❏3
   Intermittent nausea with dry heaves ❏4
   ❏5
   ❏6
   Constant nausea, frequent dry heaves and vomiting ❏7

5. **TACTILE DISTURBANCES**
   Have you any itching, pins and needles sensations, any burning, any numbness, or do you feel bugs crawling on or under your skin?

   None ❏0
   Very mild itching, pins and needles, burning, or numbness ❏1
   Mild itching, pins and needles, burning, or numbness ❏2
   Moderate itching, pins and needles, burning, or numbness ❏3
   Moderately severe hallucinations ❏4
   Severe hallucinations ❏5
   Extremely severe hallucinations ❏6
   Continuous hallucinations ❏7

6. **TREMOR**
   Arms extended and fingers spread apart.

   No tremor ❏0
   Not visible, but can be felt fingertip to fingertip ❏1
   ❏2
   ❏3
   Moderate, with patient's arms extended ❏4
   ❏5
   ❏6
   Severe, even with arms not extended ❏7

7. **AUDITORY DISTURBANCES**
   Are you more aware of sounds around you? Are they harsh? Do they frighten you? Are you hearing anything that is disturbing to you? Are you hearing things you know are not there?

   Not present ❏0
   Very mild harshness or ability to frighten ❏1
   Mild harshness or ability to frighten ❏2
   Moderate harshness or ability to frighten ❏3
   Moderately severe hallucinations ❏4
   Severe hallucinations ❏5
   Extremely severe hallucinations ❏6
   Continuous hallucinations ❏7

8. **PAROXYSMAL SWEATS**

   No sweat visible ❏0
   Barely perceptible sweating, palms moist ❏1
   ❏2
   ❏3
   Beads of sweat obvious on forehead ❏4
   ❏5
   ❏6
   Drenching sweats ❏7

9. VISUAL DISTURBANCES

Does the light appear to be too bright? Is its color different? Does it hurt your eyes? Are you seeing anything that is disturbing to you? Are you seeing things you know are not there?

Not present ❑0
Very mild sensitivity ❑1
Mild sensitivity ❑2
Moderate sensitivity ❑3
Moderately severe hallucinations ❑4
Severe hallucinations ❑5
Extremely severe hallucinations ❑6
Continuous hallucinations ❑7

10. ANXIETY

Do you feel nervous?

No anxiety, at ease ❑0
Mildly anxious ❑1
❑2
❑3
Moderately anxious, or guarded, so anxiety is inferred ❑4
❑5
❑6
Equivalent to acute panic states as seen in severe delirium or acute schizophrenic reactions ❑7

11. HEADACHE, FULLNESS IN HEAD

Does your head feel different? Does it feel like there is a band around your head?
Do not rate for dizziness or lightheadedness. Otherwise, rate severity.

Not present ❑0
Very mild ❑1
Mild ❑2
Moderate ❑3
Moderately severe ❑4
Severe ❑5
Very severe ❑6
Extremely severe ❑7

12. AGITATION

Normal activity ❑0
Somewhat more than normal activity ❑1
❑2
❑3
Moderately fidgety and restless ❑4
❑5
❑6
Paces back and forth during most of the interview or constantly thrashes about ❑7

13. ORIENTATION AND CLOUDING OF SENSORIUM

What day is this? Where are you? Who am I?

Oriented and can do serial additions ❑0
Cannot do serial additions or is uncertain about date ❑1
Disoriented for date by no more than 2 calendar days ❑2
Disoriented for date by more than 2 calendar days ❑3
Disoriented for place or person ❑4

14. Total Score:

Maximum Possible Score=67 ___
Patients scoring less than 10 do not usually need additional medication for withdrawal.

Instrument taken from Sullivan JT, Sykora K, Schneiderman J, Naranjo CA, Sellers EM: *Assessment of Alcohol Withdrawal: the Revised Clinical Institute Withdrawal Assessment for Alcohol Scale (CIWA-Ar), Br J Addict* 84: 1353–1537, 1989.

11

Suicide and Suicidality

Isaac Sakinofsky

INTRODUCTION

The possibility of suicide occurring in a patient engenders considerable anxiety in the clinician. Predominantly with patients whom we know to be depressed or acutely distressed, it casts an apprehensive shadow over our clinical evaluation and treatment of them. Although suicide will, thankfully, occur in only a minority of patients, fully half of those patients who come to psychiatric emergency rooms (ERs) admit to suicidal ideation along with their other symptoms. Suicidal behavior is usually noted in the presence of a formal psychiatric diagnosis of some kind, but to predict which among those persons we see in clinical practice will kill himself is extremely difficult. Suicidal persons collectively add up to formidable numbers, and the problem should be considered against the wider backdrop.

Suicide as a phenomenon is commonly classified into those in which persons intentionally take their lives (*completed suicides*), those in which persons injure themselves deliberately with at least "nonzero" intent to cause serious bodily harm or their own death (*attempted suicide*), and those in which persons have "zero" intent to take their lives but who take overdoses or otherwise harm themselves deliberately to achieve strong expression of feelings or to influence a person or persons with whom they are closely connected (*deliberate self-harm, parasuicide;* also confusingly referred to sometimes in the literature as *attempted suicide*). Self-injurious behavior intended only as a private expression of feelings that would lead to emotional relief is called *self-mutilation.*

In a randomized survey of a very large sample of Ontario, Canada, householders in 1990, 11% stated they had seriously thought of taking their lives at some time during their lives, and 3% said they had attempted it one or more times. These are staggering figures. Three percent of roughly 8,000,000 householders in Ontario equals 240,000 persons. Around the world, an estimated 1 million people commit suicide every year. More than 30,000 persons in the United States annually take their lives, and in Canada the number exceeded 4,000 in 1999. One quarter of the world's suicides happen in China where, unlike in Western countries, they tend to be among rural, younger females, mainly because of the readier availability to them of toxic pesticides than the less lethal substances preferred by their counterparts in the West. Suicide is the eighth leading cause of death in the general population in the United States for all ages, and the third largest in the under-30 age group. On the North American continent, four times as many males commit suicide as females. In Ontario, the conservatively estimated ratio of suicide attempts to suicides during the year 1990 was 26:1. Whichever way you look at it, suicide constitutes a major problem in the world. Disturbing as are the suicide numbers, we cannot fully envisage the toll in human grief among the families and friends who are left behind (estimated to be, on average, six persons for each suicide), not to speak of the economic burden to society. If we are to prevent such tragedies in our patients, we must ever be watchful to the possibility of suicide in them, beginning with the first assessment, and be perpetually vigilant for hints of contemplated suicidal behavior, often needing to read between the lines. Above all, we must try to understand the complex circumstances that underlie and play a specific role in pushing each such patient over the precipice.

Box 11-2. Terminology

- Completed* suicide: An intentional death by the person's own hand.
- Suicide attempt: Survival from an act with at least some degree of intention to take one's own life; the degree of intent may vary from low to very high, and often fluctuates before, during, and after the act is completed.
- Deliberate self-harm or parasuicide: An act simulating a suicide attempt with little or no intent to kill oneself, for the purpose of interpersonal advantage, short-term relief, expressing intense feelings to others, or bettering one's psychosocial predicament. (However, some authors use this as a generic umbrella term for all forms of suicidality.)
- Self-mutilation: Specific form of deliberate self-harm consisting of self-injury by cutting or burning oneself or by other means; not at all intended to threaten one's life but to relieve one's distress or feelings of numbness (possibly caused by dissociative mechanisms). Whereas other forms of deliberate self-harm are directed toward others in the person's social network, self-mutilation is intensely private and the wounds are often concealed from others.

*Completed suicide is becoming the preferred term for what used to be known as committed suicide, considered to be more pejorative and suggestive of criminal behavior, which suicide is not (although in many legal jurisdictions, assisting suicide is considered a felony).

Key Point:

Your most suicidal patients will conceal their lethal intentions from you, whereas those who in reality wish to live will seek your help to better survive their predicaments and will be more ready to disclose their suicidal thinking to you. Building a therapeutic rapport during the initial interview is critical to a working alliance, not only with you but with the health care team.

by his previous life experiences, coping style, and cultural and personal values. But make no mistake, establishing the clinical diagnosis and the best way to treat the current illness is also critically important. Predicaments may lead into psychiatric illness (as in adverse life events triggering psychiatric illnesses that have neurobiological dimensions), or the illness may itself bring them about secondarily. We cannot help our patients unless we tackle both their predicaments and their illnesses (i.e., practicing comprehensive care). Addressing one aspect alone will not necessarily cure the other after both have gained a foothold in your patient.

ASSESSING SUICIDALITY IS INVASIVE

Determinedly suicidal people know full well that the clinician's training mandates an attempt to dissuade them or even thwart them from taking their lives. Expect, therefore, that your most suicidal patients will conceal their lethal intentions from you, whereas those who in reality wish to live will seek your help to better survive their predicaments and will be more ready to disclose their suicidal thinking to you. If you hope for the right of access into the seriously suicidal person's psyche, the challenge for you is to earn it by engaging the patient in an empathetic discourse that addresses the predicament, while at the same time trying to fathom the persona of the person in the quandary.

Leston Havens, a noted psychiatrist, calls this *finding the patient*.[1] This process is the only way to get behind the defensive barriers the person has thrown up and will often release strong emotion in a patient that he previously denied to himself and others or suppressed. The expression of this outburst of feeling (or catharsis, if you like) to the empathetic listener (you) usually generates intimacy, often referred to as *rapport*. If you have succeeded in winning your patient's trust in this way, you may be rewarded, when you ask, by disclosure of the person's suicidal intentions, which means that he has bestowed considerable trust in you. However, our primary objective as clinicians is certainly not that of merely extracting from the patient the secret of whether he is a serious suicide risk, but rather that of diagnosing what ails him in its context, evaluating its treatability, and deciding what degree of urgency and safety measures should be put in place.

The inpatient staff wondered about the suicidality of a young man who had been admitted for treatment of long-standing depression. Seasoned psychiatric ward staff sensed intuitively that he might be suicidal, but the young man and his parents emphatically denied this and wanted him released from hospital. Avoiding questions about his suicidality until late in the interview, and instead engaging him in an empathetic exploration of his predicament, brought forth a flood of tears. He told me he had been unable to cry for a very long time and admitted that he was desperate at the prospect that his chronic condition might deteriorate to the point where he would have to be indefinitely confined on a psychiatric ward. His feelings of hopelessness and mental pain, he said, had inculcated a strong intention to kill himself that he tried to conceal from others, at times even from himself. The revelation of his serious suicidality resulted in the recognition of his suicidal plight by himself and his family and permitted his being given more urgent and aggressive treatment.

As this example shows, even in the most seriously suicidal person there may be a fragment of ambivalence about dying with which you can work clinically. No one truly understands how it works, but in almost everyone there seems to be a natural instinct to want to live, sometimes in spite of dire misfortune. The opposite is equally true: some people seem to become suicidal for reasons that appear trivial to us unless we are able to discern the personal meaning that the event or complex of circumstances has for the suicidal person. Emile Durkheim, the 19th-century sociologist, was struck by this conundrum, which launched him into his classic study of suicide, *Le Suicide* (1897).[2]

Key Point:

Even in the most seriously suicidal person there may be a fragment of ambivalence about dying. You can certainly assume this is the case when a suicidal patient voluntarily consults you; you have a more difficult task before you if someone is brought to you not of her own accord. Reinstilling hope and morale will be an important action that begins in the initial (assessment) interview with the patient.

INTERVIEWING THE PATIENT

It is astonishing that the same general rules for interviewing suicidal persons apply (or should apply) throughout clinical medicine. In the core volume of the book series to which this volume belongs, *Pediatric Clinical Skills*, Richard Goldbloom listed them as follows:[3]

1. Establish a warm, friendly atmosphere.
2. Maintain privacy and eliminate distraction.
3. Sustain eye contact.
4. Continue a steady, logical flow of content and conversation to nudge the most and the best out of the interviewees.
5. Listen carefully.
6. Observe carefully.
7. Season your conversation with regular expressions of empathy and support.

Elsewhere, Richard Goldbloom also advises not to have a desk between you and the patient and not to take verbatim notes but just to jot down points, so as not to interfere with the building of rapport between you and the patient. These rules hold as true for interviewing psychiatric patients as they are valid for interviewing sick children and their parents.

In my own psychiatric practice, when I am seeing someone for the first time and taking a lengthy case history, I do have a writing tablet on my lap and take "shorthand" notes for later dictation so as not to forget details that might subsequently prove important. However, I try not to let my note-taking obtrude on the interview, and I do my best to keep the focus of the interview on my interaction as a professional human being with the patient as a human being who is in a predicament that I must try to understand and

help him with. If you are taking notes, you should remember that if you selectively jot down points during the interview the patient will take note that this aspect is important, and it may reinforce behavior during the interview accordingly. After the history-taking phase, in subsequent meetings with the patient, I rarely take notes right at the time but get the substance of the interview down on paper as soon as possible afterward. I do, however, know of several colleagues who are able to take notes during all their interviews and sometimes even use their note-taking to underline emerging points or insights for the patient's attention. I suppose neither style is necessarily "correct," and you must find the one with which you are most comfortable. For my part, even though I was trained as a resident to take verbatim notes of interviews (for later supervision sessions), I discarded this method along the wayside because I found it interfered with my rapport with my patients.

Human beings have a craving to be understood; they thirst to be validated by others. Years ago, as a postgraduate student in London, the research project I designed required that I interview 50 consecutive psychiatric patients from a waiting list of those seeking psychological counseling. The experimental interviews included "concordant feedback," during which I supportively paraphrased and fed back to the patient his own account of his predicament. The interviews also included random "discordant feedback" sequences in which the predicament seemed clearly misunderstood by me, although my tone remained supportive. Both the patient and the interviewer were harnessed to psycho-galvanometers (measuring galvanic skin response, a peripheral measure of central brain arousal analogous to anxiety or agitation). During concordant feedback periods, the measures of arousal subsided, and during discordant periods, they rose (indicating agitation) in both the patient *and the interviewer*.

Just as much as the patient feels the need to be understood, so does the interviewer/therapist need to feel that you are understanding, in other words, that you are in a position to place the patient's predicament relatively accurately in a coherent, explanatory framework that accounts for his actions and reactions and allows you to formulate a plan of treatment. When this conceptual schema coincides with the patient's own understanding or elicits his own "Aha!" recognition; we call this *empathy*, and empathy leads to mutual bonding. Leston Havens[1] would agree:

Nor is it enough for the clinician to grasp both the patient's suffering and his or her strengths. That understanding must be *communicated back to the patient* for the alliance to begin; the patient needs to feel heard and seen—that is, *met*, by another person . . . which is the beginning of the affective bond.

Understanding the Predicament

Begin the interview by setting the scene as suggested above. Remember that your goal is first of all to understand this fellow human being a few feet away from you and what circumstances have brought him or her to this sorry pass. After covering the identifying information, such as age, marital and employment status, means of livelihood, living arrangements, etc., proceed next to the question of how the person came to be brought toward this interview. Do not be hesitant to interrupt during any gap in the flow of conversation to recapitulate (summarize) in a nonjudgmental, supportive, yet professional, tone of voice your understanding of the development of his predicament. You should be attempting to provide concordant feedback, but at the same time you are trying to confirm for yourself that you are getting it right and to test out your constantly changing working hypotheses. This will not only convey to the patient your sense of empathy but will also allow him to correct, if necessary, your understanding of his situation.

Try to get a sense of how the key players in the patient's life (e.g., parents, siblings, girl- or boyfriends, spouse, supervisor, children) have contributed to the predicament or buffered it for him. From the current situation, when that seems exhausted, move backward in time to ask about the circumstances of his birth and childhood, the experience of growing up in the parental household (or elsewhere), his perception of his parents and other family figures, whether there was any abuse (verbal, physical, or sexual), whether it was a dysfunctional home, and so on. Next, you will want to get an idea about his development through childhood to adolescence and adulthood, in school and subsequent educational and work situations. Was he sociable or withdrawn? What was his disposition through childhood and adolescence? Was he moody, anxious, depressed, or antisocial? Did he work hard or loaf? Did he use street drugs or alcohol, and when and how? How did he do in his schooling and work? What were his strengths and weaknesses? What about his psychosexual development? If he was in relationships, with whom, how did they work out, and why? How did he cope with losses, humiliations, rejections, and disappointments? Was he confident, or shy and diffident, passive or active, indolent or energetic, aggressive or timorous, etc.? Your own curiosity should prompt you to ask these questions in an unobtrusive way that should make the story flow almost of itself, as if you were reading through a rich, detailed, critical biography of someone interesting. As the two of you proceed through the narration of his life experiences, his dreams, needs, and desires and how they panned out, as well as his reactions, you will begin to understand how this person came to think of suicide (i.e., his particular SILC equation). During this phase of the exploration, inquiry into symptoms such as depressive mood will suggest itself quite naturally. For example, *"Did this [these traumatic experiences] eventually get you down? Did you find yourself becoming saddened, despondent, or hopeless?"*

Follow this train of thought along (it is suicidal logic, but you have not yet labeled it as such) until you are satisfied that you have an idea of the complete mental state of the patient during his ordeal. Once you are in this area, it is natural to delve into depression, degree of despair, hopelessness, helplessness, anxiety, degree of any obsessions, unusual symptoms such as perceptual or cognitive distortions, the perceived locus of threat (internal guilt and self-blame, or external paranoia), and so on. However, be sure to return to your exploration of the patient's predicament in its psychosocial context if your inquiry is incomplete. An assessment interview must flow naturally, exactly like a conversation between two intimates, one of whom is confiding in the other. The order of them does not matter, but the topics to be discussed along the way are pre-set and must each be covered even if the conversation returns to them. You will indeed be carrying out what is known as a *semi-structured interview*. You can come back to the points you are uncertain about, but you should try to cover them all, as well as others that suggest themselves to you.

For a multidimensional comprehension of the patient, you cannot bypass the formative influences of family, cultural and educational environment, and of course, psychosexual development, including peer and sexual relationships. Exposure to a home atmosphere of substance abuse, violence, or abuse of the person, for example, would need to be elicited. Inquire into each of these areas as you would when taking the history of any psychiatric patient but always with the aim of trying to understand the person's suicidality, how it arose, where it sprang from, and how sinister it can be.

Sooner or later, the moment will come when you feel that it would be appropriate to plumb the patient's level of suicide intent that you have refrained from doing until now. At this point, you yourself have learned enough about the story and the person to hazard your own informed conclusions. But only if you are certain you feel the presence of a therapeutic bond (and it is palpable) can you begin to test your theory about the genesis of suicidality in the patient. One approach might be the following:

- *"I suppose that was when you started to see suicide as a solution to your problems (or way of settling the score, etc.)? But did you think you had truly exhausted all the alternative solutions? And did you really want to cease to exist, to end up buried in the ground or cremated? Or was there any part of you left that cried out for an alternative to dying?"* This is asked to get some idea about the degree of ambivalence.

Or, if you are seeing a person because he has just recently made a suicide attempt or act of self-harm:

- *"It seems you have been in a difficult predicament. I suppose this was why you tried to take your life/injure yourself like this. Will you tell me how it all came about that you concluded that this was the thing to do under the circumstances?"*

If you do not already know whether the patient has been having suicidal ideation, the questions might be alternately rephrased as follows:

- *"Did this (these) problem(s) ever bring you down to the point where you wondered if it was worthwhile going on? Did you ever experience thoughts of ending your life? How often? How strong were they? How persistent? Who did you tell about these thoughts? How did you cope with them? What form did they take? Have they become more or less urgent or irresistible? Did you actually consider any ways or plan by which you might take your life? What steps did you take to implement these ideas? What has stopped you so far from acting on these drastic thoughts? What changes in your circumstances do you think it would take to restore your desire to go on living again?"*

The last question is important because you need to discover *what changes in his life's circumstances it would take to keep this person alive.* This will help you to design treatment strategies as well as assist in prognosis.

Always inquire carefully about any previous suicidal behavior, ideation, acts of self-harm, and attempts carried out or aborted along the way. The last category (e.g., someone sitting in the car in a closed garage but not turning on the ignition, or "playing with a noose around his neck") could be token rehearsals for the real thing, efforts to get up the courage to do so.

The questions you ask will suggest themselves appropriately according to the individual circumstances of the case and the stage you have reached in the narrative. They are probes designed to find out how much ambivalence toward death exists; that is, the degree of seriousness of the patient's suicidality is inversely related to the level of his ambivalence about dying. Your questions should never be asked in a barrage; rather, wait for each answer and help the patient to flesh out his attempt to answer each one. Study his face and mannerisms carefully when he answers. His life may hang on whether you are an accurate judge of his candor. Avoidance of eye contact or even trembling lashes or flushing of his cheeks may indicate an effort to conceal or dissimulate suicide intent. It might also just mean that he is feeling intense emotion while he tries to

answer your question or respond to your comment. Knowing this patient so far, which of these interpretations do you think it is? Do not hesitate to probe the answers to your questions until you are satisfied that you know what the answers truly are, so long as you do so in the same friendly, inquiring, logic-seeking tones. You should never become sharp or cajoling in your manner of speech because the patient seems not to trust you as much as you would like him to. After all, you are the one intruding into his deeply private space, albeit with the best intentions and in what you believe are his own and his family's interests.

Weighing the Psychological Strength of the Patient's Suicidality

Weighing the strength of a patient's suicidality is a mixture of applying clinical judgment and considering the known risk factors for suicide. Edwin Shneidman,[4] who practically put suicidology on the map in North America, postulated "psychache" as the core factor from which suicidal thinking stems. *Psychache* is his term for mental pain or suffering, not necessarily synonymous with clinical depression. It includes hurt, anguish, shame, humiliation, loneliness, murderous rage, dread of growing old or dying badly, and other such painful emotions. The overtone clearly has much in common with the symptom of depression as found in clinical depression, but it may not necessarily be part of a formal diagnosis of major depressive disorder. Psychache arises from the thwarting of some basic human need, such as the need for self-respect and respect by others or the need for loving and being loved. As you get to know your patient with suicidal ideation during the interview, try to gauge the intensity of this person's mental pain or suffering. If you like, you can even put it on a scale in your mind or on your page, say somewhere between 0 (absent) and 10 (intolerable depths). Now consider the patient's level of *perturbation,* that is, how upset or agitated he is together with the mental pain he is suffering. It is perturbation that may drive him to do something drastic about his suffering. If you like, put this on a scale from 0 to 4. Next consider the element of *adamance,* which indicates the degree of steely resolve the person is showing toward refusal to accept the problems with which he is beset but cannot change. Put this also on a scale if you wish. Try to judge the degree of objectivity the patient has left to him in appraising his own situation. Lack of such objectivity (i.e., seeing from outside the box) is *constriction* (another Shneidman term). The person is immersed in his problems and cannot be distracted for long before returning to them. Although we call this *rumination* in psychiatry, constriction implies really more than this; it is an inability to see beyond the issues and the paucity of possible solutions selected so far. He will, in fact, curtail exploration of alternative solutions, frozen into a position of *helplessness*. *Hopelessness* is soon likely to descend on him as he contemplates his personal predicament with little or no possible solutions in sight, or those that might get him out of his difficulties appear too formidable to undertake in his present condition. One needs to try to fathom the depths of this hopelessness as with all the other psychological factors one is assessing.

Eventually, when one comes to discuss the nature of the suicidal ideation that is present itself, one can better gauge *intended lethality*—whether the patient is moving to the conclusion that his life should cease, or rather whether he should rather try to *escape* from the predicament in some other way short of the cost of his life. This might be through an act of deliberate self-harm that might even endanger life, but from which he hopes or intends to be rescued. Here, taking into account the assessment of his predicament and psychological state that you have been making, choice of method becomes important in estimating intended lethality. Violent methods such as gunshot, hanging, jumping, or drowning are clearly more deadly methods, and therefore more sinister, than an intended drug overdose. Carbon monoxide inhalation is also more suggestive of higher intended lethality. The level of knowledge the patient has about lethal methods of suicide and the availability to him of such must, of course, qualify your judgment.

Although distressed adolescent females may choose over-the-counter medications like aspirin or acetaminophen, both because of their ready availability and the belief that they will survive the overdose, these are in fact dangerous drugs that carry significant mortality risk. In urban areas, most persons who have ingested over-the-counter or psychotropic drugs and are brought to hospital in time are more likely to survive because of sophisticated (and expensive) treatment. In the United Kingdom, allowable quantities for sale of these drugs have been controlled since 1998 by an act of Parliament. Because of lack of knowledge, a patient with lower intended lethality may mistakenly choose a method more dangerous than aimed at, and vice versa. So try to gauge the level of knowledge your patient has.

Evaluating a patient's level of rashness or tendency to fly off the handle, known as *impulsivity*, is important because impulse could trigger a suicidal act that, to an outsider, the predicament does not warrant. Impulsivity will also cause the person to choose the method closest at hand, which could be more deadly than he would otherwise intend. (Alcohol intake and other substance use fuel impulsive action, so be sure to inquire about such habits.) The principle of preventing suicide by restricting the means, such as by erecting barriers on bridges and subway stations and making it more difficult to purchase firearms, depends on this axiom. Doing so will not likely stop a long-planned suicide but may save the lives of angry or humiliated, possibly intoxicated, and impulsive youngsters.

If the patient has access to a firearm, you must not neglect to arrange (with family or friends) that it be dismantled and placed in safe custody out of the patient's reach and house. Note and date on the patient's record that you have done so for your own medicolegal protection.

It is unrealistic, of course, to eliminate all opportunities for the person to use the other methods that are readily available, but if you believe that a person is potentially, but not imminently, suicidal and a clinical decision has been made not to hospitalize him, for whatever reasons, the immediate family or friends must be warned about possible means of suicide. Drug supplies that could be lethal should be sorted and those no longer in use disposed of. Drugs the patient is using that are potentially lethal in overdose should be placed in the hands of a caretaker. It is probably prudent to have nonlethal drugs left in place in the bathroom or kitchen cabinet. If you think that the patient is "imminently" suicidal (a vague term that means something like over the next couple of weeks), that is another story involving whether to hospitalize him and what other action to take. It will be considered separately in a following section.

Finally, there is a psychological quality that is really difficult to assess. This is the patient's *acceptance*, or resignation to suicide. It is the reason why clinicians are sometimes dumbfounded when a patient has appeared to be doing better and then surprises everyone by taking his life. Be suspicious of an abrupt change in mood and attitude for the better when nothing has really changed in the predicament scenario or the patient's fundamental adjustment to it, and the treatment had not been appearing to have a significant impact so far. This deceptive calm may manifest even during your early assessment phase.

An acutely paranoid and agitated middle-aged man with delusions that the mafia were hunting him down was admitted to a psychiatric ward and placed under close observation. A couple of hours later, he appeared to have settled and relaxed and was noted by a nurse to be polite and behaving socially correctly in the television room. Within an hour of this observation, he was found hanging in a closet on the ward. He had decided to foil his demons by taking his life, and the decision to do so had briefly brought him the appearance of calm and normality.

WEIGHING THE PROTECTIVE FACTORS AGAINST SUICIDE

Figure 11-1 shows the tension between the negative factors discussed in the previous section and the positive factors that defend the patient from his suicidal drives. Apart from whatever is left of his natural survival instinct, we must rely on his personal qualities such as his ability to bear

SUICIDE OR SURVIVAL

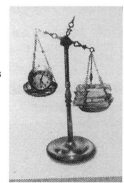

Suicidality	*Survivality*
• Adamance	• Stoicism
• Perturbation	• Adaptability
• Hopelessness	• Alternative-seeking
• Constriction	• Abhorrence
• Lethality	• Anchorage
• Acceptance	• TREATMENT

FIGURE 11-1 *The balance of vectors.*

misfortune (*stoicism*), capacity to *cope with or adapt* to adverse circumstances, and his willingness to continue to seek *alternative solutions*. Not least is his readiness to cooperate with treatment. It is important to try to get an idea whether this patient is likely to comply with medication and psychological treatment, both so this can be dealt with proactively and also as a prognostic indicator. If the patient is suicidal and not likely to be compliant, you would be more inclined to hospitalize him.

Abhorrence indicates the level of the patient's intrinsic resistance to suicide as an action. This may be for religious reasons, not so much determinant on which religion he is formally identified with, but with his faith in a deity whom he sees will protect or rescue him from his troubles or whom he fears offending by taking his life. In some cases, it may be peer pressure against suicide within a community. (The opposite was true in Jonestown, Guyana, when the followers of the Reverend Jones committed mass suicide in 1978.)

Besides religious abhorrence, many suicidal people hesitate to take the risk of maiming themselves in a suicide attempt without taking their lives. *Anchorage* is an important protective factor. If the person is ensconced within a loving and relatively harmonious family and also has responsibility for little ones, she is less likely to take a step that would seem irresponsible. However, there are many exceptions. Women with postpartum depression are sometimes at risk for suicide (and infanticide followed by suicide). Psychotic mothers have been known to drown their little ones before making an attempt on their own life. It is believed that a pregnant woman will not commit suicide, but in practice this does not hold true. Fathers have forgotten their love of and responsibilities to their families and taken their lives. Nonetheless, it is important to explore the patient's reasons for living.[5] Finally, one of the most important factors that may keep the patient alive is going to be the efficacy of *treatment*, which makes it important that

this be adequate and sustained and that the patient be compliant.

RATING SCALES

There are a number of self-report or interviewer-administered scales in existence attempting to delineate suicidal ideation and strength of the suicidal drive. They have been well reviewed for the U.S. National Institute of Mental Health by Brown[6] and fall under the following categories: (1) suicidal ideation and behavior, (2) lethality of suicide attempts (brief screening measures), (3) hopelessness, (4) reasons for living, (5) care provider attitudes and knowledge concerning suicide, and (6) measures in development. Many of these scales have satisfactory internal consistency, inter-rater reliability, test-retest reliability, and concurrent validity, but they are all extremely poor at predicting which specific person that you will see will take his own life. One of the best of these is the Scale for Suicide Ideation, a 21-item rating scale that is administered by the interviewer. Patients who score in the higher category are seven times more likely to commit suicide than those in the lower category. Such an estimate of relative risk covers over high proportions of false positives and false negatives. Calculations of predictive validity tell the story more exactly and show that it lies between 1% and 3% for the best of the scales.

This has meant that clinicians have been discouraged from using these instruments by authoritative sources, for example, the American Psychiatric Association.[7] Personally, I would modify this injunction to suggest that appropriate scales may be used as an ancillary to an overall assessment *after* you have directly interviewed the patient and broken through the patient's reserves. They should not be used *instead* of spending time with the patient directly because then their results will be meaningless to you. In my clinic, I use some of the scales because they are systematic inventories that will corroborate the interview findings. I am as much interested in how the patient answers the individual items as in the overall scores. I evaluate the answers against the careful opinion that has been forming in my mind during the interview. The patient is asked to fill out the scales one by one, always in the same sequence and in my presence, while I review any preexisting hospital charts and watch the patient out of the corner of my eye. As each scale is completed, it is handed to me and gone through immediately. I can then interrupt the patient to amplify or question his answer to any item on the scale. For obvious reasons of time limitation, I have included only the following self-report inventories in my assessments of suicidal persons, and for almost all of them I am indebted to A.T. Beck, another one of the fathers of research into suicide. There are other scales I would also have liked to have included or substituted for one or the other of them, but to make the exercise practicable and also to gather data that can ultimately be analyzed, I have stuck with the following:

Beck Depression Inventory: I use the earlier 21-item version, which gives a score ranging from 0 to 63. Each item has four possible degrees of severity, and the patient is asked to choose the one that is closest to how he feels. Thus, the suicide item includes the following:

1. "I don't have any thoughts of killing myself."
2. "I have thoughts of killing myself, but I would not carry them out."
3. "I would like to kill myself."
4. "I would kill myself if I had the chance."

I take an overall score of 16 or greater as indicating clinical depression. However, above this level I find the numbers do not seem to really discriminate between lesser and greater degrees of clinical depression. This is due to subjectivity on the part of the patient. As always, the patient is using the scale as a tool for communicating with the doctor. I know that some patients demonstrate very high scores above 40 to let me know that they are subjectively hurting and are calling loudly for my help and attention, whereas others with as great or greater depressed mood tend to play down their misery. I have known one young man with a score of 12 on the Beck Depression Inventory who committed suicide within a relatively short time span. However, in spite of his low depression score, we were able to recognize his high suicide risk because of his perturbation, hostility, adamance, and high-risk behaviors. His depression did not take the form of what is usually understood as clinical depression but may have better conformed to Shneidman's concept of psychache. Since its publication, I have included the Shneidman scale in my battery, which measures psychache (generic psychological pain) on a Likert scale and uses postcard-like pictures as checks on a person's tendency to exaggerate or underplay the answers. The battery I currently use in my clinic includes the following:

- Psychological Pain Assessment Scale.
- Beck Anxiety Inventory: This is a 21-item scale, and it measures symptoms associated with tension and anxiety (Shneidman's perturbation).
- Beck Hopelessness Scale: This is a 20-item scale of true/false choices. Scores above 10 have been shown to greatly increase the risk of suicide in follow-up studies of psychiatric patients.
- Beck Scale for Suicidal Ideation: This is another 21-item scale that details the presence and characteristics of suicidal ideation and planning. Although one can compute

an overall score on this scale, I prefer to scrutinize the answers and use them as discussion points with the patient (e.g., exploring any suicide planning that may be present).

- Modified High-Risk Construct Scale: This inventory (Figure 11-2) is interviewer based and not a self-report. It arose out of the less structured clinical assessment process I have described above and encompasses those dimensions of appraisal. An earlier version was tested in a busy psychiatric ER against several of the self-report inventories used in my clinic as well as the Modified Sad Persons Score and was found to be the best predictor of admission to hospital by blinded physicians, followed by the Beck Scale for Suicidal Ideation.[8] No psychometric properties of this scale have been established as yet, nor are there as yet data on predictive validity. Therefore, the scale should only be used by you (if you wish) as a means of organizing your clinical observations and contributing to your thinking about the patient as a suicide risk.

EVALUATING SUICIDE ATTEMPTS

Both the degree of dangerousness to life or person of the attempt as well as the degree of lethal intention behind it must be carefully assessed. If the patient is receiving medical care in the hospital (the medical or surgical intensive care unit, for instance), the medical seriousness is usually self-evident. Ask yourself what would have happened to the patient had she not been brought to the hospital in time. Potential or actual medical seriousness is not, however, always correlated with lethal intent at the time of the act, which depends on the patient's level of knowledge about the risk to life posed by the method chosen. Some patients may not, for instance, be sufficiently aware of the electrolytic or hepatic dangers of salicylates or acetaminophen in overdose and perceive them as ordinary household remedies that ought not to endanger their lives. You can ask the patient, *"Did you really mean to kill yourself? Or was it that you had to get out of an impossible situation but wanted somehow to go on living?"*

The circumstances of the attempt mean even more. If the method that was chosen was a violent one with a high degree of probability of resulting death (e.g.. firearm, jumping, attempted drowning or hanging) or the patient ingested a large quantity of substances she knew to be potentially lethal, this is a serious indication. Whatever the motivation, medically serious attempts should be viewed as bad prognostic factors for future suicide attempts. If the patient took precautions to minimize the likelihood of interference with the plan, that is also a very serious indication. The precautions subscale on the Beck Suicide Intent

Figure 11-2 Modified High-Risk Construct Scale

Name: _____   Date _____

Place estimated score for each item on right of vertical line on a scale of 0–4, where 0 = absent, 1 = mild, 2 = definite, 3 = severe, 4 = intolerable.

1. *Psychache* (subjective mental pain, including sadness, anger, hurt, humiliation, sense of loss, dread, etc.)
2. *Perturbation* (sense of tension or agitation, anxiety, restlessness, psychomotor arousal)
3. *Adamance* (steely resolve not to bow to circumstances of current adversity or to accept any humiliation that may be necessary in order to deal with problems)
4. *Helplessness* (feelings of weakness and powerless to deal with the problems, which might include his illness)
5. *Hopelessness* (feeling there will be no effective rescue from the outside)
6. *Lethality* (The person has been considering violent, aggressive, or potentially lethal ways of ending his problems. In addition to firearms, jumping from a height, or hanging, this might also include "less violent" methods such as suffocation by carbon monoxide gas or drowning or taking a large overdose in a secret location.)
7. *Impulsivity*
8. *Resignation and acceptance of SILC equation* (Suicide Is the only Logical Conclusion for me)
9. *Alcohol or narcotic abuse problem*
10. *Primary psychiatric disorder playing major role in suicidal ideation* (e.g., command hallucinations, depressive or persecutory delusions, or hallucinations)

_____ **Subtotal for Negative Items**

Using the same scoring system, place estimated score for each of the following protective factors.
1. *Stoicism* (Patient shown a capacity for fortitude and making light of misfortune)
2. *Adaptability and coping capacity* (shows willingness and ability to bend with the blows and deal with the resultant emotions; social problem-solving ability demonstrated)
3. *Alternative solution-seeking* (taking positive initiative in exploring alternative ways out of impasse other than suicide)
4. *Abhorrence* (either strong religious beliefs or fear of an unsuccessful attempt resulting in severe bodily injury)
5. *Anchorage* (significant others are in same home as patient and are well-informed, responsible people and extremely positive to the patient)

_____ **Subtotal for Positive Items**

Negative Score = 0–40 = _____

Positive Score = 0–20 = _____

Net score = _____

FIGURE 11-2 *Modified high-risk construct scale.*

Scale is the only part of that scale found to be associated with an increased risk of suicide in a 10-year prospective follow-up of suicide attempters, not the questions that ask the patient about subjective intent.[9]

One system of thinking about the intentionality behind a suicide attempt was developed by Neil Kessel[10] and based on Ed Shneidman's classic paper, "Orientations towards death: A study of lives."[11] Points to consider include the following:

- Intended cessation
- Subintended cessation
- Intended interruption
- Intended continuation

By combining your estimation of the person's intent to take his life with your evaluation of the presence or absence of intended rescue in the plan that was carried out, you may be able to categorize the true level of seriousness of the attempt. *Intended cessation* is the absolute "failed" suicide attempt, where the patient is alive purely for fortuitous reasons.

Either the degree of suicide intent, the choice of method, or the combination of both indicate absolute seriousness. It is only by some miracle that your patient is alive. Only a small minority of living suicide attempters will fall into this category. In a sample of 228 suicide attempters who were studied and followed up for over 1 year, 7% fit criteria for cessation intended. A somewhat larger group (15%) were termed *subintended cessation*, that is, ambivalently hoping for death, possibly turning their suicide attempts into a "trial by ordeal," being prepared to accept the verdict, life or death, either way. Larger groups of suicide "attempters" did not really want to die at all; 40% fell into the group of *intended interruption* (seeking relief from the pressures in their lives by temporary oblivion through overdose and hoping things would be better when they woke up). Finally, 37 % were identified as *intended continuation*, making sure by arranging their acts that there was little risk of dying even though they might present "a pantomime of suicide" for the express purpose of making interpersonal gains.[12]

Weighing the Statistical Risk Factors for Suicide

Now that you have a fairly good idea of the patient's personal predicament and of the psychological strength of his suicide logic and intentions, you should ask yourself where he ranks against the statistical risk factors that are known to make a suicidal act more likely (i.e., to "predict" suicide). Statistical factors help one to have a general idea about suicide risk, but when faced with the individual, these can easily go by the wayside. You must judge your patient on his own merits, not as part of a potentially suicidal group. In Western countries (with rare exceptions like Finland), males outnumber females among suicides as much as 3:1. Figure 11-3 shows the effect of *age by gender* on suicide rates in Canada. You will note that in recent years the suicide rates in young males rises quite steeply during the 20s and early 30s. There is another peak during middle age and again a sharp rise in late old age. The picture is quite different for female persons. The overall rates are much lower, and the same peaks can be discerned, but are shallower. The rate in young women peaks earlier than in men, and the highest risk seems to be during the 50s with another small rise during late age.

One of the strongest of the statistical risk factors is a *previous suicide attempt*. Half of completed suicides have

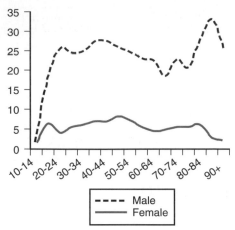

FIGURE 11-3 *Suicide rates by age and gender (1998). Note the immediate rise in suicide rates in adolescent and young adult males. It is only exceeded in late old age. Females show a similar rise but at a lower level and reach peak suicide rates in middle life. (Constructed by the author from data available in the Statistics Canada database.)*

made a previous suicide attempt. Be sure to inquire whether the patient has deliberately injured himself before in his life in what may have been a suicide attempt. When did this take place, and what were the circumstances? Was it an act considered over time or impulsive? What were the means, and what would the lethality have been if the patient had not received prompt treatment? (This last point is something you will have to decide for yourself after you have ascertained the precise means that were employed.) Persons who have previously used lethal methods should always be considered at risk, but the corollary does not apply—use of a low-lethality method does not imply that the next time it won't be lethal—it rather depends on the person's acute state of mind and desperation at the time of the next attempt. Ask where the attempt took place and how and by whom it was discovered. It is more serious if someone has taken precautions to conceal the attempt from potential rescuers, for example, by going off alone to a cottage in the country or checking into a hotel and putting the "do not disturb" sign on the door. Some patients change their minds as they begin to lose consciousness and call someone for help. Ambivalence to death fluctuates. Others are enacting "a cry for help" and try to set up discovery they hope will be in time. But this can be playing Russian roulette, since nothing like that can be foolproof.

In *The Savage God*, Alvarez tells the story of the 1963 suicide of the famous poet and feminist cult figure of her day, Sylvia Plath. Sylvia's husband, Ted Hughes, had left her for someone else. Plath lived in a house in London with their children. Sylvia had suffered previous bouts of depression, had made at least one suicide attempt, and was under treatment for depression. She arranged for an Australian au pair girl to arrive early in the morning after she intended to turn on the gas taps in her bedroom, first sealing the room off from that of her children. The au pair would rouse the concierge, who would smell the gas and discover her and the children in time. Unfortunately, the Australian girl was late, and by the time she arrived, gas had seeped through the floorboards and knocked out the concierge who lived downstairs. It was too late to save Plath, but her children survived, as did the concierge.

It is impossible to determine retrospectively with certainty whether a part of Sylvia Plath wished to be rescued. She had taken steps to protect her children but ought to have known that she could not hermetically seal off her room from the other occupants, nor could she prevent the gas from seeping through the floorboards to her neighbor below. Hughes said afterward that he had been attempting reconciliation with Sylvia but that others had been getting in the way. We can only speculate whether this was true, or indeed whether Sylvia wanted to reconcile. Her suicide intent may well have been mixed, including the possibility that she had deliberately put her life on trial.

The example of Sylvia Plath illustrates that if your patient has just made a suicide attempt or has recently made one, you will also be able to gather fresh, valuable circumstantial information helping you to infer the seriousness of the attempt from the objective facts of the attempt. These facts should be taken into account in conjunction with what the patient tells you about his intent at the time of the attempt, necessarily a subjective retrospective judgment. Has your patient taken precautions to prevent a rescue, or has she created conditions for interruption of the attempt? In most cases, people who call their significant others after they have taken overdoses have either changed their minds or not intended to die in the first place (i.e,. parasuicide, deliberate self-harm, "attempted suicide"). On the other hand, the most chilling stories I have heard are those of middle-aged women who check into a hotel without telling anybody, arrange with the concierge not to be disturbed, and then take a large overdose of drugs. The choice of method is another indicator—men tend to prefer violent methods depending on availability, whereas women prefer to use overdoses. The picture appears to be changing, with hanging becoming more common in both sexes. In the United States, where firearms are more freely obtainable, women are using these weapons far more often than is done in Canada. Firearms, hanging, or jumping from a height are unequivocal suicide methods, irrevocable once used, but overdoses will allow leeway for rescue if the person is reached in time and brought to the hospital. This last state-

ment must be qualified (as earlier stated) in countries where agricultural pesticides and other such poisons are used in suicide attempts with great frequency. The Right to Die movement has been promoting the use of overdoses combined with alcohol and suffocation by plastic bags over the head that are tied at the neck. Unfortunately, these have not only been used by hopelessly terminal patients but also by people with recoverable psychiatric conditions.

Having a *psychiatric illness* is an important risk factor for suicide. There have been a number of psychological autopsy studies of suicide samples, some of them controlled and blinded, and they all demonstrate that only a small minority of suicides occur in the absence of a concomitant psychiatric diagnosis (5% to 7%). The biggest proportions are those with a depressive illness (roughly 40% to 65%), alcoholism or other substance abuse disorders (25% to 50%), schizophrenia (10%), and personality disorders (10% to 25%). There is a high degree of comorbidity between these diagnoses, and this compounds the higher risk of suicide. The presence of a major depressive illness comorbid with "psychic anxiety," for instance, as manifested by agitation, restlessness, and panicky feelings was a predictor of suicide within the first year after the diagnosis in one study.[13] Diagnosis should always be considered a vulnerability factor, not the potential primary cause of suicide, because suicide arises out of a logical (i.e., cognitive) equation in the patient's mind. A triggering life event may set off the (il)logical process in a patient who has been weakened by having the psychiatric disorder. Some psychiatric disorders, such as psychotic depression, melancholia, or schizophrenia, create the conditions for delusional suicidal thinking.

Case Example 1

A middle-aged family man, at a time when he was having business difficulties, began to suffer insomnia, agitation, and depression. His doctor considered that the symptoms could be explained by his circumstances and that it was therefore "situational" depression. He was prescribed a low dose of antidepressant medication but did not comply. Over the following months he spoke about his stress, the difficulties in his business, and the decline in public respect he was receiving, as well as from his family. His thinking was very negative, and he spoke of failure. He could not see solutions to any problem—there was no answer, and he would lose everything, he thought. His insomnia continued, but he did not want antidepressants, and he did not want to see a psychiatrist. He told his doctor that he would not kill himself. Nevertheless, after an abortive attempt to gas himself the night before, he hanged himself the next morning. After his death, members of the family reported that his perception of business difficulties had been greatly exaggerated. It was his depressive illness (that had gone on virtually untreated), and the negative outlook that flowed from it, that had made him lose perspective.

Schizophrenia is associated with suicide deaths in 4% to 13% of cases, and the lifetime prevalence of attempts is 30% (50% in schizoaffective disorders). Suicide occurs at any time during the course of the illness, but the risk is especially high during the first 6 months of the first episode, probably because the patient clearly understands the possible prognosis for control of his mind and the probable loss of many of his life's goals. The precipitation of a suicidal act seems less related to an adverse life event and more related to the simultaneous presence of depressive symptoms and an acute flare-up of the positive symptoms of schizophrenia. Suicide in a schizophrenic patient seems often to be impulsive but could have been at the command of a hallucination.

Case Example 2

Eva had clearly been suffering from a psychotic illness for at least 5 years, with the possibility that it might have developed already during her middle teens. Persecutory phenomena featured prominently, with ideas of reference, passivity experiences, and her belief that some evil individual spoke to her through the mouth of her mother and other people; these features were reminiscent of the Capgras syndrome. She constantly questioned whether her mother was her real self or an illusion. She interpreted all her encounters with others in a paranoid way, transforming them into self-fulfilling prophecies of persecution by others. The formal diagnosis was clearly schizophrenia, but there was also an important component of hostile depression, which seemed her driving force toward taking her own life. There was a vague possibility, impossible to confirm, that her plan could include harm to others. Her brother's mood disorder suggested that there might be an important familial component toward affective loading. Eva was at very high risk for suicide. There was high lethality in the methods she was considering, several of which involved violence. Her suicidality was fueled by perturbation, constriction of thinking processes, furious anger, adamance, and minimal anchorage to her family. It was likely that she might postpone an active attempt until after she learned of the results of her university examinations. However, she could move on suicide earlier if circumstances indicated to her that she would not be successful or if her paranoid experiences escalated. I did not think that there was a basis of trust that would make it possible for her to honor a "no suicide contract" with a caregiver.

Eating disorders also carry a high suicide risk, especially *anorexia nervosa*, whereas *bulimia nervosa* seems more associated with self-harm and suicide attempts and is not infrequently concomitant with borderline personality disorder. *Panic disorders* are associated with suicide attempts, and when concomitant with depressive illness or substance abuse, they carry suicide risk. Medical illnesses may be associated with depression and lead to suicidal ideation and acts. In older patients especially, perceived physical illness has been shown to be the most significant factor in the suicides of a sample of persons 50 and older, after the presence of all active mental disorders was controlled for.[14] *Delirious* patients, such as those experiencing alcoholic withdrawal syndromes, may take their caregivers by surprise and jump out of hospital windows to escape from their imaginary demons. *Epilepsy* is associated with excess mortality from suicide. All these and more need to be considered when one is assessing the patient.

The disorder may or may not of itself be a necessary condition for suicide, but it is rarely sufficient because suicide is almost always multifactorial. Treatment, however, needs to be directed at the psychiatric disorder that is promoting the suicidal logic as much as at the adverse life events that have triggered or are perpetuating it. Therefore, you will need to carry out a systematic examination of the mental state (see Chapter 1) much as you require doing a physical examination after you have taken the history of a medical or surgical patient. Be sure to ask about any previous hospitalizations and outpatient treatment and evaluate previous treatment critically for its adequacy, persistence, and effects.

Family history of suicide or suicide attempts is another important risk factor. A growing body of evidence supports the heritability of a predisposition to suicide in some families together with heritable predisposition to psychiatric disorders such as major depressive illness. Therefore, one should inquire about different degrees of kin who may have behaved suicidally or had a psychiatric or "nervous" disorder or a problem with substance use. It is always difficult in such cases to disentangle heritability from following the example of others in the family. Suicide attempters have been found to have a higher proportion than expected of other suicide attempters or suicides in their social networks, not just family members. Therefore, if your patient admits to suicidal ideation or attempting, it could be useful to ask whether he knows or has heard of anyone else who has thought of or acted suicidally. In some circles there may even exist a "culture" of suicidal behavior.

Case Example 3

Mike is a man in his 50s whose businesses are failing. He has a history of recurrent depressions with associated panic attacks. His father died when he was in his teens and was said to have had manic-depressive illness. His older brother suffered depression and took his life. Mike's suicidal ideation seemed to be pointing to a means of escape from his considerable mental pain as the result of his business failures and depression. He had made two suicide attempts by hanging. Since this was a potentially lethal method and the second attempt was taken even further than the first, there was a good chance that the next time he might really take the plunge. He stated that the desire to kill himself during both attempts was high. The hope of preventing his suicide seemed to lie in treating his depressive episode urgently and effectively, and then maintaining him in a depression- and panic-free condition. Given his family history, I advised electroconvulsive therapy (ECT) and then maintenance with antidepressants, lithium, or ECT. He needed to be kept safe in hospital during treatment until his illness was brought under control.

Alcohol and other substance misuse are frequently present in the histories of suicide attempters and completers. Alcohol misuse disinhibits violence, depresses the person, and facilitates impulsive actions such as suicide. Alcohol and other substance misuse are often also an attempt to medicate depression (not uncommonly in persons with bipolar affective disorder), and the combination of depression and released impulsivity is a prescription for suicidal ideation and behavior. I have many times seen someone drunk admitted to emergency for suicidal ideation (and also attempts) who loses all suicidal inclination on sobering up next morning. Such a person needs to be distinguished from a suicidal person who takes alcohol before the attempt to give him the courage and who will not lose his depression and suicidality on recovering from the intoxication. The patient with an alcohol abuse problem may not always be candid, either—one of the reasons why collateral information from a partner or friend is always something you should try to arrange. If you are seeing someone in the ER, do not let the accompanying persons, if any, leave before you or your colleague has had a chance to speak with them.

Case Example 3 (continued)

After her husband completed suicide, Mike's widow sought help to understand the tragedy that had occurred to her family and to deal with her grief. She revealed that after his death she had found dozens and dozens of empty wine and liquor bottles in the attic where he used to go when he wanted to be alone. Although staff on the ward where he had been treated knew about his alcohol problem, they did not know of its extent and continuation after he had assured them he was abstaining from alcohol.

Persons who misuse cocaine and opiates often attempt or complete suicide, too. Frequently, they do so either because their lives are in a mess or because they believe they cannot shake off their drug dependency. A careful history of alcohol and other substance use should be taken, therefore. While you are asking about this is also a good time to find out about tobacco, marihuana, MDMA (ecstasy), and so on.

Childhood abuse has been shown to be associated with suicidal behavior, particularly self-harm or attempts. Sexual abuse in childhood is often uncovered in such patients, not just in women but also in men. It leaves them with distrust of others, a guilty secret, poor self-esteem, and often a desire for punishment. Adolescent girls who mutilate themselves by cutting their wrists, torsos, or legs superficially with razor blades frequently give such a history. They seem to get relief from their angst by the mild pain they inflict on themselves and the sight of their blood and often conceal the wounds under their clothing. To elicit such an explanation, one might ask the patient, *"What did you feel just before you cut/burned/etc. yourself on your arm/breast/leg/etc.)?"* The answers may be that the person felt intense pressure of emotion, shame, low self-esteem, or similar dysphoria. Sometimes the person may tell you that she felt numb and needed to feel "real" again. When you ask how she felt immediately after cutting herself, she may tell you she felt a flood of relief and emotional discharge. Sometimes self-mutilation will take the place for the patient of an alternative form of maladaptive behavior (e.g., binge eating or taking illicit substances). One of my patients has done this sometimes rather than swig cough syrup, having become addicted to the dextromethorphan such syrups contain.

Abuse history may be seen in conjunction with dissociative behavior and in borderline personality disorder. Of course, inquiries about a history of abuse need to be made delicately, if the patient has not already brought it up: *"Some persons that I have seen in circumstances similar to yours have told me that they were abused or molested as children. That didn't happen to you, by any chance, did it?"*

Verbal and physical abuse during childhood is usually found in a dysfunctional home atmosphere of parental discord as well, and I have found it associated with high levels of anxiety or agitation in the patients that I have seen. There also may be hatred of those stereotype figures who remind them of the perpetrators. These could be supervisors at work, for instance. Unfortunately, persons who have been physically abused during childhood often exhibit explosive tempers and repeat the pattern with their offspring or partners.

Key Point:

To properly gauge a patient's suicidal risk, you need to understand his predicament, estimate his psychology (attributes promoting and protecting from suicide), estimate his values, diagnose his psychiatric status on all parameters, know his family background and genetic loading, and determine where he fits within the context of statistical risk factors for suicide.

Weighing the Decision to Admit or Not to Admit

Deciding whether to admit a patient is possibly the most daunting of clinical dilemmas for the psychiatrist, let alone the medical student, psychiatry resident, or other mental health professional who sees the patient in the ER. This is where you weigh up all the findings you have come to during your painstaking exploration of the patient so far. Clearly, if you are dealing with a psychotic person with insistent suicidal ideation, whether psychotic because of severe depression or schizophrenia is no matter; you cannot depend on his ability to control his actions. He requires admission both for his safety and urgent treatment. However, many patients with suicidal ideation resist being admitted and are not amenable to persuasion. To admit them, it would be necessary to use the legal force of mental health legislation that authorizes involuntary assessment and admission, which some clinicians may be understandably reluctant to do. The treating physician in private practice is especially averse to involuntarily detaining a patient he has known for some time and with whom he has a professional relationship of trust. It comes down to whether you think the patient is likely to kill himself in the near-immediate future. Here are some of the situations that would make it *more likely that you would admit* the patient with his agreement or in spite of his resistance:

- The patient is acutely psychotic and has suicidal ideation or has made a suicide attempt.
- The patient has recently made a suicide attempt that might have been lethal had he not aborted it or been frustrated in his attempt.
- The patient is depressed (or has psychache) and has active suicidal ideation and a feasible plan with availability of means.
- The patient has psychache or depression, and you have assessed the suicidal drive as strong and difficult for him to control.
- The patient has psychache or depression; you have assessed the suicidal drive as strong and difficult for him to control, and he is unlikely to comply with treatment, a trial of which is necessary to determine his responsiveness.
- The patient has strong suicidal ideation and no anchorage.

Regarding the second situation mentioned here, I have noted sadly on a number of occasions how persons who have just aborted a potentially lethal method have been sent home from ERs only to complete suicide within a short while. One example would be the middle-aged man previously described who aborted an attempt at carbon monoxide poisoning and hanged himself the next morning. What I did not say was that after the abortive gassing he was taken to a hospital ER, where he convinced the emergency physician that he had dissipated his suicidal impulses and was sent home.

Case Example 4

Susan was a troubled young woman in her early 20s who came from a chaotic, unstable, dysfunctional, physically and sexually abusive family background where alcohol intoxication was frequent. She was also dyslexic and had inner ear problems of balance. Not surprisingly, as a child she was disruptive, violent to other children, and defiant to authority figures. From her middle teens she was placed in institutional settings for troubled youngsters, where she continued her disruptive behavior. Documented self-harm began at 19 (probably much earlier) with repeated impulsive overdoses (at least six) usually precipitated by an argument or by drinking. These resulted in frequent admissions to the hospital, where she continued her unruly behavior. Her most consistent diagnosis was borderline personality disorder, and she exhausted a number of treatment programs, including anger management groups and abuse counseling.

On a holiday weekend before her death, she presented several times at ERs complaining of vomiting and diarrhea and claiming that she had been sexually assaulted. She agreed to follow up with a sexual assault team after the weekend. However, Susan returned to different ERs over the next few days with these gastrointestinal symptoms or sublethal overdoses of her psychotropic medication. On one of these occasions, she carried a suicide note asking that she be buried together with her teddy bears. She complained that nobody believed her story about the rape or was taking it seriously. Over the next few days, her acute suicidal crisis continued. She was briefly admitted to the hospital and was discharged when she behaved disruptively. She called the police that afternoon on her cellular phone to tell them that her friend was sitting on the train tracks, when in fact Susan was. The police went down to the tracks and fetched her and brought her to the ER. At the hospital, Susan reversed her statements and said that she had no intention of going through with her plan, and that her suicidal feelings had improved since yesterday. She said she had given most of her tablets to a friend for safekeeping. She promised to follow up with the hospital, contracted for safety, and was discharged from the ER.

Hours later, Susan was killed instantly after she returned to the railway line and walked in front of an eastbound train traveling at 40 km/hr. The engineer and conductor stated their opinion that she knew what she was doing because she was looking right up at the engineer's cab of the train, and her expression vacant and without emotion. Afterward, the police recovered a suicide note in her purse. The note, in her handwriting, stated that she was "fine at the hospital and again I'm not." She wrote that someone had raped her and nobody believed her, and she hoped to die. She instructed that she was not to be resuscitated. The people in her address book were to be informed of her death, and she was to be buried with her teddy bears. No intoxicants were found at the forensic autopsy.

Susan's case shows us how a person's motivation for suicide can be as a form of revenge rather than simply the result of deep sadness, although sadness, despair, hopelessness, and other such feelings must inevitably be compounded with the urgent desire for vengeance. Her death may be viewed as a loud reproach directed at those who would not take her story about the alleged rape seriously. Her clinical career was marked by impetuosity and extreme, erratic reactivity. It is not surprising that the clinicians who sent her home took her stated reversal of suicidality at face value. She made it difficult for clinical evaluators and caregivers to connect with her, and thus her denial of suicidality seems to have been readily accepted, when it is likely that she intended the opposite communication to them. Her language was difficult to translate and was simply not understood.

Collateral Collaboration

Whenever you admit a suicidal patient, it is important that you contact the spouse or parents to make sure that you are on the same page. If the spouse or parents refuse to have the patient admitted, and the patient does not want to be admitted, you should have everyone involved sign a release. It is not enough for the lawyers that the suicidal patient makes the decision on his own and, unfortunately, you always have to bear in mind the medicolegal possibilities. This is another reason why *documentation* of your examination is so important. Make sure that you specify on what grounds you evaluated the patient's suicidality (or lack of it) and how you came to your conclusions. This becomes even more important if you decide against admitting.

Of course, the issue of patient confidentiality arises when contacting the family or significant others if the patient does not wish his family to know he is planning to take his life, which, fortunately, is not often the case. When I am assessing a patient for the first time, I refuse to enter into any such collusion because of the primacy of intervening to prevent suicide. I assume that I am seeing the patient because there is a shred of ambivalence against suicide, or that the balance of circumstances that brought the patient to me indicates the presence of ambivalence whether or not the patient subsequently denies it. It is an ethical issue, and ethics are indeed value judgments made by a group at a particular time in the life of a particular society—that is,

ethical positions are not based on science but on opinion. My value judgment is that it is unethical to deprive a family (if they love the patient) of information that could help to prevent a disaster. Also, it is a medicolegal issue, and I know of civil lawsuits having been laid against psychiatrists for not informing the parents when a teenager or spouse is actively suicidal. The difficulty only really arises in practice when a suicidal patient is established in therapy with a caregiver, and the therapist is afraid that he will lose the confidence of the patient and be unable to help him any longer if suicidal intent is disclosed to the significant other. I have seen some of these caregivers lose their patients anyway, occasionally to suicide. If the significant others are available, I generally try to preempt the problem by making it clear to the patient at the time of the initial interview that preserving his life overrides confidentiality. By involving the family during the assessment interview, with the patient present, one can bring the conversation around to the issue in such a way that the patient will himself reveal his suicidal ideation. Or, if they are not present at the first interview, they should be brought in very soon afterward together with the patient if he is not to be admitted. If one assumes treating responsibility as well as doing the initial assessment, it is more complicated to personally see the family after a therapeutic alliance (with *transference* phenomena) has developed.

One would be *less likely to admit* a patient if any of the following are true:

- The patient has full insight into the fact of his illness; he is hopeful that with help he can overcome his personal predicament, and his suicidal drive is not strong. He agrees to cooperate with treatment and to contact you (or the ER) or come to the hospital if his suicidal feelings grow stronger and more irresistible.
- His spouse, parent, or significant other is fully in the picture and assumes some responsibility, and you have assessed this person as capable of fulfilling this responsibility.
- None of the factors (as mentioned above) is present that would make it more likely that you would admit the patient.

Key Point:

Strongly consider admitting for protection and treatment psychotic patients with active suicidal ideation, patients who have just made or aborted a potentially lethal attempt, acutely suicidal patients with a strong suicidal drive who have a feasible plan, and those who have a strong suicidal drive that is beyond their control, especially if they have no strong support system.

Contracting for Safety

The last two cases illustrate the real risk the ER physician or psychiatrist is taking when you send someone home who has just carried out or aborted a potentially lethal suicidal act. They also demonstrate the pitfalls in so-called *no-suicide* or *no-harm "contracts."* Such a contract with someone with whom one does not have a very strong therapeutic alliance is useless, wish-fulfilling for the physician, and self-deceiving for the patient. The literature documents a number of suicides in inpatients and suicide attempters who made verbal or written no-harm agreements shortly before they took their lives. So-called contracts of this kind have no place in the assessment stage but retain some value when the agreement is made with a patient who has been in psychotherapy for some time in the presence of a clearly strong therapeutic alliance. The agreement can be depended on to have only a short half-life, a matter of a few days, since an upset patient will quickly forget all else but what is upsetting him at the moment. The agreement is valid only between the person and his therapist, not between the patient and a proxy caregiver or an institution such as a hospital; in my experience, patients make relationships with people, not buildings.

The Do's of Suicide Assessment

- Do try to form a positive alliance with the patient during your assessment.
- Do wait until you feel there is trust before you plunge in to assess suicidality.
- Do try to get collateral information from significant others and to share your concern about the risks, and involve them in the management and responsibility of care.
- Do make sure a suicidal person you are assessing is under direct vision at all times from you or another staff member. (I know of a person who hanged himself behind drawn curtains in an ER cubicle when nurses took a meal break.)
- Do carry out a thorough evaluation of the biopsychosocial background of the patient as well as a thorough examination of his mental state.
- Do not hesitate to consult your colleagues if you are in any doubt.
- Do document your findings and your assessment of suicide risk and the reasons for your conclusions.
- Do try to remain objective and not allow your personal feelings about the patient (e.g., like or dislike, wishes for the patient) influence your judgment that should be based not on intuition but on the facts of the case.

LOSING A PATIENT TO SUICIDE

Losing a patient with whom one has formed any kind of relationship, even that during an initial assessment, is very hard for the mental health professional. It is difficult for a veteran psychiatrist of many years' experience but even worse for a trainee who has not yet built up his professional self-confidence and other patient success stories to fall back on to balance the score. The tendency is to wonder whether it is your fault, wonder how you could have prevented it, or even to imagine that you are a bad doctor, nurse, etc. In a U.S. study, one third of therapists who experienced a patient suicide admitted severe distress and concern over their own possible role.[15]

In most cases nothing could be further from the truth. We have to remember that psychiatric disorder carries a mortality risk just like in any other form of medical practice. Sometimes suicide in a patient is unavoidable no matter what we do because the person's underlying illness and mix of biological and self-destructive personality attributes grimly propel him forward to his destiny in spite of all our efforts to the contrary. Sometimes, during the treatment of chronically and intractably suicidal persons, you are forced to take risks for ethical reasons because no human being ought to be confined indefinitely or permanently kept in custodial care because he is ill, which in any case would be impractical and self-defeating. With patients suffering from borderline personality disorder, you often need to move the focus of their attention away from their suicidality to give them a chance to learn less maladaptive coping devices. Otherwise, suicidal behavior (most often parasuicide) becomes the only currency of your therapeutic dialogue with them. Some experts in the treatment of borderline personality disorder strongly recommend against admitting these patients except to acute units for brief periods during crises—never for lengthy periods of hospitalization. (Always consult, consult, consult if you think your patient is moving inexorably toward suicide.)

Losing a patient to suicide happens most often to those who fight in the frontline, that is, those who work on inpatient units (where the sickest patients congregate) and in ERs and crisis units. Trainees in psychiatry and allied mental health professions will find themselves in these clinical environments. A Canadian study of graduates from a psychiatry residency program found that 50% of respondents to a survey had experienced at least one patient suicide during their careers, which is compatible with other findings. Sixty percent of these patient suicides occurred when they were medical students and residents.[16]

If you should lose a patient to suicide, *do not withdraw* to lick your wounds (a perfectly natural tendency); rather, seek out your colleagues (peers as well as supervisors) and (it may take some courage) speak to them about what has happened to your patient as well as your own reaction to it. It could so easily happen to them as well (and in all probability will). Unfortunately, there is a tendency on the part of colleagues, if they are not directly approached, to avoid speaking to you about the topic because they want to spare your feelings, and they think that you don't want to be reminded about it. Do not be afraid to speak to your supervisor (he should have approached you, if he is worth his salt). The difficult part for you will be to approach the bereaved family and offer counsel (not necessarily from you personally), to offer condolences, and to feel out whether you should attend the funeral (only if this was a patient you treated, not merely one you assessed). These things must be done because they are the right things to do. You will usually find the family is grateful for what you tried to do. Remember that if you are to treat really seriously ill psychiatric patients their risk of suicide will be greater, analogous to the rest of medicine. Treating such suffering people can really make a difference; anyone can treat "the worried well."

REFERENCES

1. Havens L: The best kept secret: how to form an effective alliance, *Harv Rev Psychiatry* 12:56–62, 2004.
2. Durkheim E: *Suicide*, New York, 1966, Free Press.
3. Goldbloom RB, Ed. *Pediatric Clinical Skills, 3rd Edition*. St. Louis, 2003, WB Saunders.
4. Shneidman ES: *Suicide as psychache: a clinical guide to self-destructive behavior,* London, 1993, Jason Aronson, pp 51–60.
5. Linehan MM, Goodstein JL, Nielsen SL, et al: Reasons for staying alive when you are thinking of killing yourself: the reasons for living inventory, *J Cons Clin Psychol* 51:276–286, 1983.
6. Brown GK: *A review of suicide assessment measures for intervention research with adults and older adults,* 2002, National Institutes of Mental Health. www.nimh.nih.gov/suicideresearch/adultsuicide.pdf
7. Jacobs DG, Baldessarini RJ, Conwell Y, et al: *Practice guidelines for the assessment and treatment of patients with suicidal behaviors*, Washington, DC, 2003, American Psychiatric Association, pp 83–84.
8. Cochrane-Brink KA, Lofchy JS, Sakinofsky I: Clinical rating scales in suicide risk assessment, *Gen Hosp Psychiatry* 22:445–451, 2000.
9. Beck AT, Steer RA: Clinical predictors of eventual suicide: a 5- to 10-year prospective study of suicide attempters, *J Affect Disorder* 17:203–209, 1989.
10. Kessel N: The respectability of self-poisoning and the fashion of survival, *J Psychosom Res* 10:29–36, 1966.
11. Shneidman ES: Orientations towards death. In Shneidman ES, Farberow NL, and Litman R, editors: *The psychology of suicide,* Northvale, NJ, 1994, Jason Aronson.
12. Sakinofsky I, Roberts RS, Brown Y, et al: Problem resolution and repetition of parasuicide: a prospective study, *Br J Psychiatry* 156:395–399, 1990.
13. Fawcett J, Scheftner WA, Fogg L, et al: Time-related predictors of suicide in major affective disorder, *Am J Psychiatry* 147:1189–1194, 1990.
14. Duberstein PR, Conwell Y, Conner KR, et al: Suicide at 50 years of age and older: perceived physical illness, family discord and financial strain, *Psychol Med* 34:137–146, 2004.
15. Hendin H, Haas AP, Maltsberger JT, et al: Factors contributing to therapists' distress after the suicide of a patient, *Am J Psychiatry* 161:1442–1446, 2004.
16. Ruskin R, Sakinofsky I, Bagby RM, et al: Impact of patient suicide on psychiatrists and psychiatric trainees, *Academic Psychiatry* 28:104–110, 2004.

RECOMMENDED READINGS

Bongar B, Berman Al, Maris RW, et al, editors: *Risk management with suicidal patients,* New York, 1998, Guilford.

Hawton K, Van Heeringen K, editors: *The international handbook of suicide and attempted suicide,* Chichester, England, 2000, John Wiley & Sons.

Leenaars AA, Wenckstern S, Sakinofsky I, et al, editors: *Suicide in Canada,* Toronto, 1998, University of Toronto Press.

Maltsberger JT: *Suicide risk: the formulation of clinical judgment,* New York, 1986, New York University Press.

Maltsberger JT, Goldblatt MJ, editors: *Essential papers on suicide,* New York, 1996, New York University Press.

12

Assessment of Patients with Somatization

Susan E. Abbey

INTRODUCTION

Patients with bodily symptoms or somatic preoccupation are common in both primary care and psychiatric settings and yet receive little attention, relative to their prevalence and the severity of their illnesses, in medical school curriculum and postgraduate residency training.[1] For decades they have been treated pejoratively by both medicine and psychiatry and labeled "crocks," while those who study and work with them have been called "psychoceramicists." The past decade has demonstrated the seriousness of their clinical conditions[1] and has offered new hope for treating them.[2-4]

The patients pose special challenges to psychiatric interviewers for a number of reasons. They do not form a single group. Rather, different patients bring different challenges, including medically unexplained symptoms, difficult interpersonal behavior, and reluctance to be seen by mental health professionals. This chapter will provide an overview of the most important issues related to interviewing this highly diverse group of patients and a context that you can use when faced with these patients.

Case Example 1

Martha is a 44-year-old recently divorced librarian and mother of three teens who was referred by her internist for psychiatric consultation. She has been evaluated for 6 months of unremitting fatigue accompanied by nonspecific aches and pains. She has also reported hypersomnia and described her sleep as nonrefreshing. The internist has "worked her up completely" with no findings on physical or laboratory examination. The internist has raised the question of depression—particularly in light of Martha's recent divorce and the stresses in her life—but Martha insists that

while her mood is "somewhat lower than usual, yours would be too if you were so fatigued." She is angered by the idea of seeing a psychiatrist for "something that is so clearly a physical problem."

Case Example 2

Zach is a 39-year-old civil engineer, currently on short-term disability. He is married with a 2-year-old son. He has a 5-year history of increasing physical symptoms and psychological preoccupation with them. His symptoms include palpitations, lightheadedness, a presyncopal sensation, and vague gastrointestinal upset. Two cardiologists, three neurologists, and four gastroenterologists have evaluated him, all with negative findings. There is marital strain from his preoccupation with his symptoms. He charts the symptoms on a daily basis and spends many hours on the Internet investigating potential obscure etiologies. He has been unable to work for the past year because he is so preoccupied with his symptoms. His family physician is referring him for psychiatric assessment after attending a recent continuing medical education session on anxiety disorders and wonders whether he may have panic disorder. Zach is perplexed by the referral to psychiatry and is concerned that his "overworked" family physician is "dumping him because she is not up to the challenge of sorting out this diagnostic dilemma."

Case Example 3

Moira is a 32-year-old married dental assistant referred for assessment because of her repeated and protracted absences from work related to a diverse range of somatic complaints. She has been "sickly" most of her life. Menstruation has always been problematic. She averages a minimum of 2 days off of work because of her period "on good months" and has had 64 of the preceding 104 weeks off of work for a diverse range of "serious" physical complaints, although no objective medical pathology has been documented. Over the years, she has had a wide range of symptoms, each of which has been the primary concern for a period of time. The family physician that was asked by the employer to forward a letter summarizing her medical history noted, "She is a 'thick-chart' patient and I can only say that she has seen everyone and had everything done." Her most recent problem is back pain. She is insulted by seeing a psychiatrist but is delighted with the opportunity to describe her symptoms at length.

Welcome to the world of the bodily preoccupied patient! It is a complex world with a wide variety of patients who pose a range of challenges to the psychiatric interviewer.

BACKGROUND

A lengthy discussion of somatization and somatoform disorders is beyond the scope of this chapter and is contained in a number of recent reviews.[1-4] These areas receive little emphasis in both medical and psychiatric curricula despite their severity,[1] so it is worth describing a few basic concepts that help to guide you.

Somatization is a concept with a long and convoluted history, and there are a number of critics of the concept.[2,4,5] Initially, *somatization* referred to the production of bodily symptoms by the putative mechanism of a deep-seated neurosis. For the past 20 years, the term has been used descriptively for patients who have a tendency to experience and communicate psychological and interpersonal distress in the form of physical suffering and medically unexplained symptoms for which they seek help.[4] Three components to this definition of *somatization* include: (1) the experience/perception of somatic distress (e.g., "funny feeling in my chest"); (2) a cognitive attribution as to the meaning of the symptom (e.g., "This has to be a heart attack even though my family doctor says it's anxiety. This is real!"); and (3) behavioral action in response to the symptom (e.g., call 911 or demand that a family member drive the patient to emergency). The broad term of *somatization* has been used at various times to encompass a variety of different symptom patterns, including hypochondriacal preoccupation, where the focus is fear and worry about a bodily symptom or disease, the somatic presentation of psychiatric disorders, and medically unexplained symptoms that account for 40% to 74% of visits to medical practitioners.[2]

In the past few years, there has been the call to abandon the term *somatization* and to instead describe patients in terms of dimensions including whether symptoms can be medically explained; the quality of the patient's help-seeking behavior(s); the degree to which there is health-related anxiety; and the quality of the patient's interaction with the health care system, including the degree to which he or she is interpersonally difficult. Similarly, there have been recent critiques of the diagnostic classification of somatoform disorders that have included the mind-body dualism implicit in these diagnoses; inconsistency of coding physical symptoms on both axis I and axis III; lack of sufficient data regarding reliability, validity, and utility for many diagnoses; the essentially dimensional nature of many phenomena related to these diagnoses; and the arbitrariness of setting diagnostic thresholds.[5]

Key concepts for you to keep in mind in working with these patients include the following:

- Somatosensory amplification: This is defined as the tendency to experience bodily sensations as intense, noxious or disturbing, and consisting of hypervigilance to bodily sensation, as well as a predisposition to select out and concentrate on weak or infrequent sensations and to react to sensations with emotions and thoughts that intensify them.[4] Somatosensory amplification is associated with mood and anxiety disorders, among other factors.

- Illness behavior: This refers to the ways in which people behave when they feel ill, and the term *abnormal illness behavior* has been used to describe what are considered by health care professionals to be aberrant ways of behaving in response to the feeling of illness (e.g., doctor shopping, insistence on repeated investigations or treatments, disability deemed excessive to the condition). Disease is physician-defined and requires a demonstrated or inferred pathophysiology/lesion, in contrast to illness, which is patient defined.

- Medically unexplained symptoms: This is the current term in vogue for symptoms that are not attributable to or are disproportionate to identified disease. They have also been called *functional somatic symptoms*. Research is beginning to define the biological abnormalities that may underlie these symptoms.

Counter-transference to patients refers to the cognitive and affective responses of health care professionals to patients that are secondary to their own unconscious processes; *counter-reaction* refers to the same responses that are caused by conscious awareness. This diverse group of patients is commonly the target of health care professionals' counter-transference and counter-reaction. The range of responses they may elicit in you can vary from disdain and hate to overly solicitous behavior. Health professionals, because of their own personal histories, can react in very different ways to the same patient. You need to be aware of your own counter-transference and counter-reaction and manage them appropriately.

ADDRESSING THE SPECIAL CHALLENGES OF DEVELOPING A SUFFICIENT THERAPEUTIC ALLIANCE TO ALLOW FOR AN ADEQUATE ASSESSMENT

Having a sufficient therapeutic alliance to conduct a psychiatric interview is a prerequisite for assessing patients. Each type of psychiatric disorder presents challenges to alliance building, but in my experience the bodily preoccupied patient consistently raises the most challenges. Table 12-1 shows a top 10 list of interviewing do's and don'ts.

Considerations Before Seeing the Patient

Clarifying the Reason for Consultation

It is important to understand what the referring health care practitioner is requesting from the consultation in terms of both his overt *and* covert reasons for consultation. The beginning interviewer is often stymied in this regard, not having a long track record with the referral sources and not knowing the ins and outs of their referral patterns. Certain physicians refer with the statement, "Please consult on diagnosis," but I know from having seen their patients over time that between the lines they are saying, "Please take this disagreeable and difficult patient off my hands," or "I'd love you to take her, but if you won't do that, would you at least fill out all of her time-consuming disability papers for me?" It is important to know what you can and cannot offer and to make that clear both to the referral source and to the patient. It is not uncommon to have patients arrive saying, "Dr. X says that you are going to take care of me from now on since he can't help my problems." If you have no intention or ability to take the patient on, then you need to immediately frame the interview in terms of *"Well, no. Actually that isn't my understanding. I know that Dr. X would like some help but I am unable to take you on. I can offer Dr. X an opinion that will help him in his care of you."*

Over time, you will develop a somewhat "suspicious" nose for some of the potential covert reasons for consultation. Such covert reasons include extreme irritation on the physician's part with the patient perceived as "difficult," with the resulting desire to "dump" him; pending litigation in which consultation may be seen as an inexpensive way of obtaining another opinion to help to bolster the lawsuit on behalf of either the patient or the physician (of note, this usually isn't particularly helpful, as a clinical consultation is quite different from a medicolegal consultation, and there may not be adequate attention to issues that would be of concern to insurance adjudicators or the judicial process); or an attempt to pass on to the psychiatrist time-consuming tasks that are typically nonremunerative (e.g., filling out disability papers, advocating for the patient with different persons or agencies).

Table 12-1. Top 10 Do's and Don'ts for Building an Alliance with a Somatizing Patient

DON'T	DO
Assume that the patient is thrilled to see you.	Assume the patient is unhappy about being seen by a psychiatrist.
Try to smooth things over and assume that, after all, he will settle right in once the patient starts talking to you.	Anticipate the resistance. Elicit the patient's reluctance and objections to psychiatric assessment, and address them directly.
Emphasize your psychiatric credentials.	Emphasize your medical credentials.
Feel the initial interview should fit into a typical "50-minute hour."	Book the longest initial interview time that you can—80 or 90 minutes often works best.
Feel that you should be able to do an assessment in a single session.	Allow several sessions for assessment if needed; the first session is primarily about "making friends" with a reluctant patient.
Hear it all from the patient first to keep a fresh perspective and go in with a clean slate.	Prepare for the interview with review of referral materials, available medical records, and discussion with the referral source, if needed, to clarify the reason for consultation.
Get right to the heart of the matter, all that "interesting" psychosocial and psychological stuff.	Start with the patient's physical symptoms.
Try to quickly get off the topic of physical symptoms and move on to the interesting stuff.	Listen at length to the patient's physical symptoms.
Just get to the point and ask those "shrinky" questions; after all, the patient has come to see a psychiatrist.	Normalize, contextualize, and medicalize your questions and next questions about psychiatric symptoms and psychosocial factors so that they are more acceptable to the patient.
Doubt your skills—"If only I were more sophisticated this would be a breeze!"	Give yourself credit. It's hard work to engage many of these folks.

Preparing for the Interview by Reviewing the Referral Note and Records

It is essential that you read whatever referral materials have been sent along to you before seeing the patient. In some other areas of psychiatry, interviewers prefer to hear the patient's version of events first and then move on to reviewing the records after the interview. I have found this to be a very unhelpful approach with bodily preoccupied patients because a big part of developing the initial therapeutic alliance is focusing on physical symptoms and having them see me as providing advice to their doctors rather than feeling that they are being shunted off to the psychiatric system.

The amount of records that are sent varies greatly; there may be as little as a single letter or there may be a whole raft of documentation. It is important to carefully go through and read *everything* that is forwarded. Little pearls that may aid in diagnosis can be found in unexpected places in the medical record. I often feel like a detective sifting for evidence. Given my love of murder mysteries and the personal satisfaction I feel when I stumble on something that is diagnostically helpful, this is not hard for me to do. Many of you will not like digging through the chart and will yearn to just read the summaries, but you do this at your patient's peril. There are several reasons that it is important to read everything that is available.

The first is to have a clear view of what the symptoms are and what has been done about evaluating and managing them. This is particularly important because some patients who present as bodily preoccupied are so because they have an as-yet-undetected medical illness. There are many potential reasons that diagnosis of a medical illness may be obscured, including the following:

1. There is something that is atypical about the patient's presentation.
2. The patient's personality structure and interpersonal dynamics confound her ability to present her history effectively.
3. The patient's personality structure and interpersonal dynamics in some way irritate her physicians or surgeons to the point where she isn't getting a sufficiently detailed workup, and the patient's concerns are being dismissed as invalid or "crazy."

The special added value that psychiatrists bring to the management of bodily preoccupied patients is that they have their experience as medical doctors from their internship that allows them to identify when the presentation "smells" of organic pathology and when there is a clinical sense that there is more going on medically that needs to be evaluated. Sometimes the potential physical diagnosis may be clear to the psychiatrist, and at other times there won't be a clear physical diagnosis but rather a strong sense of "I don't know what he has, but I know it isn't psychiatric—so I should start looking for canaries and zebras." It is not uncommon for me to write in my consultation note back to the referral source that, although there are clear axis I or axis II issues with the patient, "My overall clinical sense is that the person truly is sick and that further medical workup is required." It is essential to remember that the psychiatrist is often the "court of last resort" for the bodily preoccupied patient, and it is essential for the psychiatrist to adequately evaluate the patient's medical status and to ensure that basic and appropriate investigations have been done.

Second, the major goal of the initial part of the interview is to establish an alliance with the person so that a comprehensive assessment can be undertaken. Being able to say, *"I have read the various reports and I understand that you have had a very difficult time with a number of really distressing/disturbing/disruptive symptoms including x, y, and z,"* gives the patient the sense that you do care about her physical problems and that you have taken the time to familiarize yourself with them. This may also help the patient feel that the referral is not a "dump" but rather a genuine attempt on the part of the referring physician to help her since the referring physician has taken the time to detail her physical concerns.

Third, the records may help to provide some sense of what psychiatric symptomatology the person has been experiencing. There are frequently comments made in referral notes, medical consultation notes, and discharge summaries about sleep, energy, and appetite. This then helps me to use my time more effectively in terms of pursuing the more likely psychiatric diagnoses (e.g., if the referral materials focus on the patient looking sad or flat and complaining of sleep, appetite, and energy problems, then I will take a more careful history for major depression and its common comorbidities). Knowledge of these symptoms also offers an easier way into discussion of the psychiatric issues. It makes it much easier to transition into this area of inquiry by beginning with a comment such as, *"Dr. X has noted that you are having a lot of trouble with sleep; can you tell me more about that?"* and moving along with questions to elicit depressive and anxiety symptomatology beginning with: *"When people are having so much trouble sleeping, they often have other troubles as well. For example, have you had troubles with your energy lately?"* or *"Often when people are having trouble with their sleep, they find it hard to pay attention and concentrate. How about you?"*

Fourth, there may be notations in the medical records about important psychosocial stressors that may have been involved in the initiation or maintenance of the somatic symptoms. These are useful to know about and can be addressed later in the interview.

CONDUCTING THE INTERVIEW

Building a Therapeutic Alliance by Providing a Context for the Interview

Patients with bodily complaints may have any one of a number of psychiatric diagnoses or may have no psychiatric diagnosis at all. You must establish an alliance with the patient sufficient to allow an exploration of the major axis I diagnoses associated with frequent bodily complaints. This is made all the more challenging for several reasons. Most patients with bodily complaints have a difficult time understanding why they are being referred to a psychiatrist. They often experience referral to a mental health setting as evidence that their primary treating professional sees them as "crazy" or is attempting to "dump" them. It is a real skill for referring primary care practitioners and medical and surgical subspecialists to be able to adequately frame the reasons for a psychiatric referral.

Why Am I Talking to a Psychiatrist?

Patients preoccupied with bodily symptoms are perplexed as to why they are being referred to a psychiatrist since, from their perspective, their problems are in their bodies not in their heads. Preparation by the referring physician is helpful in setting a context for the interview and in helping the patient to see the referral as potentially helpful rather than pejorative or negative in any number of ways. Unfortunately, many physicians have difficulty in articulating for the patient why a psychiatric referral might be helpful.

If you are asked about how best to "sell" a psychiatric referral, there are several things that are helpful. Many patients are willing to "buy" an explanation that there are psychiatrists who specialize in the care of persons with "chronic medical illnesses and physical symptoms" and in helping people with these problems to cope with their very difficult symptoms. Drawing parallels with various psychosocial supports for patients with heart disease and cancer may make it more acceptable for patients to be seen by psychiatrists. Patients who are particularly fond of highly medicalized explanations for symptoms may be willing to see a psychiatrist when the referral is framed in terms of psychiatrists having particular expertise in treating symptoms that result from long-term stress or from "dysregulation in the hypothalamic-pituitary axis." Anticipating the patient's resistance is always helpful; for example, a physician wanting to refer a bodily preoccupied patient for psychiatric referral might say, *"I would like to refer you to a colleague who I think could be very helpful to both of us in managing your symptoms. I'm worried you may not be happy, though, when you hear that my colleague is a psychiatrist. I know that many people are worried about being referred for a psychiatric consultation, but I think it would be really helpful for both of us. I have sent other patients to this doctor, and they have found the doctor helpful."* It is particularly important to emphasize the importance of the referral in helping the referring practitioner in *his* continuing care of the patient. It is important for the referring practitioner to emphasize to the patient that he is not "dumping" the patient, and that he remains committed to the patient's care. Many patients experience referral to a specialist as an act of withdrawing care by the referring physician. It is essential to emphasize that a referral to psychiatry is not evidence of disbelief in the patient's symptoms. For the particularly reluctant patient, it is often helpful to make comments about the "progress" that has been made in psychiatry as a "field of medicine" over the past 20 years and how it is a field of medicine with special expertise with respect to mind-body relationships. It is also important to openly acknowledge the potential stigma: *"It is not like the old days, when you might be worried that my sending you to see a psychiatrist was sending you off to the loony bin, although sometimes people still worry about that."* Finally, psychiatrists may be described as doctors who have particular expertise in using a number of medications, which while initially marketed for use in depression and anxiety, are also quite helpful in the management of a variety of other symptoms including sleep problems, fatigue, pain conditions, and medically unexplained symptoms. Overall, the major messages that should be given to the patient by the referring source are that: (1) their symptoms are important; (2) the referring professional is attempting to seek help both for the patient and himself in managing the patient; (3) psychiatrists are doctors who have particular expertise that may be helpful in improving the person's quality of life; and (4) although there is still public perception of stigma around psychiatric care, this is inappropriate in the 21st century with our enhanced knowledge of neuroscience.

Starting the Interview by Addressing the Patient's Reluctance to Be Seen by Psychiatry

Understanding that patients are coming to psychiatry with great reluctance means that the first intervention that needs to be made in the interview is to directly address this reluctance. I open all interviews with such patients by commenting something along the lines of, *"So, what did you think about being sent to see a psychiatrist? Did it seem like a really crazy idea to you?"* I then carefully listen to the patient's response and directly address whatever specific concerns she has raised. Some people, particularly those who have had good explanations from the referring party, will state, "No, I understand that you are somebody who specializes in this area. I was a little surprised and skeptical when my doctor suggested it, but I understood eventually why he thought that this would be a good idea." There is a wide range of potential resistances to psychiatric referral, and one needs to try to hear both the covert and overt messages in the patient's comments so that each of her concerns can be addressed directly. For example, the patient may respond, "Well, I think he just doesn't know what to do with me anymore," to which I might respond, *"So then do you think that your doctor thinks it is helpful to get another opinion? Or does it feel to you like he doesn't know what to do with you and is throwing his hands up in the air, using this assessment as a way to get you out of his practice?"* If the patient answers "yes" to the latter question, I would counter, *"That is not my understanding. My understanding is that Dr. X is committed to taking good care of you and hopes that I might have something to add to help him in his management of your situation."*

For the patients who are disparaging of psychiatry, saying something along the lines of, "Well, I was surprised. All of you psychiatrists are crazy, and I can't see what you would have to offer anyway," I might respond with the question, *"What is your biggest worry about psychiatry? I can well appreciate that different people do have worries about psychiatry and psychiatrists."* Then I would address their concern—the "crazy" psychiatrist his best friend saw, the "wacky" psychiatrist he saw in a popular movie, the boundary-violating psychiatrist he read about in the newspaper, etc. If the question did not elicit a clear response, then I might offer a multiple-choice checklist for people, for example, *"There are a lot of reasons that people might think psychiatrists are crazy. Sometimes if people have had a past difficult experience with psychiatry or have had a family member or friend who has had a difficult experience with psychiatry, that can be upsetting. Is that the case for you? Often people don't know exactly what psychiatrists do; maybe it would be helpful if I explained. Psychiatrists are medical doctors who do full medical school training and internships, where they do further training in internal medicine and emergency medicine and then do specialty training in psychiatry. This training offers us the opportunity to be well trained in both medical diseases and emotional reactions to them."* You will note that this comment keeps the focus on the bodily experience rather than trying to prematurely move the patient into the cognitive or affective domains which may initially be more threatening to patients. *"Do you have other fears about seeing a psychiatrist? For example, some people are concerned about confidentiality or insurability."* I would then deal directly with those concerns. Many patients will state, "Well, you will just end up saying that I am crazy," in which case I will reassure them that this is not the case. I'll say something along

the lines of this: *"I don't think that you are crazy. You clearly have had a very difficult time with your symptoms and seem to have struggled along quite bravely with them. My hope is to try to find something that may be helpful to you in dealing with this very difficult situation that you find yourself in."*

Contextualize, Normalize, and Bridge

It is essential to provide context throughout the interview, beginning with why and how the interview is taking place, then moving through each stage of the interview to provide an explanation so that the patient can understand the relevance of your questions. As the first step in setting this context, after I have addressed a patient's concerns about coming to see me, I provide him with an overview of how the interview is going to progress. I will give him some estimate of the amount of time that we will be able to spend together in the interview today, and how many interviews I think we are going to need for me to be able to adequately assess him. It is rare to be able to do an adequate assessment with these patients in a single 50-minute consultation. I tell him that I am unlikely to be able to give him a clear opinion at the end of the first interview but that I will certainly explain to him what I think when I have enough information and before he goes back to see his referring physician. I let him know that the interview is going to cover a number of different areas and that all of the things that I am going to ask are going to be relevant to my understanding of his problem. I emphasize to him that it is quite common for people to not understand why some questions may be relevant, and that if he has concerns about any of the questions that I am asking or feels as though I am in some ways being "too shrinky," he needs to let me know so that I can explain to him why I am asking those questions and why his answers are important to me. I tell him that we are going to begin by hearing about his physical concerns so I can understand their impact. For me to do that, I need to know a little bit about his current life circumstances and also about his earlier life so that I can understand and appreciate the unique person he is, with his own unique stories and unique challenges that the current symptoms pose for him. I emphasize that I believe that he has symptoms that are distressing to him, and that if at any point my questions suggest that I am dismissing his symptoms, he needs to let me know this.

Along with repeatedly returning to the context of my questions, I "normalize, normalize, normalize" and "bridge, bridge, bridge." By this I mean that it is important to repeatedly emphasize that it is "normal" to experience symptoms, worries, etc., and to make explicit connections between various areas of questioning and the patient's presenting concerns. Focusing on normalizing experience can take many forms, but I always emphasize that symptoms and challenges are "normal." For example, in trying to move the interview into the emotional realm I might say, *"Most people with difficult bodily symptoms have emotional reactions to the symptoms, although different people may have different emotional reactions. What kind of emotional reactions are you having to your symptoms?"* If life stressors are described, I'd comment, *"That must be very challenging for you. It is normal for people to have bodily and emotional reactions to that type of stress, although different people have different reactions. Can you tell me about the kinds of bodily reactions you have had to these kinds of stresses? Can you tell me about the kinds of emotional reactions you have had to these kinds of stresses?"* When I attempt to do the psychiatric equivalent of a "review of systems" in terms of asking screening questions about a variety of psychiatric disorders, I'll introduce each area by saying, *"Many people who have symptoms like yours have trouble with X. Has that been a problem for you?"* If cognitive testing is required as part of the assessment, I will again normalize it: *"When people have all of the physical problems that you have described and the life stresses and emotional reactions that go along with them, it often takes a toll on their ability to pay attention, concentrate, think clearly, and remember things. I'd like to ask you some questions that I ask all patients describing the kinds of troubles that you have. Some of the questions will seem very easy, maybe even so easy that they seem ridiculous—and I don't want you to be insulted by them. Some of the questions may be harder for you, and that's OK, I just want to understand how things are for you today. The purpose of doing this testing is to understand the impact of all of these physical symptoms, life stresses, and emotional reactions on your thinking and memory."* If I am doing a Folstein Mini-Mental State exam, rather than starting with orientation questions (unless this really seems like it might be an issue), I will start by asking the patient to memorize the three words as this seems like a more "normal" question given the preamble and is less likely to offend than starting off with orientation questions. I will raise the orientation questions with some explanation, *"The next few questions may sound odd to you, especially since you have gotten yourself to this appointment today, but I need to ask them in order to make the test we are doing valid as it requires me to ask these questions. I hope they won't bother you. The test includes these questions because some people do have trouble with them, and if you do then that would be important for me to know."* Similarly, asking directly about suicidality without a "lead in" seems "weird" and out of context to most patients. I usually start with asking about a wish for hastened death (e.g., *"Many people with symptoms like yours sometimes wish that they could just fall asleep at night and die in their sleep and not wake up in the morning.*

Have you ever wished for that?"). If there is a positive answer, you can then move up the ladder of suicidal ideation. If the patient answers emphatically "no," then I would stop the screening there unless I had other reasons for concern (e.g., a clear major depressive episode, a family history of suicide, a past personal history of suicide). If he endorsed the wish to die in his sleep or if his denial of this wish struck me as ambivalent or lacking conviction, I would then work through the suicidal risk assessment process (see Chapter 11) until I felt I had a clear enough understanding of his current risk to guide my management planning.

Start by Focusing on Physical Symptomatology

A premature attempt to bring in emotions, thoughts, and other aspects of the traditional psychiatric interview *always* backfires in patients with somatic preoccupation. They are already suspicious of coming to psychiatry because they have "real physical symptoms," and they need for you as the interviewer to listen to their detailed recounting of their physical symptoms. When you listen to this detailed (and often, from our perspective, over-detailed) accounting of symptoms, patients begin to feel understood, so that when you do try to raise issues around their current social context and their emotional and cognitive symptoms, these are seen as part of comprehensive history-taking and holistic care rather than a premature attempt to "psychiatrize" what the patients perceive as a medical or physical problem. Listening to this detailed subjective recounting of physical symptomatology is often difficult for many interviewers, as one of the reasons that they have chosen to work in the psychiatric area is that they aren't particularly interested in physical symptomatology. Alternatively, as a trainee on a psychiatry rotation, potential interviewers are interested in mastering aspects of psychiatric history-taking and mental status examination focusing on cognitions and affects; they don't want to hear every detail about the shape, size, texture, and floating or lack of floating capacity of stools in a patient with bowel complaints.

It is also important to get a detailed history of the patient's physical symptoms and to attempt to establish some chronology to the symptoms because your other task is to exclude undiagnosed medical disease. This can be challenging when the patient is overly dramatic or vague. As well as being an important tool in building an alliance with patients, it is essential that you have a clear understanding of the physical symptomatology and an open mind as to whether physical symptoms that may be discounted by the physicians and surgeons referring the patient are in fact evidence of an undiagnosed physical disorder. As previously noted, psychiatry is truly "the court of last resort" for patients with complex or unusual presentations of physical disorders.

You should know both the medical and psychiatric side of human beings. Psychiatric interviewers are the only ones who are fully grounded in both medicine and psychiatry and have had the experience of what "medically sick" looks like and what "psychiatrically sick" looks like. In general, we are better at mastering our counter-reaction or counter-transference to patients, and this may help us to more clearly hear the complaints of physical symptoms that the patient is reporting rather than being overly swayed by aspects of the patient's presentation that can sidetrack medical specialists (e.g., interpersonally dramatic behavior, circumstantiality, vagueness).

I always begin interviews by telling the patient that I have read the referring materials from her doctor. I tell her that the information that her doctor forwarded is helpful to me, but that I really need to hear directly from her about her physical symptoms because "doctors don't always get it right" and a doctor's "shorthand" for describing symptoms doesn't always fully convey the patient's experience. I tell her that my goal in today's interview and subsequent interviews will be to really understand in a detailed way what is happening to her.

Establishing the Impact of Physical Symptoms on Daily Life

It is essential to understand how symptoms affect daily life. This can be achieved in several different ways. An open-ended question such as, *"How do your symptoms affect your day-to-day life?"* may be sufficient in less resistant patients, whereas more complicated patients or patients who continue to be suspicious of psychiatry may resist answering this question, feeling that in some way it is an attempt to "psychiatrize" their symptoms. In these groups, it may be necessary to take a detailed history of daily activities, beginning with the time that the patient rises in the morning through to how she showers and toilets, prepares meals, and spends her day. An hour-to-hour review of the day can be helpful in getting a clear idea of how her physical symptoms affect her ability to do basic activities of daily living, such as physical self-care, toileting, and food preparation. The interviewer needs to know the impact of physical symptoms on aspects of day-to-day social function. In other words, are the physical symptoms affecting work life if the patient is working? How do they affect role function of the patient as a spousal partner, parent, sibling, or child?

Careful listening to a description of the impact of physical symptoms on daily life may suggest psychologically meaningful material that can be explored later in the interview.

Establishing the Impact of Physical Symptoms on the Patient's Emotions

In trying to establish the effect of physical symptoms on a patient's emotional state, we enter dangerous waters; attempts to explore the emotional realm typically meet with immediate resistance on the part of bodily preoccupied patients. They are very concerned that their symptoms are going to be discounted as psychiatric in nature, and, although we may ultimately ascribe them to psychiatric disorders, we need to obtain the information in a way that is either etiologically neutral or implies that the physical symptoms are causing a negative impact on the emotions. One approach would be to say, *"These physical symptoms sound very difficult. Dealing with them would be quite difficult emotionally for most people, although different people would have different reactions. What has it been like for you?"* It is helpful, again, to return to the notion of contextualizing and normalizing questions about emotional symptomatology and to always begin with questions suggesting that physical symptoms lead to emotional symptoms. For example, *"This pain must be very difficult to live with. Most patients that I talk to say that the pain has had quite a negative impact on their emotions, for example, causing them anxiety or to be down or blue at times. Certainly, that would be quite normal given all that you have described. Has that been part of your experience at any point in time?"* Eventually with this approach, a clearer picture of the patient's emotional life emerges, and you may also begin to see relationships between emotional and physical symptoms that may be bi-directional or unidirectional from emotions to physical symptoms.

It is essential to *not* engage in premature interpretation of such a unidirectional link between emotions and symptoms. If I thought that I had some therapeutic alliance with the patient and had given him enough time to talk about his physical symptoms, I might then move to trying in a gentle way to explore the impact of emotional life on those symptoms. This can be done in several ways. With a less guarded patient, I might say something like, *"The link between your physical symptoms and your emotional life seems very clear. You know that there is a lot of new research that shows that stress and emotions affect body function and that stress and emotions act through physiological mechanisms on bodily functions to increase physical symptoms. Have you ever noticed a relationship between stress and your physical symptoms?"* Connecting putative emotional stressors with physical symptoms is most successful when a "three-stage explanation" is used that links emotional stressors to physiological responses to stress, which in turn gives rise to physical symptoms.[2] For example, suggesting to a patient that his headaches are due to a difficult marriage may be a hard sell and heard by the patient as you saying that his headaches are not real or are evidence of malingering. An easier sell is to suggest that he is under a lot of stress in a difficult marriage, and the brain and body respond to that stress through muscle contraction in the head, scalp, and neck, as well as in the smooth muscle in the blood vessel walls, and these changes result in headaches.

In the patient who is more dismissive of psychiatry and emotional symptoms or unwilling to engage in discussion, I will try to "prime the pump" and further contextualize and normalize things by bringing in an example that has either been in the news recently or from my own life, emphasizing a bona fide cause of physical symptoms that affects emotions. For example, for a number of years after I had a dry socket from a wisdom tooth extraction, I would say, "*Well, in my own life, I had a dry socket from a wisdom tooth extraction, and I found that as the days went on and the pain didn't settle down, it did take a toll on my emotions. I felt worried about whether I was going to have the pain forever, and I also felt sort of down and blue because I couldn't do what I wanted to do because the pain limited me. The pain was easier to cope with during the day, when I had things to occupy my attention and when I could call my dentist or easily go to the emergency room if the pain got a lot worse. But the nights were hard, when I had nothing else to think about and was worried about the pain. Do you think that anything like that has happened with you and your pain?*" There is a subset of patients that I consider "the worst offenders" (an example of the use of black humor to manage my counter-reaction and counter-transference to their attempts to thwart my therapeutic zeal) who are completely resistant to making any relationship between their emotional life and physical symptoms. For this group, it is best to try to keep an open ear to hear these connections as they discuss their situation and to file this information in your notes and in your brain for future reference in working with the patients or making recommendations to their referring physicians.

Understanding the Patient's Current Social Context and Stressors

Again, we are treading into difficult waters in inquiring about the psychosocial situation of many bodily preoccupied patients and patients with somatoform disorders. They are quite concerned about us blaming symptoms on social factors; at some level in our society, this has the implication that they are responsible for their symptoms and that their symptoms are not real. This is particularly true when a "two-step" explanation is used in which the stressor "causes" the symptoms rather than a "three-step" explanation, as described above, where there is a plausible psychophysiological mediating variable between the stressor and the symptom.

It is useful to initially take a very matter-of-fact approach and again link the desire for information that you are requesting in the interview back to understanding the impact of the physical symptoms. Some interviewers choose to get basic demographic data at the start of the interview, and this certainly offers a greater context for the information that follows. In a bodily preoccupied patient, this may be less effective than in some other types of psychiatric interview because of the patient's reluctance to have connections made between social, emotional, and physical factors. If people are reluctant to provide basic demographic information at the start, I will try to incorporate it later in the interview. Again, I always start with their physical symptoms: "*Having these headaches must be very difficult. I am wondering how it affects the people around you. Maybe you can tell me just a little bit about your life because I don't really know anything about you. Do you live with somebody?*" I would try in this way to learn something about the patient's current living circumstances, who is in her immediate social world, and what the reactions are of those persons to the patient's physical symptoms. To find out about the social reinforcement of symptoms, I often ask questions such as, "*Having symptoms like you are describing has an impact on most partners/families/friends, although the type of impact varies. What is it like for your partner/family/friends? How do they respond to your symptoms? How do you deal with their response?*" This may then elicit a variety or responses that are usually quite telling, varying from "Well, they don't seem to care very much, and it doesn't seem to show an impact on their lives," to "It has been quite amazing! He has never been very caring before but now he is so solicitous. He has managed to change his shifts at work so that he can be there for me at night, and he does absolutely everything around the house. You know, he never used to do anything, but now he cooks and cleans and takes care of me." Certainly in the latter case, one begins to wonder about the secondary reinforcing effects of illness behavior. In developing a management plan, you need to flag the importance of speaking directly with the partner/family/friends, if possible, to obtain collateral information so that you understand exactly what is going on and begin to develop an alliance that will allow subsequent work with them to change the social contingencies around the patient's symptoms.

Interviewing to Rule In or Rule Out the Various Somatoform Disorders

With the bodily preoccupied patient, the likelihood of a somatoform disorder is increased. The common feature of all of the somatoform disorders is that patients describe the presence of physical symptoms that might otherwise suggest a general medical condition, and yet these symptoms are not fully explained by a general medical condition, substance use, or another psychiatric disorder (e.g., the patient who is hypochondriacal about palpitations and has a diagnosis of panic disorder). The *Diagnostic and Statistical Manual of Mental Disorders,* Fourth Edition, Text Revision (DSM-IV-TR)[6] describes seven somatoform disorders. The diagnoses are shown in Box 12-1. This chapter will review the major criteria and the questions one needs to ask in order to make each of these diagnoses. A more complete discussion of these diagnoses can be found in a number of standard psychiatric textbooks, including in the full edition of the DSM-IV-TR[6] and in more in-depth reviews.[4]

Common Elements of the Somatoform Disorders

All of the somatoform disorders share some common elements. The first is that the symptoms that somatoform disorder patients experience cannot adequately be explained by a known general medical condition or the direct side effects of a substance—either a drug of abuse or medication. The diagnoses all require that appropriate medical investigations have been done. It is easy to see how this can at times be a problematic criterion. One physician's appropriate investigation may be another physician's inadequate investigation or another physician's overzealous, excessive investigation. As already mentioned, often these patients have difficult relationships with their doctors, and it is incumbent on the psychiatric consultant to ensure that appropriate medical investigations have been done.

The world would be much simpler if somatoform disorders only occurred in persons without physical pathology, but there is a substantial group of persons in whom the somatoform disorder coexists with a general medical condition or substance use. In these cases, clinical acumen is required to sort out whether the physical complaints or the psychosocial impairment associated with the complaints is in excess of what one would expect based on documented pathology.

All of the somatoform disorders require that the physical symptoms cause significant distress or impairment in life func-

---

Box 12-1. Somatoform Disorders Defined by DSM-IV-TR*

1. Somatization disorder
2. Undifferentiated somatoform disorder
3. Conversion disorder
4. Pain disorder
5. Hypochondriasis
6. Body dysmorphic disorder
7. Somatoform disorder not otherwise specified

*Data derived from American Psychiatric Association: *Diagnostic and statistical manual of mental disorders,* ed 4, text revision, Washington, DC, American Psychiatric Association, 2000.

---

tioning. Depending on the individual, this impairment may be more prominent in one area rather than another. You need to ask about the impact of the symptoms on interpersonal and social functioning as well as occupational functioning.

All of the somatoform disorders require that the symptoms not be intentionally produced for unconscious reasons, as occurs with factitious disorder, or intentionally feigned for conscious gain, as occurs with malingering. With somatoform disorders, there is also a requirement that the diagnosis not be "better accounted for by another mental disorder." This often requires a higher level of clinical judgment, and most junior interviewers will typically want input from more senior clinicians. Many axis I disorders present with physical symptoms, and at times it can be difficult to sort out when one is simply dealing with an axis I disorder such as a mood disorder, anxiety disorder, psychotic disorder, sexual dysfunction, etc., and when the symptoms are sufficient to merit an additional somatoform diagnosis.

Somatization Disorder

In asking questions to make a diagnosis of somatization disorder, you are looking for a pattern of recurring physical symptoms involving *multiple* areas of the body over time. The physical complaints should be of a level that has been termed in the DSM-IV-TR as "clinically significant." This means that the symptoms are associated with one or more of the following: (1) medical help-seeking; (2) the taking of a medication because of the symptom; (3) significant impairment in some aspect of life (i.e., social, occupational, or other areas of functioning). In history-taking, the interviewer needs to both elicit symptoms and also assess whether the symptoms meet the definition of "clinical significance."

Age at onset is another important component of the disorder. By definition, somatic complaints must begin before the age of 30 and occur over a period of several years. In classical cases, young women experience multiple somatic symptoms beginning shortly after menarche and occurring throughout adult life. There are persons who present looking as though they have a somatization disorder, but their age of onset is after age 30, and this is a problematic group that psychiatric nosologists have not adequately studied. Based on the DSM-IV-TR criteria regarding age of onset of 30 or younger, they cannot be diagnosed with somatization disorder. My own clinical experience is that these persons, who are disproportionately women, often present with a panoply of poorly explained medical diagnoses, including fibromyalgia, chronic fatigue syndrome, and a variety of pain conditions that have begun midlife.

Over the years, psychiatric nosologists have required different numbers of symptoms to make the diagnosis of somatization disorder. At the present time, persons are required to have had, over their lifetimes, four pain symptoms, two gastrointestinal symptoms, one sexual symptom, and one pseudoneurological symptom (Box 12-2). In each case, the symptom cannot be fully accounted for by a medical condition or the direct effects of a substance after appropriate medical evaluation. The trickier issue arises when there is/are a related general medical condition(s) and a clinical decision needs to be made as to whether the physical complaint or the degree of reported impairment is in excess of that expected for the condition(s).

Patients with somatization disorder are extremely likely to meet criteria for other axis I and axis II disorders. Up to 75% have comorbid axis I disorders, most commonly major depression, dysthymia, panic disorder, simple phobia, and substance abuse. On axis II there are increased rates of cluster B diagnoses in patients seen in psychiatric settings and cluster C and paranoid personality diagnoses in patients seen in primary care settings.[4] There has been extensive debate in the literature as to whether this represents a real increase in the prevalence of these other disorders or whether it is artifactual and reflects a tendency for patients with somatization disorders to spontaneously over-report symptoms and overendorse symptoms when questioned. The best evidence at this point suggests that somatization disorder patients do in fact have increased rates of other axis I II disorders and that these other disorders bring with them increased psychosocial morbidity.[4] Identification of comorbid axis I disorders is especially important in the patient with somatization disorder. In clinical practice, I have found that being able to identify and successfully treat a comorbid major depressive episode or a panic disorder can be helpful in "turning down the volume" on the somatic symptoms that the person is describing and in decreasing her medical help-seeking and psychosocial impairment (see Case Example 3).

Conversion Disorder

Conversion disorder was in many ways the birthplace of modern psychiatry in the latter half of the 19th century. Patients, particularly women, presenting with "deficits" that affected their voluntary motor or sensory function and that suggested a neurological or other general medical condition perplexed psychiatrists in the 19th century and attracted a great deal of interest. Conversion symptoms are related to voluntary motor or sensory function, and they are thus referred to as "pseudoneurological" (Box 12-3). The type of symptom may be partly related to the degree of medical sophistication of the patient. More medically naïve persons (e.g., children, those of lower socioeconomic status, the more poorly educated, immigrant patients, and persons in relationships with a profound power imbalance precluding direct communication) may present with more implausible symptoms. Conversion diagnoses are particularly difficult to make in more sophisticated persons who often present with more subtle symptoms such as sensory

---

Box 12-2. Symptoms of Somatization Disorder*

- There is a history of many physical complaints.
- Onset occurs before age 30.
- Physical complaints have resulted in medical help-seeking or significant impairment in an important area of functioning (e.g., social, occupational).
- Patient meets criteria for four pain symptoms, two gastrointestinal symptoms, one sexual symptom, and one pseudoneurological symptom, with the symptoms having occurred at any time over the course of the disturbance (i.e., they don't all have to occur together at this point in time).

Four Pain Symptoms (different locations or functions)
- Head
- Abdomen
- Back
- Joints
- Extremities
- Chest
- Rectum
- During menstruation
- During sexual intercourse
- During urination

Two Gastrointestinal Symptoms (other than pain)
- Nausea
- Bloating
- Vomiting other than during pregnancy
- Diarrhea
- Intolerance of several different foods

One Sexual Symptom (other than pain)
- Sexual indifference
- Erectile dysfunction
- Ejaculatory dysfunction
- Irregular menses
- Excessive menstrual bleeding
- Vomiting throughout pregnancy

One Pseudoneurological Symptom (not limited to pain)
- Impaired coordination or balance
- Paralysis or localized weakness
- Difficulties swallowing or lump in throat
- Aphonia
- Urinary retention
- Hallucinations
- Loss of touch or pain sensation
- Double vision
- Blindness
- Deafness
- Seizures
- Amnesia
- Loss of consciousness other than with fainting

*Based on American Psychiatric Association: *Diagnostic and statistical manual of mental disorders,* ed 4, text revision, Washington, DC, American Psychiatric Association, 2000.

symptoms. An argument has been advanced that much of what we now label as *fibromyalgia* and *chronic fatigue syndrome* may actually be sensory conversion rather than the motor conversion symptoms of the 19th century.

Case Example 4

Eva is a 21-year-old who suddenly developed profound bilateral leg weakness at age 18 and underwent extensive neurological investigation, including several detailed neurological exams and neuroimaging (i.e., computed tomography, magnetic resonance imaging). The only findings on neurological examination were nonorganic—a loss of sensation in a stocking distribution on the legs and nonorganic leg weakness. Multiple consultations with a wide variety of medical specialists ensued, and a tentative diagnosis of chronic fatigue syndrome was made. At age 21, she was referred for psychiatric assessment and was ultimately hospitalized because of her profound weakness and inability to care for herself. A sodium Amytal interview revealed the onset of symptoms was 2 days before going away to a friend's cottage with her first boyfriend. She anticipated he would "push" her to have intercourse for the first time. She also discussed her highly ambivalent feelings about sexuality, which were based on childhood experiences observing her parents having sex while sharing a hotel room on vacation.

Making the diagnosis of conversion disorder requires a detailed assessment of the symptoms and ruling out a general medical condition as the cause of the symptoms. It is essential to assess for "psychological factors" and to determine whether psychological factors can be "judged to be associated with the symptom or deficit" because the initiation or exacerbation of the symptom or deficit is proceeded by conflict or other stressors. This requirement for temporal association of

---

Box 12-3. Symptoms of Conversion Disorder*

MOTOR SYMPTOMS
- Impaired coordination or balance
- Paralysis or localized weakness
- Aphonia
- Difficulty swallowing or a sensation of a lump in the throat
- Urinary retention

SENSORY SYMPTOMS
- Loss of touch or pain sensation
- Double vision
- Blindness
- Deafness
- Hallucinations
- Seizures or convulsions

*Based on American Psychiatric Association: *Diagnostic and statistical manual of mental disorders,* ed 4, text revision, Washington, DC, American Psychiatric Association, 2000.

---

the psychological factors can make this diagnosis quite challenging. The assessment of psychological factors being associated with the symptom must involve positive findings and not be the fall-back position in a diagnosis of exclusion.

Hypochondriasis

The hallmark of hypochondriasis is the belief that one has a serious illness or is preoccupied with the fear that one has a serious illness (see Case Example 2). This preoccupation is based on a misinterpretation of bodily signs or symptoms. The preoccupation in hypochondriasis can be focused on a variety of different issues. Patients with hypochondriasis may be preoccupied with normal bodily functions (e.g., heart rate, sweating, peristalsis). They may be preoccupied with a minor physical symptom (e.g., occasional cough, a small skin lesion such as a freckle or pimple). Alternatively, the preoccupation may be with physical symptoms which they have a difficult time articulating, and their descriptions may be vague and ambiguous. Whatever the physical symptom preoccupation is, all hypochondriacal patients then make cognitive interpretations that these bodily experiences are symptoms or signs of a serious disease. Some persons may be preoccupied around a single, central disease theme such as heart disease or cancer, and other persons may be concerned about different diagnoses reflecting various bodily symptoms (Box 12-4).

In making the diagnosis of hypochondriasis, it is assumed that the patient has received "appropriate medical evaluation and reassurance." As discussed earlier, it is easy to see the potential problems associated with this criterion. Often, physicians can feel that they have appropriately explained symptoms, but it is clear that patients have not understood their physician's explanations. Occasionally, the psychiatric interviewer can "cure hypochondriasis" during an assessment interview by providing a clear explanation for symptoms, that the patient can understand. Trying to come up with an explanation that suits and can be understood by a particular patient can be intellectually challenging. I personally enjoy the creative task of trying to

---

Box 12-4. Symptoms of Hypochondriasis*

- The patient has a preoccupation with the fear or the belief that he has a serious disease based on a misinterpretation of bodily symptoms.
- Appropriate medical evaluation and reassurance have been provided to the patient without there being a diminishment in the preoccupation.
- The patient's belief that he has an illness is not of delusional intensity.

*Based on American Psychiatric Association: *Diagnostic and statistical manual of mental disorders,* ed 4, text revision, Washington, DC, American Psychiatric Association, 2000.

size up a particular patient and then figure out what type of explanation or metaphor is going to be most helpful to him.

Body Dysmorphic Disorder

Body dysmorphic disorder has a long history in psychiatry and was first known as *dysmorphophobia*. It is characterized by the belief that there is a defect in one's appearance that then becomes preoccupying and results in significant disruption in daily functioning as well as significant distress.

Case Example 5

Isabella is a 26-year-old single medical secretary. She became increasingly nonfunctional at work, and her physician employer encouraged her to seek a psychiatric consultation. She was diagnosed with major depression in the context of life stressors, including a recent breakup with a long-standing boyfriend whom she had hoped to marry and worries about her elderly parents' ill health. In her initial assessment interview, she reported that one of the factors in the breakup with her boyfriend was her "difficulties with her skin." The psychiatrist was perplexed because she had a beautiful, unblemished face. Isabella proceeded to describe a 10-year history of preoccupation with her facial skin; her belief that it was dry, flaky, and susceptible to infections; and 3 hours of showering daily to clean and moisturize her face. The psychiatrist sought a second opinion with a specialist in somatoform disorders as to whether Isabella had "some type of somatoform disorder." She was relieved to be seen by a specialist in somatoform disorders because she had been "investigating" on the Internet and believed she may have either "body dysmorphic disorder, obsessive compulsive disorder, or hypochondriasis."

Occasionally, there may be a slight physical anomaly present, and the diagnosis can be made when the patient's concerns are deemed markedly excessive. In trying to sort out whether a patient is preoccupied, it is helpful to ask her about checking and grooming behavior. Persons may spend many hours a day checking their defect or scrutinizing it. They may also use additional aids in scrutinizing their defect, including using magnifying glasses or high-contrast lighting. Rather than decreasing anxiety, their checking behavior increases it. They may also do a variety of things to try to overcome or improve the defect, such as attempts to camouflage it through plastic surgery. Isabella, in the preceding case example, was taking long showers to hydrate her skin; this is in contrast to germ-phobic patients with obsessive compulsive disorder, who might shower for hours to clean themselves of germs. People with body dysmorphic disorder usually have very poor insight into their situation, and it is often challenging for the clinician to sort

out whether their symptoms are at a delusional level. They may also report ideas of reference and believe that people are talking about their flaw or mocking it behind their backs. Body dysmorphic disorder patients are over-represented in cosmetic surgery practices. Systematic research into body dysmorphic disorder has developed over the last decade with the finding of significantly increased point and lifetime prevalence of major depression, delusional disorder, social phobia, and obsessive compulsive disorder.

Pain Disorder

Pain disorder is a diagnosis that has had a variety of different names in various editions of the DSM. In the past, it has been called *somatoform pain disorder* and *psychogenic pain disorder*. At the present time, it is referred to as *pain disorder*.

The major feature of pain disorder is preoccupation with pain that causes significant distress or impairment in functioning; psychological factors are judged to play an important role in the onset, severity, exacerbation, or maintenance of the pain. The pain cannot be explained by a general medical condition or, if a general medical condition exists, then the pain is judged to be disproportionate to the underlying medical pathology. The essential aspect of pain disorder is that psychological factors are important in the onset, severity, exacerbation, or maintenance of the pain.

Case Example 6

Robert is a 52-year-old engineering technician who is married without children. He was injured in a minor workplace accident 4 years ago with a "back strain" and has been preoccupied with mid and lower back pain since that time. He is extremely angry with his employers and has been on disability insurance since the time of the accident. The other three employees who were also injured were all back at work within 6 to 10 weeks. Over the years, he has seen a number of musculoskeletal specialists from both surgical and medical perspectives and has attended several pain clinics without success. Numerous practitioners have commented on the disproportionate nature of his pain relative to objective findings on musculoskeletal and neurological examination. There is no clear organic pathology. Two years ago he convinced an orthopedic surgeon to do a fusion but had no pain relief from the procedure; in fact, he has had a worsening of his pain over the past 6 months. His family physician has found him difficult to engage because of the level of his anger and his insistence that "there must be a cure if someone just cared enough to use their brain and figure it out!" Recently, there have been significant marital troubles, with this wife threatening to leave the marriage "if he doesn't get help for his anger."

There are two essential tasks for the psychiatric interviewer in evaluating for the diagnosis of pain disorder. The first is to ensure that there has been an adequate workup to rule out a general medical condition or to demonstrate that the general medical condition is only accounting for a small proportion of the pain. The second and most important task of the psychiatric interviewer is to assess the presence and role of psychological factors with respect to the pain. This is often an extremely challenging task because most patients with pain do not want psychological factors to be identified as they feel that it devalues and demeans their suffering. They see the invocation of psychological factors as equivalent to saying the pain is "all in your head," and along with that comes a variety of negative consequences. These consequences include lack of care from physicians, high social stigma, and the widespread belief that the person is somehow morally culpable for his pain and thus is to be blamed. This contrasts with being seen as a victim of external forces over which he has no control, which is how we usually see persons with pain associated with a general medical condition.

Undifferentiated Somatoform Disorder

This is a residual diagnostic category that is used when persons do not meet full criteria for another specific somatoform disorder. The diagnosis requires one or more physical complaints present for at least 6 months that have caused significant distress.

Somatoform Disorder Not Otherwise Classified

This is a grab-bag diagnosis that includes a variety of disorders with somatoform symptoms when the person does not meet the criteria for any other somatoform disorder. An example would be hypochrondriacal or unexplained physical symptoms that are of less than 6 months' duration. Interestingly, pseudocyesis or the false belief of being pregnant that is associated with objective signs of pregnancy is also included in this diagnostic category.

Identifying Other Axis I Disorders

The most common axis I disorders in patients with bodily preoccupation or unexplained physical symptoms are shown in Box 12-5. It is important to screen for other axis I diagnoses for two reasons. First, the patient with bodily preoccupation may have one or more of these other axis I disorders rather than a somatoform disorder. This is good news because most other axis I diagnoses are easier to treat than somatoform disorders. Although psychiatrists privilege thoughts and emotions, most axis I disorders have a strong somatic or bodily component, and this is what most patients focus on, especially in primary care and general medical settings. Patients who come to mental health clin-

ics or other psychiatric settings with major depression are more likely to be willing to talk about their low and depressed mood, amotivation, and anhedonia, but the majority of patients with major depression seen in primary care settings and in specialty medical and surgical clinics focus on their low energy, sleep and appetite disturbances, and a variety of aches and pains.

Second, it is important to identify these other axis I disorders because they can occur comorbidly with a somatoform disorder. When there is a comorbid axis I diagnosis in a patient with somatoform disorder, it typically makes the bodily preoccupation of the somatoform disorder patient more prominent and more distressing for the patient and significantly adds to the psychosocial impairment experienced by the patient.

Other chapters in this book talk about interviewing patients with these various diagnoses, but they typically do so from the perspective of psychiatrists working with non–bodily preoccupied patients. The real key in screening for other axis I diagnoses in patients with somatic preoccupation is to try to normalize and contextualize the questions and to *always begin with the physical symptoms*. For example, if I were screening for mood disorder in someone whose chief complaint is prominent fatigue, I might say something along the lines of: *"When people are as fatigued as you are, they sometimes have other symptoms as well. Could we talk about your sleep? How about your appetite? What does the fatigue do to your concentration? Are you finding that with this fatigue that your self-esteem is lowered? It would make sense that fatigued people might have troubles around their motivation; have you noticed changes? Have you noticed that when you are fatigued you have less ability to experience pleasure and less of a sexual drive? Is it harder to get a laugh out of you?"*

Clinical judgment needs to be used in terms of which other axis I disorders you screen for. As noted in Box 12-5,

---

Box 12-5. DSM-IV-TR Axis I Diagnoses Other than Somatoform Disorders that Are Commonly Associated with Unexplained Medical Symptoms and Bodily Preoccupation

---

Major Depressive Episode

Anxiety Disorders

  Panic disorder
  Generalized anxiety disorder
  Post-traumatic stress disorder

Substance Abuse and Dependence

Psychotic Disorders

  Schizophrenia
  Delusional disorder

there are several diagnoses that are most commonly associated with somatic preoccupation, and a cursory screen of each may or may not be useful, depending on the "flavor" of the patient's presentation. If there were no evidence of psychosis in either the referral materials or during the interview to suggest that it is in the differential diagnosis for a given patient, I would not do a psychosis screen. If there were soft evidence or a suspicion, then I would leave the psychosis screen to the end because it sounds the most like one is saying the patient is "crazy," and this is most likely to lead to resistance and anger on the patient's part.

Relevance of Other Components of the Psychiatric History to the Somatizing Patient

Past personal and family medical history may be informative in terms of identifying other persons with somatoform diagnoses or related axis I comorbidities or a family history of significant medical diagnoses that may be feared by the patient and stimulate bodily preoccupation or provide a template for the patient's medically unexplained symptoms. A detailed review of current medications is important because many of these patients are taking multiple medications and have iatrogenic symptomatology (e.g., rebound headaches with excessive opiate use, difficulties in attention and concentration with excessive benzodiazepine use). The substance use history is important to evaluate caffeine consumption that may be the cause for bodily symptoms (such as tachycardia or tremors) and to assess the use of other substances such as alcohol, recreational drugs, and cigarettes that may be used to self-medicate emotional distress or play a role in symptom presentation.

Developmental history is important for many reasons but is another potential landmine for the therapeutic alliance. A standard developmental history is likely to lead to irritation and scorn from the bodily preoccupied patient. The most useful approach to obtain relevant information is to normalize and contextualize the developmental history. The most important elements of developmental history are shown in Table 12-2. I contextualize the developmental history by making comments such as, *"You have clearly had very difficult symptoms. Anyone would find these challenging, but their impact typically differs depending upon people's earlier life experiences. I would like to better understand a little bit about your background so that I can better understand the current impact of the symptoms. Maybe we could start with me getting some sense about your childhood and teen years, what your health was like, and what your family's health was like during this time? Often people with physical symptoms in adulthood have had medical problems in childhood—did you? Often people with physical symptoms in adulthood have had stressful early lives, and the impact of these stressors has changed their physiology and their own response to stress. Were you ever subject to severe stressors as a child—things like physical, verbal, or sexual abuse when you were younger? The other thing that I find that is hard for people who have difficult symptoms is that sometimes they have had earlier bad experiences with health care professionals or with other people, such as parents, teachers, or religious figures, who everyone would expect would treat them well but didn't. Have you had bad experiences with anyone in a position where they should have been taking care of you but instead were treating you poorly?"*

Table 12–2. Key Elements of the Developmental History in the Bodily Preoccupied Patient

Element	Clinical Implications
Childhood experiences of illness in either the patient or family	Provides information as to models of illness on which current symptoms may be patterned and gives a sense of the value that the family placed on somatic symptoms and distress versus emotional distress.
Difficult early environment with poor parenting and verbal, physical, or sexual abuse	Associated with numerous difficulties in identification and regulation of affect and disturbances in the psychological experience of the body. This increases risk for somatoform disorders and may also increase risk of other mood and anxiety disorders.
Attachment style	Does the patient see others, particularly those in authority, as trustworthy and dependable? Does she see herself as capable of taking care of herself effectively?
	Disturbance in either domain is associated with heightened risk of problems in the health care professional–patient relationship.
Level of education	Assists in framing explanations to patient and in determining the most useful ways to deliver psychoeducational interventions.

Mental Status Examination

Formal mental status examination and formal cognitive testing should be based on the symptoms that the patient presents rather than being conducted in a rote manner. As discussed earlier, there is a greater need in this patient group to set a context for each component of the interview, and this is as much or even more the case with mental status questions.

RATING SCALES AND STANDARDIZED INSTRUMENTS

The use of rating scales and standardized instruments is less common in the area of somatoform disorders than in many other areas of psychiatry. It can help to review instruments like the Structured Clinical Interview for DSM-IV (SCID) to see how to frame questions to elicit each of the somatoform diagnoses. There are a number of rating scales that assess dimensions associated with bodily preoccupation, somatization, hypochondriasis, and abnormal illness behavior, but these are primarily used in the research context.[2]

ENGAGEMENT AND ONGOING CARE

The effort expended in building an alliance during the assessment interviews paves the way for effective ongoing care by either the referring source or the psychiatrist. Primary care physicians or specialty physicians effectively manage most bodily preoccupied patients. Some patients require ongoing care with a psychiatrist—these are typically patients with multiple axis I and II comorbidities.

The general principles of ongoing care are shown in Box 12-6. The key issues are providing the patient with a clear, positive diagnosis rather than inferring one by exclusion; providing an explanation for symptoms as described below; undertaking further medical evaluation only when it is clearly indicated; treating axis I disorders that can be treated; and helping the patient to return to full functioning. If social reinforcers are a prominent part of the picture, then these need to be addressed. Regular follow-up by the primary care physician helps to contain the patient's distress and removes the contingency of needing to present a symptom in order to access the physician's care and concern. Consultation letters to referring physicians should include specific recommendations, as shown in Box 12-7.

Each of these components of ongoing care raises different challenges depending on the individual patient. The key first element in ongoing care is conveying the diagnosis to patients in a way that is useful to them. The confidence

---

Box 12-6. Principles of Ongoing Care for the Patient with Bodily Preoccupation

1. Explanation and education are important. Help the patient to understand your medical model for his symptoms by giving him an explanatory model for his illness that is informed by the patient's personality style, educational background, and interests.
2. Regularly scheduled follow-up appointments are essential. Make them frequent enough so as to avoid as needed appointments, which encourage symptom reporting as the "ticket of admission."
3. Identify and aggressively treat mood or anxiety disorders that are primary or secondary diagnoses.
4. Rationalize polypharmacy. Determine an "ideal" pharmacotherapy regimen, and then slowly and carefully work toward it. Careful, slow tapering of unneeded opiates and benzodiazepines is a first priority.
5. Target symptoms that can be treated, and provide specific therapies where indicated.
6. Identify and attempt to modify social dynamics that are maintaining symptoms.
7. Optimize physician–patient relationship, and resolve difficulties in the relationship when they invariably arise.
8. Counter-transference and negative counter-reactions must be identified and managed by the physician.

Box 12-7. Elements to Include in a Letter Back to the Referring Physician

1. A clear description of the psychiatric diagnoses: If a somatoform diagnosis is made, there should be a clear description, with minimal jargon, about the diagnostic criteria for the somatoform diagnosis and common psychiatric comorbidities that may develop.
2. Recommendation of regularly scheduled appointments: The aim is to remove the contingency of needing to present symptoms in order to see the doctor. Set the frequency based on current frequency. Very slowly increase the time between appointments as the patient's condition stabilizes or improves.
3. Further assessment of physical symptoms if required to rule out medical cause(s) for symptoms.
4. Recommendation that further diagnostic procedures, hospitalizations, treatments, etc., be avoided unless there are clear medical indications to do so.
5. Review and optimization of pharmacotherapy: Polypharmacy, particularly with opiates and benzodiazepines, should be rationalized and slowly tapered over a number of months. Encourage the referring physician to not prescribe new medications unless clearly medically indicated.
6. Suggestions with respect to working with patient over time: These should include whatever model/explanation the consulting psychiatrist has used with the patient as well as general cautions regarding communicating with bodily preoccupied patients (e.g., starting with the physical symptoms, using "three-step" explanations of stressor, intervening pathophysiology, and unexplained medical symptom).

that a clear diagnosis inspires cannot be underestimated. Explanations regarding diagnosis need to emphasize the physical aspects of the diagnosis, and developing an explanation that includes some combination of neurotransmitters, neuromodulators, and the autonomic nervous system is usually helpful. Trying to find concrete metaphors or analogies is also helpful. It is helpful to review the pathophysiological mechanisms that underlie medically unexplained symptoms and somatization.[2]

For example, in crafting an explanation for Zach who was described in Case Example 2 and who has a diagnosis of panic disorder, I would be cognizant of the fact that he is an engineer, and therefore a detailed, mechanistic explanation would be most likely to be helpful to him: *"The good news is that we can make a definite diagnosis for you. You have a disorder that results from an imbalance of neurotransmitters in your brain. Because of this chemical imbalance, the alarm center in your brain is set off inappropriately with no or minimal stimulation. We all need the alarm center to go off when we are in danger, but yours is like a faulty smoke detector that goes off every Sunday morning when you cook breakfast. The result of the alarm firing is that there is a release of stress hormones and chemicals, including adrenaline or norepinephrine, that in turn acts on the heart and causes the palpitations or racing heart beat. The lightheadedness and fainting feeling are also related to the alarm going off—people aren't sure exactly how it works but think that there is a very slight increase in your rate of breathing which you might not even notice. This changes the pH, or acid-base balance, in your blood, and this change in pH then shifts the oxygen dissociation curve for the blood in the cerebral circulation so that less oxygen is available to the brain, leaving you feeling lightheaded and as though you might pass out. The gastrointestinal symptoms are also related to this alarm misfiring. You have had to go from doctor to doctor trying to get a diagnosis, and their difficulties in diagnosing you have, I believe, led you to spend more and more time trying to document and investigate your symptoms in the hope that with more detailed explanations your doctors will be able to make a diagnosis. The good news is now we do have a clear, positive diagnosis, called panic disorder, so you don't need to be vigilant in monitoring your body anymore. We have all the information we need to make the diagnosis. We know what you have, and we know how to treat it. The other good news is that even though the symptoms can be scary, they in fact are not going to damage your body in any way, and you are not going to have a heart attack or pass out or vomit. There are a variety of different treatments we can offer you that will help to control the symptoms and to help you get your life back. Now that is a lot of information. Why don't you tell me what you have heard me say, and I'll fill in any blanks for you before you go today."* A patient who wasn't as educated or detail-oriented might suffice with an explanation that the symptoms are the result of changes in brain chemistry and can be treated.

Specific therapies, including both pharmacotherapy and evidence-based psychotherapies, have a role to play in the management of mood and anxiety disorders and somatoform disorders. Abbey[4] reviews the recent literature on management of somatoform disorders.

CONCLUSION

Although bodily preoccupied patients pose many challenges to physicians and historically have been devalued and ostracized within both medicine and psychiatry, the past decade has seen a number of advances in their assessment and treatment. They present with severe symptomatology that markedly impairs quality of life and deserve skilled care. Building effective interviewing skills is the crucial first step for success in working with this patient population.

REFERENCES

1. Bass C, Peveler R, House A: Somatoform disorders: severe psychiatric illnesses neglected by psychiatrists, *Br J Psychiatry* 179:11–14, 2001.
2. Abbey SE: Somatization and somatoform disorders. In Wise MG and Rundell JR, editors: *The American Psychiatric Publishing textbook of consultation-liaison psychiatry: psychiatry in the medically ill*, ed 2, Washington, DC, 2002, American Psychiatric Publishing, pp 361–392.
3. Looper KJ, Kirmayer LJ: Behavioral medicine approaches to somatoform disorders, *J Consult Clin Psychol* 70:810–827, 2002.
4. Abbey SE: Somatization and somatoform disorders. In Levenson JL, editor: *The American Psychiatric Publishing textbook of psychosomatic medicine*, Washington, DC, 2005, American Psychiatric Publishing, pp 271–296.
5. Mayou R, Levenson J, Sharpe M. Somatoform disorders in DSM-V [editorial], *Psychosomatics* 44:449–451, 2003.
6. American Psychiatric Association: *Diagnostic and statistical manual of mental disorders*, ed 4, text revision, Washington, DC, 2000, American Psychiatric Association.

RECOMMENDED READINGS

Page LA, Wessely S: Medically unexplained symptoms: exacerbating factors in the doctor-patient encounter, *J Royal Soc Med* 96:223–227, 2003.
Sharpe M, Mayou R: Somatoform disorders: a help or hindrance to good patient care? *Br J Psychiatry* 184:465–467, 2004.

13

Forensic Assessment

PHILIP KLASSEN AND PERCY WRIGHT

INTRODUCTION

At first glance, forensic clinical skills may be seen to be very much the province of psychiatrists and other mental health professionals who specialize in this area. However, there are important process and content issues in the practice of forensic psychiatry that are broadly applicable to the practice of general psychiatry. Knowledge of these skills will not only enable you to feel more comfortable seeing patients who present with behavioral or clinical issues related to forensic psychiatry, but also will assist you with respect to a variety of concerns equally applicable to other domains.

Through this chapter, you will become familiar with process skills germane to forensic patients. We also expect that you will gain knowledge of certain content issues that will allow you to successfully complete interviews of patients presenting with a history of violent behavior, sexual misbehavior, or dissimilation; most students will have the interview skills to deal with forensic patients but will lack the content knowledge to know what to ask. Finally, because of difficulties with accurate self-report in forensic patients, it is common for forensic practitioners to utilize other avenues of obtaining information about patients to accurately formulate a diagnosis and prognosis. We will introduce you to modalities of forensic assessment that complement direct clinical interview skills.

OVERVIEW OF FORENSIC PRACTICE

Although forensic mental health professionals may be asked to assess persons presenting with a wide array of symptoms and concerns, most commonly we are asked to assess patients' risk of violence to others, to give a sexological diagnosis, and/or to perform a critical appraisal of a patient's mental health history at the behest of a third party. In each of these situations, the patient or subject of the assessment may be disinclined to engage in full and open disclosure of her difficulties. In addition to external motivators for limited or slanted self-disclosure, these subject areas inherently involve describing thoughts, feelings, and behaviors that are socially undesirable. As well, people may be asked to recount aspects of their history about which they may feel shame or guilt. As a result, forensic clinicians typically employ a methodological approach to data gathering that is different from that used when patients present for no reason other than a wish to remedy their own difficulties.

In addition, many persons who present for a forensic assessment either have been or may be currently subject to an adversarial process, where their interests or wishes are being challenged. This also has an impact on self-disclosure.

BEFORE YOU SEE THE PATIENT

As with all mental health consultations, the forensic clinician will be asked, through the consultative process, to respond to certain questions. These questions may be posed by the patient, by a third party, or both. It is important to identify, before initiating the process of clinical interviewing of the subject of the assessment, what questions need be answered and to whom those answers should be provided. This, in turn, will direct the course of your assessment, both in terms of consent for disclosure and the subject areas considered.

If you are asked to see a patient with forensic mental health difficulties, and he faces a judicial or quasi-judicial proceeding (e.g., facing charges, or under investigation by the Children's Aid Society), it is important to determine whether the patient is represented by legal counsel. If the patient has a lawyer, then that person should certainly be aware that the assessment is taking place; if you have reason to believe that counsel is unaware that the assessment is taking place, the patient should be given the opportunity to reschedule the assessment or to inform counsel immediately of the proposed assessment. Well-meaning referral of a patient by another mental health professional, without notification to patient's counsel, may have the unfortunate effect of jeopardizing the patient's status before the court; this issue is best addressed by direct communication between you and the patient's counsel. Patients sent for assessment by counsel, however, are protected from inadvertent or self-defeating self-disclosure by means of extension of the privileged lawyer-client relationship to the assessor.

Flowing from the foregoing, it is important that you as a forensic clinician caution the patient vis-à-vis your legal obligations as a forensic clinician and the anticipated use of your opinion. In addition to issues related to involuntary hospitalization, it is important that the patient be made aware that as a clinician, you may have to disclose certain information to child welfare authorities, a disclosure that cannot be vitiated by any relationship with the patient, including a privileged relationship (see above). It is also appropriate, given that forensic clinicians are often asked to assess risk for violent behavior and/or sexual misbehavior, that the patient be advised that you may have a duty to inform others, including the police or an intended victim, if you believe that the patient represents an immediate and substantial threat to others' safety. The prudent clinician will also engage in an assessment of a patient's capacity to consent to, or refuse consent for, the assessment (and treatment) process, as well as an assessment of his capacity to manage finances and fitness to operate a motor vehicle. Although different jurisdictions may have different legal expectations of assessors in these different domains, it is always wise to consider all of the foregoing and to advise the patient of the fact that you will be considering these issues. Finally, if the subject of the assessment is an inpatient, it is also prudent to consider whether the patient is capable of consenting to, or refusing consent for, sexual activity because this does take place on inpatient units, and staff may be held liable for the sexual activity of severely compromised patients (be they perpetrators or victims). In all of the above-noted areas, there is case law to suggest that there is an onus on clinicians to perform these functions.

Many forensic clinicians, when our relationship with the patient is purely evaluative and not therapeutic, will advise the patient of this. Given that we encourage disclosure, it is important that the patient be aware that her relationship with the clinician is not a typical clinician-patient relationship.

It is also prudent for you as a forensic clinician to advise the patient, or the referring source, that forensic consultations tend to be lengthy; it is not uncommon for patients to arrive expecting a 30- to 60-minute interview, when a good deal more time is required. In the same vein, it is helpful to advise the patient that it is typical, in forensic mental health, to request collateral information from a variety of sources to aid in formulating a clinical opinion. Although some patients may see this as intrusive, they should simply be advised that such breadth of assessment is the accepted standard in this domain of practice. Information requested may include, but is not limited to, information relating to prior mental health assessments, prior offenses, and prior investigations of the subject (e.g., by the child welfare authorities); information from collateral sources who know the patient well; and information gleaned by means of psychological or laboratory (e.g., phallometric) testing. You should become familiar with statutory obligations and safeguards in your jurisdiction regarding transmission of clinical information. That being said, we believe it is not the province of forensic psychiatry to engage in police work; when a capable patient declines the assessor the opportunity to obtain third-party information, the forensic clinician should simply articulate this in the report. If insufficient information is available to answer the questions posed to the forensic clinician, this should be stated in the forensic report; the person or body requesting the report then carries the onus for assisting the clinician in obtaining the necessary information. Finally, the issue of transmission of your clinical opinion should be broached with the patient at the beginning of the first session. If the patient or subject of the assessment declines to give you permission to communicate your findings to the referring source, there is frequently no purpose to continuing the assessment process. In this circumstance, we recommend that you simply report to the referring source that consent for disclosure of your opinion was not obtained from the subject of the assessment. Again, the onus for obtaining that disclosure then falls on the referring source.

Forensic patients will at times ask to have a third party sit with them during the interview process. We do not permit this unless the patient suffers from significant cognitive compromise, such that the patient is unable to answer most questions. The presence of a third party introduces a source of response bias that the evaluator will likely not be able to measure or fully understand; for example, the patient may have given a very different account of the events in question to a spouse or union representative and thus may feel awkward making full disclosure to you, even if he wants to.

Forensic clinicians are also at times asked to videotape or audiotape the interview. We do not have strong feelings one way or the other about this and leave determination of this issue to your preference. We do strongly suggest that you keep very careful notes of what is said in the interview; these are often subpoenaed and should be a detailed and accurate description of what was said. Never dispose of your handwritten notes; they are the only truly original source material that you have. Quoting the patient in your report is recommended in key areas; this way you can make it clear that you are not simply making assumptions about what the patient thinks. If you quote the patient in your report, though, you should have the patient's statement in quotation marks in the handwritten notes as well. For certain critical areas of inquiry, you may also want to record the question(s) posed to the patient.

Forensic clinicians are at times asked to see patients in a jail or correctional setting. Insist that you see the patient in a private interview room. Telephone interviews through glass are inadvisable; inmates know that at times these are recorded by the authorities, and even if your interview won't be, some patients may be reluctant to be open with you.

THE EVALUATION PROCESS

Before offering a forensic mental health opinion, you should be cognizant of the empirical literature in the area or areas in question. In many content domains typically seen in forensic practice, empirical research suggests that personality and its disorders, as opposed to intercurrent axis I disorders, are typically the most salient factor, as regards, for example, risk for violent offending, risk of sexual reoffense, and risk of other problematic behavior, albeit with some exceptions. As a result, we suggest that forensic clinicians, in terms of their mental framework for the assessment, begin with an assessment of personality. Specific axis I diagnoses may be pursued later because these typically are embedded within the matrix of personality, and the expressions of diagnoses, behaviorally, may be shaped by characterological variables. Accordingly, we recommend that you begin your evaluation of the patient by asking about the person's childhood and family history, educational history, occupational history, and relationship history. Not only does this provide a longitudinal context for understanding problematic behavior, but this approach also tends to deal with neutral material first, before proceeding to more emotionally charged material relating to offending behavior, underlying sexological issues, and so on. Subsequent domains of inquiry include a person's medical history, substance use history, legal history, mental health history, history of the difficulties leading to the referral, and functional inquiry.

Given that persons subject to a forensic clinical assessment at times may present as somewhat guarded in their self-disclosure for reasons articulated above, it is often best not only to begin with neutral material, but to begin with relatively open-ended questions. Particularly if they are intellectually capable and have been subject to prior forensic assessments, subjects of a forensic mental health assessment may be looking for "cues" as to what the evaluator is seeking and may respond accordingly. The early portion of the assessment should seek to minimize such cueing of the patient.

We do recommend, however, that the forensic clinician, later, confront inconsistencies or improbabilities in the patient's history. We strongly recommend that this take place near the close of the assessment; the patient may become sufficiently defensive over these lines of inquiry as to mitigate against any further self-disclosure and may even discontinue the assessment. Having some collateral information as regards the subject of the assessment available prior to beginning the clinical interview is at times of some assistance, as inconsistencies in the information provided, or disparate viewpoints, may become evident at the interview unfolds. In the absence of such collateral information, the opportunity for data-gathering through gentle and later more persistent confrontation of the patient may be lost. The use of multiple interviews may also reduce defensiveness.

At the close of a forensic assessment, the subject of the assessment may ask you your opinion, with respect to diagnosis, prognosis, or other questions that are foci of the evaluation. In choosing whether to respond to such a query, you should consider where your duty of disclosure rests; it may not rest with the subject of the assessment. As well, the clinical evaluation of a forensic patient often leads to a clearer understanding of what additional collateral information or investigations may be required in order to form a fulsome opinion of that patient—your provisional opinion at the close of an interview may change substantially upon receipt of further information. If you think that there is important information outstanding, you should refrain from offering a provisional opinion to the patient. If your duty of disclosure lies primarily within the context of the clinician-patient relationship, the patient can always be invited back for a subsequent interview. This provides the patient with an explanation of your final opinion and the reasons for same. Given that it is often difficult to be exact or unequivocal in the behavioral sciences, and given that you may have received information from various sources that are not completely consistent, we suggest, parenthetically, that you frame your response to questions posed as a conditional probability rather than in absolute terms.

A template for the clinical evaluation of a forensic patient and for generation of a forensic report is available at the close of this chapter, as Appendix 13-1.

THE ANGRY PATIENT

The evaluation of angry patients warrants special scrutiny in this chapter because the forensic clinician may be uniquely predisposed to seeing angry patients, both by virtue of the fact that the patient may be frustrated and upset by legal or quasi-judicial proceedings and because forensic clinicians are asked to assess risk of violence. An evaluation of the angry patient benefits from a particular approach.

First and foremost, you need to be aware of your own anxiety in dealing with an angry or potentially angry patient. Your best yardstick to measure the extent to which you are in danger—not only of being physically assaulted but also of performing a substandard assessment—is anxiety about your own well-being or fear of asking certain questions. This will tend to limit the scope and depth of your assessment, thus increasing the potential for errors in diagnosis and treatment recommendations. When you detect that you are becoming anxious, consideration should be given to stopping the interview and restarting the process in a setting that is more secure and where your anxiety can return to baseline or near-baseline levels. It is appropriate, in most circumstances, to advise the patient of your anxiety and the reasons for that anxiety as a segue to suggesting changes in the interview process.

When confronted with an angry or potentially angry patient, you should determine whether the source of the patient's anger is organic, psychotic, or characterological/situational. Patients who are aggressive for organic reasons (e.g., underlying medical illness or intercurrent substance intoxication) will tend to be least responsive to verbal interventions. Psychotic patients who are angry may be more responsive to verbal interventions, and those who are nonpsychotic and angry for nonorganic reasons typically may be most responsive to verbal efforts to de-escalate tension. You should be alert, however, to escalating stages of agitation and anger. As patients become more agitated, they become progressively more defensive and less able to incorporate verbal interactions between the evaluator and themselves. Increasingly, such patients will be responsive to nonverbal communications by the evaluator. As a general rule, if the patient remains verbal, the evaluator can consider verbal interventions to de-escalate anger. Once the patient begins to act out in a physical fashion, however, by means of, for example, aggressive gesticulation, aggressive behavior toward property, or other indicia of translation of anger into physical action, then a physical response is typically required, and efforts at verbal de-escalation should be abandoned. First meetings with potentially violent patients should not take place "after hours" or in physically isolated spaces; institutional settings are typically preferred due to the availability of security personnel.

When a situation with a patient begins to escalate, you should be nonconfrontational. Keep a respectful distance from the patient and attempt to sit, or stand, at an angle from the subject; facing the subject directly may be seen as more confrontational. The exit from the room should be equidistant from both you and the patient, so that either of you can leave without physically confronting the other.

Transference and counter-transference issues are also important to monitor with an angry patient. Frequently, anger that is directed toward the forensic clinician may be transferential in origin or displaced. A useful verbal de-escalation strategy, to avoid becoming a "lightning rod" for patients' cumulative difficulties or resentments, is to redirect their anger, verbally, toward persons they perceive to have caused difficulty for them previously. This deflects the patient's anger "out there" as opposed to toward you. For example, when a patient complains about mistreatment by the police, rather than asking the patient "What did you do" that led to the attention of the police, you may choose to redirect the patient by asking *"The police said what?"* or *"What did the police accuse you of?"*

You also need to be conscious of the fact that violent patients, patients with sexological diagnoses, dissimulating patients, and other patients who are frequently seen in forensic contexts may arouse strong counter-transference feelings, including counter-transference hate. It is critical that you be well aware of—and manage appropriately—negative counter-transferential feelings toward forensic patients, particularly angry ones. In our opinion, starting the interview with a personal and developmental history allows you to see the subject of the assessment, no matter how problematic the behavior, as a human being subject to the vicissitudes of temperament and development. In our opinion, this mitigates against the counter-transferential feelings that otherwise may flow from beginning to understand the patient as an offender, or simply as a person who makes "evil" choices.

VIOLENCE RISK ASSESSMENT

As with any psychiatric assessment, lines of forensic questioning are substantially derived from the question that you are being asked to answer. With respect to violence risk assessment, an important distinction is whether you are being asked to assess short-term risk of violence (i.e., the potential for violent behavior over hours to days, or at most, weeks) or intermediate or long-term risk of violence (i.e., over weeks to years). Research has shown that most clinicians are reasonably adept, and approximately equivalently adept across disciplines, in the appraisal of short-term risk of violent behavior.

Although there is no universally accepted algorithm or guide to the assessment of short-term risk of aggressive behavior, the following are some generally accepted indicators with respect to same, as articulated by Robert Feinstein.[1] The clinical interview, accordingly, should seek out information with respect to these domains.

Violent Ideation

In both psychotic and nonpsychotic patients, violent ideation is an important risk factor. You should also ask about variables that promote and forestall acting on violent ideation, or that escalate or de-escalate such ideation.

Recent History/Past History of Violence

With respect to both this area of inquiry and the point to follow, you should ask specific questions about verbal aggression, threats, property damage in anger, self-harm behavior in anger (including sublimated aggression such as substance abuse, risky driving, etc.), physical assaults, using or carrying of a weapon, use of a vehicle as a weapon, displacement of aggressive behavior toward vulnerable persons (e.g., pets or children), aggressive sexuality, and partner violence. Particularly with respect to partner violence, you will need to ask very specific questions because this is an area where patients tend to show considerable guardedness in their self-disclosure. You should specifically ask whether the subject of the assessment has slapped, punched, kicked, choked, bitten, restrained, or stalked a current or prior partner. Due to strong societal sanctions against violence toward women, most patients will reflexively answer "no" when asked if they have been aggressive to a partner; many will later acknowledge specific acts, though, when asked directly.

Behavior During the Interview

To the extent that a patient is demonstrably and observably angry and agitated, he may be at increased risk of aggressive behavior in the short term. As patients become progressively more agitated and angry, their ability to generate options, in terms of their behavior, and to utilize options provided by others, diminishes. You should gently probe patients for their willingness to consider nonviolent options and for their willingness to accept assistance.

Support Systems/Treatment

The interest, availability, and competence of a support system, as well as the capacity of the patient to participate in a therapeutic process, may be risk-reducing with respect to short-term risk of aggressive behavior.

Substance Abuse History

To the extent that a patient is intoxicated or demonstrates a probability of intoxication with potentially disinhibiting agents in the near future, that person may be at increased risk of aggressive behavior. Accordingly, a careful substance use history is imperative. Familiarity with street drug jargon and quantities regularly used is of help; for example, a quarter ounce of marijuana generates approximately 25 "joints."

Neurological/Medical History

To the extent that a person suffers from mental retardation, brain injury, or other illness affecting cognitive function, she may have diminished problem-solving capacities and a diminished capacity to accept risk-reducing interventions; thus, such persons may be at increased risk of aggressive behavior, over the short term, when they present as angered.

Other Factors

Other variables that may contribute to risk of aggressive behavior include association with criminal peers/living in a high-crime neighborhood, residential instability, active psychosis (particularly with associated angry or negative affect), financial stressors, and a lack of a structured daily routine.

With respect to risk of violence over the longer term, research has consistently shown that structured or actuarial methods of assessment tend to predict risk as well as, and generally better than, clinical assessments, in no small measure as a result of the propensity of clinical evaluators to overestimate risk, thus generating significant false-positive opinions in this area.

The clinical questions that should be asked in such circumstances are in turn driven by the structured or actuarial tools you might use. One parsimonious way of addressing which tool to use is to decide on the basis of whether the subject of the assessment has ever been convicted of a criminal charge or charges. If a person has not been convicted of any criminal charge, we suggest appraisal of personality-derived risk using the Psychopathy Checklist: Screening Version (PCL:SV)[2] and the assessment of violence risk using the Historical Clinical Risk Management-20 (HCR-20).[3] Both of these instruments assess a person's history and current state in various domains; to assist you, information required by these tools is provided in Appendices 13-2 and 13-3. We suggest using multiple structured or actuarial tools in the service of convergent validity. Both of these tools may be used for males and females.

In cases when your patient has been convicted of a criminal charge or charges, we recommend the use of the Psychopathy Checklist–Revised (PCL-R),[4] the parent instrument to the PCL:SV (Appendix 13-4). When a patient has been convicted of a "hands-on" violent offense, we suggest the use of the Violence Risk Appraisal Guide (VRAG; Appendix 13-5),[5] and when that offense has been sexual, the use of the Sex Offender Risk Appraisal Guide (SORAG; Appendix 13-6)[6] and/or the Static-99 (Appendix 13-7).[6] Information required by these instruments is provided in the appendices. The VRAG, the SORAG, and the Static-99 are for use with male offenders only.

You should note that administration, scoring, and use of the PCL:SV and the PCL-R require special training. It is strongly recommended that persons who anticipate working in the forensic domain with any regularity receive such training. Although the administration and scoring of the PCL:SV and the PCL-R may seem deceptively simple, the reliability and validity of the ensuing scores depend heavily not only on obtaining appropriate and sufficient information but also on rater training.

The same essentially holds true for the other risk assessment tools; these are, variously, more or less "manualized." Evaluators using the VRAG, SORAG, HCR-20, or Static-99 will be guided regarding the information necessary to allow for accurate scoring of the items contained therein.

CLINICAL ASSESSMENT OF ANGER MANAGEMENT DIFFICULTIES

In addition to interviewing persons for the expressed purpose of appraising their risk, forensic clinicians also are asked to provide anger management treatment for persons. The following clinical interview items are useful in understanding the origins of aggressive behavior, as well as perpetuating and precipitating factors. They are also helpful in assessing the extent to which aggressive behavior has been persistent as opposed to isolated and in identifying treatment readiness.

Infancy, Childhood, and Adolescence

We typically ask about the presence of fetal or perinatal problems, difficult temperament, availability and constancy of caregivers, methods of discipline utilized, evidence of early aggressive behavior (i.e., in childhood), and the presence or absence of formal diagnoses of attention deficit disorder or a learning disability. Aggression is, once consistently evidenced in childhood, a relatively stable behavioral trait.

We recommend that you subsequently ask about aggressive behavior in childhood, including bullying (a particularly sensitive predictor of conduct disorder) and weapons use. School sanctions vis-à-vis aggressive, defiant, or limit-testing behavior are important to address; placement in behavioral classes, psychological or psychiatric assessment in childhood, and school suspension or expulsion (and the ages at which these took place) are salient predictors of future aggressive behavior.

It is important to also canvass all of the diagnostic criteria for conduct disorder, as defined by the *Diagnostic and Statistical Manual of Mental Disorders* of the American Psychiatric Association, Fourth Edition, Text Revision (DSM-IV-TR).[7] Early onset of conduct-disordered symptoms and the presence of many conduct-disordered symptoms (i.e., many in excess of those required to make the diagnosis of conduct disorder) are predictors of adult antisocial behavior. Gang membership, while infrequent, is a salient predictor of later violence and of values and attitudes promoting aggressive problem solving. Juvenile arrests and convictions are similarly predictive of future difficulties, to the extent that if a person was subject to custody, particularly secure custody and/or training school, he may be at increased risk of future aggressive behavior.

Adulthood

We favor using a cognitive-behavioral model to understand aggressive behavior in adulthood. Typically, the affect when aggressive behavior is expressed tends to be anger. However, it is worthwhile asking whether antecedent affects include anxiety, depression, and affects other than anger; anger may be used to "mask" other unpleasant emotions, and patients can be helped with their anger when they can begin to recognize, tolerate, and deal with these other feelings.

When intense angry affect is generated, and as the patients' behavioral options diminish as a result of increasing intense affect, patients tend to respond to provocation with avoidance or antagonism. Persons will not infrequently cycle through numerous instances of avoidance before engaging in direct antagonism toward the perceived source of the provocation. It is important to recognize and point out to the patient how avoidant behavior tends to drive later antagonism, as a result of failure of adaptive problem solving.

As indicated in a previous section, given the social undesirability of aggressive behavior, it is generally necessary to question persons very closely on behavioral indicia of anger. Asking the subject of the assessment to present, in detail, recent aggressive incidents, will facilitate understanding the cognitive distortions leading to avoidance or antagonism, will assist in understanding the extent to which these persons are ready to engage in the change process, and will assist in identifying specific conflict-laden situations.

We typically ask patients to develop an inventory of both positive and negative aspects of anger. Although anger clearly can have a negative impact on relationships, can lead to aggression and social censure, is personally disorganizing for the subject, can contribute to low self-esteem, and may be used to mask other emotions, anger should also be recognized as an energizer, a facilitator of action, a facilitator of communication, and a "cue" to incipient difficulties. Helping the patient to identify positive and negative aspects of his anger promotes careful contemplation of his psychology and circumstances. The foregoing and the list of cognitive distortions that follows rely heavily on the work of Raymond Novaco and Donald Meichenbaum, and we recommend that students who plan to work with angry patients in treatment avail themselves of information on their stress inoculation training treatment methods.[8]

Cognitive distortions typically found in angry persons, and which contribute to the expression of aggression, include the following:

- All or nothing thinking: The patient will tend to see things in black and white categories.
- Overgeneralization: The patient assumes that future experiences will evolve exactly as those in the past have, with an anticipated adverse outcome.
- Mental filtering: The patient may identify a single negative detail and dwell on it exclusively, such that his perception of reality becomes inappropriately colored by it.
- Disqualifying the positive: The patient may reject positive experiences and maintain the negative beliefs that produce anger.
- Mind reading: The patient may erroneously conclude that others are reacting negatively to him without investigating the truth of this.
- Catastrophization: The patient may inappropriately exaggerate the importance or relevance of an issue, generating intense affect.
- Emotional reasoning: The patient may assume that his negative emotions reflect the way things really are.
- "Should" statements: The patient may generate intense negative affect through self-criticism.
- Labeling: The patient may label others in a reductionistic fashion, producing angry affect.
- Personalization: The patient may see otherwise benign or innocuous external events as targeting him.
- Blaming: The patient may displace responsibility for an event on others, then target that other, rather than taking personal responsibility for his behavior.
- Hostile misattributions: Persons who are often angry tend to perceive the world, perhaps as a result of childhood antecedents, as a hostile place, thus justifying the conclusion that they may respond aggressively in kind.
- Hypermasculinity: Some patients may harbor a unidimensional view of how males "should" respond to perceived provocation, not through discussion but by means of antagonism.

Patients presenting with anger management difficulties may initially describe themselves as at a loss to cope without the use of aggression as an interpersonal tool. You will need to emphasize with the patient the fact that anger management treatment promotes skills acquisition, to replace those "skills" lost. Many patients who present as habitually angry or aggressive profoundly lack the capacity for healthy assertiveness, resulting in avoidant and ultimately antagonistic behavior. Enhancing capacity for healthy assertion, as opposed to passivity and then aggression, is an important part of anger management treatment.

INTERVIEWING SEX OFFENDERS

The objectives of the clinical interview in this area are to identify sexual behavior patterns and to determine whether the patient has an underlying paraphilia.

Early History

We believe it is useful to begin a sexual behaviors assessment by asking about any history of sexual abuse during the patient's formative or even adult years. This allows the person to begin discussing sexuality in a fashion that may be more easily tolerated than discussion of offending behavior. Also, however, the patient's attitudes toward his own history of abuse, if present, may be telling in regard to the way he perceives abusive behavior. To the extent that persons discount or minimize the impact of their own history of abuse, they may also be predisposed toward minimizing harm to others when they abuse them.

It is also useful to identify the onset of sexual behavior of a consensual nature. Early onset sexual behavior tends to correlate with conduct problems and may be a proxy for a disturbed early rearing environment and/or history of sexual abuse.

Sexual Function/Outlets

You should ask the male subject of the assessment about erectile or ejaculatory sexual dysfunction. Persons with an underlying paraphilic sexual preference not infrequently manifest some degree of sexual dysfunction during "normative" sexual activity; paraphilic persons may not be aroused enough by "normative" sexual activity to achieve erection and/or ejaculation. At times, it is useful to ask these patients whether they have to fantasize about paraphilic activity during "normative" sexual activity to maintain an erection and to achieve ejaculation.

You should ask patients to identify their preferred sexual object by age and gender (male/female, adult/pubescent/prepubescent). Relative interest in various ages and genders of sexual partners should be identified; we suggest the use of a 10-point ranking scale, anchoring that scale by assigning a score of 10 out of 10 to the preferred age/gender.

You should inquire as to the number of sexual partners the patient has had; late onset of sexual activity and a low total number of age-appropriate sexual partners is not infrequently seen in paraphilic persons (e.g., persons with pedophilia). Conversely, early onset of sexual activity and a large number of casual sexual relationships have been reported in persons who have a coercive sexual preference.

Some measure of total sexual interest is also an appropriate subject for evaluation. Typically, we ask patients how many orgasms, by any means, they seek per day, week, or month. This includes autoerotic activity but also includes use of prostitutes, massage facilities, telephone sex contact, etc., as well as sexual contact with partners. Use of ancillary erotic material, be it print, video, or Internet-derived, is also useful to identify. Persons should be questioned as to the specifics of the ancillary materials they use, particularly if that material is Internet-based; specific chat rooms, newsgroups, or Web pages can give important information about a person's underlying sexual preference. Autoerotic fantasy, similarly, is useful to identify; whereas sexual behavior is the product of a host of convergent influences, masturbatory fantasy is entirely the product of underlying sexual preference and provides important information with respect to the same.

Review of Paraphilias

Paraphilias are, by definition, deviant sexual preferences. They are described as deviant either because they interfere with dyadic, mutually satisfying sexual behavior (e.g., the transvestite who is disinterested in sexual relations with partners because he is really only aroused by wearing women's clothing) or because they involve coercive sexual activity (e.g., pedophilia, sexual sadism). The diagnosis of a paraphilia may be made by any one of three means. Persons may be diagnosed as paraphilic when they self-report such a preference, although patients do not typically volunteer this information, and careful questioning will be required. Patients may be diagnosed as paraphilic when they generate a positive phallometric test result for same from a reputable phallometric laboratory with published or available sensitivity and specificity data (see discussion to follow). Persons may also be diagnosed as paraphilic when they engage in behavior that cannot reasonably be accounted for by any other psychiatric diagnoses.

There are a number of specific paraphilias that have been identified. Research has shown that when persons suffer from one paraphilia, they typically will suffer from multiple paraphilias; on average, a paraphilic patient will suffer from two or three paraphilias, although one will typically be the central organizing paraphilia.

It is not, in practical terms, possible to ask a patient questions about every possible paraphilic preference. We suggest that in essence the most common and most troublesome or troubling paraphilias be the subjects of routine investigation for persons who are alleged to have engaged in sexual misbehavior. Many paraphilias will typically present with specific cognitive distortions; we suggest that in addition to the sexual interest, patients be asked about the presence or absence of these cognitive distortions because these will become targets of treatment.

Paraphilias are found almost exclusively in males. When a female is alleged to have engaged in problematic sexual behavior, nonparaphilic explanations for that behavior should be sought.

Exhibitionism is defined as a sexual preference for exposing one's genitals. Exhibitionists will typically attempt to engage in this behavior in a fashion that can be explained away; for example, they may later claim they were urinating in public rather than exposing their genitals, or they may claim that their bathrobes fell open just at the moment they opened the front door. Exhibitionists typically engage in this behavior frequently and repeatedly. Often, the critical issue for exhibitionists will be observing the facial expression of their victims. At times, exhibitionists will state that they enjoy seeing surprise or shock on the face of their victims. At other times, they will profess that the expression seen on the faces of the victims was one of admiration of the exhibitionists' genital organs. The cognitive distortion or distortions that typically accompany this behavior include a belief that the victim will be impressed with the exhibitionist's organs and will wish to have sexual relations with him.

Exhibitionists may also suffer from pedophilia; you should question the exhibitionist as to the age and gender of his victims and should note whether the exhibitionist was engaged in this behavior near a park, playground, school, etc.

Voyeurism is defined as a sexual preference for observing others, typically adult females, engaged in intimate activity (e.g., bathing, undressing, or engaging in sexual behavior). Not infrequently, voyeurs will have an interest in erotica in its various forms as well. They may use sophisticated technology to achieve their aims and should be questioned about this (e.g., video recording equipment installed in bathrooms, shoe-mounted fiber-optic cameras). One of the critical issues in the evaluation of a voyeur is whether the voyeuristic behavior was the primary interest of the perpetrator, or whether in fact the voyeur has an underlying coercive sexual interest and his covert observation(s) of females took place in the context of preparing for coercive sexual behavior ("rape planning").

Frotteurism and *toucheurism* are related nonconsensual sexual preferences; the frotteur has an interest in rubbing his body, typically his genitals, against a nonconsenting, usually adult female, victim. Typically, the frotteur will rub his genital region against the behind of an adult female, and this will usually take place in a relatively tight space, again, where the action may be rationalized (e.g., on a crowded subway train). Toucheurs have a sexual preference for nonconsensual sexual touching of another person, typically an adult female. Most frequently they will, again in a crowded or tight space, brush their hand against the buttocks or the breasts of a female. A significant minority of frotteurs and toucheurs have an underlying coercive sexual interest; they should be questioned regarding this.

Persons who present with a history of donning female clothing may have an underlying gender identity disorder or may have transvestitic fetishism. A review of the evaluation of gender identity–disordered persons is beyond the scope of this chapter. These persons do not suffer from a paraphilia. Transvestitic fetishists are persons whose sexual preference involves masturbating while wearing women's clothing. These persons are typically heterosexual males but are usually hyposexual in terms of relations with others. They achieve sexual arousal through the feel of wearing women's clothing, frequently undergarments, lingerie, or pantyhose. Transvestism may occur in persons who also have masochism or sadism; transvestitic fetishists should be questioned about these paraphilias.

Pedophilia is defined as a sexual preference for prepubescent children. *Hebephilia* is defined as a sexual preference for pubescent children. The majority of pedophiles and hebephiles prefer opposite sex minors; a significant minority will prefer same sex minors, and another significant minority will in fact be bisexual in their preference. Pedophilic and hebephilic persons will not infrequently involve themselves in activities that bring them in contact with children; they should be closely questioned with respect to vocational or avocational activities such as involvement in Big Brothers, the Scouting movement, driving a school bus, camps, day care, youth organizations, etc. Cognitive distortions typically found in pedophiles or hebephiles include the belief that the victim was interested in, enjoyed, or experienced sexual pleasure as a result of the sexual contact. Pedophiles and hebephiles will at times relate that they felt controlled or seduced by the child or youth and may even believe that their behav-

ior was helpful to the child. Pedophiles and hebephiles should also be questioned as to their relations with adult females; not infrequently, these persons will seek out single mothers who have children within the pedophile or hebephile's preferred age range, so as to obtain access to those children.

Persons who engage in sexual violence with adult females are a heterogeneous group. These patients fall along a continuum, from those who offend largely for reasons of antisociality or psychopathy, at times facilitated or disinhibited by high levels of expressed anger and/or substance intoxication, to persons who are fundamentally paraphilic. To the extent that patients who have engaged in coercive sexual behavior with adult females lack evidence of antisociality or psychopathy, evidence of an underlying paraphilia should be sought. A number of cognitive distortions have been noted in persons who engage in coercive sexual behavior with adult females; these individuals typically harbor adversarial attitudes regarding male–female relations, tend to evidence substantial suspicion and mistrust toward females and their intentions or verbalizations, and/or engage in victim blame (e.g., suggesting that because the victim was wearing a short skirt or was out late at night, she was in fact seeking such sexual interaction). At the paraphilic end of this spectrum are patients with *sexual sadism* (at times with accompanying *necrophilia,* a sexual preference for sexual interaction with a deceased person). Persons who engage in coercive sexual behavior with adult females should be questioned as to their interest in power and control over their victims and the infliction of pain, humiliation, or suffering. Specifically, the arousal value of the aforementioned should be the subject of questioning; sexual sadists will at times lose their erection when the victim experiences insufficient pain, humiliation, or suffering. Some sexual sadists will inflict pain, humiliation, or suffering on a victim without engaging in any overt sexual behavior—they may choose simply to masturbate to thoughts of their actions later. Sexual sadists should also be questioned regarding their sexual behavior with "consenting" partners; not infrequently, these persons will engage in sexual behavior with their partners in a manner that is described by the partners as unduly rough or impersonal. Persons with a coercive or sadistic sexual interest frequently, for reasons that are unclear, favor anal sexual activity. They not infrequently also wish to engage or do engage in bondage or related activities with consenting partners. An interest in binding, cutting, burning, penetration, and manual or ligature strangulation should also be investigated. Persons with a necrophilic interest may have a vocational or avocational interest that will bring them into contact with deceased persons (e.g., employment at funeral homes), and this should be assessed.

PSYCHOPATHY

For many years, *psychopathy* and *sociopathy* were largely lay terms, poorly operationalized and often misunderstood. Over the past several decades, due largely to the work of Dr. Robert Hare and his colleagues[4] in the construction and repeated validation of the PCL-R and related instruments, our understanding of psychopathy has been greatly enhanced. Psychopathy is the personality dimension most related to offending behavior, both in criminal and mentally disordered offenders. The "gold standard" for the measurement of psychopathy (in criminal samples) is the PCL-R. The PCL:SV[2] is the preferred instrument for noncriminal psychiatric or civil samples. A youth version is also available. Much of the information needed to score these instruments will be obtained in a standard psychiatric/forensic interview, although it should be noted that file information from persons or institutions with whom the subject of the assessment has had contact is mandatory for scoring these instruments.

However, there are areas of clinical inquiry that are important to the scoring of these instruments and may not typically find their way into a standard psychiatric interview. Psychopathic persons are egocentric, exploitive, behaviorally unstable, and sensation seeking, and some additional lines of inquiry are often helpful in assessing for psychopathy.

Restlessness and sensation seeking should be the subject of clinical inquiry. Psychopathic persons frequently are easily bored; they will describe engaging in criminal behavior, high-risk recreational behavior, changes of partners, changes of jobs or residences, changes in geographic locale, and substance-abusing behavior, in part out of a wish for excitement or relief of boredom. Psychopathic persons are frequently duplicitous and manipulative. They should be questioned as to whether, at times, they have engaged in lying simply for the exercise itself, as opposed to for material gain. Persons with psychopathy are frequently parasitic; they should be questioned as to the extent to which they engage in self-supporting behavior, as opposed to asking others (e.g., the state or partners) to support them. Psychopathic persons generally have superficial relationships with others. Their sexual behavior tends to be promiscuous, and they typically have no interest in shouldering the responsibilities of a relationship; rather, they are simply interested in sexual contact for hedonistic reasons alone. These persons may readily admit that they have no interest in goal setting or long-term thinking, and they should be questioned about this. The irresponsibility manifested by psychopathic patients is not infrequently displayed in their parenting or financial behavior; these persons typically are not involved as parents, and their financial history should be questioned in detail. Patients' attitudes and behavior regarding sex and money may say a great deal about how they comport themselves in relationships.

MALINGERING

The DSM-IV-TR defines *malingering* as intentional production of false or grossly exaggerated physical or psychological symptoms, motivated by external incentives. It is indicated that malingering should be strongly suspected if any combination of the following is noted:

- Medicolegal context of presentation
- Marked discrepancy between the person's claimed stress or disability and objective findings
- Lack of cooperation during the diagnostic evaluation or with treatment
- Presence of antisocial personality disorder

Malingering should be differentiated from a factitious disorder, which may present with physical symptoms, psychological symptoms, or both. Factitious-disordered persons are attempting, by means of intentional production of symptomatology, to enter into or remain in the patient role. At times, intentional symptom production may be due to both malingering and a factitious disorder.

Persons may attempt to malinger a wide variety of psychiatric or psychological symptoms, depending on the context in which they finds themselves. In this section, we will focus on those symptoms that are perhaps most frequently malingered: psychotic symptoms and amnestic symptoms.

Professionals evaluating patients in a medicolegal context should always be alert to the possibility of malingering. Because malingering, by definition, is driven by an external incentive, you need to establish whether there is a motive for malingering. You must also bear in mind that, for various reasons, persons with bona fide symptoms may minimize those symptoms to appear "normal." Patients with major mental illness may have little or no insight into their illness or may not wish to be stigmatized as suffering from a mental disorder. It is certainly not uncommon for persons with a mental disorder, even when charged with serious offenses, to minimize their symptomatology or deny it altogether. Perhaps most singularly challenging is the person with an established major mental illness who also has a comorbid antisocial personality disorder. Discerning the symptom burden that such a patient was experiencing at any given time can be difficult because these persons may concurrently present with real and malingered symptoms.

Before attempting to discern whether presenting symptoms are malingered, you should be familiar with the phenomenology of major diagnostic categories in psychiatry, usual patterns of symptom presentation, and the longitudinal course of illnesses; seeing many patients with real psychiatric illnesses is very helpful in discerning malingering because this will provide you with a clinical sense of usual symptom sets.

A more complete overview of the assessment of malingering is available from Rogers,[9] including excellent chapters by Phillip Resnick and Cercy et al.

Psychotic Symptoms

Persons who attempt to malinger psychotic symptoms present with varying degrees of knowledge of or exposure to individuals truly experiencing psychosis. An effort should be made to determine the extent to which the subject of such an assessment may have had exposure to psychotic symptoms.

A number of features of malingered psychosis may assist in differentiating such symptomatology from real psychotic symptoms. Persons who attempt to malinger psychotic symptoms will generally present with a dense history of polymorphous psychotic symptoms; they typically attempt to present with a vast array of symptoms to suggest that they are profoundly psychotic. Their reported symptom burden is frequently in excess of what one sees in persons who truly suffer from psychosis. The evaluator should refrain from taking a judgmental stance when hearing this, and indeed should present herself as interested in hearing all about the multiplicity of symptoms.

Not infrequently, malingerers will describe hallucinations as continuous, as opposed to persons suffering from, for example, schizophrenia, who more frequently describe their hallucinations as intermittent. Persons who attempt to malinger psychotic symptoms typically also describe vivid and dramatic visual hallucinations; these are relatively less common in persons with a primary psychotic illness. Those who attempt to malinger psychotic symptoms will often draw attention to their illness and may even present, clinically, as having insight into their disorder; it is not unusual for a malingerer to immediately inform the evaluator that "I am delusional!" Persons who attempt to malinger psychotic symptoms, even if they have had exposure to psychotic patients, may have little knowledge of the taxonomy of mental disorders, and their malingered psychotic symptoms may not easily fit within a diagnostic category, at times giving rise to a diagnosis of "atypical psychosis" or "psychotic disorder not otherwise specified" by evaluators less familiar with the vicissitudes of malingering. Rapid onset and offset of psychotic symptoms should arouse suspicion that the symptoms are malingered, as should reports of continued symptomatology in the absence of observable evidence of same; malingerers often feel that they need to *continue* to present as psychotic, in the service of exculpation.

Persons malingering psychotic or other symptoms will at times present with approximate answers to questions (e.g., $2 + 2 = 5$). What becomes clear in such cases is that the malingerer is able to discern what is being asked for or about and has the capacity to slant her answer in a pathological direction. When pressed as to the specifics of her profuse symptomatology, she may be unable to offer detail. We are reminded of a patient who claimed to hear the voices of both Eva and Zsa Zsa Gabor, identical twin actresses. When asked how he made the distinction between their voices, the patient could offer no response.

Persons who attempt to malinger psychotic symptoms will most typically focus on the core or positive symptoms of schizophrenia. They may be able to, with considerable facility, express delusional thinking or the experience of auditory or other hallucinations. However, their affect may not be congruent with what they describe. For example, someone may describe seemingly tormenting persecutory delusions or horrifying visual and auditory hallucinations but present as relatively neutral affectively. You must bear in mind, however, that persons with schizophrenia will present as most affectively disturbed by problematic symptoms early in the course of their illness; after many years of suffering from schizophrenia, persons with this diagnosis may later present as somewhat inured to even the most troubling delusions and hallucinations.

As well as asking about delusional thought content and accompanying affect, you should examine for the presence or absence of thematically consistent behavior. Persons who appear to be behaviorally undisturbed by delusions and hallucinations, except where it serves the purpose of exculpation, should be suspected of malingering. Malingerers are not typically seen laughing or talking to themselves.

Even persons who are well able to malinger delusions or hallucinations have a good deal more difficulty malingering thought form disturbance or negative or deficit symptoms of schizophrenia. Their histories also typically do not reveal the functional decline seen in persons who suffer from an ongoing primary psychotic illness.

In terms of the clinical evaluation of malingered psychotic symptoms, it is always preferable to begin exploration of such symptoms in a very open-ended manner. Later, your questions should become progressively more directive as you seek to increase elaboration of symptoms from the suspected malingerer. You may also attempt, later, to suggest highly improbable psychotic symptoms to malingerers; vigorous and enthusiastic affirmative responses to highly improbable suggestions vis-à-vis delusions and hallucination provide strong evidence for malingering.

In the final analysis, one of the best ways of determining whether psychotic symptoms are malingered is by means of inpatient hospitalization. It is very difficult for a nonpsychotic person to maintain a truly psychotic presentation for extended periods of time; he will fatigue of attempting to maintain these symptoms and will experience an ongoing pull, through his daily interactions, toward reality-based responding. The authors recall such a person who was remanded to our inpatient assessment unit having been charged with numerous robberies (the charges themselves aroused suspicion because a delusional motivation for robbery, particularly when not acting alone, is uncommon). After several weeks of assiduously maintaining a presentation that suggested both psychotic symptoms and brain damage, the person in question was ultimately overheard discussing, with one of the cooks serving the inpatient unit, the nuances of preparation of a béarnaise sauce; collateral information ultimately revealed that not only the patient but his wife and his immediate family members were all participants in an elaborate scheme to both avoid criminal responsibility for the predicate offenses and defraud an insurance company. The absence of a preexisting history of significant mental disorder should also arouse suspicion. That being said, we once evaluated a person who had previously been admitted to over 50 psychiatric facilities throughout North America, claiming a variety of psychotic symptoms on each occasion in the service of avoiding criminal prosecution and obtaining free lodging.

Malingered Amnesia and Memory Impairment

Persons may attempt to malinger ongoing cognitive impairment, discrete periods of retrograde amnesia, or both.

When assessing patients who present with amnesia or cognitive impairment, it is of course essential that you rule out the existence of an underlying central nervous system disorder or psychiatric disorder that could account for it. Many central nervous system disorders present with cognitive impairment, as do numerous psychiatric illnesses (e.g., schizophrenia). The temporal lobes are the anatomical sites that correspond most closely with memory deficits; biomedical investigations should focus particularly on disorders or lesions affecting these areas.

When assessing persons suspected of malingering cognitive impairment, you should be aware that most individuals who malinger cognitive impairment tend to *overestimate* recognition memory deficits, attentional deficits, and immediate recall deficits they assume to occur in truly brain-injured persons. The cornerstone of the assessment of malingered cognitive impairment lies in comparing the reported deficits with the real deficit experience of persons known to have traumatic brain injury or other central system processes. A number of psychometric measures can assist in this regard (see discussion to follow). In addition,

persons who attempt to malinger cognitive impairment may show inconsistencies in terms of the nature of the impairment over time and across testing or evaluative situations, and with respect to the putative anatomical location of their deficits. Persons who attempt to malinger cognitive impairment will need to remember, so to speak, which deficits they manifested on the last testing occasion; therefore, it is advisable to test these persons, clinically or psychometrically, on two or more distinct occasions, preferably separated by a substantial period of time. As well, since those who attempt to malinger cognitive impairment may not be aware of the functional correlates of given deficits, evaluation of their level of function (particularly on an inpatient unit) may show behavior or abilities inconsistent with deficits evidenced on testing.

Periods of isolated, retrograde, and dense amnesia are only infrequently found to have an underlying neurological basis. The principal differential diagnosis, in this case, includes malingered amnesia and dissociative amnesia. Much has been published on dissociative amnesia, although much of this literature is psychodynamic and based on case studies. Dissociation and dissociative amnesia continue to be some of the most vigorously contested phenomena within the field of psychiatry.

Making a clinical distinction between malingered and dissociative amnesia is very difficult. At the very least, you should ask about prior traumatic experiences, prior episodes of dissociation, and the presence of precipitating trauma. As with malingered psychotic symptoms, the more pressing the identified motive for the amnesia, the more strongly malingering should be suspected; when episodes of amnesia correspond only with socially undesirable events, serious consideration should be given to the diagnosis of malingering.

COLLATERAL INFORMATION/AUXILIARY INVESTIGATIONS

Obtaining information from other sources is critical in the practice of forensic psychiatry. In part, this is due to fact that the patients seen in a forensic practice may be reluctant to disclose information about themselves that they perceive to be socially undesirable. It is also the expectation of referring sources that forensic clinicians will engage in a thorough evaluation of the patient, including verifying aspects of the patient's self-report by means of information from another source or sources. Three principal vectors of corroborative information are typically sought or used in the practice of forensic psychiatry: direct collateral information from persons or institutions with whom the patient has had contact, phallometric testing, and psychometric testing.

Collateral Information

It is routine in the practice of forensic psychiatry to interview persons who know or have known the subject of the assessment well. The specific questions asked will depend on the nature of the presenting problem. We typically recommend that the forensic evaluator interview those who have good knowledge of the patient's past, as childhood and adolescent history is germane to, for example, violence risk assessment and sex offender risk assessment. Interviewing a patient's siblings or parents or reviewing school records may be of use. It is also useful to attempt to interview a person who has intimate knowledge of the person's adult life, which may be a family member or close friend, but most typically will be a spouse or ex-partner. Given that the two principal domains of expression of characterological maladaptation are the social and occupational domains, it is not uncommon to ask to speak to a work colleague. Given that individuals may relate very differently to peers and supervisors, you may wish to speak to both a coworker and a supervisor.

Frankly, it is our experience that women tend to provide better collateral information than men; women not infrequently present as more psychologically minded and may also be more forthright because criminal men typically associate with criminal peers, and there is a strong sanction among criminal peers against speaking to authorities about friends.

The date and time of the in-person or telephone interview with collateral sources should be recorded. All collateral sources should be advised, before the interview, of the limits to confidentiality vis-à-vis the assessment and reporting process. They should give their (informed) consent to proceed. The length of the interview should be recorded. Subjects of the interview(s) should be questioned as to whether the patient attempted to influence their responses in any way. When interviewing a collateral source by telephone, you should ask whether she is alone in the room, or whether she can be overheard by others.

Information should be sought from institutions where the patient was seen before the onset of the adversarial process, for example, hospitals, individual treatment providers, child welfare authorities, correctional facilities, and the like. Patients may be more willing to disclose information when that disclosure is not temporally linked to a process they perceive as adverse to their interests. This information may also be critical in understanding prior behavior in treatment and why prior efforts at treatment did or did not help, for both patient- and provider-related reasons. Information immediately antedating or postdating a critical event (e.g., police officers' notes or jail records) may also provide very important information about mental state .

Phallometric Testing

Phallometric testing is laboratory testing of underlying sexual preference. Phallometric laboratories are relatively widely distributed throughout North America, although there is admittedly little standardization of the phallometric testing process at present; as a result, you should choose a phallometric laboratory carefully based on reputation, publications, and availability of information regarding sensitivity and specificity of their tests. Phallometric testing involves exposing a male patient, in a laboratory, to visual stimuli, narratives, or both, while measuring penile blood flow. Phallometric testing is most typically used to determine whether a person is experiencing pedophilia, hebephilia, or a violent or coercive sexual preference. Phallometric testing has been shown to have good discriminant validity and, at least with respect to pedophilia and hebephilia, excellent predictive validity. All persons who are to be assessed clinically for sexual behavior alleged to involve minors, or coercive sexual behavior with an adult partner, should be evaluated phallometrically. Reputable phallometric laboratories will achieve sensitivity levels (with respect to tests for an inappropriate age preference or a coercive sexual preference) in the range of 0.6 to 0.8, with specificity values above 0.9. Because there is a clear need for robust specificity (it would be highly inappropriate and unethical to generate significant false positives in this form of testing), persons who have an underlying paraphilia may at times not be captured by these tests. For this reason, you should bear in mind that the positive predictive value of a nondeviant phallometric test is nil.

Psychometric Testing

There is a very large number of psychological tests available to assist in the evaluation of patients; a full discussion of the tests available is beyond the scope of this chapter. Certain tests, however, are particularly useful in forensic evaluation. Most prominently, these include personality tests (typically also including tests of response bias) and tests designed to detect malingering.

The most widely used personality test is the Minnesota Multiphasic Personality Inventory-2 (MMPI-2).[10] This test has a lengthy history and robust psychometric properties and can be very helpful in providing information about personality traits and affective states that may not have been clear to the examiner on the basis of a clinical evaluation. In our opinion, exposure to the MMPI-2 will provide the student with a much better working knowledge of personality than the DSM-IV-TR. The MMPI-2 also has robust validity scales that provide important information with respect to response bias. Response bias is frequently an issue in forensic evaluation. The MMPI-2 (and other personality inventories with measures of response bias) can be of great help in corroborating the clinical impression a person is attempting to present in a particular fashion. Some persons attempt to look more virtuous than they really are; the MMPI-2 and other personality inventories can provide information about defensive or "fake good" presentations. Some persons attempt to present themselves as more ill or disturbed than they truly are; the MMPI-2 and other personality inventories can also provide information about negative impression management.

Psychometric tests addressing the issue of whether a person is malingering may also be of some utility. The Miller Forensic Assessment of Symptoms Test[11] and the Structured Inventory of Reported Symptoms[12] may assist in determining whether a person is malingering psychiatric symptoms, particularly psychotic symptoms. The Test of Memory Malingering[13] is a very useful test in evaluating whether a person is attempting to malinger memory deficits.

CONCLUSIONS

We hope that this chapter provides you with some of the tools necessary to master the evaluative process with forensic patients. For those of you who do not plan to engage in extensive clinical work with aggressive, dissimulating, or sexually problematic patients, the information in this chapter provides insight into and allows for recognition of forensic presentations (e.g., psychopathy). We tend at times to think of forensic patients as denizens of the specialized settings, for example, correctional facilities or forensic inpatient units. However, patients presenting with the behavior disorders discussed in this chapter are regular users of the health care and mental health care system long before they are seen by specialized forensic professionals; family practitioners, psychiatrists, and other health care professionals are likely to see these behavior disorders before the forensic psychiatrist, and they should have the knowledge and skills necessary to complete a diagnostic evaluation and arrange for referral of the patient to a specialized service as required.

REFERENCES

1. Feinstein RE: Clinical guidelines for the assessment of imminent violence. In van Praag HM, Plutchik R, Apter A, editors: *Violence and suicidality*, New York, 1990, Brunner/Mazel.
2. Hart SD, Cox DN, Hare RD: *Manual for the Hare psychopathy checklist: screening version (PCL:SV)*, Toronto, Ontario, Canada, 1995, Multi-Health Systems.
3. Webster CD, Douglas KS, Eaves D, Hart SD: *HCR-20: assessing risk for violence, version 2*, Vancouver, BC, Canada, 1997, Simon Fraser University.
4. Hare RD: *Manual for the Hare psychopathy checklist–revised (PCL-R)*, ed 2, Toronto, Ontario, Canada, 2004, Multi-Health Systems.
5. Quinsey VL, Harris GT, Rice ME, Cormier CA: *Violent offenders: appraising and managing risk*, Washington, DC, 1998, American Psychological Association.
6. Hanson RK, Thornton D: *Static-99: improving actuarial risk assessment for sex offenders. User Report 1999-02.* Ottawa, Ontario, Canada, 1999, Department of the Solicitor General of Canada.
7. American Psychiatric Association: *Diagnostic and statistical manual of mental disorders*, ed 4, text revision, Washington, DC, 2003, American Psychiatric Association.
8. Meichenbaum D, Novaco R: Stress inoculation: a preventative approach. In Spielberger C, Saranson I, editors: *Stress and anxiety*, vol 5, New York, 1977, Halstead Press.
9. Rogers R: *Clinical assessment of malingering and deception*, New York, 1997, The Guilford Press.
10. Ogloff JR: The legal basis of forensic applications of the MMPI-2. In Ben-Porath Y, Graham J, Hall G, Hirschman R, Zaragoza M, editors: *Forensic applications of the MMPI-2*. Thousand Oaks, CA, 1995, Sage Publications.
11. Miller HA: *Miller forensic assessment of symptoms test professional manual*, Lutz, FL, 2001, Psychological Assessment Resources.
12. Rogers R, Gillis RJ, Dickens SE, Bagby RM: Standardized assessment of malingering: validation of the SIRS, psychological assessment, *J Clin Consulting Psychol* 3:89–96, 1991.
13. Tombaugh T: *Test of memory malingering*, New York, 1996, Multi-Health Systems.

Appendix 13-1. Interview/Report Structure

Identifying data
Sources of information
Personal and development history
- Childhood and family history
- Education history
- Employment history
- Relationship history

Medical history
Alcohol and drug history
Mental health history
Legal history/history of community supervision
History of the predicate offense(s)
Review of collateral information
Functional inquiry and mental status examination
Psychiatric impressions and recommendations
- Fitness to stand trial (where appropriate)
- Capacities
- Diagnosis
- Risk assessment
  □ Assessment of static/actuarial risk
  □ Assessment of dynamic risk factors
  □ Composite estimate of risk
- Risk management suggestions

Appendix 13-2. PCL:SV Items

1. Superficial
2. Grandiose
3. Deceitful
4. Lacks remorse
5. Lacks empathy
6. Does not accept responsibility
7. Impulsive
8. Poor behavioral controls
9. Lacks goals
10. Irresponsibility
11. Adolescent antisocial behavior
12. Antisocial behavaior

Appendix 13-3. HCR-20 Items

1. Previous violence
2. Young age at first violent incident
3. Relationship instability
4. Employment problems
5. Substance abuse problems
6. Major mental illness
7. Psychopathy
8. Early maladjustment
9. Personality disorder
10. Prior supervision failure
11. Lack of insight
12. Negative attitudes
13. Active symptoms of major mental illness
14. Impulsivity
15. Unresponsive to treatment
16. Plans lack feasibility
17. Exposure to destabilizers
18. Lack of personal support
19. Noncompliance with remediation attempts
20. Stress

Appendix 13-4. PCL-R Items

1. Glibness/superficial charm
2. Grandiose sense of self-worth
3. Need for stimulation/proneness to boredom
4. Pathological lying
5. Conning/manipulative
6. Lack of remorse or guilt
7. Shallow affect
8. Callous/lack of empathy
9. Parasitic lifestyle
10. Poor behavioral controls
11. Promiscuous sexual behavior
12. Early behavioral problems
13. Lack of realistic long-term goals
14. Impulsivity
15. Irresponsibility
16. Failure to accept responsibility for own actions
17. Many short-term marital relationships
18. Juvenile delinquency
19. Revocation of conditional release
20. Criminal versatility

Appendix 13-5. VRAG Items

1. Lived with both biological parents to age 16
2. Elementary school maladjustment
3. History of alcohol problems
4. Marital status
5. Criminal history of nonviolent offenses prior to the index offense
6. Failure on prior conditional release
7. Age at index offense
8. Victim injury
9. Any female victim
10. Meets DSM-III criteria for any personality disorder
11. Meets DSM-III criteria for schizophrenia
12. Psychopathy Checklist score

Appendix 13-6. SORAG Items

1. Lived with both biological parents to age 16
2. Elementary school maladjustment
3. History of alcohol problems
4. Marital status
5. Criminal history of nonviolent offenses prior to the index offense
6. Criminal history of violent offenses prior to the index offense
7. Number of previous convictions for sexual offenses
8. History of sex offenses only against girls younger than 14 years
9. Failure on prior conditional release
10. Age at index offense
11. Meets DSM-III criteria for any personality disorder
12. Meets DSM-III criteria for schizophrenia
13. Phallometric test results
14. Psychopathy Checklist score

Appendix 13-7. Static-99 Items

1. Prior sex offenses
2. Prior sentencing dates
3. Any convictions for noncontact sex offenses
4. Index nonsexual violence
5. Prior nonsexual violence
6. Any unrelated victims
7. Any stranger victims
8. Any male victims
9. Young age
10. Single

14

Emergency Assessment

JODI LOFCHY

INTRODUCTION

The emergency room (ER) is a unique environment in which to assess a patient with a possible psychiatric illness. Whether in a general hospital ER or in a psychiatric hospital setting, you will be acutely aware of the sense of time urgency to complete a focused assessment and quickly come to a decision about disposition. This is not the typical 50-minute outpatient office assessment, carefully booked weeks and even months ahead. There may be more referrals lined up for you to see; the patient may be volatile and unable to tolerate an in-depth interview approach; or it may be the middle of the night, and both you and the patient are tired and reluctant to prolong the assessment any longer than necessary. These systemic patient and clinician variables color all emergency assessments and must be understood clearly before an appropriate decision can be made regarding clinical management.

Patients come to the ER on their own, with their families or friends, and at times with their therapists and doctors or even the police. All patients, regardless of the nature of their problems, are triaged in the ER as to the level of urgency of their presenting complaint. Psychiatric problems are triaged with the same principles in place; life-threatening issues—suicide, acute psychosis, violence—are assessed quickly by the nurses and referred directly to the ER physicians and then to the psychiatric team on call. Less acutely psychiatrically ill patients are seen by the ER staff and not necessarily referred on to psychiatry. They may be given referrals to outpatient psychiatric services or discharged with no prescribed follow-up. It is very important to remember that the others accompanying the patient often have the most details about the recent events or the best appreciation of the severity of the situation at hand. How the collateral information is collected and incorpo-

rated into the history and the plan will be discussed in this chapter.

Psychiatric emergencies can be assessed in two different types of ERs—the general hospital or the more specialized psychiatric hospital. Clearly, there are two different cultures present in these settings. In the general hospital, strong feelings may be evoked in health care workers, more comfortable with medically ill patients, who are now confronted with bizarre, difficult, and at times frightening patients with mental illness. These patients may be seen as taking valuable time and resources away from the acutely medically ill emergency population. In the psychiatric hospital, the atmosphere may be more understanding and supportive of the psychiatrically ill patient, but medical backup will often not be available to you on-site; your patients must travel to the closest general hospital for emergency investigations and medical consultation.

Some ER settings are designed with the potentially violent patient in mind. Unlike an outpatient setting where an office might include artwork, a desk full of papers, books, and knickknacks, the ER provides a rather "sterile" setting that is safe by its lack of decorative accessories. You should approach the ER assessment with that potential for violence in mind. This affects the way the interview is conducted— the positioning of the chairs, the decision whether to include another staff or security member in the room, and the need to be aware of the safety features in the room and how to use them (e.g., alarm buzzers, video monitors, doors that cannot be barricaded). Flexibility is the key to approaching an interview in the ER: you can leave the room at any time if you are uncomfortable, and there is no set amount of time that you must be in the room with the patient.

In the ER, you must be constantly aware of the risk aspects of every case. Important questions to ask yourself include the following:

- What if the patient leaves precipitously?
- Can I detain the patient against his will? Do I have enough information to do so?
- What if there is an acute medical problem that needs to be attended to immediately?

There is no time for a detailed personal or family history in the face of such immediate concerns!

There is a significant comfort in working as part of a multidisciplinary team in the ER. Nurses, clinicians, social workers, and psychiatric assistants, together with the house staff of medical students, residents, and staff psychiatrists, may all take part in the assessment process. Each group brings a particular expertise to the process, which is to the patient's benefit. And most importantly for you, there is group support and input into often-difficult decision-making about patient management. The team provides a great sounding board when dealing with challenging patients; others can be a good check when strong feelings are evoked with particular patients. As well, team members can be invaluable in assisting in the gathering of collateral information.

Working in a team is the most time-efficient and safe way to practice emergency psychiatry.

Case Example 1

The Fed-Up Young Woman. A 23-year-old woman presents in the general hospital ER after having had a fight with her boyfriend. She states she is "fed up." She is threatening to overdose on all her medication at home "to end the pain." She has a long history of multiple ER visits with sublethal suicide attempts and many years of self-harm in the form of cutting and burning herself. She has recently finished a group therapy and sees her family doctor sporadically to renew her medications, which "do nothing to help." She has been prescribed a number of psychotropic medications, which she does not take regularly. She uses alcohol and cannabis weekly. She would like to come into hospital to get more help for her depression and sort out her medications. Emergency has referred this patient to you for a risk assessment.

Case Example 2

The Traffic Teen. You are in a psychiatric hospital ER, and the police have brought in an agitated 19-year-old man in handcuffs after they found him walking in traffic shouting nonsensically at the cars and pedestrians. They are concerned he has a mental illness and want him assessed. They find some identification on him, and you are told he has never been to this hospital before.

How are you going to proceed with these assessments? What are the factors that will determine your ultimate disposition? What questions do you need to ask yourself along the way? What are the risks involved in each case (Box 14-1)?

THE ER INTERVIEW: THE HISTORY

Identifying Data

Gathering identifying data is one of the most important parts of the interview, both for you and the patient. This is where the interview begins—with you introducing yourself and getting to know a bit about this person of whom you will be asking many questions, often of a most personal nature. Even if you know some demographic information from the emergency registration form, it is still worthwhile going over this with the patient. This part of the interview feels the *least* like a psychiatric interview and can serve as an opportunity to put the patient (and yourself) at ease and establish an alliance. As well, certain diagnostic alarm bells may go off if you hear your patient is a 36-year-old, recently arrived immigrant who is unemployed, with no family in this country, living on the streets. Compare your associations to an alternate scenario of a married 76-year-old retired teacher who is a mother of three and grandmother of seven, living with her husband in their own home. I am not suggesting you make pejorative assumptions on learning of a patient's social and demographic status; rather, you start thinking immediately about the particular risks and diagnoses to which that the patient is vulnerable.

Components of the Identifying Data

- Name: Get the patient's full name and ensure proper spelling. Ask, "How would you like me to address you during the interview?" and assume the proper title Mr./Mrs./Ms. applies unless you are instructed otherwise.
- Age
- Marital status: Is the patient single, married, divorced, separated, or in a common-law relationship? It is worth-

---

Box 14-1. Before You See the Patient

✓ Chart
✓ Level of agitation/sedation
✓ Safety: setting, self, others
✓ Visual MSE
✓ Accompanying others
✓ Route of referral
✓ Voluntary or involuntary?

while to find out the duration of the current marital status.

- Children: Ask, even if the patient is single, how many children there are, where they are, and whether contact with them is maintained. You will need to keep in mind whether there are any children at risk if the patient is a single parent and/or ill.
- Living situation: *NFA* means "no fixed address." Does the patient live in a hostel, rooming house or group home, apartment, or house? Who is in the home with the patient?
- Employment: Find out precisely what the patient does for a living. If the patient is currently unemployed, you should ascertain what was the last job, when it ended, and why.
- Source of income: You should determine whether the patient is receiving public assistance or is on disability; if it is the latter, it is worthwhile clarifying whether it is for medical or psychiatric reasons, and whether it is short-term or long-term disability.
- Country of origin: "*Are you from [your current city]? How long have you been here?*" This will tell you whether there are immediate acculturation stresses to expect.
- Is the patient previously known to the ER?

Reason for Referral

What is the reason for referral? Who is referring this patient for a psychiatric assessment, and what is the question being asked? The ER physician often has a very specific question to ask you, and it is worthwhile clarifying this before you start your assessment. If the question is one regarding acute suicide risk, you may choose to avoid a detailed past psychiatric history and an elaborate differential diagnosis. What the ER physician would like to know is whether this patient is safe to discharge or if immediate hospitalization required. At other times, a more general question is being asked, such as, could a psychiatric diagnosis explain the patient's presentation to the ER at this time? Sometimes it is the family physician in the community who has sent the patient to the ER to see a psychiatrist. If you have not spoken directly to the family doctor and no note accompanies the patient, it is important to clarify the reason for the referral before starting your assessment. Patients may have a very different understanding as to why they have been told to go to the ER by the doctors who have sent them. If the patient is being detained as an involuntary patient and there is a request for a psychiatric assessment as a result of potentially dangerous behavior, this should be documented on the appropriate legal document. You should read the document to clarify this and to ensure that it has been completed appropriately.

Referral Sources

Possible referral sources include the following:

- ER physician
- Other medical service (e.g., internal medicine, neurology, surgery)
- Family doctor
- Community or outpatient psychiatrist
- Police
- Family
- Justice of the peace (e.g., after concerned family/others have sought involuntary assessment)

Common Reasons for Referral

Common reasons a patient may be referred are as follows:

- Assess suicide/violence risk.
- Does this patient need admission?
- Could there be a psychiatric explanation for this unusual presentation?
- Is this patient capable enough to refuse this surgical procedure? We would like a second opinion.
- Does this person have a mental illness?
- Can you find this patient psychiatric follow-up and housing?

Chief Complaint

The chief complaint is the patient's subjective complaint and the duration it has been a problem. Questions that elicit this include the following:

- "*What brings you to the hospital today?*"
- "*What has been the problem that led up to your coming here?*"
- "*Why is your family/Dr. X so concerned about you?*"
- "*How long has this been going on?*"

"My whole life," is not a helpful response. You are trying to get a recent time frame so that you can focus your history. Try to help the patient be more specific: "*I understand that you have been feeling badly for a while, but what happened today that made you decide <u>now</u> was the time to get help?*" You should document verbatim what the patient says, even if it is bizarre or irrelevant. There are times when the patient denies a problem but concerned others have intervened to access help. Again, at these times, using the patient's words is helpful. "There is nothing wrong with me, I am fine," will still serve as a chief complaint of sorts. If the patient does not give a chief complaint, you may want to incorporate the versions of others (e.g., "The patient was mute, but the police describe the patient standing naked in traffic saying, 'Jesus will save me.'").

History of Presenting Illness

The history of presenting illness (HPI) is the crux of the emergency assessment. Why now? The focus is on the here and now. Why did the patient come to ER at this particular time, either alone or at the insistence of others? What are the stressors that have contributed to the patient feeling ill? What are the psychiatric symptoms? After initially letting the patient tell his story, you need to be thinking of ruling in or out a provisional diagnosis. You need to go looking for symptoms and duration if they are not described spontaneously. Given the time urgency in the emergency assessment and the acuity of the presentation, you must be very focused. You may choose to ask about relevant comorbid conditions if you feel they may contribute to the recent history. It is especially important to ask about substance use because it may be contributing to the current presentation. When a patient is referred for a risk assessment, it is essential to explore all the known risk factors for suicide and violence within the HPI.

The patient may be rambling or disorganized and not making sense. Sometimes you can get helpful responses when you keep your questions short and close-ended:

- *"What do the voices say?"*
- *"Why do they want to hurt you?"*
- *"Have you been feeling this scared for days or weeks?"*

When the patient is severely psychotic or mute, you may have to rely on the collateral sources for all of the history and proceed directly to the mental status examination when with the patient. The Traffic Teen in Case Example 2 may not be able to attend to an interview and will have little insight into his bizarre behavior. The identification of the patient provided by the police may help you locate family or other collateral sources of information.

Be sure to describe the recent events in sufficient detail to understand the risks involved; if there has been dangerous behavior or a recent suicide attempt, you will need to pursue this in depth. If there are persecutory delusions, it is extremely important in the ER to explore the patient's response to these questions:

- Has she sought revenge?
- Is someone at risk?
- Is she at risk herself for suicide as a result of her extreme distress?

The chronological preceding stressors and symptoms are the context for the recent decompensation, and your questions will help the patient describe what he has been experiencing over the last number of weeks or months. It is important to use the patient's words when describing the history. The style of documentation takes the form of "The patient describes electrodes being placed in his brain by the neighbors upstairs," or "The patient states that . . ." or ". . . claims that . . ." This helps to keep the history neutral and does not implicitly support or challenge his story.

Components of the HPI
- Time frame
- Stressors
- Symptoms, diagnostic criteria
- Risk factors for relevant dangerous behavior
- Substance use/abuse: When was the last use?
- Current medications: Is the patient taking them? If not, why not?
- Current supports
- Psychiatric support: When is the next appointment?
- Coping strategies

Past Psychiatric History

The focus of the past psychiatric history is to understand past and current contacts with the psychiatric system. If there has been an extensive history of admissions, it is most relevant to document the most recent admissions in some detail. You should try to obtain an overview of when the patient first became ill and how many admissions there have been in total. You would like to know if past presentations to the hospital are similar to the presentation you are seeing today. For the purposes of the ER assessment, you will not learn about every admission in detail; you may want to request records from other hospitals to fill in the details later, but you should try to determine whether there have been patterns in the circumstances of admission or discharge—did the patient leave against medical advice and not follow up with the recommendations? Were these involuntary admissions? You should explore the history of suicide attempts, legal history, and history of substance abuse in this section of the interview. In terms of past treatments, you may get an overview of the various medications tried and if anything has been particularly helpful. The patient may also be able to tell you the diagnoses made over the years; this is worth asking about. You should also ask about community supports and other resources that may have been useful on an outpatient basis (e.g., Alcoholics Anonymous, case manager, home care, self-help groups).

Components of the Past Psychiatric History
- Most recent admission
- Number of admissions, and at which hospitals
- First episode of psychiatric illness and first psychiatric contact

- Treatment overview: Medications, psychotherapy, electroconvulsive therapy, etc.
- Suicide attempt history: Lethality, outcome, intent
- Legal history: Any pending charges? Incarceration? If there is a history of assault, were weapons involved?
- Substance abuse: With street drugs, what was the route of use? Any history of alcohol abuse? Abuse of prescribed or over-the-counter drugs? What has been the longest period of abstinence? What have been the sequelae? Have there been periods of abstinence? Has the patient received any treatment?

Past Medical History

Past medical history describes any current medical problems and notes past hospitalizations or surgeries. You should routinely screen for any neurological conditions that may account for the presentation with note of head injury and seizure history.

Social History

Social history is very important in the ER assessment. It is quite different from the detailed developmental history that you would pursue in a general assessment. In the ER, you are most interested in the patient's highest level of functioning, so that you can place the present episode in some perspective. You should ask specific questions about school, past relationships, and occupational history to understand function prior to the onset of illness. As well, you should inquire about the patient's optimal functioning while having a psychiatric illness. You should be interested in the patient's current support system and the quality of the relationships at this time. You may have already explored this in the HPI if this is a part of the current presentation; perhaps a relationship has just ended, and the patient is devastated, hopeless, and having trouble coping with the loss. In this case, you would spend time understanding the quality of the relationship and the reasons for its ending as part of your initial history. The social history might be spent looking for patterns of previous reactions to ended relationships and understanding how the current reaction is similar or different. You may choose to incorporate family history into this section by drawing a pedigree and noting any major mental disorders in biological relatives.

Components of the Social History
- School: What was the highest level of educational attainment, and at what age was it reached?
- Relationships: Have there been intimate relationships in the past? If not, what is the patient's understanding of why not? What is the longest previous relationship? If

relevant, ask the patient to describe a current relationship; is it a supportive one?
- Occupational history: What types of jobs has the patient had? What was the longest period of employment? Why have previous jobs ended? Are there any concerns with current job?
- Family history: This could be a separate category, but document if positive.

MENTAL STATUS EXAMINATION

The mental status examination (MSE) is the definitive component of the emergency assessment. It begins with your observations the moment the patient walks through the door. When a patient is unable or unwilling to provide a history, the MSE is crucial. Your detailed observations of the patient's mental state serve as a key reference point for this current assessment and for future presentations to the ER. The more clearly you are able to describe the specifics of the psychopathology in phenomenological terms, the better the chances are for future caregivers to know in what way this patient has been ill in the past. A comparison of the MSE in the ER prior to inpatient admission to that at the time of discharge shows how the patient has improved with hospitalization. The MSE can change throughout the interview, and your job is to document as best you can what you are observing over the course of your assessment (Box 14-2).

Components of the MSE

- Appearance: Describe in detail how this person looks, is dressed, and any distinguishing characteristics. Is she dressed appropriately for the weather? If not, why not?

Box 14-2. Elements of the Mental Status Examination

Appearance
Behavior
Attitude to examiner
Speech
Mood
Affect
Thought process/form
Thought content
Suicidal/homicidal ideation
Perception
Cognition
Insight
Judgment
Impulse control
Reliability

In the ER, patients' appearances can provide crucial clues as to self-care ability and judgment. Bizarre or eccentric dress could indicate mania or schizophrenia; neglect and lack of self-care could lead to consideration of depression, substance abuse, or cognitive dysfunction.

- Behavior: Are there any tics, noteworthy mannerisms, or movement disorders? Psychomotor agitation or retardation? If the patient has an acute and severe movement disorder (e.g., dystonia), you will intervene immediately and not proceed with a full history. It is important to note the specifics of any agitation because this may quickly progress to a violent outburst unless you de-escalate the situation.

- Attitude to examiner: The patient's manner towards you should be noted. Is it hostile, seductive, pleasant, suspicious, etc.?

- Speech: Note the rate, rhythm, volume, prosody, fluency, quantity, and spontaneity. You may be looking for signs of intoxication in the ER and speech may be altered. Loud and pressured speech should lead you to think of mania.

- Mood: Note the patient's subjective description of her emotional state in her own words.

- Affect: Give an objective description of the patient's emotional state, including the quality, range, appropriateness, and intensity. In the ER, if the patient describes a significant history of depression but appears euthymic during the interview, this would not fit—the affect would be inappropriate to the thought content, and you may question the severity of the depression.

- Thought process/form: This is the way in which the person thinks, how ideas are put together internally, and the form in which they are expressed: coherence, logic, and stream. Patients can be incoherent or grossly disorganized when acutely psychotic and may demonstrate other variants of thought disorder (e.g., tangentiality, circumstantiality, derailing, clang associations, perseveration) that require you to help redirect the interview back to the topic at hand.

- Thought content: This covers a broad spectrum from ideas, themes, and worries all the way to obsessions and delusions. In this portion of the MSE, describe what the patient is thinking about and the focus of the concerns. You may be screening for particular phenomena if you are concerned about psychosis and would need to mention ideas of reference, thought insertion/withdrawal/broadcasting as well as any delusional themes, with examples you have obtained in your history. You want to comment on both the pertinent positives and negatives as to what you might expect with this patient and this diagnosis. The only time you cannot comment on thought content occurs when the patient is mute!

- Suicidal/homicidal ideation: This is an essential and important part of the emergency MSE. You should deter-

mine and document whether there is active or passive ideation, plan, and intent. With homicidal ideation, you may want to determine and document whether it reflects an intended victim or a nonspecific threat. The suicidal and homicidal ideation or attempt may already have been discussed in the history with more detail (e.g., access to means, lethality), but in the MSE you are commenting on the current ideation during the interview.

- Perceptions: You are looking for unusual sensory experiences: illusions, hallucinations, depersonalization, and derealization. These are most often associated with psychosis but also occur in substance intoxication and withdrawal, severe personality disorders, and medical conditions such as seizure disorders. If hallucinations are of a command nature, it is important to explore the response to these; is the person able to ignore them or distract himself, or does he comply with potentially dangerous orders? The patient may not be able to verbalize what he is experiencing but may appear to be responding to internal stimuli, either auditory or visual hallucinations, and you can make note of this in your MSE.

- Cognition: This includes orientation, attention, concentration, memory, and intelligence. You can comment on all of these dimensions of cognition from your observations during the history-taking without formal testing. A full Folstein examination is not indicated for every ER patient, but if you are concerned about dementia or delirium it would be essential. As well, you would perform the "clock test" in these situations to test for ideomotor dyspraxia. You can often comment on intelligence from listening closely to the use of language and syntax as well as general knowledge. Memory and concentration are evidenced in the recall of dates and the details of past history.

- Insight: This refers to understanding of the illness and appreciation for the need for treatment. Do patients see themselves as having an illness and appreciate the factors that have contributed to them being ill? Many psychiatric patients in the ER deny that they are ill and minimize the concerns others voice. They may externalize the causes for their problems and blame others. Lack of insight together with impaired judgment may contribute to dangerous behaviors that result in violence to others or themselves. Your description of insight into illness and appreciation of the benefits and risks of proposed treatment will form the basis of a capacity assessment for treatment.

- Judgment: This refers to recent behaviors and future planning. Over the course of the history-taking, look at the person's ability to make socially appropriate judgments that do not lead to trouble. A confused person may be leaving the stove on repeatedly, putting people at risk from inadvertent fire setting. An impulsive overdose after an argument with a boyfriend may reflect poor judgment in a young woman, but her subsequent ability to access help and quickly visit the ER may demonstrate good judgment. Standardized tests of judgment (e.g., What would you do if you were in a crowded theater and someone shouted "Fire!"?) are not that helpful in the ER. You are looking for realistic examples from the patient's life to assess judgment.

- Impulse control: Is this patient impulsive? Has there been evidence of this during the interview, as reflected by losing control or even running out? Does the impulsivity carry a likely risk of dangerous consequences?
- Reliability: How reliable is this person in giving a history? This aspect of the clinical evaluation is often evident immediately in obtaining the identifying data. If the patient is an unreliable historian, everything that follows may be suspect. The incorporation of collateral history is essential in these cases.

IMPRESSION

Once you finish documenting the history and MSE, you then summarize the case briefly before moving toward your *Diagnostic and Statistical Manual of Mental Disorders*, Fourth Edition, Text Revision (DSM-IV-TR) multi-axial diagnosis. The "impression" of the ER case should highlight a number of important aspects. When describing the ER presentation, you want to stress why the patient is here now. "In summary, M.C. is a 29-year-old gay HIV-positive Asian male who presents to the ER after an impulsive overdose of 10 clonazepam (2.5 mg) this evening. His suicide attempt occurred after learning of the death of a close friend from AIDS today. He has no other symptoms of depression and no past psychiatric history. He is currently not suicidal and is regretful of his actions. He is medically stable."

Your summary should always include a risk assessment for suicide and violence (if relevant) and should discuss whether hospitalization is needed. To continue with the above case: "M.C. now wishes to return home and is agreeable to outpatient follow-up in the crisis clinic. He has a close friend who will be spending the night with him, and both are aware of the emergency services available should the suicidal ideation return or should he have any further distress. He is at low risk of suicide at this time, given his remorse/guilt about the attempt, lack of depressive symptoms, and strong support system. He is not currently in need of hospitalization, not certifiable, and can be discharged from the ER."

Whether the patient is being admitted to hospital or discharged in spite of your feeling an admission might be helpful, it is important to discuss in your assessment whether the patient meets criteria for involuntary detention. A patient can be admitted to hospital as a voluntary patient, agreeing to come in and understanding the need for the admission. Alternatively, the patient may choose to leave. If you have concerns about the patient's self-care abilities or his physical safety risk to self or others, you need to be aware of your legal responsibilities and act accordingly. If a patient wants to leave, you should document why the patient is not being detained involuntarily. An example of this kind of case would be someone with a treatment-refractory depression who is not suicidal, who may benefit from an inpatient stay to reassess medications or consider electroconvulsive therapy, but is ambivalent about being admitted and chooses to go home and follow up with an outpatient psychopharmacology consultation.

When making a diagnosis, it is important to try to make a provisional diagnosis, even if you are not exactly clear about what is going on. Often, it is too early in the course of the illness with a first presentation to have a definitive diagnosis. Commonly, substance abuse makes the presentation complicated by either being the primary cause of the symptoms or meeting criteria for a second comorbid condition. To venture a "best guess" as to what is going on gives your colleagues a starting place to work from—either on the inpatient ward to which the patient is being admitted or the next time this patient presents to the ER. It is helpful to make a differential diagnosis, again, to broaden the thinking about the range of diagnostic possibilities and to allow for a full workup. If you are seeing diagnoses in old charts you do not agree with or do not understand, you do not have to perpetuate the labeling in this way; you may document, for example, "? Post-traumatic stress disorder—as per old chart—no evidence at this time."

There remains ongoing concern about noting axis II personality disorder diagnoses in the ER. It is difficult to make the diagnosis of a personality disorder on the basis of one assessment, *but* if a patient has a long history on file with recurrent behaviors and symptoms that meet criteria for a personality disorder, and you are seeing evidence of the disorder on your assessment, you can venture on to axis II with a "rule out: borderline or antisocial personality disorder." And even if you do not have an old chart or a detailed past psychiatric history, you are always able to comment on the personality *traits* present in your emergency assessment. Again, you are communicating with your colleagues who will see the patient at the next ER visit, and your thoughts about diagnosis are always appreciated.

Components of "Impression"

- Summary statement: emphasis on "why now"
- Risk assessment: suicide/homicide
- Need for hospitalization: If not, why not?
- Certifiability
- Capacity to make treatment decisions
- Diagnosis: DSM-IV-TR

findings (when possible), either by yourself or with colleagues. This gives you an opportunity to process the family's input, the information received from other treatment facilities or persons, and old records from your hospital. You have talked to the other members of your team to compare histories and observations. You may have called the staff psychiatrist on call to review the case. With all this input, you have made a decision about the best management plan for this patient and his family. When you enter the room, you may bring in any other clinicians who have been involved with the case. Rather than starting off enthusiastically with "Here is what we are going to do!", it would be helpful to go back to the patient and explore his idea of the treatment plan and what he thinks would be helpful. Then you can take the elements of the plan that may have some overlap with yours and present your version: *"I agree that in some ways you feel fine and you do not want to be in the hospital. But from what you and your family have told us, you are not doing so well at home. People are scared for you and worried about your safety. We think being in the hospital is the quickest way for you to feel better, and you told us you want to be able to go back to work, etc."*

Even if you are planning to detain the patient involuntarily, you should always explain the need for the admission and hope that he can perceive that your holding him there is based on concern and caring, not as a punitive means. Literature and experience tell us that patients do not typically experience the involuntary detention as coercive once they are well, and at times they may return to the psychiatrist to thank her for holding them in hospital when too ill to make the decision themselves.

With ambivalent patients, you may want to help them look at the pros and cons of coming in to hospital or being treated as an outpatient. Often this exercise can help the patient better understand your decision-making process.

Closing Phase

You need to have a clear way of indicating the ER assessment is over. You may be very busy with cases lining up in the ER, and your pager may be going off repeatedly. You do not want to abruptly stand up and say, "Goodbye, good luck, gotta run." Ideally, you would like to be able to give warning that the interview is coming to a close. You may announce that you are going to take a break and explain that you will be talking to the other members of the team who may have spent time with the family, or that you want to go and call Dr. Smith, the patient's family doctor or psychiatrist.

At times, you may have to use body language to indicate that the interview is coming to a close by standing up and opening the door. Before doing this, you should ask the patient whether she has any questions, but there will be a time where you will make the decision to end the interview. Once you have presented the plan and are wrapping up, you may say, *"We need to stop now, but I just want to go over the plan again..."* It is helpful to ask the patient to play back the plan as she heard it, to see how much has actually registered and to give you some insight into the likelihood of her following up with your recommendations. As you end, you want to positively frame the ER visit: *"It is great that you knew to come here when you were so upset. All ERs are open 24 hours a day, there is always a doctor here to talk to should things get bad again."*

I tell the patient we will be putting a full note on the chart about today's visit that will be helpful should she need to come back again. The team will already be aware of the details of the story from tonight, and she will not have to go through everything again. This is often reassuring for the patient who experiences the medical system as large, impersonal, and at times fragmented with minimal communication within and between hospital settings. Continuity of care, as demonstrated by you through documentation and phone calls to the other community physicians after the ER assessment, is good care and is appreciated by the patient.

ER INTERVENTIONS

Biological

There are times in the emergency assessment you may need to offer the patient medication. It is preferable for you to complete your history and MSE without medicating the patient, as any sedating agent will mask or remove symptoms and create challenges in making a diagnosis—or the patient will fall asleep and you will be unable to complete your interview. But clearly there are circumstances when medication is essential for the acutely ill psychiatric patient. The two most common situations are agitation and psychotropic side effects (e.g., acute dystonia, akathisia). With the agitated patient, you may want to offer medication orally or sublingually if verbal de-escalation has been unsuccessful. *"Would you like some medication to help you feel more settled? You seem to be awfully upset."* If the patient refuses medication and continues to escalate, threaten, or exhibit signs of overt physical aggression, you may need to change your approach slightly. Now the patient has a more limited choice because you have decided chemical restraint is essential for safety reasons. *"Would you like the medication under your tongue or in needle form?"* In other words, the medication will be given, and the patient can help to choose the route of administration.

There will be times when the patient is unable to choose because the psychosis, anger, or intoxicated state precludes making that decision, and you will move to stabilize the patient and the situation at hand and choose the medication and route without further patient participation. In Case Example 2 with the agitated young man in traffic, the patient may need immediate sedation with psychotropic agents if he remains agitated when coming out of the police handcuffs. Usually, there are no difficulties medicating the patients who are experiencing drug-induced adverse effects. They are eager to obtain relief and grateful for your swift recognition of their state and your immediate intervention.

Investigations for the emergency patient are specific and are ordered to ensure a medical condition is not causing or contributing to the psychiatric presentation. Most commonly, we order toxicology screens; these are most helpful when we do not know what the patient has ingested in an overdose or what substances contribute to a state of intoxication or withdrawal. Computed tomography scans are now done routinely in the general hospital ER and may have already been done before the patient has been referred to psychiatry if this is a new presentation of psychosis or dementia, or if a neurological condition is being ruled out. When you have doubts about the indications for blood work or further investigations, it is always helpful to see the emergency physician as a consultant to you; she can help you clarify the medical situation or suggest further input from the perspective of internal medicine or neurology.

Psychological

There are many opportunities during the ER assessment to incorporate therapeutic interventions that will help the patient to engage, settle, and trust you. Empathic interviewing is the most important skill you can learn in your training in psychiatry. The ability to enter the patients' worlds and to do your best to appreciate their life experiences and current situation from THEIR frame of reference is not to be underestimated. It is difficult, at times, to suspend judgment and not rely on your own life view in listening to others, but the kindness, openness, and curiosity you bring to the inquiry of the anxious, confused, angry, or distressed patient in crisis are very much heard, even when you do not think the patient is listening. Tone is essential— you can ask any question you need to, no matter how sensitive the subject matter, as long as you have a matter-of-fact and respectful tone.

Empathy is not to be confused with reflexive pat comments such as, *"Your father died? That must be very upsetting for you."* Does the patient look or sound upset? A more open and not presumptive question might be: *"Your*

father died? What was that like for you?" or *"You don't look particularly upset. What was your relationship like with your father?"* It is empathic to address the patient's affect if it is clearly evident during the interview. *"You say that losing your job is no big deal, but you sound very angry when you talk about your boss."* or *"You speak about being glad that the relationship is finally over, but tears are running down your face as we speak; perhaps there is some sadness there as well as relief."* The woman in Case Example 1 is clearly very angry, although she presents as wanting to overdose and will frame her distress in terms of sadness. It can be helpful to point out her frustrations with the system and the treatments she has received thus far. Use your observations in a way that will help you better understand the patient and her particular way of experiencing the world.

For many patients, coming to the ER is the culmination of weeks and months of difficulties mounting. Although they may fear the hospital, on some deeper level, many wish for admission. For some, it is disappointing to be told that they are not "sick enough" to require a bed; others are immensely relieved. Either way, it is reassuring to be given a plan of action for when they leave the ER. In many other areas of medicine, the patient may leave the office or ER with a prescription, an instruction sheet, or an outpatient referral form. This acts as a concrete reminder of the visit to the doctor and evidence that he cares—what we call a *transitional object*.[1] The child's blanket or stuffed animal is an example of the early transitional object, serving as a substitute for maternal comfort, before the capacity to self-soothe becomes internalized. In psychiatric assessments, we can give patients similar comforting reminders: we can write down the plan for the patient to take, or we can give a brochure for community supports or a card with the phone numbers of distress lines and the ER. All of these items represent a piece of ourselves from the assessment that the patient can hold onto as a source of assurance that there is hope and help available. Some patients will find your words serve the same effect, but the "souvenir" from the ER will tide them over until they connect with the outpatient resource to which you have referred them.

Some psychiatric patients can be experienced as "difficult" by all who have contact with them—usually these are the patients with personality disorder diagnoses. You may find it difficult to sit in a room with a patient who is hostile, rude, abusive, needy, controlling, or entitled. You may have strong reactions to any or all of the above types of personality styles. It is not unprofessional to dislike the patient, but it would be unprofessional to not question *why*. Is this a reaction specific to you, or does everyone have similar feelings about this patient? Does this patient trigger a gut reaction in you, based on your own life experiences and relationships? This type of counter-transference response can be extremely helpful in understanding patients and the effect they have on others in their lives and perhaps the feelings they are experiencing as well. For example, the impotence you may be feeling in terms of not knowing what to do may very much resemble their own sense of futility about their lives. The better you know yourself and your own reactions, the better a position you will be in to make an accurate diagnosis and treatment plan.

Conversely, patients may have strong feelings toward you based on past relationships with significant people. This transference may take the form of seeing you as the powerful authority figure who has the ability to make important decisions about their lives for them. It is important to remember that even though it might feel good to be idealized, however briefly, your fall from grace can come quickly when you or the system disappoints them in some way, and the anger and devaluation will be close at hand. The key point to remember is that when there are strong feelings emanating from either you or the patient during the assessment, you should pause, take a step back, and question what is going on. This way, you ensure that a professional relationship is maintained, and ultimately you will have a deeper understanding of yourself and the patient.

Social

Social interventions in the ER involve helping the patient to access support. The majority of patients present alone to the ER, and it is a part of every assessment to understand the presence or absence of family and community. Times of crisis can be used to establish new relationships with family members. It can be a sign of strength to ask for help. Offering the patient a telephone to call a family member can lead to reparations in a previously conflicted or estranged relationship. Patients can call friends or family to come to the ER or to provide temporary shelter while they are in crisis. Members of the team can make these calls as well, but it is much better if the patient is the one to initiate the contact, whether with a family member or a community agency. The person in need is motivated to ask for help, and you are not making any assumptions about what he wants. When the patient is too ill to ask for help, this is when we intervene and do all we can to access whatever support is available. Typically, the medical house staff will speak to the family doctor to get collateral information and to arrange follow-up. If there is any concern whatsoever about children's safety, there is an obligation to notify the Children's Aid Society or the appropriate service in your area.

HIGH-RISK PATIENTS

The Suicidal Patient

A risk assessment for suicide is a part of every ER assessment. Some patients may not be initially forthcoming with the hopelessness of their thoughts, and it will be a relief for you to ask directly about suicidal ideation. It is a common misperception of medical students that asking about suicide creates ideas of suicide that may not have been there to start with. This is not the case; you may be helping them put into words distressing thoughts that they had been unable to share up to that point. Concerned and direct questioning can offer relief to the covertly suicidal patient. Remember, asking, *"Have you had any thoughts of wanting to hurt yourself?"* is not the same thing as asking about suicide. There are many patients who have chronic histories of self-harm, and they can tell you very clearly they want to hurt themselves but have no intent to die.

Key Point:

Harm self ≠ Kill self

You need to specifically ask, *"Have you had any thoughts of wanting to end your life, to commit suicide?"* Be sure to clarify as well what the patient means by the use of the word *suicide*—the patient may be using this term to describe the desire for self-harm.

Key Point:

Asking about suicide does not increase risk of action; it is a relief for patients to talk about these feelings

---

Questions for *Every* ER Patient About Suicide

1. Ideation: passive versus active
   a. *"Do you have thoughts about ending your life?"*
   b. Passive suicidal ideation: "I'd rather not wake up in the morning," or "I wouldn't mind if a car hit me when I was crossing the road."
   c. The patient would rather not be alive but does not admit to an idea that involves an act of initiation.
   d. Active suicidal ideation: "I do think about killing myself," or "I feel like throwing myself into the face of oncoming traffic."
2. Plan
   a. *"Do you have a plan as to how you would end your life?"*

3. Intent
   a. *"You talk about wanting to die, and have even considered taking pills, but are you planning to do this?"*
   b. There are patients who have significant suicidal thoughts and have fantasized about the ways in which they would end their lives but can tell you very clearly they have absolutely no intent of putting these plans into action: *"Oh, no, I could never do that, I have children."* Fantasizing about suicide can provide some comfort to those in distress to know there is always a way out. Your job is to assess who is at risk of acting on those fantasies. If intent is ambiv*alent* or unclear, it is helpful to ask, *"What has stopped you from ending your life at this point?"* You are looking for protective factors.
4. Past attempts
   a. Patients who have had past suicide attempts are at a higher risk of completing suicide in the future. The highest risk period of past attempt is within the past year. You must explore the lethality and outcome of each attempt, noting if medical intervention was required.

Key Point:

Suicide attempt within the past year puts a patient at a higher risk.

Additional Questions for the ER Patient Presenting with Suicidal Ideation

1. Lethality of plan: *"What is your perception of the lethality?"* Some people think five sleeping pills will kill them; others think a bottle of acetaminophen is not dangerous because it is available over the counter.
2. Access to means: If the patient says he would shoot himself, *"Where would you get a gun? Exactly how would you go about procuring one?"*
3. Time/place: *"Have you picked out a place in which to carry out your attempt? How isolated is it? What arrangements have been made?"*
4. Final arrangements: Inquire about suicide notes, settling affairs, and communications to others.
5. Protective factors: *"Do you have family, pets, religion, and/or a therapist?"*
6. Ambivalence: All patients presenting with suicidal ideation in the ER are ambivalent; the nonambivalent ones act without seeking help. You have an opportunity; address this ambivalence during your assessment, and try to instill hope. *"There must be a part of you that wants to live; you came here tonight for help."*

7. Homicide: Is anyone else in danger of violence? This is of note especially with psychotic depressions, delusional jealousy, and postpartum depression/psychosis.

Emergency Assessment of a Suicide Attempt

If a patient is being referred to you after already having made a suicide attempt, you must assess the current suicidal ideation as above, but explore in great depth the attempt that has just occurred. Areas to explore include the following:

1. Setting: Was the setting isolated? In the woods? Out of town or in the family home?
2. Others present: What was the likelihood of being found?
3. Impulsivity versus premeditation: Was the act performed in the heat of anger, or was it well thought out with the day and time picked in advance?
4. Intoxication: Substances disinhibit, and intoxicated people act in ways they may not otherwise when not drinking or using drugs.
5. Medical attention: How was this accessed? Did the patient take an overdose and then pick up the phone and call 911, or did someone find her unresponsive and call an ambulance?
6. Expectations of dying: What did she think would happen if she cut her wrists? Did she truly think she would die?
7. Time lag from attempt to arrival at the ER: The longer the time lag, the higher the risk—if he has not told anyone about this attempt and presents a few days later, this is more concerning than picking up the phone immediately to call for help.
8. Feelings about survival: Does the patient feel guilt or remorse? Determine the level of embarrassment versus disappointment and self-blame: "I couldn't even get this right and kill myself properly."

The SAD PERSONS test (Box 14-3)[2] is a good screening acronym in the ER, but the scoring should not be used as the sole guide to your clinical management. The patient who presents with a number of suicide risk factors should be referred for a psychiatric assessment, and it is on the basis of that assessment in consultation with the staff psychiatrist that decisions about management are made for each individual case.

The Violent Patient

Assessing an agitated patient is one of the most anxiety-provoking aspects of emergency psychiatry. Recognizing early the progressive stages of violence and intervening

---

Box 14-3. SAD PERSONS Screening for Suicide

Sex: male
Age: <19 or > 60
Depression
Previous attempt
Ethanol (alcohol) abuse
Rational thinking loss (i.e., psychosis)
Social supports lacking
Organized plan
No spouse
Sickness (especially if chronic or uncontrolled pain)

---

appropriately are skills that are essential parts of training (Table 14-1). Agitation occurs along a continuum and will progress unimpeded unless you intervene to de-escalate the situation.

Before you begin any assessment, you should observe the patient to determine the level of agitation present. The setting in which you conduct your interview needs to be safe. The patient who is anxious or agitated may be pacing and need more space than the tiny interview room allows. The noise and stimulation of an ER waiting room may create more distress for the patient, and it is helpful to triage quickly to a quiet interview room equipped with safety features such as video cameras, silent alarm buzzers, staff in close proximity, bolted furniture, and two doors of exit. You should feel comfortable in asking for a team member or psychiatric assistant to be in the room with you during your assessment. You want to make sure both you and the patient have access out the door. Feel free to call "time outs" during the process if at any point you are concerned. Before you take the patient into the room, look for potential weapons—both on yourself and in the room. No ties, identification tags hanging from the neck, or dangling jewelry should be worn during psychiatric assessments. The room should be free of loose objects such as garbage cans or telephones.

If police brought the patient to hospital, you should discern whether handcuffs were necessary. It is not recommended to assess the patient in cuffs because it is difficult to engage with the patient and develop a trusting relationship when she is bound in this way. If the patient is too agitated to safely assess without handcuffs, you should move to the medical equivalent of handcuffs: mechanical

restraints. The police can assist you and your team in transferring the patient from cuffs to restraints.

The agitated patient may settle when you speak calmly, softly, and with respect: *"Mr. Brown, I realize you have been waiting a long time, I apologize for the wait. Can you tell me about what is upsetting you at this time?"* The suspicious patient may need specific reassurances about safety: *"We are here to help you, and you are safe here. You are in the hospital."* As verbal threats become more evident, you need to use skills of verbal de-escalation to help the patient. The patient may be unable to sit down and may be physically intimidating. You should not make yourself vulnerable by sitting when the patient is towering above you. If the patient is unable to sit, you should stand as well and attempt to gently set limits while still attempting to understand what is of concern: *"I cannot understand how to help you when you are yelling or threatening me."* You should not make sustained direct eye contact with the patient, especially if he is paranoid. Rather, a nonthreatening stance, angling your body away from the patient, is preferable. If the patient's state continues to escalate, you should anticipate overt aggression and be vigilant about potential assault. At this point, you will be making decisions about the types of physical interventions—mechanical and/or chemical restraint. Once the anger is spent, the resolution phase is one in which you can often reengage with the patient to explain what will be happening at this point (e.g., admission to hospital, police involvement).

With the disorganized psychotic or intoxicated patient, this spectrum of violence can move very quickly from one stage to the next, and it may be almost impossible to de-escalate the patient when he is not able to hear you and appreciate the meaning of your reassurances. You will have to think quickly and be observing for signs of psychosis and disinhibition (e.g., ataxic gait, incoherent or slurred speech, response to internal stimuli) quite early on in the process because these are all signs that the patient is distracted and may not be able to respond to your preliminary interventions. When you need immediate assistance, you may choose to call a "Code White," which is the hospital's code indicating an agitated patient. Often, a psychiatric code team will arrive and be able to assist you in restraining and medicating the patient. Having medication close at hand is a good idea even if you do not need to use it. The most important principles are those of safety—for you, the patient, and the setting.

Table 14-1. An Approach to the Agitated Patient

Stages of Violence	Stages of Intervention
1. Anxiety/agitation	1. Safety
2. Verbal threats	2. Verbal de-escalation
3. Overt aggression	3. Physical interventions
4. Resolution	4. Medication

OTHER CHALLENGES

The Medically Ill Patient

"Have they been medically cleared?" This is a most familiar question to both psychiatry and ERs. But what constitutes medical clearance? When patients are referred for a psychiatric consultation in the ER, they are usually seen first by the ER physician. The ER doctor will determine the primary reason for the presentation. Based on the clinical picture at hand, a physical examination and investigations may have been ordered. The controversial cases typically involve an intoxicated or cognitively impaired patient. Toxicology screens are not indicated on every intoxicated patient in the ER if the substances are known and the presentation is in keeping with the expected effects; however, if there is an unusual presentation or unknown substances may be contributing, the toxicology screen can be helpful. The challenge in doing the psychiatric assessment occurs if the patient is still intoxicated or sedated. Optimal assessment may involve letting a patient sleep off the effects of the drugs and alcohol in the ER before you begin.

It is not always clear what service should be consulting to the patient with cognitive impairment. Delirium is a medical emergency; dementia can be managed by either medicine or psychiatry depending on the presentation. Each case should be discussed with attention paid to the acuity of the medical presentation and the resources available in each of the services.

When you are not comfortable with the patient's medical status, you should document your concerns as part of your consultation note and discuss this with the referring source. It will then be up to the ER to consult another service to clarify the diagnosis or assist you in this process.

The Difficult Patient

In the ideal emergency assessment, by the time you finish your assessment, meet with the patient and family, and review the disposition plan, everyone involved is pleased, grateful, and understanding of your explanations and recommendations. There are cases, however, where the patient and/or family have very different expectations from you and the system in terms of what you should be providing. Commonly, this takes the form of hoping for an inpatient stay and treatment in hospital. It is important to realize that your clinical judgment regarding appropriate management, while incorporating the patient's values and preferences, is the primary determinant of outcome. In the ER, "consumer satisfaction" is not always about giving patients what they want. The skill is trying to explain the reasoning behind your thinking in a way the patient and concerned others will understand. There are times when you will be discharging angry and even threatening patients; this is difficult to experience, but it does not mean you have done a bad job. You have done what is best for the patient, but for many reasons, he may not be able to understand your reasoning at that time. Your documentation will support your decision-making process for future reference.

The Patient Who Does Not Speak English

There will be times you will need to use the assistance of an interpreter in taking your history in the ER. Ideally, the interpreter should not be a friend or relative of the patient and should be trained as a translator. A professional translator will allow you to speak to the patient directly as you normally would, and then she will answer in the patient's words, in the first person. Thus, you are not saying, "Ask her if she is sleeping," and the interpreter does not reply, "She says. . . ." Rather, this should be a seamless interview where eye contact is maintained with the patient with the translator's voice accompanying. In the middle of the night and in busy ERs, it is difficult at times to get an interpreter, and we are often left requesting help from the hospital employees who might speak the language in question. Issues of confidentiality should be explained, and then you can help them to interpret in the way described above. It is very frustrating to ask a question and then observe a long, heated dialogue between the patient and the interpreter with the final translation being, "She says, 'no.'" Clearly, a lot more has been said than that, but you are at a loss to understand what has transpired. Only under extreme circumstances should you use family members as interpreters; sensitive aspects of the psychiatric history will be biased with a family member in the room. That being said, there may be situations where this is your only alternative, and you must do your best to understand the patient's story with the help of whoever is available.

Returning to Case Example 1, "The Fed-up Young Woman," the following are questions to ask:

1. What do you want to ask ER staff before seeing the patient?
   a. Has she been searched?
   b. Is she capable of harming herself in the ER while she is waiting?
   c. Is she intoxicated now?
   d. Did she overdose on any meds today?
   e. Is she being held involuntarily at this point?
2. How do you want to focus your assessment?
   a. Intent: suicide versus self-harm
   b. Are there psychiatric symptoms?
3. How do you feel in the room with her?
4. Collateral: boyfriend, general practitioner, old chart
5. Has admission been helpful in the past? If not, why not?
6. Has her chronic risk of self-harm and suicide changed from baseline in any way?
7. How can you optimize her outpatient follow-up and offer her a plan that instills hope?

Ideally, this patient will leave the ER feeling she has been understood and willing to follow up with her family doctor for supportive therapy. She remains at chronic risk for self-harm but was not suicidal at the end of the assessment—she called her boyfriend from the ER and was returning home to stay with him that night. You suggest calling the family doctor with feedback about the ER visit and recommendations for a psychiatric consultation to assess the medications, and she is agreeable to this plan.

In Case Example 2, "The Traffic Teen," the following issues should be addressed:

1. What do you want to ask the police before they go?
   a. Has he been searched?
   b. Violence en route: What was the need for handcuffs?
   c. Are there signs of intoxication?
   d. Is there a legal record? Have they checked?
2. How do you want to focus your assessment?
   a. Assessment of violence risk, agitation: Should I bring in extra staff?
   b. Will he need mechanical and/or chemical restraint?
   c. If he is disorganized and unable to answer coherently, why is this?
3. Is there a need for medical clearance?
4. Collateral: Can we locate family through the identification on the patient?
5. If this is a first episode of psychosis, can family offer a history that helps with your differential diagnosis?
6. Prepare for psychiatric admission, complete forms for involuntary hospitalization, assess capacity to consent to treatment, inform the nurses of the patient's level of agitation, and ensure that the patient is settled and safe for transfer to the ward when a bed is available.

You are concerned that this young man is at risk for a first episode of psychosis and may be at the early stages of a schizophreniform illness. You feel that he is at risk to himself and others given his bizarre and dangerous behavior that day. You detain him on an involuntary basis and order toxicology screens and routine blood work. He requires both mechanical and chemical restraint. You admit him to the psychiatry holding unit for a longer observation period once he is sedated and resting.

SUMMARY

The ER is an exciting and potentially volatile setting in which to work. It is a significant portal of entry for many patients into our medical and psychiatric systems. We have the ability to make this introduction to our health care system a positive and therapeutic one for patients and their families. With an organized and focused approach to the emergency psychiatric assessment, the clinician is able to form a diagnostic impression that will offer an acutely ill patient an individualized treatment plan and address the most immediate concerns. It is important to keep in mind the variables at play in the emergency assessment: the patient, system, and clinician factors that contribute to the impression reached and the ultimate management plan. All staff working in ERs should have an appreciation for the risks and challenges in assessing the psychiatrically ill patient. By keeping psychiatric emergency assessment skills finely honed, clinicians will be able to safely, efficiently, and empathically evaluate and treat the patient in acute distress.

ACKNOWLEDGMENTS

The author would like to thank Drs. Justin Geagea and Jillian Sussman for their thoughtful review of this chapter and their helpful suggestions.

REFERENCES

1. Winnicott DW: Transitional objects and transitional phenomena, *Int J Psychoanal* 34:89–97, 1953.
2. Patterson WM, Dohn HH, Bird J, et al: Evaluation of suicidal patients: the SAD PERSONS scale, *Psychosomatics* 24:343–349, 1983.

RECOMMENDED READING

Dubin WR, Weiss KJ: *Handbook of psychiatric emergencies*, Springhouse, PA, 1991, Springhouse Corporation.
Groves J: Taking care of the hateful patient, *N Engl J Med* 298(16):883–887, 1978.
Kaplan HI, Sadock BJ: *Pocket handbook of emergency psychiatric medicine*, Baltimore, MD, 1993, Williams and Wilkins.
MacKinnon RA, Michels R: *The psychiatric interview in clinical practice*. Philadelphia, 1971, WB Saunders, pp 401–427.

15

Assessment of Medical/Surgical Patients

Jarret D. Morrow, Mark R. Katz, and Gary Rodin

INTRODUCTION

The psychiatric assessment of the medical and surgical patient presents unique challenges related to the physical condition of the patient, the involvement of multiple medical caregivers, the frequent unsuitability of medical settings for a confidential assessment, and the multiple interacting factors that contribute to psychiatric morbidity in this population. The subspecialty of consultation-liaison (C-L) psychiatry developed to ensure appropriate psychiatric expertise to assess and treat psychiatric disorders, which may be present in more than 25% of medically ill populations,[1] and to address the associated problems that affect health care use and compliance with medical treatment in such patients.[2]

Key Point:

Psychiatric illness has high comorbidity (>25%) with medical/surgical patients.

PREASSESSMENT CONSIDERATIONS

A variety of issues may be important to consider when a medical or surgical patient is referred for psychiatric consultation, even before the clinical assessment takes place. These include the reason for the consultation, the medical state of the patient, and the setting of the interview.

The Reason for the Consultation

A request for a psychiatric consultation on a medical or surgical patient may originate from the patient or from con-

cerns of the medical team. Common reasons for the team to initiate the request include concerns about the presence of a psychiatric disorder, concerns about the contribution of psychological factors to physical symptoms, or questions about patient competence to provide informed consent to a medical or surgical treatment or to be discharged from hospital. In some cases, psychiatric consultations are initiated because of concerns of family members. The concerns of these parties may differ and, as a psychiatric consultant, you may need to distinguish in such assessments the perceived interests of each. You may also need to judge the urgency of the consultation, giving priority to cases in which there is agitation, psychosis, suicidal/homicidal ideation, or threats made by the patient to leave against medical advice. Discussion and negotiation with the person consulting you at the time of referral may allow a mutually agreeable time frame for the consultation to be established.

It is important for you to respond to the stated reasons for the consultation, although other important issues can also be addressed at the time of the consultation. The most common reasons for psychiatric referral in a tertiary care service, in order of frequency, are depression, behavior management, agitation, judgment, informed consent, discharge against medical advice, and suicidal risk assessment.[3] The most common psychiatric disorders diagnosed by psychiatric consultants are organic mental disorders (OMD; delirium followed by dementia and substance-induced OMD), depressive disorder, and substance-use disorder.[3] However, referrals may not be representative of the problems and disorders in medical patients because only a small minority of medical patients with psychiatric comorbidity are referred for psychiatric assessment, and most often such referrals occur late in the hospital stay.[4,5]

Medical State of the Patient and Setting of the Interview

The psychiatric assessment of medical and surgical patients is often made more difficult by their physical illness and by the circumstances in which the consultations must take place. Sedation, confusion, and physical symptoms such as pain, shortness of breath, or profound fatigue may limit the length of time of the interview. In some cases, brief, frequent sessions are necessary to complete the assessment, and there must be prioritization in the data-gathering effort. The opportunity to conduct private interviews in medical inpatient settings is often limited. Often, interviews must be conducted in shared patient rooms in which other patients and health care staff enter and exit the room frequently during the interview. With patients who are not bed-ridden, conducting the interview in a private room on the ward or in another office within the hospital may allow more privacy. When this is not possible, you may need to find practical solutions to create as much privacy as possible, including drawing a curtain around the patient's bed, speaking in quieter tones, or asking the patient's roommate or roommate's family to leave the room.

CONDUCTING THE ASSESSMENT

Chart Review

Psychiatric assessments in medical settings usually must take into account information obtained from multiple sources. It is important first for you to clarify with the patient's treatment team what are the specific questions that they want answered. Before interviewing the patient, it is also valuable to review the patient's chart thoroughly; this will help you to play an integrative role in the patient's management and to arrive at an accurate and complete psychiatric opinion. Information from the nursing staff and from the nursing notes can also provide important clues to the patient's mental status at different times of the day.

Clinical Interview

In introducing yourself to the patient, it is important to clarify whether the patient is aware that a psychiatric consultation has been requested and to offer the patient the

opportunity to discuss this with the treating team if this has not already occurred. Visual inspection at this time may provide important clues about agitation, depression, anxiety or restlessness, pain or other physical distress, labored breathing, or weakness. Furthermore, clues about the integrity of cognitive functioning may be revealed by observing whether the patient has been reading a book or magazine, staring vacantly at the wall, or apparently responding to hallucinations.

Safety Issues

Agitation or other behavioral disturbances are common reasons for psychiatric consultation in the hospital setting. Delirious patients who become aggressive or pull out their intravenous lines may represent a danger to themselves, and some patients may pose a risk to others. With patients who are obviously agitated or aggressive, it may be wise to have other staff in the room while the interview is being conducted. However, distinguishing behavior that is disruptive to the ward from that which is truly dangerous is also important. Chemical restraint may not be justified if it is only being used to reduce disruptions to the hospital staff. When safety is a concern, the interviewer should arrange his chair closer to the door than that of the patient, without blocking the patient's access to the door. Sensitivity to the patient's need for physical space may also be important. For example, sitting too close to or offering to shake the hand of a paranoid patient may be interpreted as threatening.

Mental Status Examination

The initial interaction with patients may provide a wealth of information about their mental state. The interviewer should pay close attention to both verbal and nonverbal communication and to what they reveal about social judgment, cognition, and affect. With patients who are confused, the focus will need to be more on the mental status evaluation than on history-taking. In such cases, formal tests of attention and cognitive functioning may be performed early in the interview. When patients are defensive about revealing cognitive impairment, it may be most feasible for you to evaluate this informally through questions about the details of hospitalization, medical illness, and treatment. When cognitive impairment is not revealed by such questions, there is less likely to be gross impairment in the formal testing of their mental state. You may normalize the process of testing cognitive functioning by explaining that problems with attention and memory are common in the setting of acute medical illness.

Building an Alliance with the Patient

Some patients are reluctant to be assessed by a psychiatrist or other mental health professional for fear they will be regarded as "crazy," that their physical symptoms will be dismissed, and that their medical practitioners will abandon them. Patients who have not been told by their attending physicians about the psychiatric consultation may be resentful about it. It is important for you to clarify your role and the reason you were asked to assess the patient. This might be explained, for example, by saying, *"I was asked to see you by your doctor because he was concerned about your mood."* It is also important to address the patient's concerns about the psychiatric consultation early in the interview and to attempt to identify a common goal. Most often, the interview should begin with a focus on the patient's medical condition because this is most likely to be an area of shared concern.

Confidentiality

Patient confidentiality is an important issue to address directly with the patient. You must make clear your role with regard to both the patient and the person requesting the consultation and what information, if any, may be kept confidential from the medical team. You should make it clear that you must report to the patient's attending physician. Some personal information may or should be withheld by you to protect the privacy of the patient, but other information—particularly homicidal or suicidal ideation—must be disclosed. It is generally unwise to promise confidentiality about issues related to the medical illness or its treatment since you must be able to collaborate with the rest of the team. In any case, absolute confidentiality is unrealistic to promise in this setting because multiple medical caregivers are involved in the patient's care and have access to the medical record.

The Consultative Process

The key to being an effective C-L psychiatrist is to be accepted and integrated into the medical or surgical service. This means being a member of the team rather than an outsider who drifts in from the psychiatry department to offer an opinion and then leave. Being a member of the team requires considerable time, energy, resources, and means, among other things. Other elements include the following: (1) participating in patient-centered team rounds; (2) contributing to the educational development of medical-surgical house staff, nursing, and allied health professionals; (3) being involved in programmatic planning; and (4) developing academic linkages.

An effective liaison psychiatrist understands in a detailed way the medical and surgical issues facing patients and comfortably communicates that understanding both to the patient and consulting party. As a rule, the more the C-L psychiatrist is involved in indirect (nonclinical) activities such as education, research, and programmatic planning, the busier he will be in terms of receiving clinical referrals.

For example, providing a seminar on alcohol withdrawal delirium to a medical service may increase the number of referrals as the expertise and availability of the psychiatric consultant are highlighted.

One by-product of a strong liaison relationship may be that the psychiatric consultant is asked to see patients at a much earlier point in the hospitalization or the course of the illness, offering the potential for prevention of and early intervention with psychiatric difficulties. Some patients may be referred prematurely, such as when there is an expectable emotional response to the receipt of bad news. Such "inappropriate referrals," however, may help to build the alliance with the treatment team and may provide an opportunity to demonstrate the differences between normative and pathological distress states.

The optimal behaviors of the C-L psychiatrist may be summarized in the following list of do's and don'ts.

DO:

1. Familiarize yourself with the common medical or surgical illnesses and treatments on the consulting service.
2. Become involved in the weekly rounds/team meetings where you can provide input into the care of all patients and pick up preventative or early intervention referrals.
3. Become an active teacher of staff physicians, house staff, and other members of the health care team.
4. Develop joint academic endeavors with consulting services; nothing strengthens the relationship better than being academic collaborators.
5. Provide timely assessments and practical management recommendations to the consulting party.

DON'T:

1. Convey a negative attitude about the appropriateness of referrals or about recommendations not being followed. Instead, use these referrals as opportunities for teaching.
2. Provide psychiatric opinions that are excessively detailed or technical in terms of psychodynamic jargon or diagnostic terminology.
3. Overstep your role as consultant. You are not the attending physician—you should not usually be providing new information to the patient about the medical condition or providing treatment recommendations to the patient directly without discussing these issues with the consulting physician.
4. Be overzealous as an advocate for routine assessments, unless this is requested by the consulting service. In other words, don't be a busybody!

Neurocognitive Evaluation

Particular attention will be paid in this chapter to the neurocognitive examination, which, in medical populations, may often reveal impairment. Before cognitive testing, it is important to ensure that the patient has appropriate sensory aids, such as glasses or hearing aids. Alterations in the level of consciousness may be the first clue to the presence of neuropsychiatric impairment. The patient's failure to maintain alertness despite repeated attempts to rouse or engage him may be the first sign of delirium. Attention can be tested formally by the forward digit span test, that is, by asking the patient to repeat five numbers listed forward (the minimum for a normal score) or four numbers backward. Backward recall tests both attention and short-term memory. An additional test of attention is the vigilance test, which involves saying one letter per second and having the patient respond when the letter *a* is spoken. A single error on this test is considered abnormal. Speech abnormalities may be evident in slurring, which is common with intoxication. Language is assessed in terms of rate, rhythm, and fluency and with tests of naming, reading, writing, and verbal comprehension. Recent memory can be assessed by orientation to person, place, and time and by asking the patient to recall three objects immediately and again 3 minutes later after having conversed with the patient. More remote memory can be difficult to assess because of the difficulty distinguishing between fact and confabulation. However, asking historical questions that are part of common general knowledge can help you avoid this difficulty.

Standardized mental status examinations, such as the Folstein mini-mental status examination (MMSE) can be used to screen for cognitive dysfunction.[6] In particular, serial use of this exam can provide an objective marker for changes in level of cognitive impairment in patients. The MMSE involves a series of questions that test cognitive features, such as orientation, memory, attention, calculation, language, ability to follow commands, and reading and writing. It can be administered in about 5 minutes, and scores of 23 or less are considered indicative of impairment. Low scores can result from a variety of causes, including delirium, dementia, mental retardation, and lack of cooperation. The draw-a-clock-face test is another test of cognitive impairment and visuospatial constructional ability, which can be useful in screening for delirium and early dementia. These tests are sensitive for the presence of impairment but do not necessarily help identify its cause or differentiate between acute and chronic confusional states.

Case Example 1

Agitation/Confusion/Psychosis. Mr. M was a 65-year-old man who was admitted to hospital with a chronic obstructive pulmonary disease exacerbation. While on the medical ward, the patient rarely left his room, ate very little, and seemed to have very little interest in life. The internist suspected that the patient might be suffering from depression, and a referral to psychiatry was made. Preliminary discussion with the patient's wife, who was present at the time of assessment, revealed that the patient was no longer able to recognize some family members and seemed intermittently confused about where he was. There was no history suggestive of cognitive impairment prior to 4 days before admission.

When Mr. M was seen in his hospital room, he presented as a somewhat disheveled, elderly man receiving oxygen via nasal prongs. His face was expressionless, and he exhibited a moderate degree of psychomotor retardation. The psychiatrist suspected cognitive impairment in view of the patient's age, medical condition, presentation, and reports by the nursing staff that he was often asleep during the day and awake at nighttime.

When interviewed, the patient had difficulty answering questions and was unaware of the reasons for hospitalization or how long he had been an inpatient. The consultant shifted to tests of orientation, attention, and cognition. These tests, together with a Folstein MMSE score of 15/30, suggested that the patient was severely cognitively impaired. A diagnosis of hypoactive delirium was made.

Management of the patient involved treating the patient's underlying medical condition, ruling out other medical causes such as electrolyte disturbances, and optimizing the patient's environment. A clock and calendar were placed in the patient's room to improve orientation, and the patient was moved to a room near the nursing station for closer supervision. A review of the patient's medication revealed that a benzodiazepine was prescribed for sleep, which may have exacerbated his cognitive impairment. This medication was subsequently discontinued and replaced with a low dose of an atypical antipsychotic. Support and education about delirium were provided to the family, who were very concerned about the marked change in the patient's mental state.

It has been estimated that delirium is present in 10% to 30% of patients on medical and surgical wards and is even more common in intensive care unit settings. It is most common in patients who are postsurgery, older than 60 years of age, have prior central nervous system disease (e.g., dementia), or have been drug dependent. Common causes of delirium include urinary tract infections, pneumonia, metabolic disturbances such as hyponatremia or hypercalcemia, hypoxia, and medication-related effects. A mnemonic that helps to remember causes of delirium is provided in Table 15-1.

Table 15-1. Differential Diagnosis "I WATCH DEATH"

Infection	Encephalitis, meningitis, HIV, syphilis
Withdrawal	Alcohol, sedative-hypnotics
Acute metabolic	Acidosis, alkalosis, electrolyte disturbance (especially hyponatremia and hypercalcemia), hepatic/renal failure
Trauma	Closed-head injury, postoperative, burns
CNS pathology	Hemorrhage, stroke, tumor, abscess, subdural hematoma
Hypoxia	CO_2 poisoning, hypotension, anemia
Deficiencies	Vitamin B_{12}, folate, niacin, thiamine
Endocrinopathies	Hyper-/hypoglycemia, hyperparathyroidism
Acute vascular	Hypertensive encephalopathy, stroke
Toxins or drugs	Medication, illicit drugs
Heavy metals	Lead, manganese, mercury

Delirium differs from dementia in that the former is associated with more acute onset and more marked fluctuation in course. Although all spheres of cognitive functioning may be affected, the hallmark of delirium is impaired capacity to maintain attention.[7] The mental state of patients with dementia, in contrast to that of delirium, is usually more consistent, with little diurnal variation. However, a "sundowning" phenomenon has been described in some dementia patients, particularly with Alzheimer's disease, in which an exacerbation of behavioral symptoms occurs in the afternoons and evenings. Other neurocognitive functions affected in delirium include consciousness, memory, orientation, language, and perception. Delirium may be of the hyperactive type associated with agitation, aggressive behavior, hallucinations, and delusions; or the hypoactive type, with decreased reactivity, motor and speech retardation, and facial inexpressiveness.[8] The latter is commonly mistaken for depression in medical settings.

Factors you must consider in the assessment of a patient with delirium include safety of the patient—the most appropriate focus of the interview—and the need for corroborative information. Some agitated delirious patients may require either chemical or physical restraint to prevent them from harming themselves or others. When clear cognitive impairment is present, you should shift to assess its extent rather than proceeding with a full psychiatric assessment. It is also important in such cases for you to establish whether the patient has sufficient understanding of the illness and treatment situation to make capable treatment decisions. In these circumstances, much of the information required for a comprehensive psychiatric history will need to be obtained from other sources such as old charts, family, and the patient's treatment team.

When impaired attention is suspected, formal testing can include tests of digit span recall, vigilance, constructions, and handwriting. The Folstein MMSE is also quite useful in this regard. Since levels of consciousness may fluctuate, it is important for you to examine the patient more than once daily and to review the observations of the regular nursing staff. The presence of emotional lability and visual hallucinations or rapidly changing delusions, especially of a paranoid nature, should also raise your suspicion of an organic or delirious state. Such patients may also exhibit formal thought disorder with loosening of associations or illogicality.

Case Example 2

Depression/Demoralization. Mrs. H was a 62-year-old woman referred by her cardiologist for psychiatric assessment. She suffered from a mild but progressive abnormality of her mitral valve, but her disability far exceeded what might have been expected based on her physical findings.

When Mrs. H arrived for psychiatric assessment, she presented as a well-groomed middle-aged woman who appeared somewhat anxious and moderately depressed. Despite this appearance, the patient initially did not report any symptoms of depression. She commented on how difficult it was for her to attend the appointment due to her physical condition and that she might have to leave the appointment if her "heart acts up." She reported a progressive deterioration in her physical functioning such that she had quit her job 1 year ago and was currently having difficulties managing her home. However, she believed that her problems were physical, and she was surprised when her surgeon had referred her for psychiatric assessment.

Soon after the interview began, Mrs. H began to cry. She reported numerous recent stressors including the loss of her daughter in a car accident 2 years earlier, a cousin who passed away 6 months prior to the interview, and difficulties with her finances. Mrs. H. tended to ruminate over these events, and, although she tried to smile during questioning and to deny emotional problems, she admitted to feeling depressed for the past year. She also reported a loss of interest in her hobbies of cooking and knitting, as well as difficulty concentrating and reading her favorite books. She expressed strong feelings of hopelessness regarding her medical condition and treatment options. As well, she endorsed passive suicidal thoughts and described profound feelings of guilt about her inability to take care of her physically disabled mother-in-law.

The psychiatric diagnosis in this case was that of a major depressive episode. Treatment involved a combination of supportive-expressive psychotherapy to help her adjust to the multiple losses she had endured and a trial of an

---

Key Point:

Assessment of delirium in patients requires tests of attention and cognition.

antidepressant medication to reduce depressive symptoms and improve her functional adjustment.

There is an increased risk of depressive disorders in most medical illnesses, although they are frequently undiagnosed in medical and primary care populations.[9] One explanation for this underdiagnosis is that many symptoms of depression, such as changes in sleep, energy, concentration, and appetite, may be attributed to the underlying medical condition rather than to depression. Depression may also be missed when it is incorrectly assumed that a patient's mental state is a "normal" reaction to the situation, or when patients are reluctant to disclose their feelings to their treating physician. Realistic feelings of sadness or hopelessness in a terminally ill patient can be difficult to distinguish from the despair of a depressed patient. However, if the symptoms of sadness, loss of interest, and the vegetative symptoms of depression, particularly those less likely to be due to the associated medical condition, are persistent and are affecting the person's functioning, you should consider a diagnosis of depression. Persons who have a past history of depression, low social support, and more severe medical illness are most at risk. Depression may also be overdiagnosed in medically ill persons when symptoms of medical illness or hypoactive delirium are mistakenly attributed to depression.[9] In that regard, the apathy of patients with dementia or with metabolic abnormalities, such as uremia, must be distinguished from that of depression. Similarly, the facial immobility and psychomotor retardation that is common in patients with Parkinson's disease may mimic that of depression. Cognitive testing will help you to differentiate patients with dementia from depression. Although severe depression may be associated with impaired attention and memory, dementia is more likely to be associated with confabulation and with scores below 23 on the MMSE.

Key Point:

Depression, in particular, is common in the medically ill, and the diagnostic criteria that are most sensitive and reliable include depressive symptoms regardless of whether they overlap with medical symptoms.

Different diagnostic strategies have been proposed to deal with the lack of specificity for major depression of vegetative symptoms in patients with medical illness. The *Diagnostic and Statistical Manual of Mental Disorders,* edition 4, text revision (DSM-IV-TR) suggests an "etiologic" approach, in which symptoms judged by the clinician to be etiologically related to a general medical condition are excluded from the diagnostic criteria for major depres-

sive disorder. However, this distinction may be difficult to determine in practice and raises the likelihood of excluding depressed patients who may be candidates for antidepressant treatment. A study by Koenig et al.[10] suggests an inclusive approach, in which all symptoms are included without making a judgment as to whether they may be related to a comorbid medical disorder. This system was found to be the most sensitive and reliable approach in their study.

Case Example 3

Anxiety. Mrs. A was a 56-year-old woman who was recently diagnosed with lung cancer. Her oncologist referred her to psychiatry for difficulty with sleeping.

Mrs. A presented as a relatively well-groomed, pleasant middle-aged woman who appeared to be somewhat restless and agitated. She mentioned that she felt uncomfortable in hospitals and doctors' offices. She noted that she had been having difficulty with sleeping for the past 2 weeks, which coincided with her diagnosis of lung cancer. As well, since her diagnosis, she acknowledged that she had become increasingly irritable and had difficulty concentrating and also reported feeling like she was "walking around in a daze." Although she tried to avoid talking about her condition, she admitted that she often felt somewhat detached from the world and from herself except when she had reexperienced receiving the diagnosis in the form of dreams and flashbacks.

In this case, the consultant diagnosed the patient with an acute stress disorder. The patient was administered an antidepressant to help resolve her anxiety symptoms and difficulty with sleeping. She was also referred to a psychologist for cognitive behavior therapy.

Anxiety symptoms are a common reason for psychiatric consultation in the hospital setting, and hospitalization itself may be anxiety provoking. In evaluating anxiety in the medical/surgical patient, it is important for you to determine whether it is associated with a preexisting psychiatric condition or related to the current medical situation. Although anxiety is a common response to a threatening diagnosis or to treatment or to complications of their medical condition, some medical illnesses or medications can induce many of the symptoms of anxiety directly on a physiological basis. These include hyperthyroidism, pheochromocytoma, and medications, such as corticosteroids, antiemetics, bronchodilators, caffeine, and withdrawal from benzodiazepines or alcohol. Features that suggest that anxiety may have an organic basis include onset of anxiety symptoms after age 35, lack of personal or family history of anxiety disorder, lack of avoidance behavior, poor response to anti-panic agents, absence of a significant event generating or exacerbating the anxiety symptoms, or lack of childhood history of phobia or separation anxiety disorder.[11]

Key Point:

Many medical conditions may cause anxiety, especially respiratory and endocrine disorders.

Depression may present with anxious features or may occur concurrently with an anxiety disorder. Panic disorder has been demonstrated to occur at much higher rates in the medically ill than in normal populations. Patients with generalized anxiety disorder, a condition that is underdiagnosed in the medical setting, have often been known as "worriers" by their friends and family. As well, generalized anxiety disorder often occurs comorbidly with panic disorder, social phobia, depression, and alcohol abuse. Acute stress disorder may occur in the hospital setting with patients who have been told that they have a terminal illness. Patients with specific phobias that lead to refusal of diagnostic investigation may be referred for psychiatric consultation when this problem interferes with medical management.

Case Example 4

Treatment Refusal/Incapacity. Mr. L was a 40-year-old man with type 1 diabetes mellitus who presented to the hospital with cellulitis of his right foot. His primary physician told the patient that his foot would require amputation because of complications of the infection. The patient was extremely upset when informed of this news and became agitated and angry toward the hospital staff. As well, the patient refused to undergo the procedure, despite being informed of the consequences. Psychiatry was consulted to assess his capacity for informed consent.

Despite appearing agitated and upset, Mr. L presented as an attractive, athletic, well-groomed man. He began the interview by questioning the psychiatrist about his credentials and demanded to see the "head of psychiatry," who he felt would be the only person who "could understand me." He also voiced concern that a junior member of the staff had conducted his medical assessment. The psychiatrist worked to form a therapeutic alliance with the patient, which included discussing some of the patient's feelings he had toward his medical staff.

It became apparent that the patient felt helpless and frightened by the situation and felt that his concerns about being disabled by the amputation were not being taken seriously enough. His anger diminished as he began to understand the reasons for the proposed amputation and the consequences of refusing the surgery. He clearly stated that he did not want to die, but felt that he had to do something to slow down a process in which he did not feel like a partner. The psychiatrist deemed the patient to be capable to consent to the treatment and made a psychiatric diagnosis

of a narcissistic personality disorder. The psychiatrist helped the treatment team to understand that the patient's low self-esteem contributed to his need to be regarded as important, and that the patient's fears of dependency heightened his need for control of his environment. As a result, the team spent more time with him explaining the procedure and the potential for improved quality of life with a prosthesis after surgery. The patient ultimately consented to the procedure and was referred for psychotherapy after this intervention.

Informed consent in a competent patient involves a process that is voluntary and specific and requires that reasonable information be disclosed to the patient. Information that should be provided[12] includes the following: (1) the diagnosis and a description of the medical condition; (2) the nature and purpose of the proposed treatment; (3) the risks and benefits of the proposed treatment; (4) alternatives to the proposed treatment, including risks and benefits; and (5) projected outcome with and without treatment. The most common context in which the question of capacity is raised is treatment refusal, although incapable consent is as problematic as incapable refusal. The capacity to consent to treatment is not a global concept, and patients may be capable to consent to some treatments but not to others. It includes the ability to engage in a dialogue about the risks and benefits of a treatment option and to apply the discussion meaningfully to one's present situation.

To assess the patient's capacity to consent to a specific treatment, you should ascertain whether the patient understands the information communicated to him about the illness and treatment and whether he appreciates the consequences of treatment decisions. Questions such as, *"What has the doctor said is wrong with you?"* or *"What treatment has she proposed?"* or *"What are the side effects of treatment?"* or *"What do they think might happen if you refuse treatment?"* help to clarify the patient's comprehension. In contrast, questions such as, *"What do you think might happen to you if you accept or refuse the treatment?"* or *"How might the treatment affect your quality of life?"* or *"What will happen to you if you don't get the treatment?"* address the ability to appreciate the consequences of accepting or refusing the proposed treatment. Patients must also be able to communicate their treatment decisions verbally or nonverbally. If a patient is deemed to be incapable, he must have a substitute decision-maker such as a family member or previously assigned power of attorney. In the case of an emergency, health care legislation typically allows for temporary treatment of the incapable person without consent. One study of patients referred to psychiatry for competency assessment found that patients deemed incompetent were more likely to be male and to have an organic brain syndrome, whereas patients deemed competent were more likely to have an adjustment or personality disorder or no psychiatric diagnosis.[13]

Key Point:

Assessment of competence or capacity to make treatment decisions is commonly requested of psychiatrists and involves assessing the patient's ability to understand the diagnosis, treatment options, risks and benefits of consent and of refusal, and the ability to communicate a decision.

Not all patients who refuse treatment are incapable. Further, treatment acceptance by patients should be considered in terms of a gradual process instead of an immediate response. Treatment refusal often reflects a breakdown in the physician-patient relationship when patients feel angry with or abandoned by a health care provider. In these cases, your role may be to facilitate better communication between the patient and the primary care physician. Some patients may feel they have little control or say over their treatment or feel they have been provided with too little information.

Noncompliance with recommended treatment is another perceived problem in the medical setting. Such noncompliance may include missed appointments, not filling prescriptions or taking prescribed medications, not following a recommended diet, or not adhering to lifestyle changes. Asking questions about compliance in ways that minimize shame can improve the accuracy of assessment. For example, your inquiry may begin with a normalizing statement, for example, *"Many patients have difficulty following their doctor's advice or taking their pills. Many of the reasons for this are quite understandable. Do you ever have difficulties with this?"*

Factors that affect compliance include understanding and acceptance of the illness, depression, or feelings of hopelessness or ineffectiveness. Manic or hypomanic patients may tend to deny their illness or the need for treatment. Psychotic disorders, obsessive compulsive, anxiety, or personality disorders, or substance abuse may also affect compliance in different ways.

Case Example 5

Medically Unexplained Illness. Ms. C was a 35-year-old woman who was referred for psychiatric assessment because of chronic unexplained symptoms of extreme fatigue. These symptoms began after a flulike illness and were exacerbated by physical exertion. However, extensive medical investigations failed to reveal a physical cause for these symptoms. Ms. C described herself as a perfectionis-tic person who had begun to feel overwhelmed by escalating work pressures in her position as a marketing executive. She had suffered from chronic symptoms of dysphoria and at least one apparent episode of major depression. However, she regarded her symptoms of fatigue as distinct from those of depression and believed that one set of symptoms did not necessarily trigger the other.

Ms. C believed that her devotion to work had interfered with her ability to form a relationship and to have a family. She had difficulty setting limits on the expectations she placed on herself and often found herself working to the point of exhaustion. Ms. C was also highly sensitive to emotional injury and tended to experience dramatic fluctuations in her affect states. Although she desired help, she objected to assumptions by medical caregivers that her fatigue was caused by psychological factors and, as a result, several previous experiences with psychotherapeutic treatment had been unsuccessful.

Ms. C began weekly psychotherapy sessions with a therapist who focused on helping her to identify and tolerate affect states, to attend to her own subjective experience, and to modulate her activity based on her symptoms. This treatment was associated with a gradual reduction in her symptoms and a greater sense of agency. She resigned from her former employment and obtained a part-time position in a community agency whose goals felt more consistent with her own. Her symptoms of fatigue gradually improved, although she experienced periodic exacerbations after excessive exertion. Her symptoms of dysphoria also subsided, although she was still prone to experience mood fluctuations, which were not necessarily explained by environmental circumstances.

Ms. C's fatigue might be regarded as an example of medically unexplained somatic symptoms. Although she had a history of chronic dysphoria, perfectionism, and major depression, her symptoms did not meet criteria for a somatoform disorder. It was important for her that her therapist accepted the validity of her symptoms, whatever their etiology, and not assume that they were psychogenic in nature. She benefited from a psychotherapeutic approach that was focused on empathy and responsiveness to her experience and from help in making decisions more compatible with her own interests and needs.

Frequently, a medical or surgical team requests a psychiatric consultation for somatic symptoms that seem to lack an organic basis. Such patients may have an undiagnosed medical condition, a somatoform disorder, or a tendency to *somatize,* that is, to communicate psychological distress in the form of somatic distress.[14] Somatic symptoms may also be associated with depression, anxiety, or personality disorders. Transient somatization can also occur in response to an acute medical event such as a myocardial infarction.

Somatization disorder is characterized by medically unexplained symptoms that affect many organ systems. Often, the onset is in early adolescence, with a waxing and waning course subsequently. Patients with this disorder have a high comorbidity of axis I and II disorders, including substance abuse. Hypochondriasis has, as its core feature, the fear of disease despite negative medical investigations and repeated physician reassurance. Conversion disorder involves symptoms that are involuntary and affect motor or sensory functioning. Common symptoms include paralysis, aphonia, seizures, and double vision. Pain disorder is characterized by physical pain that has a psychological component associated with its onset, severity, or maintenance. The hallmark of body dysmorphic disorder is the preoccupation with an imagined defect in appearance.

Key Point:

Patients with somatic symptoms may have a medical illness, a somatoform disorder, or a variety of psychiatric illnesses, or they may somatize transiently in response to stress.

It is important for you as a consultant to consider the possibility of factitious disorder and malingering as a cause of unexplained somatic symptoms. Factitious disorder involves consciously feigning symptoms for the purpose of assuming the sick role. Patients with factitious disorder may work in medical professions, such as nursing or medical technology. Malingering differs in that it involves conscious feigning of symptoms for secondary gain, such as financial rewards or narcotic medication. Malingerers may be more reluctant than those with factitious disorder to have underlying painful or invasive diagnostic testing, although there can be an overlap between the two diagnoses. Diagnoses of factitious disorder are often difficult to make because these patients attempt to deceive their physicians. Factitious disorders may include self-induced infections or the unnecessary taking of medication such as insulin. In many cases, the diagnosis is based on unusual laboratory data, as well as observations made by hospital staff.

There is a category of symptoms that include chronic fatigue and fibromyalgia, which are regarded as medically unexplained. Those patients have symptoms that do not meet criteria for either traditional medical or psychiatric diagnoses although they often suffer from prominent symptoms of depression.

Case Example 6

Personality Disturbance. Mr. R, a 45-year-old man with Wegener's granulomatosis, was receiving hemodialysis for renal complications arising from this disease and had a tracheostomy for upper respiratory tract involvement. While admitted to the hospital for medical complications, the patient made frequent requests for consultations to otolaryngology (ENT) to assess his tracheostomy and for his nursing staff to come to his room. The nurses observed that the patient seemed to become anxious when he was left alone. Despite several visits from ENT and an eventual revision of his tracheostomy, the patient continued to make demands to be seen by the ENT service and for staff to attend to many other requests. The medical treatment team was concerned that there might be some cognitive impairment and consulted psychiatry.

When interviewed, the patient appeared older than his stated age and was bedridden, though well groomed. His oxygen saturation was within normal limits on room air, and he did not exhibit any respiratory impairment. He was orientated to person, place, and time and scored 29/30 on the MMSE. No abnormalities of attention, memory, and abstraction were detected. His mother, who was present, complained of feeling burdened and overwhelmed by his requests and by his need for advice in decision-making. The patient noted that he felt the treatment team seemed to avoid him and limit their interaction with him.

The patient was diagnosed with narcissistic and dependent personality traits. The staff acknowledged feeling frustrated and burdened by his excessive demands. Counter-transference feelings and issues were discussed with the staff, and suggestions were made to create a schedule of nursing visits to diminish his feelings of uncertainty and helplessness. Steps were also taken to enhance the therapeutic relationship with his primary treatment team; he was also referred for psychotherapy.

Patients with personality disorders tend to have histories of behavioral and relationship problems that often recur in their relationships with medical staff. Medical staff may blame such patients for problematic behavior that they view as willful. Such negative reactions to these patients may interfere with collaborative relationships and result in psychiatric consultation. Your efforts to help physicians and staff to understand what it is about a particular patient that makes them feel uncomfortable can help them better tolerate these feelings and maintain an empathic posture. To facilitate the therapeutic alliance, you may need to address the transference of the patient and/or counter-transference of the staff.

Key Point:

Frequently, patients with personality disorder engender counter-transference reactions in their medical treatment team, which often results in psychiatric consultation.

COMMUNICATING RESULTS OF ASSESSMENT

A consultation note that effectively communicates treatment information to the primary treatment team is a vital part of the psychiatric assessment of the medical/surgical patient. In such notes, it is important for you to clarify and address the question posed by the treatment team and to write concisely in language that the treatment team will clearly understand. You should avoid including unnecessary personal information about the patient in the consultation note, but should convey sufficient information to help the primary treatment team to understand the etiology and nature of the problem.

Addressing the question posed by the treatment team involves offering an opinion on psychiatric diagnosis as well as treatment recommendations. Some of the recommendations will include treatment that can be implemented by the primary treatment team, and in other cases, patients may need to be referred for more specialized treatment. Biological interventions include medication or electroconvulsive therapy, and the specific names of suggested medication and appropriate dosage information should be offered. Supportive psychological interventions may be performed by the patient's primary care physician along with a liaison role of the consultant, who may attempt to enhance that therapeutic alliance. If these measures do not work, patients may require more specialized treatment from a psychiatrist including supportive-expressive therapy or cognitive behavioral therapy. Environmental interventions may also be helpful in caring for cognitively impaired patients, including recommendations on lighting and placement of visible clocks. Consultation with social workers to address issues of finance/employment is also often very useful. It is important to emphasize the importance of an integrative approach to the treatment of medical/surgical patients.

SUMMARY

Patients in medical settings often demonstrate psychological or psychiatric problems related to underlying psychological, biological, and social factors. Reactions to medical illness, complications of medical treatment, noncompliance or refusal of treatment, impaired capacity to consent, and medically unexplained somatic symptoms are common reasons for referral. Psychiatric clinicians in medical settings require particular flexibility due to the need to collaborate with multiple caregivers and to conduct assessments in settings that are often less than optimal. In many cases, problems in the relationship of the patient with the medical team are important underlying causes of the presenting problem. You must be able to diagnose psychiatric illness, identify the complex interrelationship between medical and psychiatric factors, and contribute to the successful provision of appropriate medical care. The biopsychosocial model is now widely accepted, and it is an essential element of daily psychiatric practice in medical settings.

REFERENCES

1. Silverstone PH: Prevalence of psychiatric disorders in medical inpatients, *J Nerv Ment Dis* 184:43–51, 1996.
2. DiMatteo MR, Lepper HS, Croghan TW: Depression is a risk factor for noncompliance with medical treatment: meta-analysis of the effects of anxiety and depression on patient adherence, *Arch Intern Med* 160:2101–2107, 2000.
3. Diefenbacher A, Strian JJ: Consultation-liaison psychiatry: stability and change over a 10-year period, *Gen Hosp Psychiatry* 24:249–256, 2002.
4. Schwab JJ: Psychiatric illness in medical patients: why it goes undiagnosed, *Psychosomatics* 23:225–229, 1982.
5. Huyse FJ, Herzog T, Lobo A, et al: Detection and treatment of mental disorders in general health care, *Eur Psychiatry* 12(Suppl 2):70s–78s, 1997.
6. Folstein MF, Folstein SE, McHugh PR: "Mini-mental state": a practical method for grading the cognitive state of patients for the clinician, *J Psychiatric Res* 12:189–198, 1975.
7. Lipowski ZJ: Delirium (acute confusional states), *JAMA* 258:1789–1792, 1987.
8. Camus V, Burtin B, Simeone I, et al: Factor analysis supports the evidence of existing hyperactive and hypoactive subtypes of delirium, *Int J Geriatric Psychiatry* 15:313–316, 2000.
9. Rodin G, Craven J, Littlefield C: *Depression in the medically ill: an integrated approach*, New York, 1991, Brunner/Mazel.
10. Koenig HG, George LK, Peterson BL, Pieper CF: Depression in medically ill hospitalized older adults: prevalence, characteristics, and course of symptoms according to six diagnostic schemes, *Am J Psychiatry* 154:1376–1383, 1997.
11. Rosenbaum JF, Pollack MH, Otto MW, Bernstein JG: Anxious patients. In Cassem NH, Stern TA, Rosenbaum JF, Jellinek MS, editors: *Massachusetts General Hospital handbook of general hospital psychiatry*, ed 4, St Louis, 1997, Mosby–Year Book, pp 173–210.
12. Simon RI: *Concise guide to psychiatry and law for clinicians*, Washington, DC, 1992, American Psychiatric Press, pp 23–55.

13. Katz M, Abbey S, Rydall A, Lowy F: Psychiatric consultation for competency to refuse medical treatment: a retrospective study of patient characteristics and outcome, *Psychosomatics* 36:33–41, 1995.
14. Lipowski ZJ: Somatization: the concept and its clinical application, *Am J Psychiatry* 145:1358–1368, 1988.

RECOMMENDED READING

Levenson JL, editor: *The American Psychiatric Publishing textbook of psychosomatic medicine,* Arlington, VA, 2004, American Psychiatric Publishing.

16

Assessment of Patients with Neurological Disorders

ANTHONY FEINSTEIN

INTRODUCTION

The assessment of patients with neurological disorders presents a particular set of challenges for mental health professionals and students. With the emphasis shifting from the phenomenological components of psychiatric evaluation to the cognitive assessment, you will require additional skills that complement the standard mental state examination. Furthermore, ancillary investigations such as neuroimaging take on added relevance in the presence of neurological disease and, together with a detailed cognitive examination, may provide valuable insights that help account for behavioral abnormalities. This chapter will outline the basic principles you must follow in completing a cognitive examination, provide a template for the assessment, and highlight common misconceptions and diagnostic pitfalls. Finally, the utility of neuroimaging in conjunction with cognitive testing will be briefly discussed.

BASIC PRINCIPLES OF COGNITIVE TESTING

There are some essential principles that must be followed for the assessment to retain validity. First and most obviously, if a neurological disorder is present or suspected, the patient must initially be seen by a neurologist. A neurological examination may not necessarily provide the diagnosis at that point, but notwithstanding will facilitate the subsequent mental state assessment in a number of important ways: (1) It will provide confirmation of neurological illness, an essential prerequisite in the case of patients whose primary difficulty may be a somatoform ill-

ness; (2) It may furnish valuable clues as to cerebral localization, which can then be explored further with the cognitive assessment and neuroimaging; (3) It can provide pointers to whether the pathological process is essentially cortical or subcortical, with implications for the cognitive profile of the patient.

With the neurological examination completed, the following points should be adhered to when assessing cognition:

- The cognitive assessment follows a standard mental state examination that addresses the patient's appearance and behavior, mood and affect, thought form and content, perceptual experiences, judgement, and insight.
- Patients with a neurological disorder may not be aware of any deficits, be they physical or cognitive. This "anosognosia" means they may not be able to direct you to the presence of any problems.
- Fatigue may frequently be an issue in cognitive testing. In more acutely ill patients admitted to hospital, testing may therefore require repeat sessions of short duration.
- In performing a cognitive assessment, you should always be aware of the patient's level of education and cultural background and take these factors into account when interpreting the results.
- You should stick to a set order of testing. Thus, your examination proceeds sequentially through the following areas: consciousness and orientation, attention and concentration, language, memory, visuospatial and constructional abilities, and finally, frontal lobe tasks. Failure to follow this sequence can lead to difficulties when interpreting data. For example, if memory testing

precedes the language assessment in an aphasic patient, deficits in recall may represent a failure to understand or respond correctly to a question instead of a failure in memory.

- Furthermore, within each cognitive domain you should start with the easiest questions and, depending on the response, move on to the next level of complexity. This basic premise is followed throughout the protocol outlined in further discussion.
- Access to an informant is often invaluable as an adjunct to the assessment, providing additional insight into the presence and severity of deficits.
- A cognitive assessment by itself is not diagnostic of any disorder. It is always completed as an adjunct to the history and formal mental state examination and complements other ancillary investigations like neuroimaging and biochemical indices.
- The cognitive assessment lacks the sensitivity of formal neuropsychological testing. However, the latter is more time consuming, expensive, and often not readily available. Guidelines for deciding whether a patient needs more detailed testing are provided in the Neuropsychological Testing section to follow.

THE COGNITIVE ASSESSMENT

There is a plethora of tests from which to chose when it comes to completing cognitive testing. Although the choice is most often dictated by the preference of examiner, tests do vary in their sensitivity. A useful rule of thumb is that tests that tap into more than one aspect of cognition are particularly useful in teasing out deficits. A good example is the Controlled Oral Word Association Test (COWAT)[1], also known as the Verbal Fluency or FAS test. This paradigm probes a patient's attention, the ability to sustain attention (termed *vigilance*), and semantic memory, which collectively enhances its utility as a screening measure for cognitive deficits.

Before beginning testing, you must note the patient's age, her level of education, the time of day, and cerebral dominance. The latter will lie along a continuum, but for the purpose of this examination asking the patient whether she is right- or left-handed will suffice.

Premorbid IQ

In patients who are fluent in English, this can be assessed rapidly with a reading test, such as the National Adult Reading Test.[2] This consists of a list of 50 words that range from easy to difficult in terms of the correct pronunciation. All the patient has to do is read out the words while you score the responses according to phonetic accuracy. The test is based on the premise that reading skills are fairly resilient to the deleterious effects of an acquired brain disorder and will therefore provide a marker for what the intellect was like before the patient took ill. Given the tests cultural bias, different versions have been developed for British and American subjects.

Consciousness

In a general hospital setting, a psychiatric assessment is not infrequently requested for a patient whose level of consciousness is reduced. Under these circumstances, testing higher-order cognitive functions like those subserved by the frontal lobes will not be possible. However, some information may be still gleaned from patients whose consciousness is impaired. Here the help of an informant like a nurse or family relative is useful. Issues you should consider include the following:

- Is the patient continent?
- Does the patient spontaneously open her eyes?
- Does the level of consciousness fluctuate according to time of day?

Such simple assessments can shed light on the degree to which consciousness is impaired, thereby providing a marker to judge future improvement or deterioration. Fluctuations according to time of day may suggest a delirium, particularly if a patient's mental state worsens as nightfall approaches.

Orientation

This is tested in three domains: time, place, and person. In keeping with principles outlined above, the sequence of questions moves from easy to more difficult.

- Time: year ± month ± weekday ± time of day
- Place: country ± province (state) ± city ± building
- Person: name ± age ± date of birth

Attention and Concentration

There are many different ways of testing these cognitive abilities. There may have been clues from the history that the patient is experiencing difficulties in these areas, for example, an inability to watch a television program from beginning to end, or similar difficulties concentrating on a newspaper article. Two ways to probe attention are as follows:

1. Ask the patient to give the months of the year in reverse order.
2. Ask the patient to serially subtract 7 from 100.

For both these tests, record the responses and encourage the patient to keep going until no further responses are possible. In one of the most widely cited of all psychometric tests, namely the Mini-Mental State Examination,[3] the serial 7s test is done for five subtractions only. Although undoubtedly still useful, if you bail out early in this fashion, it is often not possible for you to comment on a patient's ability to sustain attention over a more prolonged period of time, the attribute of *vigilance*. Thus, it is important with the serial 7 test for you to encourage the patient's perseverance while recording the patient's responses.

A third useful way to assess attention is the Digit Span test.[4] This test makes up one of the subtests of the Wechsler Adult Intelligence Scale and is considered a sensitive index of cerebral dysfunction in a patient with an acquired brain insult. In this test, a series of digits is presented at intervals of one per second. You start by calling out three digits and asking the patient to repeat them in the forward direction. If the correct answer is obtained, the process is repeated with four digits, then five digits, etc. Patients are allowed two chances at each level. If they correctly repeat the digits on first hearing, the examiner moves on to the next level. Once a ceiling is reached for the forward repetition of digits (usually seven digits), the process is repeated, but this time the patient is asked to repeat the digits in the reverse order. For the digit span backward, you start once again with a sequence of three digits and build up as described above until a ceiling of six digits is reached. Patients are once again allowed two chances at each level. Should a patient fail both attempts at one level, the score is taken from the previous level successfully completed. There are published, age-corrected normative data for the Digit Span test.[5] It is strongly recommended that you have the series of digits written out before testing begins.

Language

Disorders of language can be broadly divided into expressive (fluent) and receptive (nonfluent) difficulties. In a Broca-type aphasia (dominant inferior frontal lobe pathology), patients have difficulty expressing themselves, whereas in a Wernicke-type aphasia (dominant posterior superior temporal lobe lesion), the problem is primarily one of comprehension. A conduction aphasia occurs when lesions interrupt the arcuate fasciculus, the tract joining Broca's and Wernicke's area. The resultant speech is fluent, with many paraphasic errors that are mainly phonemic (see further discussion). Examining language involves four stages:

- Assessment of spontaneous speech during conversation and picture description
- Naming ability
- Comprehension
- Repetition

During *spontaneous speech* by the patient, look for the following: articulation; fluency; syntax, that is, the correct use of grammar (agrammatism is associated with Broca's aphasia); paraphasic errors or word substitutions that can either be semantic (e.g., calling a pen a pencil) or phonemic (e.g., calling a pen a pin); word-finding problems that manifest as circumlocutions (e.g., when asked to name a pen, the patient hesitates and then describes the object instead ["something to write with"]); and finally, the melodic flow to speech, which is termed *prosody*.

When testing *naming* ability, you should point to some common everyday objects like a shoe, cuff, watch, strap, buckle, etc. A chart with pictures of less common objects can then be used to challenge the patient further.

Comprehension can be tested at four levels. First, can the patient keep a conversation going? Second, can the patient respond to commands that do not require a verbal response (e.g., ask the patient to point to the door, ceiling, and floor)? Third, can the patient comprehend a sentence such as *"What color is grass?"* or *"What do we cut bread with?"* Finally, if all three levels have been successfully completed, you should move on to testing concept comprehension with questions such as, *"What do we call the man who works in a fancy restaurant and creates delicious meals?"*

Repetition must be tested because it gives clues to the presence of a transcortical aphasia. Here, the lesion lies outside the primary language areas (i.e., Broca's, Wernicke's, and the arcuate fasciculus). To test repetition, begin with one-syllable words (e.g., gun, boat) and then move through two (e.g., prosper, happy), and three (e.g., enable, postulate) syllables. Finally, ask the patient to repeat a phrase such as "no if's, and's or but's." In patients with a conduction aphasia, repetition is severely affected. In a transcortical motor aphasia, however, a patient presents with expressive difficulties as in a Broca-type picture, except repetition to various degrees is spared. In the case of a transcortical sensory aphasia, the patient resembles a Wernicke-type picture, but with repetition once again intact.

Reading

Reading is a skill that most often matches language. Ask the patient to read aloud, and then test the ability to comprehend what has been written. For example, hand the patient a piece of paper that has the sentence, "Close your eyes," written on it. On a more complex level, give the patient a paragraph of text to read aloud, and then test whether the content has been understood. Pure alexia occurs but is rare.

Writing

Ask the patient to write a sentence spontaneously and then to write a dictation from you. Agraphia, suggesting a lesion of the angular gyrus, may occur with acalculia, right-left disorientation, and finger agnosia, the four features comprising the Gerstmann syndrome.

Calculations

Calculations should be tested verbally and in writing. Assess addition, subtraction, multiplication, and division. Examples illustrating the complexity would be as follows: $12 + 37$; $45 - 16$; 9×12; $64 \div 4$.

Praxis

Apraxia refers to the inability to perform skilled motor movements in the presence of normal comprehension, muscle strength, and coordination. A distinction is made between buccofacial and limb apraxia. To test praxis, ask the patient to demonstrate how he would blow out a match, salute like a soldier, and brush his teeth. If a patient cannot follow these commands, test his ability to imitate you performing these movements.

Memory

The plethora of terms describing various aspects of memory may at first glance appear confusing. One useful approach to disentangling the terminology is as follows:[6] Memory can be subdivided into that which is effortful (known as *explicit* or *declarative*) and that which is not (called *implicit* or *procedural*). The latter cannot be tested at the bedside and involves memory that arises from conditioning, priming, and the acquisition of motor skills. Explicit memory, on the other hand, demands conscious effort and can be divided according to whether it is *short term* or *long term*. There is no absolute time distinction between the two. Rather, *short-term* memory should be thought of as immediate or working memory, or to use a computer analogy, the memory that is held "online." It can be subdivided further into *verbal* and *visual* components. Similarly, *long-term* memory (which by exclusion is all that is not immediate) can be divided into *verbal* and *visual*. *Long-term* memory may, in turn, be divided into *semantic* (i.e., factual information) and *episodic* (i.e., personally experienced and temporally specific).

In addition to the above schematic representation, there are other terms that are frequently encountered. Memory may rely on *recall* (the absence of cues) or *recognition* (cues are present). Furthermore, *anterograde* memory refers to a patient's ability to *acquire* or lay down new memories, whereas *retrograde* memory refers to the ability to *retrieve* facts and events from the past.

The following template provides a method to assess memory:

- Short-term verbal memory can be tested by asking a patient to remember a name and address (seven facts in all). Record the number of trials (up to five) that it takes the patient to do this. This simple test provides a marker of anterograde memory.
- Short-term visual memory can be tested by asking a patient to remember a series of shapes. These may be complex, as in the Rey-Osterrieth Test, or simpler, as in a series of checkerboard designs.
- Long-term verbal and nonverbal memory can be tested by asking the patient to recall the above information at the end of the entire cognitive examination. Retrograde amnesia is assessed with questions that probe semantic and episodic memory. Examples of the former are a series of general knowledge questions (e.g., *"What is the capital of Canada?" "Who is the Prime Minister of the United Kingdom?"*), whereas episodic memory can be tested by autobiographical recall.

Right-Hemisphere Skills

The assessment of right-hemisphere skills centers on various aspects of neglect and agnosia in addition to constructional and spatial abilities.

Different types of agnosia are tested as follows:

- Object recognition (visual agnosia): Ask the patient to identify common objects like keys, pen, etc.
- Finger agnosia: Ask the patient to name and move various fingers.
- Disturbance of identification body parts (autotopagnosia): Ask the patient to move on command and name various body parts.
- Estimating distances (visuospatial agnosia): Ask the patient which of two objects in the examination room is nearer.
- Facial recognition (prosopagnosia): Ask the patient to identify well-known personalities (Figure 16-1).

Personal neglect can be tested by asking the patient to discriminate left from right and thereafter various mixed combinations by instruction the patient to *"touch your left foot with your right hand"* and *"touch your left ear with*

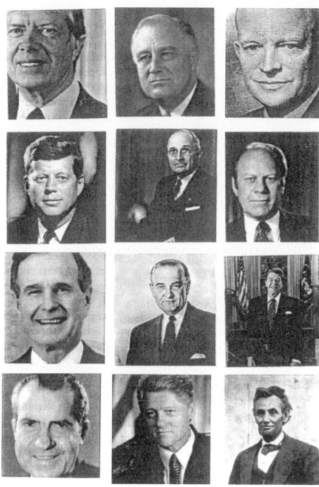

FIGURE 16-1 *Face recognition.*

the ring finger of your right hand." Hemispatial neglect can also be tested by instructing the patient to fill in the numbers on a blank clock face and mark the time at 10 minutes past 11.

Constructional ability can be tested by asking the patient to copy a series of shapes that increase in complexity from two to three dimensions (Figure 16-2).

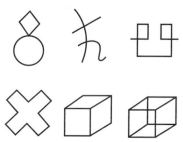

FIGURE 16-2 *Constructional ability test.*

Frontal Lobe Tasks

Before discussing a list of tests that are sensitive to frontal lobe function, a few comments on the anatomy of this region are called for. Although the prefrontal cortex is the area that subserves many aspects of cognition, an appreciation of other frontal areas is also necessary in completing an assessment:

- The motor cortex lies anterior to the central sulcus, and lesions here can result in a contralateral paralysis or paresis.
- The premotor system is important for integrating motor and sensory function with connections to the primary sensory cortex, somatosensory cortex, primary motor cortex, thalamus, and caudate nucleus. Lesions here may give rise to apraxia and difficulties with fine coordination.
- The frontal eye fields control conjugate eye gaze.
- Broca's area in the inferior frontal lobe controls the expression of speech with lesions resulting in a nonfluent aphasia.

The prefrontal cortex, pivotal in regulating mood, behavior, and cognition, contains three discrete neural circuits that run in parallel to the basal ganglia before looping back to prefrontal areas of origin:

- The dorsolateral prefrontal cortex (DLPFC) is linked to spatial and conceptual reasoning processes and plays an important role in regulating verbal fluency, attention, and certain aspects of memory.
- The ventral prefrontal cortex (VPFC) is central to behavior regulation and emotional control, including stimulus reward associations.
- The anterior cingulate prefrontal cortex (ACPFC) is pivotal in controlling motivation. Lesions here can produce varying degrees of apathy ranging from mildly reduced motivation to akinetic mutism.

The fact that these circuits run to subcortical areas explains an important clinical observation, namely that nonfrontal lesions may produce typical frontal-type behaviors through a process of disconnection (e.g., a lesion in the VPFC may give rise to disinhibited, socially inappropriate behavior characterized by an indifference to adverse consequences). Given that the VPFC circuit starts in the inferior aspect of the prefrontal cortex before relaying sequentially in the caudate nucleus, globus pallidus, substantia nigra, subthalamic nuclei, and finally certain thalamic nuclei before returning to the inferior prefrontal cortex, a lesion anywhere along this pathway may alter behavior as described previously.

There are a number of bedside frontal lobe test batteries available.[7,8] They comprise a mixture of tests that probe attention, verbal fluency, semantic memory, abstract thinking, and cognitive flexibility, the last of these referring to an ability to inhibit or modify verbal and motor responses according to changing instructions or circumstances. All these cognitive functions can be tested, and the results should be combined with behavioral observations that better reflect the functioning of the VPFC because this region defies neat psychometric correlations. Some commonly used tests that are sensitive to the functional integrity of the prefrontal cortex include the following:

- Initiation tasks: The most widely used is the COWAT or letter fluency test.[1] Here the patient is required to produce orally as many words as possible beginning with the letters F, A, and S. The patient is allowed 1 minute per letter, and at the end of the test the person's totals are added to give the final score. Patients are instructed not to use proper names (e.g., Sydney, Simon, Sue) or the same word with different endings (e.g., fun, funnier, funniest). Like the Digit Span test, there are published normative data for the COWAT.
- Analogous tests: An analogous test calls for the patient to name as many four-legged animals as possible in 1 minute.
- Abstraction
  - □ Abstraction ability is tested by asking the patient to interpret the proverb, *"A bird in the hand is worth two in the bush."* The examiner must be sensitive to education and cultural issues here.
  - □ A second way to test abstract thinking is to ask the patient a series of questions: *"In what way are the following paired items similar and different . . ."*
    - *"Car and bus?"*
    - *"Apple and pear?"*
- Response inhibition and shift testing: This can be tested as follows:
  - □ Go–No Go test: Ask the patient to raise one index finger in response to one tap on the table. The patient is not to respond when you tap twice. The patient should not see you tap, so use the undersurface of the table for this. Having completed 10 trials, switch instructions (e.g., the patient must not respond to one tap, but must raise an index finger when you tap twice). Failure to inhibit responses when none are called for is deemed pathological.
  - □ Alternating hand movements: In this test, one had forms a fist while the other has fingers extended, palm facing toward the patient. Alternate these positions between the right and left hand three times, then ask the patient to repeat what you have just done.

- □ The Luria three-step procedure: This calls for you to perform a sequence of movements with the right hand, using the left hand as a base with fingers extended and palm pointing upward.
  - Step 1: Fist strikes palm.
  - Step 2: Edge of hand with fingers extended strikes palm.
  - Step 3: Palm strikes palm.

Repeat this three times, then ask the patient to reproduce what you have just done. The patient should perform the sequence five times. Then ask the patient to repeat the process with the right hand acting as the base and the left hand completing the three-step sequence.

NEUROPSYCHOLOGICAL TESTING

Although the cognitive examination outlined above has significantly greater sensitivity than screening instruments such as the Mini-Mental State Examination,[3] it still falls short of a detailed neuropsychological assessment. The latter, however, is time consuming and expensive. Furthermore, many clinicians do not have ready access to such a service. All of this raises the question of when to refer a patient with a neurological illness to a neuropsychologist.

Indications for undertaking a formal neuropsychological assessment include the following:

- Colleagues or superiors report a decline in a person's work performance, or the person reports subjective cognitive difficulties in the absence of a prominent mood, substance use, or anxiety disorder.
- A patient is applying for a disability settlement.
- A patient is about to enter a treatment trial that may improve (or harm) cognition. A cognitive baseline is therefore required.
- A patient is entering a cognitive rehabilitation program. Once again, a cognitive baseline is needed to determine relative strengths and weaknesses.

CORTICAL VERSUS SUBCORTICAL DEMENTIA

The cognitive profile in patients with neurological disorders can differ according to whether the burden of disease is cortical or subcortical. Senile dementia of the Alzheimer type may be regarded as the quintessential cortical dementing illness, whereas Huntington's and Parkinson's diseases represent typical subcortical gray-matter dementias, and multiple sclerosis represents the white-matter equivalent. It is important to emphasize that these cortical/subcortical distinctions are not neatly defined anatomical divisions; rather, they reflect differing functional profiles. Thus, apraxia, agnosia, and aphasia are all markers of cortical rather than subcortical cognitive abnormalities. On the other hand, one of the hallmarks of subcortical deficits is delayed information-processing speed. Therefore, patients will have difficulty with timed tasks such as the COWAT. Although both groups may display prominent memory problems, cortically based disorders may result in relatively greater difficulty acquiring new information, whereas in patients with a greater subcortical burden, memory deficits may be more pronounced when *retrieval* is challenged. In more advanced disease, these distinctions can become blurred. Nevertheless, clinicians must remember that a widely used brief cognitive screening measure like the Mini-Mental State Examination is geared toward cortical cognitive deficits and lacks sensitivity for predominantly white-matter dementias like multiple sclerosis.

NEUROIMAGING

Brain imaging can be either structural (e.g., computed tomography [CT], magnetic resonance imaging [MRI]) or functional (e.g., single photon emission computed tomography [SPECT], positron emission tomography [PET], functional MRI [fMRI]). For clinicians, CT, MRI, and SPECT are the commonly available modalities. PET and fMRI are still largely limited to research protocols.

MRI has many advantages over CT when it comes to structural brain imaging. These include greater anatomical sensitivity, improved visualization of cerebral white matter, and the ability to image the posterior fossa and medial temporal lobe structures without bone artefact. MRI technology does not make use of radiation, thereby facilitating serial studies. Finally, the brain can be easily scanned in the axial, coronal, and sagittal planes. CT, on the other hand, is cheaper and, in the early stages after traumatic brain injury, may be preferred given the isodense properties of blood.

Neuroimaging is an important ancillary investigation for the following reasons:

- It may help the neurologist diagnostically.
- It may provide important clues to the neurologist and psychiatrist concerning cerebral localization. However, here is it important to remember that a lesion at one anatomical location may exert functional effects that are removed from it, a process called *diaschisis*.
- It may provide clues as to why a patient's behavior has altered. In this regard, it forms one part of a workup that starts with history-taking and proceeds through the neurological and mental state examinations, detailed cognitive assessment, and other investigations (e.g., biochemical, electroencephalogram) if pertinent. What a clinician is looking for here is a *confluence* of findings.
  - □ One example of a clinical situation in which all the data come together neatly is as follows: The history suggests stroke; the neurological examination confirms a right-sided weakness; cognitive assessment reveals an expressive aphasia; MRI shows a left frontal hemorrhage; and SPECT demonstrates hypoperfusion in the area of the lesion. In this example, neuroimaging is essentially confirmatory. However, another common clinical situation where neuroimaging carries added diagnostic weight is as follows: The history reveals subtle personality change characterized by mildly inappropriate social behavior; neurological examination is normal; so too is the formal mental state; the cognitive assessment demonstrates mildly reduced verbal fluency (e.g., fewer than expected words on the FAS test); MRI shows mild frontal atrophy; and SPECT displays moderately severe frontal hypoperfusion. The confluence of the history and neuroimaging findings points strongly toward a diagnosis of fronto-temporal dementia.

CONCLUSIONS

This chapter has provided a template for the psychiatrist, resident, and medical student to use in the assessment of patients with neurological illness. Given the high prevalence of cognitive deficits in neurological disorders, completing a clinically based cognitive assessment is mandatory to any comprehensive assessment. Furthermore, the information obtained is of considerable practical importance, for there are data linking deficits to many other real-world difficulties patients experience. These range from the workplace to relationships to the basic activities of daily living, all of which adversely impinge on quality of life. Completing an examination as outlined in this chapter will therefore not only enhance the diagnostic process, but will also assist in determining effective treatment and rehabilitation strategies.

REFERENCES

1. Benton AJ, Hamsher K, Sivan AB: *Multilingual aphasia examination,* Iowa City, IA, 1983, AJA Associates.
2. Nelson HE: *National Adult Reading Test (NART): test manual,* Windsor, England, 1982, NFER Nelson.
3. Folstein MF, Folstein SE, McHugh PR: "Mini-Mental State": a practical method for grading the cognitive state of patients for the clinician, *J Psychiatric Res* 12:189–198, 1975.

4. Wechsler D: *Wechsler adult intelligence scale–revised,* New York, 1981, Psychological Corporation.

5. Spreen O, Strauss E: *A compendium of neuropsychological tests,* ed 2, New York, 1998, Oxford University Press.

6. Hodges JR: *Cognitive assessment for clinicians,* Oxford, England, 1994, Oxford University Press, pp 5–19.

7. Dubois B, Slachevsky A, Litvan I, Pillon B: The FAB: a frontal assessment battery at bedside, *Neurology* 55:1621–1626, 2000.

8. Ettlin TM, Kischka U, Beckson M, et al: The frontal lobe score: part 1. Construction of a mental status of frontal systems, *Clin Rehabil* 14:260–271, 2000.

17

Assessment of Patients with Intellectual Disabilities

ELSPETH A. BRADLEY AND SHEILA HOLLINS

INTRODUCTION

The following Case Example introduces a man with a differential diagnosis of depression, atypical grief reaction, or dementia. He differs from the typical patient you will see in your clinic because he has moderate intellectual disability. You have probably had little, if any, experience with people with intellectual disabilities. You may be anxious and feel unskilled when presented with such a referral. We aim to help you to manage your anxiety and to prepare for your first meeting so that you will be able to provide a reliable opinion and management plan suitable for the needs and circumstances of someone with intellectual disability. We will introduce you to the ways in which your assessment and management of Mr. Jones will be similar to your usual practice and explore ways in which you may need to modify your approach. We will conclude with several vignettes that illustrate typical clinical presentations you may encounter. By the end of the chapter, you should be able to do the following:

- Understand the ways in which intellectual disabilities, and associated comorbidities, can change the presentation of psychiatric disorder
- Understand the importance of the communicative function of behavior disturbances
- Adapt your communication style for someone with limited expressive and/or receptive language, and use pictures to support communication
- Know how to work with an informant

- Understand the importance of environmental factors (supports and expectations) in the genesis of the presenting problem
- Understand the difference between the management and the treatment of behavioral and psychiatric disturbances
- Appreciate that the cause of the intellectual disability may have implications for mental health across the life span
- Create a treatment environment

Case Example 1

Paul Jones has been referred to your outpatient clinic by his concerned family physician. The physician explains that Paul is a 32-year-old man with Down syndrome living with his 75-year-old widowed mother. He has had little contact with health services in the past because he has enjoyed good health, apart from needing to have his ears syringed regularly and having annual thyroid function testing. Paul always attends appointments with his mother, who tends to speak for him, although Paul has quite good comprehension and enjoys a joking relationship with the receptionist and the clinic nurse. Mrs. Jones reports that Paul has become very withdrawn since his father died 2 years ago, and recently he has been enuretic and encopretic. His sister, a gynecologist, wonders whether he is developing dementia, knowing that this occurs earlier in persons with Down syndrome, or whether his symptoms are due to a prolonged and atypical grief reaction.

Table 17-1. Approach to Psychotherapy Assessment

Collect patient from the waiting area on time with or without his care provider.
Ask whether he would like to be seen.
Therapists—introduce yourself using your first name.

Therapist	**Patient**
"Do you know why you have come here today?"	Usually says no
"Your carer/nurse/GP said you have got some worries. She thinks you need some help to think about your worries. Is that right?"	Usually silent, sometimes a nod
"You are brave coming to see us today (said with warmth). What are you worried about?"	Often tearful: "My mother died," or "Someone hurt me," or a nonverbal movement that suggests pain or avoidance
"That's upsetting. Do you want to tell me more about this?"	

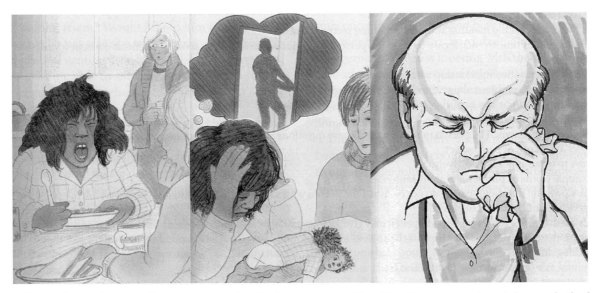

Note: This may be a good point to offer some pictures related to the presenting problem. The pictures may need a verbal prompt by the therapist (e.g., *"Have you ever felt like that?"* or *"What do you think is happening in the picture?"*)

Within 10 to 15 minutes:

"Would you like to talk to someone about this? In a group, or on your own with one other person?"	Usually able to decide quite quickly
"We will find a therapist for you. It may take some time to find the right person."	

Pictures here are taken from the Books Beyond Words counseling series of 30 books for people who find pictures easier to read than words. See www.rcpsych.ac.uk/publications/bbw. (From Hollins S, Horrocks C, Sinason V: I can get through it, London, 1998, Books Beyond Words, Gaskell Press, and St. George's Hospital Medical School; Hollins S, Sireling L: When Mum died, ed 3, London, 2004, Books Beyond Words, St. George's Hospital Medical School, and Gaskell Press. With permission of Hollins and Sinason, 2004.)

previous assessments (e.g., psychological and communication) about premorbid functioning. In the absence of such information, although the MSE provides a structured approach to observe and experience the patient, any diagnostic formulations should remain provisional.

Further guidance in modifying the psychiatric diagnostic interview for persons with intellectual disabilities and suggested questions to elicit information about abnormal experiences are available in several recent publications.[3-5]

Key Point:

Information gained from meeting with a person with intellectual disability is often insufficient to make a definitive psychiatric diagnosis. The meeting is important in establishing the beginning of a treatment alliance, and this is facilitated by attending to the person's own feelings and perceptions about the reason for the consultation and by asking about any worries or concerns.

PSYCHIATRIC AND BEHAVIOR DISTURBANCES IN PERSONS WITH INTELLECTUAL DISABILITY

Psychiatric Disorders

Persons with intellectual disabilities display the same range of psychiatric disorders as the general population, but the prevalence of these disorders is three to four times greater. In addition, some disorders (e.g., stereotypies and self-injurious behaviors [SIB]) are unique or more prevalent in this group.

A psychiatric diagnosis generally requires both an account of the person's subjective experience/symptoms (e.g., feelings and thoughts) and descriptions of the person's behavior/signs (either self-articulated or provided by an informant). Intellectual disabilities can greatly alter the clinical presentation of psychiatric disorders, partly because the subjective account is less available in lower-functioning persons and partly because the person may communicate his distress through alternative behaviors (e.g., one of our patients who was subsequently diagnosed with depression was referred because of his "annoying behavior" of swallowing batteries and coins). In general, the mental health disturbances, clinical presentation, and treatment needs of persons with mild intellectual disabilities are more closely aligned to the general population (without intellectual disabilities) than to the specific problems presented by those with more severe intellectual disabilities. However, even persons with milder intellectual disabilities have difficulties communicating their subjective experiences and inner discomforts, particularly when health care workers are unaware of the accommodations they need to make to assist. This can give rise to misdiagnoses and inappropriate treatments.

For persons with *autism*, the clinical presentation may be even more atypical. A diagnosis of autism or autism spectrum disorder usually has significant implications for the person's daily support needs. Treatment of psychiatric disorder in persons with comorbid autism and intellectual disability is unlikely to offer much benefit if these supports and understanding are not available. Not infrequently, persons with autism and milder intellectual disabilities, attempting to communicate their distress, may be perceived by caregivers as "manipulative" and "demanding," whereas those with more severe disabilities and autism communicate their distress in the form of severe aggression toward others, the environment, or self (i.e., SIB).

The clinical picture of those with intellectual disabilities (with or without autism) is further complicated by the reality that the same disturbed behavior can arise from different etiologies (e.g., medical disorder, emotional upset, or psychiatric disorder), and likewise the same psychiatric disorder (e.g., depression) can give rise to different changes in behavior (e.g., aggression or withdrawal).

Aggression

Aggression is the most frequent reason a psychiatric evaluation is sought. The differential diagnosis of aggressive behaviors is shown in Table 17-2. Multiple etiological factors may coexist, so that the contextual issues (e.g., when, where, and with whom the aggression arose) also have to be documented and understood.

Psychotic Disorders

In general terms, *psychotic disorders* are overdiagnosed in this population, and consequently, antipsychotic medication is overprescribed. It is important to determine whether psychotic-like behaviors represent behavioral decompensation in a stressful environment or a psychotic disorder (e.g., schizophrenia) because the treatment is different: the former responds optimally to changes in the environment and expectations on the person, and the latter to medication. Persons with severe intellectual disability (IQ < 50) do not have the language skills necessary for a diagnosis of schizophrenia. However, the severity of the intellectual impairment is not always recognized without more formal psychological assessment, and the apparent poverty of speech or repetitive speech noted in the acute care setting may be misinterpreted as part of the deficit state of schizophrenia.

Mood and Anxiety Disorders

Mood and anxiety disorders tend to be underdiagnosed, and consequently medications for these disorders are underused. Anxiety disorders are still poorly understood in this population, but environmental factors (e.g., environments that are stressful because they are not attuned to the specific developmental challenges the person has) are likely to be important in the etiology and therefore the treatment of these disorders. *Post-traumatic stress disorder* (PTSD) is also underdiagnosed in this group, and we need to be mindful that some of the clinical procedures used with the general population (e.g., restraints and seclusion in inpatient psychiatric wards to manage disruptive behaviors) may be anti-therapeutic for some patients with

Table 17-2. Differential Diagnosis of Aggression

Aggression Associated With:	Causes of Aggression	
	Observed or Hypothesized	*Experienced*
Health Problems	■ Pain and/or injury ■ Medical illness ■ Medication side effects ■ Seizure related ■ Dental problems	Changed experience of self giving rise to fears, anxieties, and confusion. Limited understanding will escalate fears (e.g., fear of medical procedures, fear of dying) and further distort perceptions.
Supports and Expectations	■ Inappropriate expectations and/or inadequate supports ■ Inability to express needs ■ A way to obtain positive reinforcers ■ A way to avoid an uncomfortable circumstance	Embarrassment, humiliation, shame, fear, anxiety, cognitive disintegration and psychological fragmentation, and empathic failures (i.e., perceptual and cognitive impairments not understood by care providers).
Emotional	■ Loss and/or bereavement ■ Disappointment ■ Changes in environment or daily life ■ Bullying or assault ■ Unexpected changes ■ Task-related anxiety ■ Difficulties modulating affect	Upset, confusion, loss of control, mistrust, fear, anxiety, and emotional lability.
Psychiatric Disorder	■ Reflects irritability secondary to mania, depression, or organic mental syndrome ■ Associated with psychotic experiences (e.g., hallucinations, delusions)	Changed experience of self and distorted perceptions giving rise to distrust, fear, anxieties, and confusion.

With permission from Bradley and Hollins, 2004.

intellectual disabilities (given their level of understanding) and will add to their emotional distress.

Obsessive and Compulsive Behaviors and Attention Disorders

Obsessive and compulsive behaviors and problems with *attention, impulsivity, and hyperactivity* are more prevalent in persons with intellectual disability compared with the general population (particularly so for some etiological subgroups, e.g., autism). However, it may be problematic to differentiate obsessive compulsive behaviors from ritualistic and perseverative behaviors, especially in lower-functioning persons, and to determine whether problems with attention, impulsivity, and hyperactivity, while inappropriate given the chronological age, may not be so inappropriate given the person's mental age. Therefore, a description of these behaviors as they emerge over time is important from a treatment perspective. Sometimes these behaviors meet DSM-IV-TR criteria for disorder such as attention deficit/hyperactivity disorder (ADHD) or obsessive compulsive disorder (OCD), and standard treatment

for these disorders can be tried. However, it is recommended that each behavior be carefully and separately monitored because there may be a differential treatment response.

Tics, Self-Injurious Behavior, and Stereotypies

Tics, SIB, and stereotypies are also more prevalent among persons with intellectual disability. However, these may also occur for the first time after psychotropic medication, underscoring the need to routinely screen for these behaviors before starting the administration of such medication.

Where possible, episodic/new-onset disorders (e.g., depressive, hypomanic, psychotic disorders) should be differentiated from more chronic background conditions (e.g., hyperactivity or compulsive behaviors) and disorders (e.g., ADHD, OCD). Chronic conditions may be associated with the biological circumstances giving rise to the intellectual disability or the psychological consequences during childhood of growing up with that disability. New-onset/episodic disorders and chronic conditions can also coexist (e.g., bipolar affective disorder, hyperactivity, tics, and compulsive behaviors is a pattern sometimes seen in persons with autism). In such potential complexity, it is essential to adopt a systematic assessment approach (Figures 17-1 and 17-2; see Psychiatric Assessment: Key Areas of Inquiry section) and to carefully document all such symptoms and behaviors to determine which ones may herald a new-onset psychiatric disorder and which ones may be long-standing. Clarifying these circumstances leads to more targeted intervention and better outcomes.

Diagnostic Overshadowing

Diagnostic overshadowing occurs when all the changed or unusual behaviors are attributed to the intellectual disability or, conversely, everything is attributed to a psychiatric disorder without due acknowledgment of the impact of one on the other. The phenomenon of the *cloak of competence* occurs when a person with intellectual disability, because of some relatively good skills, gives the impression of greater understanding and functioning than are actually present. Both phenomena point to the need for care providers in the health care and developmental sectors to work closely together and draw on each other's skills.

Comorbidity

In addition to psychiatric comorbidity, persons with intellectual disabilities may have other comorbidities that contribute to behavior disturbances.

Developmental

Not all persons with the same IQ (see functioning levels below) have the same cognitive/psychological challenges; differences in expressive and receptive language abilities, visual and auditory perceptual processing, and memory and learning styles, for example, can give rise to a mixed profile of skills and abilities. If not recognized, this can result in frustration for caregivers because they may gauge the overall ability of the persons on their strengths and have inappropriate expectations of them, giving rise to emotional disturbances. Sound psychological and communication evaluations are helpful in teasing out these issues.

Medical

Other disabilities such as hearing, visual, and motor impairments (e.g., cerebral palsy) are greatly increased in this population, as are medical disorders (e.g., seizure and sleep disorders, gastroesophageal reflex disorder, thyroid

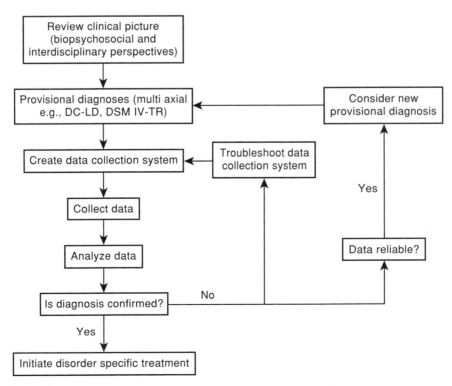

FIGURE 17-1 *The psychiatric diagnostic process.*

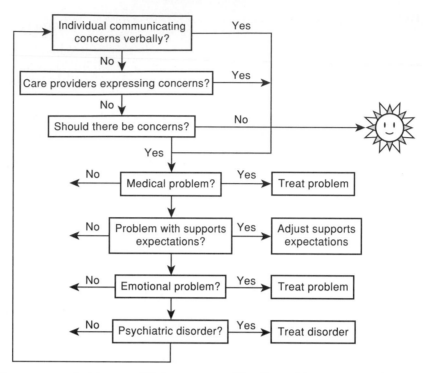

FIGURE 17-2 *Mental health assessment: decision tree. (With permission of Bradley and Summers, 2004.)*

dysfunction) and dental needs. It is essential that primary health care for persons with intellectual disabilities be proactive and preventive because otherwise many of these treatable conditions remain hidden and contribute to unnecessary discomfort and behavior disturbances. In any psychiatric assessment, these potential conditions should be looked for routinely. It is also helpful to inquire about how the person communicates physical pain and emotional upsets. This alerts care providers to the subtleties of the person's verbal and nonverbal behaviors so that they become more accurate observers of the person during the assessment and treatment phases and in monitoring side effects of medication.

Key Point:

Developmental, medical, and other comorbidities can distort the presentation of psychiatric disturbance.

Medical Syndromes and Behavioral Phenotypes

There are many medical syndromes associated with intellectual disability. Identifying these syndromes can alert the well-versed clinician to possible underlying medical condi-

tions across the life span. Behavioral phenotypes are specific patterns of behaviors associated with a genetic etiology such as Down, fragile X, Prader-Willi, Angelman, Rett, and 22q11.2 deletion syndromes. Identifying these phenotypes is important because they may be associated with specific psychiatric vulnerabilities (e.g., schizophrenia in 22q11.2 deletion syndrome). For many of these syndromes and behavioral phenotypes, practice guidelines for medical and psychiatric care across the life span are available.[6]

Levels of Dependency and Optimal Supports

Persons with intellectual disabilities are more dependent on others and their support environment in their daily existence. Unmet needs can give rise to a variety of behavior disturbances (e.g., behavior that is oppositional and aggressive) and to psychiatric disorders (e.g., depression or PTSD).

Personality Disorders

Personality disorders are reportedly higher in this population, but you should be wary of diagnosing a disorder that reflects more on the person's level of functioning (e.g., dependent personality disorder) and his legitimate need for certain supports.

DIAGNOSTIC SYSTEMS

The DSM IV-TR[2] and the *ICD-10 Classification of Mental and Behavioral Disorders*[7] are most widely used in making psychiatric diagnoses. Both are standardized on the general population. Criteria for psychiatric disorders, particularly in intellectually lower-functioning persons, are not developmentally appropriate. For example, symptom criteria are generally weighted toward verbal and complex concepts (e.g., self-reports about guilt, feeling suicidal). Also, neither system adequately acknowledges the multiple problems and circumstances that arise in the lives of persons with intellectual disabilities.

The ICD-10 Guide for Mental Retardation (ICD-10 MR)[8] recommends a multiaxial diagnostic approach: axis I, severity of retardation and problem behaviors; axis II, associated medical conditions; axis III, associated psychiatric disorders; axis IV, global assessment of psychosocial disability; and axis V, associated abnormal psychosocial situations faced by persons with intellectual disability. These are not to be confused with the five axes of the DSM-IV-TR, where mental retardation and borderline intellectual function are coded on axis II.

DC-LD: Diagnostic Criteria for Psychiatric Disorders for Use with Adults with Learning Disabilities/Mental Retardation[4] is a consensus-based (intellectual disability psychiatrists in the United Kingdom) system designed to be complementary to the ICD manuals and available for use when existing ICD-10 criteria are inadequate, as is the case for persons with moderate to profound intellectual disability. Again, a multiaxial system is used: axis I, severity of intellectual disabilities; axis II, causes of intellectual disabilities; axis III level A, developmental disorders; axis III level B, psychiatric illness; axis III level C, personality disorders; axis III level D, problem behaviors; axis III level E, other disorders; Appendix 1, intellectual disability syndromes and behavioral phenotypes; Appendix 2, other associated medical conditions; and Appendix 3, factors influencing health status and contact with health services.

In terms of understanding ICD-10 psychiatric diagnoses as they apply to persons with intellectual disabilities, and how the clinical interview should be modified, *Practice Guidelines for the Assessment and Diagnosis of Mental Health Problems in Adults with Intellectual Disabilities*[3] offers an international review of current evidence and consensus opinion from clinicians working in the field. In conducting the clinical interview, reference is made to the Psychiatric Assessment Schedule for Adults with Developmental Disabilities (PAS-ADD),[9] a semi-structured interview with both the patient and a key informant. This instrument has a three-tier structure that allows it to be adapted according to the linguistic ability of the participant. It is an excellent teaching tool because it includes questions to elicit particular features (e.g., psychosis) that can usefully be adopted in more informal clinical assessments.

RATING SCALES

There is a wealth of rating scales now available and comprehensively reviewed by Aman[10] and O'Brien et al.[11] One such scale, the Aberrant Behavior Checklist–Community (ABC-C),[12] has been shown to be a useful measure of change over time at all levels of disability after an intervention. This is an informant-based measure comprising five scales:

I. Irritability, agitation, crying
II. Lethargy, social withdrawal
III. Stereotypic behavior
IV. Hyperactivity, noncompliance
V. Inappropriate speech

Reliability and validity data are well established.

Another set of scales that identify changes in behavior over time or before and after an intervention are the Health of the Nation Outcome Scales for People with Learning Disabilities,[13] developed by the Royal College of Psychiatrists in the United Kingdom. In general terms, rating scales are best used to document behaviors against which, for example, interventions may be tracked and evaluated. They may be useful as screening tools for psychiatric disorder, but such use must be followed up by comprehensive evaluations as described above.

Key Point:

The differential diagnosis of behavior and psychiatric disturbances is outlined in Figure 17-1 and Table 17-2.

CLINICAL CONTEXT AND USE OF MEDICATION

The psychiatric assessment usually requires several meetings. Often, persons present in crises and have to be managed more urgently.[14] It is important, therefore, to differentiate between "management" and "treatment." Management deals with the immediate problem (often medications are used to manage acute distress or disruptive behaviors, and sometimes, in the short term, the problems diminish). However, without greater participation of the multidisciplinary team (providing psychological, behavioral, and occupational communication perspectives) and

Medical Status

- Ask about motor impairments (e.g., cerebral palsy).
- Ask whether hearing and vision have been tested, and request a copy of the most recent review.
- Inquire about seizures in the past and present.
- Explore for other medical problems. In particular, explore for pain-related disorders that may not be immediately apparent, such as wisdom teeth and other dental problems, headaches, problems with feet, joints and spine, bones, arthritis, upper gastrointestinal problems, constipation, diarrhea, and food intolerance. For women, be alert for premenstrual syndrome and menopausal changes.
- Determine whether the etiology of the intellectual disability is known and whether a syndrome has been identified. If identified, what are the medical problems associated with that etiology or syndrome? Does this patient have any of these associated medical problems?
- How involved is the family physician? Is proactive medical care provided? For example, is the family doctor aware of the syndrome and associated medical disorders and providing interventions for these?

Medication

- List current medication, doses, and times given.
- Inquire about past medications and any adverse response to past medications. Caregivers supporting persons with intellectual disability are usually able and willing to prepare a comprehensive medication history and will bring this to the consultation if requested to do so.
- Note history of any allergies.

Family History

- Explore for intellectual disability, emotional and psychiatric disorders (and response to any medications tried), seizures, dementia, and other systemic disorders.
- Ask about conditions that cause pain (e.g., family history of migraine, premenstrual syndrome).
- Substance misuse in families may be relevant to current illness and may be a pointer to etiology (e.g., fetal alcohol syndrome).

Social History and Circumstances

- Ask caregivers to prepare a biographical time line of the patient's past (i.e., in chronological order list an account of the events and changes that have occurred in the person's life).
- Inquire about school and work history and history of previous placements. This information gives clues to the person's behavior in other settings with different levels of supports and expectations. It also provides information on previous level of functioning and abilities.
- Ask about past and present social supports; identify current networks of both informal and specialized support (e.g., do caregivers have a clear plan of what to do when there is a behavioral crisis?).

Life Events and Trauma

- Significant life events and trauma must always be explored and considered, even if not recent.
- Explore any history of previous separations (and the client's response to these), traumatic experiences, and abuses.
- Inquire about past and present emotional relationships and supports. This information is helpful in identifying the person's emotional needs and how best to support these.

Psychological and Communication Profile

- Do you understand the person's psychological profile (cognitive, perceptual, learning style), strengths and difficulties, and capacity for receptive and expressive communication?
- Do caregivers understand the person's abilities and specific difficulties?
- Are the expectations placed on this person appropriate?
- Has there been a deterioration in his skills and abilities?
- Is further assessment required?

REVIEW OF PREVIOUS ASSESSMENTS: HELPFUL INFORMATION AND WHAT ELSE MAY BE NEEDED

Psychiatric Assessments

Exercise caution in cases where the previous diagnosis was made in a hurry (e.g., in the emergency room) or by someone unfamiliar with persons with intellectual disabilities and in the absence of a multidisciplinary assessment (e.g., generic health care setting)—the wrong diagnosis can stick for years. Any diagnosis should be supported by symptoms and behaviors that contributed to the diagnosis; otherwise, treat with caution until you become more familiar with the patient's symptoms and behaviors and his support environment. Where possible, tracking patterns of psychiatric disturbance over the years is helpful in establishing onset of first disturbance and subsequent episodic patterns. A clear description of the first episode of psychiatric disturbance is often invaluable; subsequent inappropriate interventions and adverse effects of medications often cloud the diagnostic picture. Previous assessments often have embedded gems of information (e.g., history of nasal voice and cardiac problems), which take on new meaning as new research findings become available (e.g., discovery of 22q11.2 deletion syndrome, which is associated with schizophrenia, congenital heart disease, and velopharyngeal incompetence). Multiple diagnoses for the same person covering the gamut of psychiatric disorders should alert you to a possible underlying autism spectrum disorder (see Box 17-2).

Psychological Assessment

A psychological assessment should provide more comprehensive understanding of psychological functioning (perceptual, cognitive, processing) and help to identify support needs. Often done during the person's school career, such assessments provide an opportunity to track changes in functioning over time to determine whether there has been an improvement or a decline. Better functioning while at school and a decline in later years may point to less than adequate supports after leaving school or some other cause—this can be investigated (e.g., by putting in more appropriate supports). Assessment also provides important information on a person's response to testing and expectations, response to failure, and learning style (e.g., Is learning best with visual or auditory material, or both?). Determine whether further psychological or adaptive functioning assessment would be helpful.

Psychotherapy Assessment

A psychotherapy assessment may provide information about emotional intelligence. The patient, psychiatrist, and psychotherapist working together may contribute to more attuned medication monitoring.

Communication Assessment

A communication assessment will reveal discrepancies in receptive/expressive language and point to possible auditory, visual, or language-processing problems and possible early developmental language disorder or comorbid autism (all relevant in the differential diagnosis of psychotic-like behaviors).

Occupational Therapy Assessment

Particularly helpful in the assessment of persons with autism and/or sensory integration problems (e.g., fragile X), an occupational therapy assessment can result in helpful recommendations for interventions and appropriate sensory diet.

Behavior Therapy Assessment

A behavior therapy assessment will determine what was done in the past and what worked. Has a functional analysis of the behaviors of concern been done? Is it needed? Are behavioral escalation protocols available with recommendations for interventions at each point in the escalation? Have problematic behaviors been operationally defined and target behaviors identified against which to monitor medication and other interventions? Are there protocols for crisis management and as-required usage?

Developmental Pediatric Assessment

A developmental pediatric assessment usually provides details of early behavior (e.g., autism behaviors) described when the patient was a youngster, even when the diagnosis was never made or forgotten about as an adult. These may point to a syndrome or describe physical features that are now recognized as associated with a particular syndrome, and the person can be referred for genetic/dysmorphological assessment and confirmation. These assessments may comment on early neurological vulnerability (e.g., incontinence) or other conditions that should now be followed up and given new understanding. It is always important to pursue the etiology of the intellectual disability because this may point to medical and psychiatric vulnerability across the life span, and potential conditions which, if identified, may be preventable.

> **Key Point:**
>
> A comprehensive interdisciplinary assessment usually results in better outcomes:
> - More appropriate support of developmental needs
> - More accurate diagnosis of emotional and psychiatric disorder
> - Targeted treatment (e.g., counseling, psychotherapy, behavior support, environmental alteration, support to caregivers and adjustment of expectations)
> - Less inappropriate medication and less need for medication

DIAGNOSTIC PROCESS

After meeting with the referred person and members of her support system, a provisional diagnosis is generated (see Figures 17-1 and 17-2), and recommendations are made. Implementation often requires working closely with care providers to agree on a treatment strategy and establish a treatment environment and a monitoring system (e.g., of mood, anxiety, eating pattern, sleep) to assess response to treatment (see Figure 17-2). Where the nature of the psychiatric disturbance remains unclear, treatment/ intervention trials (e.g., of medication and/or behavioral support) can be considered with careful monitoring of response as identified by operationally defined specific behaviors.

In arriving at a definitive psychiatric diagnosis (which may take several weeks or months), you need, as previously stated, to be aware of the difference between *managing the behaviors of concern* (often successfully achieved with medication or other more intrusive strategies but possibly leading to "chronic crises management") and *treating the underlying disorder* that is the root cause of the behaviors of concern (often less successfully achieved when interdisciplinary input is not available).

INVESTIGATIONS

Investigations should be done as indicated for any medical disorders suggested by the history (e.g., descriptions of occasional choking/vomiting and sleep disturbance would raise concerns about gastroesophageal reflux disorder), physical examination (e.g., reluctance to having a body part examined might point to pain), provisional psychiatric diagnosis (e.g., dementia), or presence of a syndrome (e.g., Down syndrome—thyroid testing and screen for sensory impairments). Many adults with intellectual disabilities have never been investigated for the cause of their disability, and such investigations should be offered. Others may have had some previous investigations, but with new diagnostic tools becoming available (especially for genetic disorders) these persons might also be reviewed.

TREATMENT ENVIRONMENT

An optimal treatment environment involves the following:

- Support the person according to her developmental needs; that is, provide supports and expectations appropriate to her level of functioning and specific to any comorbid disabilities (e.g., autism, auditory processing problems).
- Remember that when the person is in distress, her level of functioning may be lower, and environmental supports need to be increased as required.
- Establish clear protocols for what to do when the person escalates or gets upset (e.g., use an escalation hierarchy with clear descriptions of person's behavior along the continuum as she escalates and clearly prescribed staff interactions at each point along this continuum). This promotes structure and consistency, helps the person de-escalate, and contains anxiety (in staff members as well).

- Recognize that staff turnover in residential and day settings is often high, and written protocols and training for new staff are essential to ensure continuity of care. Where this does not occur, anxiety can escalate for both care providers and the person with intellectual disability, giving rise to crises that may mistakenly be attributed to a deterioration in the person's mental health state. In these circumstances, the person may be given further medication, giving rise to greater medication side effects, which may result in further behavioral escalation in the client. Without an adequate assessment and treatment environment, many appropriate psychiatric and behavioral interventions will be rendered useless and the person with intellectual disability labeled as violent and dangerous when in fact the problem lies more with the system of supports than with the person.
- Recognize that staff training is usually enhanced by involving patients and care providers in the training and in identifying their own support priorities.

Case Example 3

Peter, a man with intermittent severe challenging behavior who has a moderate intellectual disability and some autistic traits, was sharing his own house with a co-tenant named Mary. Mary had learned that the arrival of the postman in the morning was a highlight in Peter's day and that sorting the post was his "job." A new "sleep-in" worker picked up the post one morning and triggered a violent incident. The support team recognized that this was a failure of staff training.

Be aware that some interventions that are helpful to the patient may run counter to usual policy and vice versa (e.g., physical restraint in community settings is often seen as intrusive and therefore the last option, but for some persons restraint may be therapeutic, and the treatment goals would then be to help the person manage with less restraint). Idiosyncratic treatment needs of persons with intellectual disability are not infrequent and need to be acknowledged and worked out case by case involving key stakeholders and persons consenting to the treatment.

In addition, recognize that staff burnout is high in this service area and that staff need to feel heard and supported.

Key Point:

Psychiatric assessment involves both an assessment of the person and an assessment of his support environment to ascertain the extent to which the referral problems are located in the system of supports (e.g., inappropriate expectations) and the extent to which they reflect patient issues (e.g., seizure or psychiatric disorder), or a mix of both (e.g., seizures increase in certain stressful environments).

> **Key Point:**
> ___
> Assessment of the person's developmental support needs is the initial stage in identifying and maintaining an optimal treatment environment.

> **Key Point:**
> ___
> It is prudent to differentiate clearly between "management" and "treatment" of the referral concerns.

> **Key Point:**
> ___
> Care providers are an integral part of the treatment team, implementing intervention strategies and providing feedback about progress.

ADDITIONAL CASE EXAMPLES

Further clinical vignettes demonstrate the impact of the level of intellectual functioning on psychiatric presentation, assessment, and treatment.

Case Example 4

Mild intellectual disability. The psychiatric presentation of mild intellectual ability is more similar to the behavior and affect of the general population.

Lucy, aged 21 years, is in her final year of a modified program at school. She is living in an apartment with support from staff who visit 3 to 4 days per week. She is able to get herself up in the morning in time for school, take care of her personal hygiene, make her own meals, and make her own way to school using public transport. She has difficulty with math and money change and needs some assistance when buying groceries and clothes. Lucy grew up in a very dysfunctional family; she experienced neglect by her mother and sexual and physical abuse by male friends of her mother. Crises, when Lucy becomes agitated and violent towards family members, are triggered by interaction with her mother. At these times, she is taken to the emergency room, and in the past several years she has had repeated visits as well as involuntary short stays in crisis units.

Diagnoses have included depression with suicidal ideation, dysthymia, adjustment disorder, eating disorder, school refusal, self-mutilating behavior, oppositional defiant disorder, attention deficit disorder, impulsiveness, agitation and violence, aggressive outbursts, and obesity. She has been treated with a variety of medications including benzodiazepines (lorazepam, clonazepam) antidepressants (fluoxetine), antipsychotics (perphenazine, risperidone, olanzapine) and stimulants (methylphenidate), without apparent benefit.

Lucy was referred to the specialist team working with persons with intellectual disabilities and, after an interdisciplinary assessment, a treatment program was initiated. Components of the latter include weekly insight-oriented psychotherapy, behavioral support in school and home, supervised visits with her mother, support from the psychiatrist who works jointly with Lucy and her psychotherapist to review and rationalize her medications, and systems meetings involving her school, support workers, family, psychotherapist, and psychiatrist.

Since initiation of this treatment program, Lucy has done remarkably well and has not needed to go the emergency room. In addition, working with her psychotherapist, Lucy has developed a shared language that more accurately describes her subjective experiences. Through this shared language, she is helped to develop self-soothing strategies and is able to provide more accurate feedback about her experience of the medication. The latter has allowed changes in her medication more closely attuned to her bodily experiences and feeling states that has resulted in better compliance.

Lucy is seen as a young person with mild intellectual disability (with implications for optimal support), who has suffered significant deprivation and abuse during her early years and who now has difficulties modulating her affect particularly in the presence of particular triggers (e.g., interactions with family members). All previous attempts at psychiatric diagnoses can be understood rather better in this context, and furthermore this context provides opportunities for prevention (of future mental health disturbances) and rehabilitation (alternative less disruptive ways for her to manage her affect).

Comment. This is an example of an effective and closely coordinated interdisciplinary and holistic response to a complex set of psychosocial needs.

Case Example 5

Severe intellectual disability and comorbid autism. Comorbid autism is associated with even more atypical clinical presentations, especially when past trauma complicates the history.

Colin is 35 years old and a nonidentical twin. He has a severe intellectual disability, is on the autism spectrum, and has a high level of anxiety. His brother does not have intellectual disability but still lives at home with their widowed mother. Colin has been living in residential care for 3 years. After leaving a special boarding school, he lived at home for many years until his aggression toward his mother became more physically assaultive. He would like to live at home, but his mother will not agree. Recently, he has been "in trouble" at the day center on three separate occasions for having sex with other men in the toilet area. He has also been accused of "interfering" with an 8-year-old boy, but no charges have been pressed. His care plan requires that he always have an escort when he is neither at home (residential care) nor attending the day center. He was assessed for psychotherapy and invited to join an outpatient men's group for men with intellectual disability who display sexually inappropriate or offending behavior. He is supposed to attend weekly therapy.

The focus of work was to get to know him better in the group, to understand the effect of his comorbid autism condition on his capacity for relationships, and to explore his capacity for empathy. Psychiatric assessment was ongoing by observation in group therapy by a psychotherapist who is also a psychiatrist. His social worker maintained close contact with everyone involved and ensured that education about safe sex was offered.

In the group, Colin disclosed his own sexual abuse at about the age of 8 years by a male family friend. He described how he thought he was dying, but he didn't tell anybody about this assault because the man said Colin would get into trouble. Colin is unable to say no to invitations from other men to have sex but always becomes extremely agitated afterwards. He seems to crave the attention and physical closeness of other men, but the child within him becomes terrified, and the experience is always a negative one. The extent of his vulnerability and risky behavior has become clearer in the group, and he has shown very little capacity for insight or empathy with others. His management plan was changed to increase the support offered to him, particularly during social events, and he began individual art therapy while also continuing in the group. It is anticipated that long-term therapy and intensive social support will be needed. Psychotropic medication has not proved helpful in this case.

Comment. This case shows the importance of risk assessments, interagency working, and the support some people need to be able to attend therapy.

Case Example 6

Profound intellectual disability. Here we are entirely reliant on care providers documenting targeted behaviors to determine the etiology of the problematic behaviors. Without such systematic documentation, disorders can remain unrecognized and untreated.

A few months after birth, Maria, now 35 years of age, suffered a brain infection and has been registered legally blind since around age 2 years. Visual impairment adds complexity in determining cognitive ability. Maria participates in self-care activities (e.g., she will wipe her face with a cloth, hold her arms out to dress when prompted); she can take herself to the toilet and can feed herself with a spoon. She makes requests by approaching staff and leading them to the area where the requested item is located (e.g., to the kitchen for a food item, to the coat rack when she wants to go out). She was institutionalized at age 5 and during her late teens discharged to the group home where she is presently living. Here she was observed to engage in episodic SIB (e.g., rubbing her eyes and ears, causing extensive bruising and sometimes open sores) and stripping off her clothes.

At first, this SIB was managed by admission to the local inpatient adult psychiatry ward where she would be managed by four-post bed restraint (limbs secured to the four corners of the bed) and heavily sedated over several weeks while the SIB subsided. New care providers, upset by this treatment, decided to try and manage her at these times in her home setting and so sought psychiatric consultation. The differential diagnosis of these episodic SIBs included allergies and mood disorder. Documentation of sleep (and other behaviors) for possible mood disturbance over several months revealed a phase shift in her sleep with a 4- to 6-week cycle, such that at the beginning of this cycle she was up during the day and mostly asleep during the night, and at the end of the cycle she was up at night and mostly asleep during the day.

Melatonin was introduced at night (slowly, because of her history of allergies), and 10 mg was found to stabilize her sleep with a more normal sleep-wake cycle. With this sleep pattern, SIB reduced significantly (possibly because staff were no longer trying to get Maria up during the day when she was in her sleep phase), and when SIB did occur the clinical picture suggested an allergic response, although the specific allergens have not been identified (possible allergens include particular brands of hygiene products, some foods, and seasonal mold later identified in the outside wall of her room). Nonspecific management of these allergic reactions has been helpful. With less SIB and better management of her allergic responses when these occur, Maria appears to be happier overall, and staff members are finding her more agreeable to be with.

Comment. SIBs in persons with profound intellectual disabilities are often a means of communication about an inner discomfort (e.g., emotional upset) or disorder (psychiatric or medical, including physical pain). Engaging care providers in an exploration of what the behavior is communicating (by identifying and monitoring particular behaviors in different environments and in response to different activities during the regular day) helps them to consider the behavior in a different light (e.g., their client is "communicating" rather then "behaving inappropriately") and often results in identifying the underlying cause of the problematic behavior.

CONCLUSION

In this chapter, we have described an interdisciplinary approach to assessment in working with persons with intellectual disabilities. It is our experience that careful attention to finding ways to help the person communicate his experience and to understand the perspective of the person, through an interdisciplinary evaluation of his needs and supports, is of itself therapeutic; both the person and the caregivers feel empowered, thus promoting favorable treatment outcomes.

Acknowledgments

Thanks to Marika Korossy for scholarly support in the preparation of this chapter.

REFERENCES

1. Howlin P: *Autism: preparing for adulthood,* London, 1997, Routledge.
2. American Psychiatric Association Task Force on DSM-IV: *Diagnostic and statistical manual of mental disorders,* ed 4, text revision. Washington, DC, 2000, American Psychiatric Association.
3. Deb S, Matthews T, Holt G, Bouras N: *Practice guidelines for the assessment and diagnosis of mental health problems in adults with intellectual disabilities,* The Ironworks, Cheapside, UK, 2001, Pavilion.
4. Royal College of Psychiatrists: *DC-LD: Diagnostic criteria for psychiatric disorders for use with adults with learning disabilities/mental retardation,* Occasional Paper No. 48, Royal College of Psychiatrists. London, 2001, Gaskell.
5. Levitas A: The psychiatric diagnostic interview evaluation in patients with mental retardation and developmental disabilities, *Ment Health Aspects Develop Disabil*, Special Issue: 4(1):2–16, 2001.
6. Cassidy S, Allanson J, editors: *Management of genetic syndromes,* New York, 2001, Wiley-Liss.
7. World Health Organization: *The ICD-10 classification of mental and behavioral disorders: clinical descriptions and diagnostic guidelines,* Geneva, 1992, World Health Organization.
8. World Health Organization: *ICD-10 guide for mental retardation,* Geneva, 1996, World Health Organization.
9. Moss S, Patel P, Prosser H, et al: Psychiatric morbidity in older people with moderate and severe learning disability. I: Development and reliability of the patient interview (PAS-ADD), *Br J Psychiatry* 163:471–480, 1993.
10. Aman MG: Assessing psychopathology and behavior problems in persons with mental retardation: a review of available instruments. A report prepared for the National Institutes of Health. Washington, DC, 1991, US Dept. of Health and Human Services, Public Health Service, Alcohol, Drug Abuse, and Mental Health Administration.
11. O'Brien G, Pearson J, Berney T, Barnard L: Measuring behavior in developmental disability: a review of existing schedules, *Dev Med Child Neurol* 43 (Suppl87):1–72, 2001.
12. Aman MG, Burrow WH, Wolford PL: The Aberrant Behavior Checklist—Community: factor validity and effect of subject variables for adults in group homes, *Am J Ment Retard* 100(3):283–292, 1995.
13. Roy A, Matthews H, Clifford P, et al: Health of the Nation Outcome Scales for People with Learning Disabilities (HoNOS-LD): glossary for HoNOS-LD score sheet, *Br J Psychiatry* 180(1):61–66, 2002.
14. Bradley EA: Psychiatry Residency Year 1 (PGY1), University of Toronto, Intellectual Disabilities Psychiatry Curriculum Planning Committee. Toronto, 2002, Centre for Addiction and Mental Health. www.intellectualdisability.info/how_to/AandE_eb.html
15. Scottish Executive: Health needs assessment report: people with learning disabilities in Scotland. *Health Scotland*, Edinburgh, 2004.
16. Levitas A, Gilson SF: Predictable crises in the lives of people with mental retardation, *Ment Health Aspects Develop Disabil* 4(3):89–100, 2001.
17. Bolton P, Rutter M: *Schedule for Assessment of Psychiatric Problems Associated with Autism (and other developmental disorders) (SAPPA): informant version,* Cambridge, UK, 1994 Developmental Psychiatry Section, University of Cambridge and London, Child Psychiatry Department, Institute of Psychiatry [unpublished].
18. Krug D, Eric J, Almond P: *Autism Screening Instrument for Educational Planning (ASIEP-2),* Austin, TX, 1993, Pro-ed.
19. Schopler E, Reichler RJ, Renner BR: *The Childhood Autism Rating Scale,* Los Angeles, 1988, Western Psychological Services.
20. Nylander L, Gillberg C: Screening for autism spectrum disorders in adult psychiatric out-patients: preliminary report, *Acta Psychiatr Scand* 103:428–434, 2001.
21. Lord C, Rutter M, LeCouteur A: Autism Diagnostic Interview–Revised: a revised version of a diagnostic interview for caregivers of individuals with possible pervasive developmental disorders, *J Autism Develop Disord* 24:659–685, 1994.
22. Lord C, Rutter M, Goode S, et al: Autism diagnostic observation schedule: a standardized observation of communicative and social behavior, *J Autism Develop Disord* 19:185–212, 1989.

18

Assessment of Patients for Insurance and Disability

BARBARA J. DORIAN AND ASH BENDER

INTRODUCTION

Typically, patients first come to a mental health professional on referral from a family doctor or other specialist or by their own request or that of a family member. In this chapter, we address the special issues that arise when the patient has been required to attend for assessment by a third party. Although there are elements common to all psychiatric assessments, the unique circumstances of this type of interview require some modifications of technique and some special considerations. Many clinicians are reluctant to undertake this type of examination, believing that the skills involved are inaccessible to them and being fearful of the potential outcomes. They view the role of independent examiner as outside the traditional role of the clinician who is confident in the realms of expertise in *Diagnostic and Statistical Manual of Mental Disorders*, Fourth Edition, Text Revision (DSM-IV-TR)[1] diagnoses and comfortable in the roles of caregiver and patient advocate. The issues of functioning, impairment, and disability transcend the diagnostic categories and psychosocial formulations of illness that are so familiar to clinicians, and the stance required is often imagined to be purely that of investigator-detective ferreting out signs of deception as opposed to acting in the patient's interest. Clinicians are aware that their opinions in these matters may have far-reaching consequences and are concerned about making incorrect judgments, being publicly humiliated, or being engaged in some form of legal recourse. In this chapter, we hope to impart a simple, stepwise approach to this type of assessment that will allay your anxiety and permit you to undertake this work with increased skill and confidence.

DISABILITY BASICS

To understand disability, we want to develop some working definitions. Many exist, but for the sake of continuity, we will familiarize you with definitions from the World Health Organization (WHO) and the American Medical Association (AMA):

Impairment

- Problems with body function or structure such as a significant deviation or loss[2]
- Deviation of anatomical structure, physiological function, intellectual capability, or emotional status from that which the person possessed prior to an alteration in those structures or functions or from that expected from population norms[3,4]
  - □ Partial: Prevents, to some degree, a normal bodily function
  - □ Complete: Total loss of that bodily function

Disability

- Health-related restriction or lack of ability to perform any activity within a range of normal[5]
- Medical impairment that prevents a person from performing specified intellectual, creative, adaptive, social, or physical functions[4]
- Inability to complete a specific task successfully that the person was previously capable of completing, owing to a medical or psychological deviation from prior health status or from the status expected of most members of society[4]

- Inability or altered ability to accomplish a given task successfully[4]
  - □ Partial: Ability to perform some but not all required tasks of a job
  - □ Complete: Person can perform none of those tasks

Disability may occur due to a limit or insufficiency in many areas, including mental and physical function or lack of the development or skill necessary to perform the task. It is important to remember that the degree and extent of disability are unique to each person. As previously mentioned, psychiatric disability is not always correlated to the degree of psychological impairment (specific symptoms and severity) but is dependent on the context (type of work) and individual characteristics such as personality.

Severity of Impairment and Disability

Currently, there are no guides that provide precise measures—such as percentages—of impairment in mental disorder. This is due to the absence of objective tests for the validation of percentages of impairment and the fact that numerical statements, such as percentages, do not readily capture the multiplicity of factors that may influence psychiatric and behavioral disorders. As a result, this leaves you with the task of clinically assessing the level of disability; that is, the effect of impairment due to mental disorder on the person's ability to function in areas of activities of daily living, social functioning, concentration, and adaptation. Activities of daily living include things like eating, sleeping, dressing, sexual functioning, home care, and recreation. Social functioning is primarily concerned with interpersonal relationships, including family, friends, coworkers, and the general public. Concentration includes general cognitive abilities such as memory and attention span, persistence, and pace (i.e., the ability to maintain focus and complete tasks within a time frame). *Adaptation* refers to the ability to perform necessary tasks at work and the probability of compensation or decompensation under workplace conditions.

Below are the AMA classes of impairment. The class of impairment should be assessed in each area before determining the overall degree of impairment:

- Class 1, no impairment: No impairment is noted.
- Class 2, mild impairment: Impairment levels are compatible with most useful functioning.
- Class 3, moderate impairment: Impairment levels are compatible with some, but not all, useful functioning.
- Class 4, marked impairment: Impairment levels significantly impede useful functioning.
- Class 5, extreme impairment: Impairment levels preclude useful functioning.

Those with overall *Class 4 (marked)* and *Class 5 (extreme)* impairment meet criteria for "catastrophic impairment" due to a mental or behavioral disorder according the American Medical Association's *Guides to the Evaluation of Permanent Impairment*.[6] Other examples of catastrophic impairment include paraplegia, total loss of vision in both eyes, and severe neurocognitive dysfunction. In general, catastrophic impairment is regarded as a total disability.

Impairment may be permanent or temporary, depending on the potential for ongoing recovery, the availability of further effective treatments, and the presence of psychosocial stressors that may influence the patient's level of symptomatology. Permanent impairment or maximum medical recovery is said to occur when the patient's condition has stabilized, when all appropriate treatments have been given, and when further progress is not anticipated in the foreseeable future.

Determining Causality

Often, an evaluator is asked by the insurer to address causality when an impairment and resulting disability are present that preclude normal occupational function. Medically, causality exists when there is an association between the exposure and the medical condition (outcome) and that would not have existed without exposure. When considering compensable psychiatric disability, the outcome is a mental disorder, and the exposure is typically a workplace stressor, either physical (e.g., accident, injury, or assault) or psychological (e.g., workplace conflict, harassment, effects of personality disorder). Although these medical concepts are generally universally accepted, decisions for compensation may also be influenced by legal interpretations.

Characteristics that support a causal relationship include the following:

- Temporal relationship
- Mechanism that is physiologically plausible
- Contiguous relationship with a dose-response or duration effect
- Consistency between cause and effect
- Specificity with the absence of other explanations
- Coherent with current medical understanding

Legal Considerations

Unfortunately, no unifying definition of psychiatric injury exists to make the determination of causation (injury) and outcome (psychiatric disability) easier. A simplified legal definition of a "psychiatric industrial injury" eligible for compensation includes the following elements:

(1) a psychiatric injury that is (2) work-related and (3) precludes work.

Currently, a psychiatric injury for the purpose of worker's compensation is most clearly defined by utilizing the DSM-IV-TR, published by the American Psychiatric Association, or the *International Classification of Diseases,* edition 10 (ICD-10), which is published by the WHO. It is important to preclude any preexisting conditions such as personality, which increase vulnerability to injury, but consider carefully the arising injuries that meet the essential elements of the claim. Indeed, a work-related injury can exacerbate a preexisting condition, resulting in greater disability than expected, which should be considered as part of the psychiatric injury. This extends from the maxim that the employer "takes the worker as he is." For example, the disabling aspects of post-traumatic stress disorder (PTSD) arising from a workplace accident can be amplified by a preexisting personality disorder, for which all the elements of the PTSD constitute a work-related injury. Analogous to this example would be an overweight and poorly conditioned worker who sustains a lower back injury. Despite having several preexisting risk factors for a lumbar strain, the worker would be compensated fully for the workplace injury.

Establishing the elements of causation is less clear. There is growing recognition that "stress" from the workplace (be it psychological or physical) can result in psychiatric injury. The nature of the temporal relationship between a resulting workplace psychiatric injury and the causative factor is not well defined and is still determined by the evaluator. A ballpark range for the temporal relationship between the deemed causative factor and the defining features of the injury has been suggested to be about 6 months, which comes at the risk of excluding some cases. A longer time frame should be considered, particularly when there has been a complex mix of severe physical injuries and a subsequent psychiatric disorder that becomes manifest after the crisis of physical injury has occurred, hospital care (e.g., surgery, ICU, pain, beginning rehabilitation) has somewhat waned, and people become more cognizant of the magnitude of their losses.

Somatoform Disorders and the Concept of Malingering

Sometimes, being "sick" can be advantageous. These advantages may be overt and literal, such as the desire for compensation, avoidance of military duty, reluctance to return to previous employment, or other concrete social or financial goals. The advantages may be primarily psychological (e.g., cry for help, expression of suffering, wish for care), and these may be expressed in a conscious or unconscious manner.

Patients may magnify their symptoms as an expression of any of these wishes, and the question of symptom magnification (i.e., the reporting of symptoms at a greater severity than supported by the objective evidence) is often a directly stated or implicitly implied component of the request for psychiatric evaluation. Not infrequently, there has been a difference of opinion among previous medical examiners regarding the presence and significance of symptom magnification, and this history often heightens the tension between the patient and the third party requesting the examination.

Symptom magnification generally occurs along a continuum from completely unconscious, to partially conscious, to completely conscious and deliberate. It may manifest as a minor elaboration of current symptoms, an unconscious production of symptoms with no associated organic pathology, or the complete fabrication of symptoms and disability. Complex mixtures of unconscious needs and wishes and conscious motivations may often coexist. Somatoform disorders, including pain disorder, conversion disorder, and factitious disorder, are the diagnostic categories that capture many forms of psychologically based elaborations of illness and disability. In somatoform disorders, the motivations are believed to be unconscious and psychologically determined. In factitious disorders, the physical or psychological symptoms are intentionally produced or feigned, although the motivation is not that of compensable gain but rather to assume the sick role. Finally, issues of motivation may occur in response to psychosocial stressors in the absence of a formal psychiatric diagnosis. This is most often expressed as distress and reluctance to perform in particular work environments. Contextual issues such as conflict with supervisors or coworkers, feelings of personal or racial discrimination, a sense of betrayal by the employer, or overwhelming personal and family problems may influence a patient's ability to function. In this case, you have the task of determining whether a mental disorder is present or whether the issues relate more to personal preferences and choices.

In situations in which any incentives for illness are apparent, efforts should always be made to evaluate the authenticity of self-report. This is most critical when there is suspicion of malingering; that is, when the symptoms appear to be produced intentionally and there is a clear and obviously recognizable external goal or gain. According to the DSM-IV-TR, "[T]he essential feature of Malingering is the intentional production of false or grossly exaggerated physical or psychological symptoms, motivated by external incentives such as avoiding military duty, avoiding work, obtaining financial compensation, evading criminal prosecution, or obtaining drugs." It is suggested that malingering should be strongly suspected if any combination of the following is noted:

- Medicolegal context of presentation
- Marked discrepancy between the person's claimed stress or disability and objective findings
- Lack of cooperation during the diagnostic evaluation and in complying with the prescribed treatment regimen
- The presence of antisocial personality disorder

Other clinical factors suggestive of malingering include the following:

- Incongruent affect with mood
- Incongruence in work and recreational disability
- Overvaluation of prior functioning
- Inconsistency in self-report
- Evasiveness
- Unnatural course of symptoms
- Tenacious involvement in the claim process
- Eager and spontaneous return to subject of impairment
- Inconsistent severity of symptoms with previous assessment
- Endorsing unusual and rare symptoms

Neuropsychological testing can also provide supporting evidence of malingering and clarification of other diagnostic factors, including major mental illness, personality disorder, and intellectual functioning. Unfortunately, no test exists to absolutely rule in or rule out malingering. Instead, the diagnosis of malingering exists on a balance of probabilities, much like the assessment of risk for suicide or homicide. In general, three categories exist for malingering: definite, probable, and possible.

Definite malingering exists when there is clear and compelling evidence of exaggeration or fabrication of symptoms that is considered rational and volitional (motivation). Additionally, there must be an absence of alternative explanations for the symptoms or behavior. Criteria for *probable* and *possible malingering* are based on how much supporting evidence is available. Obviously, one of the most definitive methods to detect malingering is surveillance, in which observed behavior clearly is inconsistent with patients' self-report of functioning (e.g., an injured and depressed worker is observed spending a fun-filled day at an amusement park). Clearly, this extends beyond the clinician's role. Clinicians are, however, requested on occasion to review surveillance tapes prepared by third parties. Professional colleges have differing standards and guidelines regarding the use of such material and should be consulted before agreeing to review such tapes or provide an opinion based on information gathered by covert surveillance. It is important to note that there may be several alternative explanations for behaviors which, on the surface, suggest the diagnosis of malingering to you. Indeed, malingering may fully account for only 10% to 20% of the cases you will see in assessing disability, and alternative explanations must always be fully considered because the determination of malingering carries extensive legal, financial, and medical consequences for the disabled worker.

Now that we have covered the basics, let's move into the preparation stage.

CONSIDERATIONS BEFORE GETTING STARTED

The circumstance of the assessment for insurance and disability differs from that of the traditional clinician-patient relationship as normally defined in terms of implications for a duty of care. In other forms of consultation, the provision of care may be circumscribed and limited to the provision of recommendations to the referring physician; however, the considerations are exclusively those of the best interests of the patient. In the case of insurance and disability assessment, the interests of the third party as the client who has referred the patient must also be served. Although the third party requesting the assessment may be seen as the primary client, the clinician is still bound by the needs of compassionate and ethical behavior with respect to the patient. As a consequence, you have a number of responsibilities: to be as thorough and accurate as possible, to gather and present enough information in the report to substantiate and provide a rationale for the conclusions and recommendations, and—most of all—to remain impartial.

Human nature involves having issues of gain play into every clinical contact of this nature. As discussed, the wishes may be primarily unconscious or implicit (e.g., to validate one's experience and suffering, to maintain the sick role, to be cared for, to be freed from responsibilities). Alternatively, or even at the same time, the wishes may relate to more explicit and concrete financial and material gains such as money, not returning to work, or not being retrained in another position. Insurance companies and other third parties often emphasize the issues of gain. However, the clinician has an obligation to fully understand the experience of suffering and illness, disability, and compensation from the patient's perspective and to remain open minded while collecting data to support the ultimate conclusions and recommendations of the evaluation.

Some tips to remember are as follows:

- Maintain a professional stance, and don't become angry or critical even if patients are defensive or antagonistic—they haven't chosen to be there.
- Remain tactful and careful in inquiries about potentially sensitive subjects such as sexuality, ethnicity, religious and cultural practices, education and ability, and family dysfunction.

- Explain to the patient why discussion of any "hot topics" is relevant to the purpose of the assessment.

Negotiation of the fee for the assessment and report should be completed before seeing the patient. You may choose a standard fee for the type of assessment and report required, an hourly fee, or some combination based on a preliminary review of the file, relevant information provided by the third party, complexity of the case, and questions to be answered. Regulatory bodies in your jurisdiction can provide guidelines and standards for setting such fees. It is important, however, not to discuss your fee in the report. The report may be viewed by many different parties, including other caregivers, the insurance company, the patient, and potentially lawyers or other advocates.

The next considerations are those of informed consent, disclosures, and the parameters of confidentiality. Every patient has the right to know the clinician's training, area of specialization, and credentials. In many clinical situations, this is not dealt with in detail or in an explicit manner unless requested by the patient. In the case of an assessment for insurance and disability, however, it should be standard practice to give the patient a brief overview of the examiner's qualifications and the specific expertise on which the third party is calling. This is also an important part of the final report.

With respect to confidentiality, it must be made explicit that the report (which will be the result of the interview and a review of accompanying documentation and any psychological testing) will be released directly to the third party, who in essence owns the report. If the patient does not wish to reveal information (regarding the material issues of the consultation) as a result, then it should be clarified that a statement by you regarding incomplete information provided by the patient will be made in the report. Informed written consent addressing these issues is required before proceeding to the clinical interview. If collateral information gathered through direct contact with family members, health care providers, employers, etc. is anticipated as a component of the assessment, then written authorization must be signed by the patient for each specific contact. Patients should be informed that they may request a copy of the report from the third party and that they are entitled to view this clinical record. From a practical standpoint, you should assume that in every instance the patient will receive a copy or be made aware of the contents of the report, and you should keep this in mind when preparing the report.

Confidentiality does continue to be important with respect to the patient's right to privacy. Patients may reveal things about themselves, their life histories, and their experiences that have no material bearing on the current issues and which are normally protected by the bounds of privacy and confidentiality (e.g., details of a sexual assault, a child being given up for adoption). This information should not be included in the report or should be referred to in very general terms (e.g., patient suffered a significant loss at the age of 18).

On occasion, the third party may request that you release a copy of your report directly to the patient. If you choose to do this, it is important to ensure that there is a written request to this effect that can be appended to the patient's file. Again, you need to reflect on the contents of the report and the impact on the patient. In rare instances, it may be justified to simply release the report directly to the patient. In most cases, it is prudent to meet with the patient to review the contents of the report, to deal with reactions and feelings, and to provide explanation and translation into accessible language, ensuring that the patient understands the rationale for your conclusions and recommendations.

Some tips to remember include the following:

- Avoid making critical or judgmental references in the report regarding the patient's lifestyle, socioeconomic status, or personality or any statement that might imply a stigmatizing attitude.
- Avoid complaints by remaining sensitive and respectful, giving the patient the opportunity to ask questions, and focusing on the positive aspects of the report.
- Avoid negative comments about other health care providers or treatments.

A key issue in the assessment is actually conceptualizing the report before seeing the patient and beginning the interview. Most importantly, you need to be absolutely clear about what questions are being asked of you as an assessor and what information beyond the elements of the standard psychiatric interview will be required to answer them. The questions you are being called on to answer generally relate to the variety of circumstances under which patients are sent for psychiatric evaluations of this type. These may include the following:

- Confirmation of the diagnosis
- Evaluation of the level of impairment and disability
- Determination of causality; that is, the link between the inciting incident (e.g., accident, assault, workplace stress) and the diagnosis and level of impairment
- Evaluation of other factors contributing to the patient's presentation (i.e., a formulation of the confluence of psychological, social, developmental, and systemic issues that have caused this person to be in this circumstance at this time)
- Evaluation of the appropriateness or efficacy of previous treatments
- Evaluation of compliance with treatment

- Determination of the expected time course of recovery and factors influencing this course
- Further treatment recommendations
- Determination of the patient's ability to return to regular or alternative employment and the need for any temporary or permanent restrictions with respect to specific functions or tasks
- Determination of the capacity to perform and be responsible for the unique requirements of a profession (e.g., to drive a police car, to carry a gun)
- Evaluation of the barriers to return to work and recommendations regarding the process for facilitating vocational rehabilitation

In every case, the primary task is to assess the person's psychiatric diagnoses according to the DSM-IV-TR multiaxial system, including a statement of the primary psychiatric disorders (axis I), the presence or absence of a personality disorder (axis II), the presence of a medical diagnosis and the contribution of any interaction between the psychiatric and medical condition to the level of impairment (axis III), other sources of stress having an impact on the person's condition (axis IV), and finally, an assessment of the person's level of functioning according to the global assessment of functioning (GAF) scale (axis V).

The AMA guidelines for the review of functioning across a number of domains (i.e., activities of daily living, social functioning, cognitive abilities, and capacity to perform in a work environment) provide a framework for the specific evaluation of the severity of impairment and level of disability. An important factor in this review is the recognition that psychiatric disorders are highly variable in both their presentation and their response to treatment. The severity of symptoms, levels of impairment, and degree of disability may differ widely within diagnostic categories. A person with the same diagnosis and same level of impairment may be much more disabled than another person, and a person may manifest a greater degree of disability in one context than in another. Consideration of these issues is extremely important when answering questions about prognosis, treatment, and fitness to return to a specific job or occupation. Many adjudication systems are primarily diagnostically driven, and adjudicators may respond to a client's claim purely on this basis, to the disadvantage of the client with complex or treatment-resistant disorders.

An ideal formulation of psychiatric disability should convey the diagnoses, the severity of the symptomatology, the response to treatment, the contributing contextual and personality factors, and a statement that on the basis of these factors the person is able or unable to perform particular tasks or function in certain environments.

Note: With respect to the formulation of the person and the forces contributing to the current presentation, there are multiple factors to consider, and the interview must elucidate these issues (e.g., attachment style, roles, relationships, defensive structure, coping capacity, culture, supports for adaptation).

Setting the Tone

Simply put, in assessing a patient regarding issues of compensation and disability, you need to keep in mind the following circumstances: in this setting, there is a constant dynamic tension between the needs, interests, and motivations of the patient; the needs, interests, and motivations of the referring party; and the needs, interests, and motivations of the assessor. You therefore have the particular challenge of making an empathic engagement with the patient as dictated by the standards of clinical care and of having the patient be as forthcoming as possible, while gathering a great deal of highly specific information in a circumscribed time and evaluating the veracity of the patient's history and presentation and doing so without destroying a minimum baseline of trust or harming or enraging the patient.

Your stance as the clinician is very important. As health care providers, we normally approach the patient from a respectful, caregiving stance, not necessarily taking everything the patient says at face value, but on the whole engaging collaboratively with the patient while being alert to the issues of unconscious motivations and conflict. However, insurance companies and other third parties have an economic incentive to prove that the patient is somehow taking advantage of the system or is not fully deserving of benefits, compensation, and medical care. Often, patients are sent with an explicit or implicit message that they have not followed the expected course of recovery and reintegration into work. Some patients describe a sense of violation in this type of setting, feeling they have been "assaulted" with questions, implied criticism, and disbelief. Like all patients, those sent for disability evaluations deserve to be treated respectfully, objectively, fairly, and compassionately.

The feeling of respect may be further conveyed by the examiner's dress and manner. Many physicians currently dress in a casual fashion and adopt an easy-going, open style, including addressing the patient by first name without having first obtained permission to do so. This may be acceptable generally; however, in these assessments it is useful to set a more formal tone and to dress and greet the client accordingly. Patients should be addressed as Mr., Mrs., Dr., etc., unless the patient specifically requests otherwise. If a patient is from another culture and has a name you don't know how to pronounce, then it is helpful both in conveying respect and building an initial alliance to ask the patient for the correct pronunciation and to establish how the patient would prefer to be addressed.

Begin by reviewing the chart in a general fashion so that you have a sense of the history and issues in broad brush strokes. You should focus particularly on the questions being asked of you and any issues of inconsistency, incongruity, or controversy. Attend to key reports made by physicians or psychologists in sufficient detail so that you will be able to confront the patient with respect to inconsistencies between the history as given and information from other sources. In this way, you should have enough of a sense of the situation to direct the interview but remain open and unprejudiced in order to draw your own conclusions. It is helpful to make it clear to the patient that you have reviewed elements of the file, but that your role is that of an independent assessor, and so you will need to elicit much information directly.

Patients may become irritated if they think you are not interested enough to have reviewed the material meticulously or merely because they are asked to repeat their story after having told it many times before. We always say to the patient: *"I have reviewed the information to have a general sense of what you have been through, but I haven't looked at the details of some of the other consultants' reports as I feel it is important to hear directly from you and to make up my own mind. Before writing the report and making my final conclusions and recommendations, I will review all of the information in detail to be sure I am aware of all of the important issues."*

This stance strikes a balance between letting the patient know you are interested and concerned enough to have reviewed the important aspects of her case before seeing her, but that you also are giving her a fair hearing unprejudiced by others' opinions and are therefore willing to empathically immerse yourself in the person's experience of illness, disability, and history of relationships and interactions with other health care providers, assessors, employers, and insurance companies.

Note: Some assessors take an alternative stance, performing a detailed chart review and summary before seeing the patient. Two advantages of approach are the increased capacity to challenge the patient on inconsistencies in the history and presentation over time and the certainty that you are not missing a key area of inquiry. This may be obviated by ensuring the chart is scanned for references to frequently contentious issues such as substance abuse, legal proceedings, prior insurance claims, or any other recurring themes.

Interview techniques and psychometric evaluation combined can often distinguish issues of feigning (malingering) from what is known as "a distressed response style." Cultural considerations are also critical in this, as normative behaviors for expressing illness, distress, disability, or relating to professionals may vary considerably. It is important to be aware of the culturally determined patterns of illness behavior in the range of clients you may see and to not evaluate the client's response style from the exclusive viewpoint of the predominant North American culture.

Case Example 1

Referral. You have just received a letter in the mail from Mr. D's insurance company asking for a disability assessment. The insurer has requested for you to provide a DSM-IV diagnosis, to render an opinion regarding capacity to work and prognosis for returning to work, and to make treatment recommendations with the goal of return to work. The cover letter on the file indicates a suspicion of malingering due to conflicting reports regarding the severity of his depression, previous compensation claims, and increased symptomatology when return to work plans are being formulated.

File Review. Mr. D. is a 43-year-old divorced man currently living in his home with a girlfriend of 5 years. Mr. D.'s partner is 12 years older and has several chronic medical conditions. He has not worked for the past 18 months after sustaining a back injury. Mr. D. was working in a warehouse when he strained his lower back lifting a heavy crate.

After carefully reading the file provided by the insurer, you learn that Mr. D. is suffering from a low back strain with evidence of disk herniation at the L1 level. There are reports of minimal participation in physiotherapy and rehabilitation due to complaints of chronic and severe pain. The records from the family physician 5 months ago also suggested a diagnosis of "depression and stress" which have left Mr. D. "totally disabled." Mr. D. was started on paroxetine and maintained on a starting dose of 20 mg/day with intermittent supportive counseling from his family physician. He was prescribed Tylenol #3 for control of his pain to be taken on a prn basis.

Three months ago, Mr. D. was referred by his family doctor for psychiatric consultation and diagnosed with a major depressive disorder, single episode, mild. The psychiatrist indicated that Mr. D. did not appear to be in significant distress and, after titration of his antidepressant, he would likely be able to return to full-time work in 6 weeks with standard low back physical restrictions.

Interview. At the time of your assessment, Mr. D. reports worsening low back pain and depressive symptoms preventing him from returning to work. He reports being compliant with his medications with no significant response to his antidepressant. He is currently taking 30 mg/day of paroxetine and receives weekly supportive psychological counseling through the employee assistance program provided by his employer. He describes the counseling experience as positive but denies any discernible benefit.

Mr. D. reports that his daily functioning is quite limited and that he has become socially isolated. His relationship with his girlfriend has been strained by the current financial situation and sexual dysfunction since initiating treatment with the antidepressant. He continues to perform limited physiotherapy exercises at home but feels that his pain is too intense to cope. Mr. D. reports that he is "too weak" to do anything and is unsure if he will ever be able to return to work. As an additional stressor, Mr. D. reports conflict with his insurer over delay in payments for his psychological disability, and he received a letter from his employer indicating potential termination if he does not provide appropriate medical documentation.

Before his injury, Mr. D. reports that he was doing "great" and denied any significant conflicts or impairment. Mr. D. denies any past psychiatric history, abuse of substances, or family psychiatric difficulties. He denies any past criminal charges but had a previous short-term disability claim for a similar low back injury in the past. After the previous injury, Mr. D. reports returning to the same position with 6 weeks of physiotherapy and being otherwise healthy.

Mr. D. is the middle child in a blue-collar family. He has an older brother and younger twin sisters. He initially reported an uneventful childhood; however, on further inquiry, he reveals a sense of isolation, alienation, and conflict with his brother, whom he viewed as his father's favorite. He describes being close with his younger twin sisters and seeing them as his main confidants, although he acknowledges resentment of their special connection with his mother. He describes himself as an extremely independent loner who became a caretaker in his family but had few long-lasting friendships or intimate relationships. Despite doing "better than most" in school, he stopped after obtaining a high school diploma. Mr. D. made several unsuccessful attempts at entering the police force and the fire department and settled for unskilled jobs in shipping and receiving. He has worked as a night manager in distribution warehouse of the same medium-sized company for the past 10 years. He reports being satisfied with the "independent" nature of the job but feeling unsupported by his "greedy" employers. He describes his main interests as reading and computer work and notes that he currently spends most of his time engaging in these activities.

On mental status examination, Mr. D. presents as a thin man appearing his stated age and in significant discomfort. He has an obvious impaired gate and is wincing and grimacing as he enters the room. He is, however, able to remain quietly seated for the duration of the 2-hour interview. He is modestly dressed and groomed. Initially, Mr. D. interacts in a somewhat hostile and defensive manner but becomes cooperative and engaged with expressions of interest and concern. He speaks articulately throughout, providing a consistent and coherent history, revealing a lively intelligence and wide-ranging knowledge. He appears mildly depressed and endorses feelings of anger and frustration and hopelessness regarding his future and his recovery. He admits to passive suicidal ideation. There are no psychotic symptoms evident and no deficits in his cognitive functioning. Mr. D. describes himself as willing to engage in treatment but unsure about any positive outcomes.

Collateral. With his permission, you contact Mr. D.'s girlfriend. She reports that he has been quite isolative and spends his days alone at home. She continues to work and to take on more responsibilities at home including cleaning, shopping, and the finances; she characterizes Mr. D. as "lazy." He is able to dress and bathe himself but takes frequent naps during the day, complaining of pain and fatigue. She reports that their relationship has suffered due to his irritability and lack of interest in sex. She states he never liked his job but was happier when working there than he is at the present.

Psychiatric Rating Scales. To help determine the severity of symptoms that Mr. D. is experiencing, you have him fill out the following rating scales:

- Beck Depression Inventory
- McGill Pain Questionnaire
- CAGE questionnaire

Mr. D. reports moderate to severe levels of depression and pain, but there is no evidence of a substance abuse disorder. You note that Mr D.'s endorsement of symptoms appears greater than anticipated from your interview findings.

Psychological Testing. Mr. D. is referred to a neuropsychologist specializing in psychometric evaluation. He participates in a battery of psychological tests over 1 day which include the following:

- Wechsler Adult Intelligence Scale–Revised
- NEO Personality Inventory–Revised
- Minnesota Multiphasic Personality Inventory
- Test of Memory Malingering scale

The neuropsychologist prepares a detailed report for your review. Mr. D.'s intelligence is in the above-average range. Both personality inventories indicate that Mr. D. has narcissistic qualities and tends to be introverted and prone to somatization. The response subscales on the Minnesota Multiphasic Personality Inventory indicate a normal response style, with some evidence of psychological symptom exaggeration on a few subscales when compared to normative values. Other scores indicate that Mr. D's cognitive complaints appear to be in keeping with normative values for age, level of education, and level of psychological impairment.

FUNDAMENTAL QUESTIONS

- What is the diagnosis?
- How severe is the impairment?
- Is the psychiatric disability work related?
- How well is he functioning now?
- How well was he functioning before?
- How would you formulate the developmental, personality, interpersonal, and dynamic issues that contribute to this presentation?
- Is there an expectation for improvement? What treatments might be useful?
- What is the motivation for return to work, and what are the barriers (physical, psychological, systemic)?
- What interventions will optimize work potential?
- How are you going to explain this outcome and your recommendations to the insurance company?

ASSESSMENT

The assessment begins in the waiting room. As you go to greet the patient and introduce yourself, it is important to be observing aspects of the patient's demeanor, behavior, and interactions with others—for example, is the patient sitting comfortably chatting with the receptionist? Is the patient displaying pain-related behaviors (e.g., grimacing, sighing, wailing, lying on the couch, clinging to his spouse or accompanying person)? It is also helpful for you to be aware of the quality of the patient's interaction with the receptionist and any spontaneous statements made that reveal the patient's attitude to the examination. You should observe the initial affect state of the patient in response to the introduction. Some examples here include that the person is compliant, prickly and adversarial, withdrawn and resentful, subdued, apprehensive, anxious and fidgety, in pain, or dramatic.

You should also carefully observe how the patient walks to the consulting room and settles into the chair, especially in cases where there is comorbid physical injury and questions concerning pain and limitations in functioning. Again, you should review the gait, pain behavior, use of a cane or other support consistent with known anatomy, or exaggeration for effect. Once in the consulting room, you should determine whether the patient is comfortably seated or requires a firmer chair or other aid due to physical injury. Attention to these details will provide valuable information and greatly facilitate your ability to positively engage the patient.

As discussed, patients may consciously or unconsciously exaggerate symptoms or portrayal of disability for reasons of secondary gain (e.g., compensation), as a component of a psychiatric disorder such as factitious disorder or somatoform disorder, or merely as an expression of a wish to be understood and to have their distress and disabling experience taken seriously. The wish to impress the interviewer with the extent of suffering occurs not infrequently, especially when there has been a prolonged course of physical illness with complicating psychiatric illness, as well as conflicts with other caregivers who have felt that the patient "should be better by now." Given this, it is extremely useful to state at the beginning of the interview that you can be of most help to the patient if he if open and direct and can describe his symptoms and functioning as accurately as possible.

Initiating the Interview

"What is your understanding of why you are here and the purpose of our meeting?" serves as an appropriate opening question. Not infrequently, the answer is "I don't know, the insurance company told me I had to come here," or "You are going to decide whether the insurance company is going to pay me or not," or, in an antagonistic patient, "You tell me. You are just another one of those compensation people who just want to jerk me around."

You should always clarify your relationship to the third party who has requested the assessment, explain the specific issues you have been asked to address, give a brief explanation of your credentials, indicate why the third party has asked for your opinion, answer any questions, and have the patient sign a consent form or review the consent if this has already been done.

An example of how to handle this is, *"The insurance company has asked me to see you in order to understand how your accident has affected you psychologically, to sort out whether there is a specific diagnosis for your condition, and whether further treatments may be helpful to you. They have also asked for recommendations about your returning to work. They have asked me to see you because I am a psychiatrist with expertise in the treatment of trauma, assessment of disability, pain, etc."*

You should determine whether the patient in fact understands and agrees to the terms and is giving informed consent. Often, you have to clarify that the insurance company may use your report as a component in its decisions regarding compensation or related matters, such as eligibility for treatment, but that you are not responsible for those specific decisions. Generally, you should state that you will give some feedback about your understanding of the clinical situation at the end of the interview, but for final opinions or recommendations you have to review the file in detail and put all the information together.

You should engage the patient by listening to concerns—often complaints—about having to go through such assessments and empathizing with the patient as to how difficult it is to be in this situation. You should explain the process; that is, the approximate length of the interview, whether there will be subsequent meetings or referral for psychological testing, the approximate time to prepare the report, and the limits of confidentiality. Clarify the fact that this assessment is for the purpose of evaluation and not for the establishment of a treatment relationship.

The content of the interview ideally begins with your asking the patient to describe the inciting incident, accident, or circumstance that has led to the current assessment. Asking initially in an open-ended fashion allows a patient to tell his "story" in his own way and from his point of view and has several advantages, which are worth the time taken. The patient experiences the interest and concern on the part of the interviewer, greatly facilitating cooperation and engagement with the structured diagnostic components of the evaluation. Also, going back to the original history of the events, the context (literal, interpersonal, social, financial, etc.), and the responses of the patient and significant others often provides extraordinarily useful information about important dynamic issues that may be active in determining the course of illness and disability.

Case Example 2

You are seeing a machine operator who suffered a severe crush injury of his hand when the machine he was working on malfunctioned. The damage to his hand was so extreme that amputation was required. In listening to the story of the incident and asking clarifying questions, a number of emotionally relevant issues are revealed: the machine had been known to be unsafe; workers had been asking management to deal with this; the patient was a recent immigrant and fearful of refusing to work on the machine; his initial thought was that he was going to die; coworkers became distraught and there was a delay in the arrival of the ambulance and transport to the hospital; the patient was terrified and in severe pain for a prolonged period in the emergency department; within his culture and religion loss of a hand had a highly specific and stigmatizing meaning; his wife initially blamed him for the accident and was critical of his profound emotional reaction to amputation; the patient blamed himself on the basis of historical guilt about perceived failures in his life and a religious/cultural view that he must have deserved punishment; no one from the company came to see him in hospital or inquired about his welfare thereafter.

All of these issues, with their complex psychological and interpersonal meanings, set the stage for the development of psychiatric disorder and a prolonged course of

rehabilitation. The referring third party was questioning the seeming resistance to treatment and the lack of progress with respect to physical and functional rehabilitation and resolution of the psychiatric sequelae of PTSD and major depression. The responses to this scenario from the insurance company and other health professionals varied from an implicit or explicit questioning of the patient's authenticity and motivation for recovery to genuine puzzlement about why the patient was not recovering as would be expected. Exploring in depth the circumstance of the accident provided rich psychological material that can be seen to have contributed to the stage for the current outcome.

Typical Clarifying Questions

- *"What were your first thoughts and feelings?"*
- *"What is your belief about why this happened?"*
- *"Do you blame anyone?"*
- *"How did other workers, supervisors, or employers respond?"*
- *"How did you get to medical care, and what was that like?"*
- *"How did your family and friends respond to your injury?"*

After the inquiry about the initiating circumstances, the next tasks involve those of the standard structured psychiatric interview for DSM-IV-TR diagnoses, past psychiatric history, medical/legal and substance use history, evaluation of personality style, and developmental, personal, and family history . Other core areas of inquiry include intellect, education, and detailed work and compensation history, financial status, living situation, history of compensation, and history of interaction with employers, unions, and the medical care system. In the personal and developmental history, one should be alert to the presence of significant losses, previous trauma or abuse, capacity for attachment, and supportive interpersonal relatedness. A detailed history of treatments and treatment response is important, particularly when considering issues of prognosis.

The next task is the function-oriented assessment, in which you conduct a thorough review of the mental and behavioral effects on functioning across the four domains of impairment defined by the AMA guidelines. These include activities of daily living, social functioning, cognitive capacities (concentration, persistence and pace), and adaptation (ability to perform in work environments).

Function-Oriented Assessment Questions

Some typical types of questions for a function-oriented assessment include:

- *"Tell me what you do in an ordinary day."*
- *"How long does it take you to bathe, dress, eat, prepare a meal, etc.? Do you need help with any of these activities? What prevents you from doing any of these things?"*
- *"Do you have to lie down during the day? How often? For how long?"*
- *"Are you able to watch TV, read a book or newspaper, visit a friend, take part in a sport or hobby? How often? How long can you do these things at a time?"*
- *"How often do you go out? For what purpose? For how long?"*
- *"Are you able to do chores, shopping, finances, or pay bills? Do you need help with these things? Do you plan and coordinate tasks and decisions with anyone? Have you given up doing certain things? Do other people have to take care of you? In what way?"*
- *"With whom do you interact? How often? For how long?"*
- *"Do you get frustrated easily? Do you have trouble following instructions, being forgetful, concentrating, finishing tasks, staying focused?"*
- *"What activities make you feel worse? What kinds of activities, people, or interactions can't you cope with?"*
- *"What do you do for fun and interest? With whom? How often? For how long?"*
- *"What aspects of your work do you feel you could do? What aspects would be impossible for you?"*

Establishing a clear time course of symptomatology and, in particular, the relationship of the symptoms to the accident or injury and its sequelae is critically important. It is also essential to know whether there has been any history of psychiatric symptoms or disorder antedating the event. It is also highly relevant to determine what other factors in the patient's life may be contributing to the presentation independent of the sequelae of the accident or injury. This, at times, is a difficult judgment call; for example, a divorce or problems with a child may occur as a consequence of the effects of the accident and subsequent disability or may, for the most part, have an unrelated etiology. Most frequently, there are elements of both explanations, and the clinician must weigh these contributions when commenting on questions such as, "What is the relationship of the diagnosis and disability to the original incident?" It is extremely helpful in this formulation to always keep in mind throughout the interview the question, "How do the patient's personal, family, and developmental history; conflicts and defenses; interpersonal relatedness; and personality style shape the responses or adaptations to the current context?"

Throughout the interview, you should also be judging your experience of the patient's genuineness and authenticity. A combination of open-ended, closed, and direct questions and asking about the same facts or themes at dif-ferent points in the interview or from different angles may reveal inconsistencies over time, incongruities in response, symptoms not consistent with known syndromes, and motivations and attitudes toward compensation and return to work.

RATING SCALES AND NEUROPSYCHOLOGICAL TESTING

Standardized psychological tests and rating scales are useful adjuncts to a thorough clinical examination and relaying objective information to those reviewing a report. In Case Example 1, we made reference to some rating scales that are frequently used in disability assessments. Validated symptom rating scales, such as those for depression, pain, and alcohol, are helpful in determining symptom severity. Responses may alert the clinician to inconsistencies in self-report or convey significant information regarding the effects of treatment. Using commonly accepted rating scales facilitates report reviewers in decision-making and supports your conclusions made in the report. Typically, combinations of self-report and clinician-administered scales are recommended, particularly when a determination of symptom severity and arising impairment is in question.

Note: The GAF scales are commonly used in general psychiatric assessments to indicate a level of functioning or prognosis. The score (0–100) can be based on either functional impairment or symptom severity and is therefore less informative about specific domains of functional impairment than the AMA classes of impairment.

At times, it may be impossible clinically to determine the nature of a psychiatric disability or whether it truly exists. Neuropsychological testing is an additional tool for determining authenticity of symptoms and clarifying other prognostic features such as intelligence and personality. Neuropsychological tests may identify deliberate exaggeration of symptoms or intentionally poor performance, which is coined a *negative response bias*. These are neuropsychological descriptions of behavior but without the identification of the underlying motivation, be it conscious or unconscious, intentional or unintentional. Disorders that may be associated with these response behaviors on neuropsychological testing typically include mood disorders, somatoform disorders, and factitious disorders. Detection of negative response bias on neuropsychological testing is based on three basic principles:

1. Inconsistency between clinical observations and test results
2. Discrepancy between obtained and expected scores
3. Between-evaluation inconsistency ("test-retest variability")

Several validated neuropsychological tests exist for personality and malingering. Some with which you may want to be familiar include the following:

- Wechsler Adult Intelligence Scale–Revised
- NEO Personality Inventory–Revised
- Personality Assessment Inventory
- Rey Malingering Tests
- Structured Interview of Reported Symptoms
- Test of Memory Malingering
- Minnesota Multiphasic Personality Inventory

Let's use the assessment of memory to highlight how neuropsychological testing can support suspicions of malingering. An example of discrepancy between clinical observation and test results occurs when an examiner is able to elicit a seamless account of the workplace injury and treatment history during the interview, but the patient reports major short-term and long-term memory deficits during formal testing. Discrepancy between observed and expected scores are also seen when test scores are substantially lower than normative scores adjusted for age and diagnosis (e.g., 25-year-old woman of average intelligence scoring below scores of a validated sample with severe dementia on a cognitive test). Lastly, between-evaluation inconsistency often presents as significant deterioration in performance on testing over a short period of time, which cannot be accounted for by the mental disorder. All of these observations serve to support the determination of malingering if the negative response bias is evident in the context of significant motivations for such a response.

ANSWERING THE QUESTIONS

Answering the questions posed in the referral must be done in a systematic way wherever possible. Having a clear and methodical approach will help to bring clarity and support to your conclusions.

Diagnosis

Making an accurate diagnosis is essential for timely and appropriate treatment planning and a fair determination of compensation. Currently, the multiaxial system of the DSM-IV-TR is the gold standard used by insurers. Making a multiaxial diagnosis calls for clear thinking and good investigative work. After you have collected sufficient information, it is important to organize your database and to follow a systemic procedure:

Step 1: Determine whether there are exaggerated or feigned elements to the presentation.

- Is there evidence of intentionality?
- What is the probable motivation?

Step 2: Identify current primary diagnoses and consider recurrence and severity.

- Include all comorbid diagnoses (e.g., substance-use disorders).
- Consider adjustment disorder (excessive response to stressor).
- Remember the "not otherwise specified" (NOS) categorization (i.e., does not meet threshold criteria to allow for diagnosis of a disorder but there are still clinically significant symptoms).

Step 3: Rule out substance-induced and/or substance-use disorders (axis I) as the primary explanatory diagnosis.

- Review history of prescription and nonprescription drug use, including alcohol.
- Is the type/amount of drug likely to produce the current symptoms?
- How has the substance influenced course of symptoms?

Step 4: Rule out disorders due to general medical conditions (axes I and III).

- Review medical history and investigations.
- Are there medical conditions likely to produce symptoms?
- Consider whether medical conditions have influenced the course of symptoms, such as in the following:
  □ Pain disorder
  □ Somatoform disorder
  □ Conversion disorder

Step 5: If no specific diagnosis is present, do the symptoms represent a normal or maladaptive response to a stressor?

□ V Code diagnoses in DSM-IV-TR (e.g., adult antisocial behavior or occupational problem)
□ No diagnosis (Remember that just because someone is sent to a mental health professional, that person does not automatically have to receive a psychiatric diagnosis!)

Step 6: Look for evidence of personality traits/disorder and/or borderline intellectual functioning/mental retardation (axis II).

Step 7: Identify active, relevant, and significant general medical conditions (axis III).

Step 8: Identify psychosocial and environmental problems (axis IV).

Step 9: Assess level of functioning using the GAF (axis V).

Formulating and Providing an Understanding

The final step is a summary statement of the temporal sequence, causality, and contributions of psychological, social, physical, behavioral, and environmental factors that have resulted in the patient's current diagnosis, level of symptomatology, and level of functioning. Making an accurate diagnosis is one of the most crucial steps in clarifying disability due to mental disorder, but diagnosis alone does not explain a person's illness experience. Certain diagnoses are more likely to be associated with impairment in multiple domains of functioning; however, significantly different levels of impairment can be seen with the same diagnosis and illness severity. After going through the process of making a DSM-IV multiaxial diagnosis, the clinician then turns to the AMA classification of impairment (none, mild, moderate, marked, or extreme) and rates the patient's level of functioning in four domains—activities of daily living, social functioning, concentration, and adaptation. As discussed previously, impairment and disability can be reinforced by primary psychological gain such as fulfilling unmet dependency needs, deriving nurturance and support, or passively expressing hostility. Secondary gain such as avoiding work and receiving compensation are also powerful predictors of ongoing disability. Personality factors, substance use, pain, somatization, and motivation may dramatically influence functional capacities generally or in specific environments. Once the clinician has established ratings for each aspect of activity, an overall rating of impairment is provided, which is a summary judgment of the patient's overall level of functioning.

In Case Example 1, Mr. D. was suffering from a depressive state that he experienced as quite disabling. Despite having some control of his symptoms, his level of frustration and disillusionment appeared to be major contributors to his sense of helplessness and low level of functioning. Although Mr. D. was a capable and intelligent man, the consequences of a relatively minor low back injury become comprehensible when viewed through the lens of his developmental history, psychological makeup, and current environment. In a sense, the back injury represented a clear reminder of his shortcomings in life and accentuated his sense of failure. Mr. D. initially presented his early life in superficially positive terms. Further inquiry elicited a sense of emotional deprivation and grievance regarding not having attained the station in life to which he felt he was entitled. Mr. D. experienced deficits in early caretaking and nurturance. He was alienated from his father and brother and felt rejected as inferior, leaving him with an insecure sense of his masculinity. His mother seemed also not to be available to him, perhaps overwhelmed by the demands of home, husband, and four children but certainly with a more lively affective attachment to his younger twin sisters. Mr. D. adapted to this situation by developing a caretaking role towards his sisters and mother and a pseudoindependent, dismissive stance toward others, while retaining fantasies of his own power and special capacities. He found solace and a sense of competence through his involvement with books, computers, and other solitary activities. He avoided close connections with others but may have appeared brittle, arrogant, and sullen with authority figures. One must presume that these personality characteristics contributed to his lack of success with his initially chosen careers of firefighting and the police force. These failures were experienced as a further blow to his self-esteem and presumably enhanced Mr. D.'s underlying sense of deprivation, grievance, and entitlement.

He had had few intimate relationships with women and fled from his brief marriage when confronted with the responsibilities of having a child. He subsequently chose an older woman as a compromise between his wish for a stabilizing relationship and the need to maintain a more dependent position. Mr D.'s work in a warehouse allowed a balance between his comfort with isolation, avoidance of interpersonal conflicts (particularly with authority figures), and an opportunity for enhanced self-efficacy, in part through his job performance and in part through unrealistic fantasies of increasing wealth and power. Mr. D.'s back injury both represented a further personal failure and provided an unconscious psychological opportunity to redress his underlying sense of deprivation. Being at home, he could no longer find the same refuge that he enjoyed in his solitary job on the night shift; on the other hand, he could be cared for and benefit from the sense of legitimate need while avoiding autonomous responsibilities. Isolating himself at home would be a predictable coping pattern for Mr. D., at the expense of his relationships—his disability and lack of functioning both communicating a wish for nurturance and his anger and sense of grievance at his previous deprivation and lack of success. The possibility of being retrained in an alterative position also posed a new threat to his defenses of isolation and avoidance, both activating his anxieties and depressive frustration and thwarting his fantasies of power and wealth, exposing him to a sense of worthlessness and helplessness as he views these opportunities as beneath him. His partner, while increasingly resentful, has also unwittingly supported Mr. D.'s disabled role by assuming increasing responsibilities for their home and financial security. As a consequence of the confluence of these forces, Mr D. has increasingly been prone to somatization of his considerable psychological distress and thus become captive in a cycle of pain, depression, helplessness, and impairments in functioning with much of the origin of this situation being outside his conscious awareness. Such an analysis allows one to see that Mr. D.'s personality, defensive structure, developmental history, and current environment are all significant contributors to his depression and present barriers to his return to work. A treatment plan, to be effective, must directly or indirectly—and in particular, nonjudgmentally—address the multifaceted aspects of Mr. D.'s current state.

Determining Prognosis for Return to Work

Unfortunately, there is not a great deal of literature concerning mental disorder and the prognosis for return to work. Clearly, there are several clinical factors involved that are influenced by the complexity of the occupational health system and confounded by issues such as secondary gain, especially in relation to money. To simplify an inexact science, we have broken down the assessment into three categories: positive factors, negative factors, and barriers for return to work (Appendix 18-1). Further research is needed to clarify the weighting of these individual factors and is often based on the knowledge and experience of the examiner.

Making Recommendations

As a consultant and independent medical examiner, it is important to report your findings in a clear, comprehensible, and respectful manner, clearly answering the questions asked of you. If you are asked to make recommendations, ensure that they are comprehensive and focused with the goal of relieving impairment and fostering return to work. After all, even Freud recognized that our purpose in life is "to love and to work" (*"Lieben und arbeiten"*).

It is important to consider how disability affects not only the patient and the treating parties but also other parties involved, including the workplace, the insurer, and the home. We call this the "occupational mental health system," the system in which mental disorders affecting one's ability to work are influenced. Here are some of the other possible players besides you and your patient:

- Health care providers
  - Attending physicians
  - Occupational nurse
  - Physical therapist
  - Psychologist
  - Employee assistance program counselors
- Workplace
  - Human resources personnel
  - Occupational health and safety specialists
  - Coworkers
  - Employer
  - Union
- Insurer
  - Adjudicator
  - Case manager
  - Lawyer
- Home and community
  - Patient's lawyer
  - Family
  - Support and advocacy groups

After the parties involved have been identified, recommendations for improving work-related disability can take on several forms. The primary process through which this is achieved is by *supporting strengths* and *reducing barriers* through communication and collaboration. This role is often taken on by a case manger, but it is guided by a physician's recommendations.

Recommendations can be made by the assessor to various participants in the occupational and mental health network of the worker. These may include the following:

- Health care provider
  - Education
  - Pharmacological treatments
    - Medication/doses/titration/duration/side effects
    - Referral, if treatment-resistant
  - Psychological
    - Type/duration/frequency
    - Further cognitive or other psychometric testing
  - Physical treatments
    - Specialist consultation
    - Occupational therapy/physical therapy
    - Chiropractic
    - Medication changes
- Worker/patient
  - Abstinence from or reduction of substance use
  - Nutritional/exercise/stress interventions
  - Physical activity limitations if warranted
  - Participation in labor market retraining and academic upgrading
- Home and community
  - Education
  - Social support
  - Transportation
  - Monitoring
- Insurer
  - Case management issues
  - Suitability of labor market retraining and academic upgrading
- Workplace
  - Available duties
  - Roles and demands in accommodation
  - Union and managerial support
  - Monitoring

WRITING THE REPORT

The written report is the final product and demonstration of your expertise. Unlike many clinical records, many others besides health professionals will potentially utilize this report to make decisions based on your findings and conclusions. As a result, clarity and utility are of the utmost importance.

The general rules in writing the report are as follows:

- Its content and appearance must be professional and respectful.
- It must identify the questions asked and answer them accordingly.
- It must be fact based with stated sources.
- Its content must clearly support its conclusions.
- It must avoid legal conclusions (i.e., who is at fault).
- It must avoid direct statements or conclusions about credibility, letting the facts speak for themselves.
- It must use standardized instruments or methods, where possible, to allow comparison.

Report Content and Appearance

The preferences of the party requesting the report may vary somewhat; however, a typical structure for a medical disability report is presented below.

I. Reason for Examination
   a. Purpose and source of referral
   b. Time, place, persons involved
   c. Confidentiality exclusion
II. Examiner's Credentials
III. List of records reviewed and collateral information
   a. Date, type, source
IV. Identifying Data
   a. Individual identifiers
   b. Job description, employment history
V. Review of Records and Collateral Information
   a. Pertinent findings
   b. Missing details
VI. Interview and Examination
   a. History
   b. Mental status examination
   c. Physical examination
   d. Standardized tests
VII. Summary and Conclusions
   a. Restate objectives of examination
   b. Summary of findings
   c. Limitations and reliability, inconsistencies
   d. Findings relevant to each objective/question
   e. Formulation of contributing factors
VIII. Recommendations
   a. Treatment
   b. Work capabilities and restrictions, return-to-work process

SUMMARY AND CONCLUSIONS

We have demonstrated an approach to the psychiatric assessment of patients for the purpose of insurance and disability claims. Such assessments require not only the provision of psychiatric diagnoses but also consideration of the effects of mental illness on psychological, social, and occupational functioning and an evaluation of the psychological, physical, and environmental factors that contribute to the person's ability or inability to return to work or to qualify for compensation. These assessments are infinitely interesting, challenging, and rewarding. Although they require some special considerations, they are not outside the realm of empathic, effective, and thorough clinical care. When appropriately performed, they can be of enormous value to patients, families, health care providers, employers, and insurers.

REFERENCES

1. American Psychiatric Association: *Diagnostic and statistical manual of mental disorders*, ed 4, text revision, Washington DC, 2000, American Psychiatric Press.
2. World Health Organization: *International classification of functioning, disability, and health*, Geneva, 2001, World Health Organization.
3. Cocchiarella L, Andersson GBJ, editors, *Guides to the evaluation of permanent impairment*, ed 5, Chicago, 2001, American Medical Association.
4. Demeter SL, Andersson GBJ: *Disability evaluation*, ed 2, St Louis, 2003, American Medical Association/Mosby.
5. World Health Organization: *International classification of impairments, disabilities, and handicaps*, Geneva, 1980, World Health Organization.
6. Doege TC, Houston TP: *Guides to the evaluation of permanent impairment*, ed 4, Chicago, 1993, American Medical Association.

Appendix 18-1. Prognostic Factors for Return to Work

	Positive	Negative	Barriers

Individual	Young age
	Good premorbid
	  functioning
	Active coping
	High motivation
	Work history
	Diagnosis: mild/acute
	Less severity
	Treatment response
	Capacity to engage
	Psychological mindedness
	
	Capacity for self-reflection,
	  insight
	Education
	Transferable skills
	Adaptive defence mechanisms
		Severe physical injury
		  -Head injury
		  -Pain
		Delay to medical care
		Diagnosis: severe/chronic
		Comorbidity
		  -Substance abuse
		  -Forensic history
		  -Personality disorder
		Older age
		Past psychiatric history
		Past medical history
		Duration of illness
		Duration of disability
		Poor compliance
		Primary gain
		  -Dynamic
		  -Financial
		Secondary gain
			Education
			Language
			Lack of transferable skills
			
			Stigma
			Secondary gain
			  -Financial
			  -Nurturance/care
			  -Avoidance of responsibility
			
			Intelligence
			Transportation
			Premorbid defense mechanisms

Workplace	Vacation time "Best Practice" management Communication during leave Monitoring	Lack of policies Insufficient benefits Demand/control Effort/reward	Toxic work environment Availability of modified work positions Stigma Culture
Insurer	Comprehensive benefits Active case management	Adversarial claim process Pending litigation	Active and ongoing litigation Relationship with insurer Labor market reentry options
Health Care Provider	Psychological skills Pharmacological skills Timely communication Clear management plan Continuous monitoring to prevent relapse	Overprotective style Delayed communication Delayed treatment Collusion with the patient	Availability of treatment resources Community caregiver's stance

Home and Family	Family/social support	Culture/values inhibiting
		  use of resources
		High expectations at home
			Psychosocial/cultural support for
			  disability role
			Stigma

19

Assessment of Children

JOSEPH H. BEITCHMAN AND CORINE E. CARLISLE

INTRODUCTION

As clinicians we must recognize, diagnose, and appropriately intervene with children who have psychiatric disorders. In this chapter, we offer some guidelines on how to understand and approach the at times daunting and puzzling, but often rewarding task of bringing clarity, direction, and relief to the perplexed and distressed children and families you will encounter.

We have divided this chapter into three parts. The first is introductory and provides some context that will be helpful in understanding the clinical approach to a child and family. The section will be especially helpful for those who are new to the clinical assessment of children or who wish to have a quick refresher on the key issues. We briefly review and illustrate relevant developmental and family issues. This sets the stage for the second part, which describes the approach to the family and the child, including the questions to ask to obtain the relevant history. The third section more explicitly deals with the clinical interview of the child, how to approach it, what sort of issues emerge, and how to piece the information together into some coherent understanding of the referral question.

WHAT IS DIFFERENT ABOUT THE ASSESSMENT OF CHILDREN?

In all areas of medicine, we struggle to understand disease process in the context of an individual's biological, social, and psychological environment. This is especially true in child psychiatry, where a child's context is such a strong influence on the expression of developmental strengths and vulnerabilities. Even as advances in the basic sciences increase our understanding of fundamental illness processes, we nevertheless need to integrate this knowledge into a biopsychosocial understanding of the child. The psychiatric clinical interview of the child is uniquely designed to ascertain the necessary information about the child's current functioning, developmental capacities, and biological and social contexts so as to allow accurate diagnosis and effective treatment.

The Developmental Trajectory

Every child is an actively developing individual embedded within a family system and a wider social context. The process of development and the importance of family context are critical points of difference between the assessment of children and adults. Furthermore, it is not usually possible to review the history or symptoms with a child as one might with an adult. We depend on the child's parents to provide the history and a description of the symptoms; we look to confirm, refute, elaborate on, and understand the child's clinical picture by combining information from the direct interview of the child and the collateral information from significant adults in the child's life. Thus, the process is usually more time consuming. The pace must be adjusted to the tolerance and cognitive level of the child, and there is greater dependence on integrating information from multiple sources.

The active process of development adds several interconnected layers of complexity to achieving a thorough and accurate diagnostic understanding of the child patient. Dysfunction in children is ascertained by the degree by which they are developmentally "off course." Although there are broad general markers for normal development, there is also substantial variation from child to child. It is necessary to determine the developmental trajectory for the individual child as well as to compare the child's trajectory to the average normal developmental trajectory. For example, a 5-year-old child with autism who is not verbal but has developed rudimentary gestural communication with a primary caregiver may be "on course" for his own individual trajectory but yet far off the normal developmental course of a 5-year-old. A previously gregarious and outgoing 12-year-old who withdraws from all peer contact is evidencing a departure from both her individual trajectory and the average 12-year-old developmental trajectory.

Development is a lifelong process, but the rate and degree of change in adults are substantially less than in children. In the adult interview, it is possible to obtain retrospective information about early development and infer the impact of disrupted development on current functioning. The patient and adult both "observe" the information from "outside" of the developmental process (for the most part). In the child interview, the child is "in motion," in the midst of development. It is our task to "get onto the conveyor belt" and assess the child at that point as if moving with him. While "on the conveyor belt," we gather information about the child's ability to negotiate his physical environment, establish and maintain social relationships, regulate his internal world, and communicate internal states. It is also necessary that we stand "off the conveyor belt" and assess the progress of development and the biological and social contexts to the developmental trajectory.

Also, development is not a smooth linear process but one with irregular and intermittent progression. Just as there are physical growth spurts, so are there periods of rapid progression in other lines of development. Developmental challenges are approached and mastered in a series of trials. It is not always easy to tell whether a child is developmentally off course. For example, an 11-year-old boy who has a history of separation anxiety and behavioral inhibition is now experiencing difficulty in making and keeping peer relationships. Is this a *departure* from his developmental course? A *delay* in this line of social development? Or a *new manifestation* of long-standing anxieties and social skills deficits? In some cases, treatment options may be the same, regardless of your understanding of why the child is off course. In other cases, it is vital to have a realistic sense of the child's developmental capacities (and not overestimate them) so as to adequately support the child and family. Often, it is necessary to follow symptoms over time to adequately understand the child's developmental context.

Child Development and the Family Context

The primary caregivers and family are a critical force in shaping the child's developmental trajectory. An essential part of the assessment of the child is to understand the nature of the child's position within his family, a sense of the emotional climate in the home, the degree to which the parents get along with each other and are unified in their attitude and approach to childrearing, and their attitudes and ideas about their child. Not uncommonly, parents will have divided perspectives on the nature of their child's concerns. In this situation, you must determine the degree to which this may be having an impact on their child, and factor it into the planning and implementation of the treatment.

It is also not uncommon for the assessment to uncover that other members of the family are suffering from clinical or subclinical psychiatric distress. It may even be that the child has no clinical disorder but is reacting to dysfunction in other family members or in the family as a whole. However, keep in mind that the child's development and behavior have also shaped the family and how it functions. A family may appear at the time of assessment to be dysfunctional because of multiple adaptations to the child's difficulties. This is a reciprocal system; the child and the family affect each other. Assessment of the child aims to disentangle the elements of this reciprocal system, which may perpetuate difficulties for the child and family alike. Do not allow this information to promote the laying of blame on either the child or the family, but rather, use it as indication of the efforts of each to cope to the best of their abilities and resources.

Case Example 1

An 11-year-old girl with increasingly severe symptoms of obsessive compulsive disorder had curtailed her eating habits because of fears that the food was contaminated. Her parents were distraught to see her not eating. They agreed to order in specific food from restaurants so that she would have something to eat. By the time the girl came for assessment, the family had made multiple adaptations to the girl's increasingly restricted behaviors around eating, washing, and sleeping.

Key Point:

What may at times appear to be pathological may have originated in the family's attempt to cope with the difficulties to the best of their abilities and resources. It is important not to lay blame.

Child Development and Information Gathering

There is also complexity in obtaining information about the psychiatric symptoms and internal experiences of the child patient. The stage of development determines the capacity of the child for understanding and communicating the symptoms of psychiatric illness. The younger the child, the more necessary it is to rely on observation and play interactions, as well as on obtaining collateral information from caregivers. Furthermore, the child is seldom the one who requests psychiatric referral. Most commonly, a parent, teacher, or other adult in the child's life will initiate the assessment. In practical terms, it is then critical to get collaborative information from adults. Commonly, parents and teachers will have diverse perspectives on the nature of the child's problems. It then becomes our challenge to be thorough and comprehensive enough to clarify the issues raised and to formulate an appropriate intervention plan.

Key Point:

The parents, teacher, and child may have different perspectives on the area of concern. Incorporate each of these perspectives into the formulation of the clinical problem.

Child Development and the Expression of Psychiatric Illness

It is intuitive that development influences the onset and the expression of psychiatric illness. Psychiatric disorders have characteristic ages when symptoms first emerge. For example, separation anxiety typically presents in young children, whereas mood disorders more often present in later childhood or adolescence. Psychiatric illness does not manifest itself in children exactly as it does in adults. Some of these differences are incorporated into the *Diagnostic and Statistical Manual of Mental Disorders*, Fourth Edition, Text Revision (DSM-IV-TR)[1] criteria, as in the case of a depressive episode, where criteria permit children to have an "irritable mood" as opposed to a "depressed mood." Other disorders are usually first diagnosed in children and not in adults such as mental retardation, autism, pervasive developmental disorder, reactive attachment disorder, feeding disorders, separation anxiety, selective mutism, tic disorders, learning disorders, attention deficit hyperactivity disorder (ADHD), conduct disorder, and oppositional defiant disorder. Those assessing children must be familiar with these diagnoses and their DSM-IV-TR criteria.

You can safely assume that no child has read the DSM-IV-TR, and it is seldom that a child will come with a clinical presentation that exactly matches the diagnostic criteria found in that manual. Many children with psychiatric disorders will have more than one disorder or have subclinical symptomatology from more than one diagnostic category. For example, a child with ADHD may have comorbid symptoms of oppositional defiant disorder and conduct disorder, or a child with encopresis may exhibit symptoms of anxiety. Even when the symptoms *can* be assigned to a particular diagnostic category, it is important to identify the

issues in the child's current family circumstances, school environment, or social circle that will provide an explanation and understanding of the child's difficulties and help identify possible approaches to intervention. Look for recent changes in the child's life experience, such as a new school, parental separation, a new step-parent, and so on.

It is also true that the pattern of symptoms may evolve as the child develops. This may lead to more symptoms and more diagnoses as the child develops, or it may mean that the child's diagnosis changes over time. For all these reasons, it is vital to keep a broad differential diagnosis during the interview, to screen broadly for other areas of symptomatology, and to listen carefully to the child and family as they describe current and past areas of difficulty. Even if a child does not appear to meet criteria for any clinical diagnosis, it is important to consider that someone was sufficiently concerned about this child to prompt psychiatric referral. A thorough assessment may reveal difficulties in the child or the family that were not necessarily the reason for referral but are nonetheless the source of dysfunction and concern.

Case Example 2

A 9-year-old girl was referred for assessment of multiple severe somatic complaints and depressed mood. Assessment revealed parental discord and extreme anxiety in the girl's mother. In this case, parent-child relationship difficulties were the focus of treatment in family therapy.

Child Development and Treatment of Psychiatric Disorders

The developmental process and the child's sensitivity to environmental factors add complexity to the assessment of children but also provide you with many treatment intervention possibilities. Few of the psychiatric diagnoses in childhood lend themselves to one specific prescribed form of intervention. This is often because of psychiatric comorbidity and because the manifest symptoms can arise for many different reasons and be maintained by several different factors, as will be illustrated later in this chapter. Although it is important to seek and accurately identify (by DSM-IV-TR diagnostic criteria) clinical diagnoses, it is equally important to determine symptomatology, its meaning to the family and child, and the impact the symptoms have on both the family and the child. Each of these factors directs intervention. Our challenge is to understand the possible reasons behind the child's symptoms; this will then maximize the array of interventions available and the chances that interventions will be effective. Symptoms may be attributable to family system dysfunction, learning difficulties at school, developmental difficulties that emerge as the child is presented with increasingly complex cognitive and social challenges, or some other change in the child's life experience.

The treatment plan must address the child's perspective of the current difficulties, biological vulnerabilities, the symptom picture, the functioning of the family, and the child's wider social context. The treatment plan may be a medication, a special educational program, individual or family psychotherapy, or a combination of these or others. Each is a lever by which to return the child (and the family) to the optimal developmental trajectory.

Case Example 3

A 10-year-old boy is referred for assessment because of behavior difficulties at home and school. Assessment reveals that he is "clingy" and demanding of his mother. He requires explanation of where his mother is going and exactly when she will be back each time she leaves the house. At bedtime he takes a long time to settle and requests multiple "good nights" and reassurances from his parents. If he wakes at night, he will sometimes sleep in his parents' bed or on the floor of his parents' bedroom so as to feel safe. He has an active imagination and extrapolates his own catastrophic stories from television programs and books. At school, he has trouble paying attention and getting his work done. Homework is also a source of tension at home. He is socially immature and does not respond to social cuing appropriately. He has been the target of bullying at school. He was born prematurely by emergency cesarean section. He had difficulty breathing at first and had to stay in the intensive care unit for a few days. Otherwise, all developmental milestones were within normal limits. He lives with his biological parents and younger brother. His father is a long-haul truck driver and is often away from home. His mother is a homemaker who can feel overwhelmed by this boy, especially when her husband is away. There is a family history of anxiety disorder. This child may have a biological vulnerability to anxiety. He was a "fragile" newborn, and his parents were very protective of him as an infant.

Comment. This boy has symptoms of anxiety, inattention, and hyperactivity and poor social skills. The biological context includes premature birth and a family history of anxiety disorder. The family context is complicated by the frequent absence of his father. In this instance, combination therapy of medication for the child to address his high anxiety and family therapy to modify the now maladaptive family roles was successful in treating this boy's and his family's difficulties.

Brief Overview of Child Development

It is not the place of this chapter to attempt a complete overview of child development; however, assessing whether a child is developmentally off course requires some working knowledge of child development. For the child patient, psychiatric assessment implies developmental assessment (in the broadest sense). We provide a very brief summary of pertinent major developmental processes and milestones, and also the clinical diagnoses that are commonly made in children at certain ages. For an in-depth review of development, we direct the reader to the recommended readings provided at the end of the chapter. The material presented in this section highlights the need to consider the biological, psychological, and social determinants of dysfunction in children if we are to gain a comprehensive understanding of the clinical problem.

For example, a 12-year-old boy diagnosed with ADHD may have a history of premature birth, neonatal intensive care admission, repeated hospitalizations for severe asthma, parental conflict, and a parental separation at age 4 years. Another 12-year-old boy diagnosed with ADHD may have an uneventful pregnancy and birth and no family conflict, but a family history suggestive of ADHD in his father. The DSM-IV-TR diagnosis for these two boys is the same, but the understanding of their difficulties and the treatment plans to address them will differ in many ways.

Development is a multidimensional process that is biologically determined yet altered by environment and experience, and that also itself alters the environment through the child's changing interactions with it. We will consider the mutually interdependent biological, psychological, and social influences on development for preschool and school-aged children.

The Preschool Child: Infancy to 4 Years

The biological substrate of development begins with the birth of cortical neurons from approximately day 40 to 125 of intrauterine life. Aberrations in the subsequent division, migration, and differentiation of neurons can lead to mental retardation[2] and neurological disorders. Fetal alcohol syndrome,[3] epilepsy,[4] autistic disorder,[5] and schizophrenia[6] are postulated to be associated with abnormal neural migration and differentiation. More subtle intrauterine changes in cell organization and function may be related to vulnerability to psychiatric disorder in extrauterine life. Once the child is born, toxins such as lead and mercury and illnesses such as meningitis and traumatic brain injury can have a direct deleterious effect on neurological development.

Temperament, a child's characteristic style of responding, is an important biological factor in development. Modern concepts of temperament address the emotional, motivational, and adaptive aspects of behavior. Three broad aspects of temperament are gaining wide acceptance: reactivity or negative emotionality, self-regulation, and approach-withdrawal. *Reactivity* or *negative emotionality* refers to irritability, negative mood, and high-intensity negative reactions and can be subdivided into distress at limitations (e.g., irritability, anger) and distress at novelty (e.g., fearfulness). *Self-regulation* has two subcomponents: the effortful control of attention (e.g., persistence, nondistractibility) and of emotions (e.g., self-soothing). The *approach-withdrawal* dimension, sometimes referred to as *inhibition* or *sociability,* describes the tendency of a child to either approach novel situations or people or, conversely, to withdraw and be wary. Temperament is considered a relatively stable, biologically based intrinsic characteristic, which is nevertheless modifiable through environmental influences.[7]

Parenting does not modify temperament substantially, but temperament is a critical biological influence on the functioning of the parent-child dyad. An active, intense 2-year-old may be a "handful" for a quiet, introverted mother. On the other hand, a child with the same temperament may be experienced as lively and engaged by a mother who is herself energetic and outgoing. Relative "goodness of fit" between child and parent is an important facilitator of secure *attachment* of the child. A child's early experiences of attuned parenting influence the biological refinement of neural pathways that will in turn facilitate exploration of the environment and individuation from parents as the child grows. By 1 year of age, the child has established attachment to primary caregivers.

The movement from parental regulation of eating and sleeping to self-regulation is a major developmental task in the first year or so of life. Temperament has a bearing on the speed and ease with which a child will establish his or her own biorhythms. Motor control matures from head to foot and from proximal to distal. There is a movement from instinctual, primitive reflexes to voluntary muscle control. Interaction of the parent with the child promotes verbal and nonverbal communication, motor development, and visual and auditory processing capacities. The acquisition of mobility (crawling then walking) occurs by approximately 1 year of age. This represents a major shift toward independence and provides an ever-widening array of sensory and motor experiences for the child.

Fear of strangers and separation anxiety emerge at approximately this age. The child will retreat from people unfamiliar to her and cry at the departure of the primary caregivers. Communication moves from reflex smiles to reciprocal social interactions with primary caregivers to voluntary gestural communication to verbalizations. The child should have single word skills by the age of 1 year and speak in simple sentences by age 3. The child will usually understand more than he can say, and the parents should be alert to their 2- or 3-year-old child who seems not to understand simple two- and three-word phrases.

Symbolic thought develops and is seen in the child's ability to recognize herself in the mirror, understand the symbolic meaning of language, and engage in fantasy play. By age 4, children are independently mobile, have fine motor skills that allow them to manipulate small objects and draw pictures, and can play cooperatively with other children. At this age, they have begun to self-regulate emotions (e.g., 3-year-old boy hugs his favorite teddy bear to comfort himself when he is upset about not getting ice cream) and self-limit behavior (e.g., 4-year-old girl does not hit her little brother when he interrupts her play by taking her Barbie doll; instead, she calls her father to intervene).

Children ages 2 to 5 years old are often very curious about the sexual differences between boys and girls. Just as they are exploring other aspects of their world, they explore their bodies and the sensations that arise in them. Parenting should ideally provide children with information about appropriate public behavior while allowing them to feel good about their bodies. In the preschool years, children already demonstrate a choice of toys and patterns of play that are typical of male or female gender identity and role. Boys who prefer to wear girls' clothing, play with dolls, and avoid rough play may prompt concern in parents about the child's gender identity. Likewise, girls who dislike wearing dresses, prefer to play with boys, and who choose action heroes as role models may also prompt parental concern and psychiatric referral. There is increasing latitude in gender roles in our current society; nevertheless, children themselves may express strong feelings of wanting to be or be like the opposite sex.

Other difficulties that can prompt referral for psychiatric assessment during these early years are regulation problems (e.g., feeding and sleeping problems, shyness, aggression) and parent-child relational difficulties (e.g., issues of discipline). Fine motor, gross motor, and language skills are developing rapidly over these first 4 years, and referral may result from parental concern about lack of progress in any of these developmental spheres. Mental retardation, pervasive developmental disorders (including autism), coordination disorders, learning disorders, communication disorders, and ADHD are possible diagnoses in this age group. Tic disorders may emerge at this early age, although they more commonly present at age 7 or 8 years.

The School-Aged Child: 5 to 12 Years

Starting school is a major developmental step. The child leaves home for a substantial portion of the day. Primary caregivers are not present. New environments, new authority figures, new rules, new social relations, and new expectations for performance must all be negotiated. For children who have been in day care since a very young age, the start of school may not be so dramatic a shift from previous experience. For children not previously in day care, starting school may represent the first significant time away from parents and primary care givers. The challenges of school are also opportunities for mastery and competition.

School-aged children are curious about the world they live in and the people around them. They are eager to acquire and integrate new knowledge. They are developing reasoning capabilities and generating hypotheses about their environment. Frequently, they have incomplete information on which to base hypotheses, and their reasoning may seem comical to adults. Children of this age may be exquisitely sensitive to criticism. Their building sense of self is commensurate with their attempts to build knowledge of the world around them. Insensitive criticism of their efforts to understand the natural and social world can have a heavy negative impact on their self-esteem. Success in school can greatly promote a child's sense of mastery and spur the child to further achievement. Likewise, a child who struggles with the academic, social, or behavioral demands of school may feel defeated and have poor self-esteem.

The promotion of "multiple intelligences" within the educational system and opportunities to demonstrate accomplishment in an area of strength may be critical in sustaining a child through struggles at school. For instance, a child who is creative may derive self-esteem from artistic accomplishment at school. This may be protective during a time when the child is doing poorly in math and English. Likewise, organized sports may offer a constructive outlet for energy and aggression in a child who has attentional difficulties. This allows the child to feel good about running and jumping—things that may actually get the child in trouble in the classroom.

The birth of a younger sibling can challenge the child for physical space in the home (e.g., the child may no longer have her own bedroom), for the attention of primary caregivers, and, as the younger sibling grows older, she is a competitor in terms of skills and knowledge. Severe sibling rivalry or failure of a child to adapt to the birth of a younger sibling can prompt clinical referral.

School-aged children most often prefer same-gender playmates, and gender-specific games can be observed on the playground. Games and play become more rule-oriented, although children at these ages are still very active in fantasy play. Mastery of new skills and ideas and competition with peers are the important tasks in this age group. Success in academics, sports, and social interactions leads to self-esteem. Interest in sexual differences and sexual behaviors continues and increases as children approach early adolescence. Children may be very aware of body differences at this age. Girls may be concerned about weight and engage in dieting to obtain unrealistic and unhealthy thinness. Boys may be concerned about their physical size and strength. Children, particularly

girls, who are early to develop physically, may be subject to teasing.

The school-aged child is fully mobile, has good fine-motor control, and has good command of language. Lack of gross motor coordination, poor fine motor control, or language difficulties are concerns that may arise in these years if they have not come to clinical attention earlier. Most children have attained daytime bladder and full bowel control by this age. Enuresis and encopresis are common clinical problems presenting in this age group. The major developmental task of the school-aged child is the separation from parents and the adaptation to school life. Separation anxiety and school refusal may result in psychiatric referral. Somatic symptoms, such as frequent stomachaches and headaches, may lead to time off school and concern about the child's academic and social functioning. The structured school environment requires children to be able to attend to, comprehend, and carry out instructions. Difficulties in attention (e.g., ADHD), language processing or oppositional defiance are common reasons for the school to suggest assessment. Social problems such as difficulty making or keeping friends, bullying, or being bullied are problems that can emerge in this period. Often, problems in behavior or academic performance do not arise until the later elementary grades, when workload increases, academic material becomes more complex, and peer relationships become more sophisticated and challenging.

Key Point:

The major developmental task of the school-aged child is the separation from parents and the adaptation to school life.

OBTAINING THE HISTORY

You have received a referral request. A critical first step is to understand the reason for referral and the history of the child's problems. There are several important components involved in obtaining the relevant information: what to ask, whom to ask, and how to go about asking. We review some of these principles in this section, starting with the initial phone contact with the child's family. Although information obtained directly from the child forms an essential part of the assessment, we discuss in greater detail the interview with the child in a later section of this chapter.

Before the First Meeting

After receiving the referral request, contact the family to review their concerns and reasons for the referral and to arrange the appointment. During this initial contact with the family, you should ask who wants the assessment—the parents, the teacher, or someone else? Do both parents agree on the need for the assessment? Sometimes, parents will disagree on the need for the assessment, but one parent (most often the mother) may insist. In this situation, it is best to have both parents attend the initial interview, since the other parent may hold the key to successful intervention. If he or she is not in attendance, you will not be able to recruit him or her to assist in the implementation of your treatment plan.

Inquire about the child's attitude toward the assessment, what he understands, and what he has been told. Children can have many different ideas about the reason for a psychiatric assessment. They may assume it to be like visits to their pediatrician and will be concerned that they will get "a needle" when they arrive. They also frequently experience the assessment to be about something "bad" they have been doing, and they may fear punishment or blame. Advise the parents to tell their child the reasons for the assessment. This should be done in a way that the child will understand and so as to make him not feel blamed and to make him believe that the assessment may help him in some way. Be sure that the parents tell their child there are no needles, that they will be seeing a talking doctor who helps children with worries and problems, and who also helps families when families have problems getting along. Tell the parents how long the first appointment will take, what you plan to do, and what they might expect from the first meeting. Tell the parents that their child can bring along a favorite toy to the assessment if he wishes to do so. This can help alleviate the child's anxiety and facilitate the initial interview. Check the current custody arrangements for the child.

The Office Environment and the Use of Toys

The office must be organized to facilitate the assessment of the child and family. There should be ample space to accommodate the child and parents and any others. There should an appropriate selection of toys and materials geared to the age and sex of the child. The seating arrangement should be comfortable, including chairs suitably sized for children. A surface or small table that the child can use to color, draw, or play on should also be available, and simple play materials provided such as paper, pencil, and nontoxic crayons. Additional materials would include toy furniture; some small figures or dolls representing babies, children, and adults; some blocks; a few cars or trucks; and Lego pieces appropriate for the fine motor skills of the age of the child being seen. The room should be safe; breakable objects and scissors or other sharp objects should be out of reach of the child. Furthermore, valuable personal items

should be out of the child's reach so as to avoid potential confrontations generated by the child's interest in these personal items. It is best to include only a modest display of toys. Too many toys may overstimulate the child, or the child might be so absorbed in the toys that she is difficult to engage. Also, parents may feel bad if they believe the toys they provide their child at home do not measure up to the toys available in the clinician's office.

Toys serve several functions in the assessment of children. The presence of toys allows the child to feel welcomed in the clinician's office; it communicates to the child that it is a place for children. Toys will help the child to feel more comfortable and less fearful of being with the assessing physician. After your introductory remarks to the child and family, toys allow the younger child to be occupied while you speak with the parents. During this time, observe how the child explores the room and uses the available toys. Is the child very tentative in her exploration, never leaving the parent's knee? Or is the child "all over the place," moving from toy to toy but not settling on any one item for very long? A child's play with toys can communicate many things about the child: motor skills, outgoingness, attention, aggression, and ability to listen to and follow rules. A child's fantasy play may reveal important themes that potentially relate to the clinical difficulties. For example, one child playing with a mother and father doll identified the mother doll as a witch and had the mother doll thrown into a garbage can. You should be cautious about interpreting such displays, but it does alert you to potential areas for further inquiry.

Play materials can also be used with older children. A useful approach will be to have them draw pictures. They can be invited to draw a picture of a person and a picture of their family doing something. This can then be used as an opportunity to engage the child in some discussion about the characters they have drawn and what they are doing. The pictures may represent important thoughts, beliefs, and experiences of the child. For example, one child with a history of hydrocephalus, when invited to draw a picture of a person, drew a picture of a boy with a large body and a very small head. Once again, one must be cautious about drawing inferences; nevertheless, it suggests the importance of inquiring further about this boy's concerns about the size of his head and his mental capabilities. (This is explored further in the Interviewing Children section to follow.)

Key Point:

The child's drawings often represent her thoughts, feelings, beliefs, and experiences and offer a window into the child's mind.

It is tempting to use board games (such as checkers) or card games with older children. Although structured games allow engagement with the child and may provide a setting for conversation, they do not promote imaginative play and they do not provide the child with an opportunity to "play out" fears, concerns, or difficulties. They also promote competition with the physician, which though potentially informative, may impede the clinical assessment.

Custody and Access Arrangements

If the child is not living with both biological parents, be sure to clarify custody arrangements before booking the first assessment appointment. If it is clear that the child resides with both parents and both have custody, then the assessment can proceed even if the child attends with only one parent. If, on the other hand, the child is living with one parent, confirmation of the legal status of custody and access is required. Sometimes the child is brought for assessment by the noncustodial parent, unbeknownst to and/or against the wishes of the custodial parent; the assessment should not proceed under these circumstances. If custody and access arrangements are not completely understood from the initial telephone conversation with the parent/guardian, they must be clarified at the beginning of the first assessment meeting.

The First Appointment

Who should come for the first appointment? Ideally, the child, both parents, and all siblings should attend for the first appointment. As discussed previously, the child is embedded in the family system, is influenced *by* the family, and is an influence *on* the family. Seeing the child in the context of the whole family system can be extremely helpful in the assessment of the child's difficulties. Although this is the preferred and perhaps ideal circumstance, it is more common, however, that the child will attend the initial appointment with the mother or legal guardian. After the initial appointment, you will have a sense of the relative importance of seeing both parents together (with or without the child) and of including siblings in future appointments.

For the first appointment, whether you invite the whole family or just the child and primary caregiver, it is essential to keep in mind the goal of assessment: obtaining a thorough understanding of the child. The primary caregiver or parent(s) may be the most efficient source of information about the child's past and current functioning, birth history, and early development. It is also vital to learn about the child's role and functioning in the family; this is most efficiently and accurately accomplished by observing the whole family together. Not only will you see how the child and family members interact, but also parents and siblings

can provide information about how the child's difficulties have affected them. However, do not assume that the relationships observed in the family interview are necessarily the same as the "in vivo" experience in the daily life of the family. There should be consistency between your observations during the family interview and the information obtained on how the family members usually interact. If not, you will need to understand the reasons for the discrepancy. For instance, parents may say that their son does not care about school, yet during the course of your interview he appears especially sad and worried that he may be failing. Ask the parents how they understand the difference between their ideas and your observations.

The First Face-to-Face Contact

Greet the family and child in the waiting room. Introduce yourself to the parents and be sure to introduce yourself to the child (and siblings, if present). Invite them to come with you, and show them into your office.

Even if the parent has described the presenting problem in the initial phone contact, remind them that you had spoken on the phone, but that you want to be sure that you understand fully their reasons for the visit. Then, ask again why they have come and what they expect from the assessment. It may be that different members of the family have very different answers to these questions. Even so, each should be given an opportunity to voice an opinion, including the child. Tell the family that different perspectives on an issue are common and that it is not your role to judge which is right or wrong, but rather, it is important to hear different perspectives so as to get as complete an understanding as possible of the problems that have prompted clinical assessment. Be sure to ask the child what he understands of the reason for the visit and whether he has any questions or concerns about what is going to happen during the meeting. For example, *"Johnny, do you know why your Mom and Dad wanted you to come here today?"* Answers such as, "Because I am bad at school," or "Because I get stomachaches," or "Because my mom said I had to come," reveal the child's perspective about being at the assessment and how he feels about the area of clinical concern and also hint at the impact the problem has had on the child's self-esteem. Even if the answer to the question is "Nothing!" or "I don't know," it is an opportunity to explain the purpose and process of the assessment and to allay potential fears about "needles," blame, and punishment that the child is unlikely to voice.

After you clarify the purpose of the assessment, tell the family how you plan to proceed. For example, *"Let me tell you how I would like to proceed today. We will meet together for about 30 minutes or so. Afterward, I will meet alone with Johnny for another 30 minutes. We will take a short break during which you can find some juice or coffee in the canteen on the ground floor. After the break, I will meet with both Mom and Dad to complete the assessment and offer you some feedback."* In most instances, you will need more than one appointment to gain a sufficient understanding of the child's problems. Tell the parents that you do not know whether you will need to schedule another appointment, but it is likely that you will need to do so. Depending on the complexity of the case, you may elect to tell the parents, before the first appointment, that the assessment is likely to take more than one appointment.

Identifying Information

Some of the child's identifying information will already be known from the initial phone contact with the parent/guardian, but most will be collected at the start of the interview. Some identifying information may be left to be obtained later in the interview when areas of clinical concern are discussed (e.g., if fighting at school is the presenting problem, the information about school grade, program, and performance at school may be obtained later in the interview both to improve flow of the interview and to avoid raising high anxiety in the child very early on).

Regardless of who attends the first appointment, it is important to identify who lives in the child's home and the relationship of each of these persons to the child. There may be extended family (such as a grandparent, aunt, uncle, or other relative) living with the child who have a bearing on the child's behavior. The biological parent may be living with a new partner after separation or divorce. There may be children from a parent's previous relationship who live in the home. Be certain to determine all the persons with whom the child resides and all the significant persons in the child's life, such as an older half-sibling or cousin living in or outside of the family home.

If the child is not living with both the biological parents, it is necessary to clarify the access and visitation arrangements. This is an important legal issue in terms of which parent can authorize a psychiatric assessment of the child. Beyond these legal issues, however, it is also important to explore custody and access arrangements because they are common areas of severe and sometimes lingering conflict between parents. Furthermore, if the child lives with one parent and visits with the other parent who shares custody or has visitation access, times of transition between homes can be times of extreme conflict between parents, between either/both parents and the child, and also extreme conflict for the child. This topic is easily broached. For example, *"Mrs. Jones, can you tell me who lives in your home with Johnny?"* Mrs. Jones explains she lives alone with Johnny. This then provides the opportunity to inquire about the child's other parent and to what extent the child has contact

with that parent. Some fairly standard and straightforward questions to address this area are: *"Can you tell me when Johnny sees his father?" "How many times per month does Johnny see his father?" "What days of the week and times of the day does Johnny spend with his father?" "Is the visitation schedule regular?"* In addition, it is important to ask how the child gets to the noncustodial parent's home and how the child is returned. Ask whether there are issues that arise during the transitions from one parent to the other. It will usually be important to speak with both the custodial and noncustodial parent to make an independent judgment about the extent to which the child's difficulties are specific to one setting versus the other and/or about the extent to which the difficulties in one setting contribute to those in the other.

Clarify the nature of the child's relationship with his siblings. The child can be in a situation in which an older sibling bullies or exploits the child, provoking and otherwise contributing to the child's difficulties. Likewise, the child can in turn be provoking, exploiting, or bullying an older or younger sibling. You will need to decide whether the sibling issues fall within the normal range of sibling rivalry/conflict. Consider the intensity of the sibling conflict, whether there seems to be any parental favoritism of one child over the other, and, if so, the extent to which the child is perhaps aware of this favoritism and reacting to it. If there is evidence of physical harm to either child, recommendations must to be developed and employed to ensure safety in the home.

Once the names and relationships of the family members attending the interview have been learned and clarified (this usually takes about 5 minutes, unless the family situation is very complicated), it is often nice to ask the younger child a question or two for which he will be confident of the answer. *"And how old are you, Johnny? What grade are you in? What is your teacher's name?"* This initial verbal contact communicates to the child that you are interested in what he has to say, too, and can put the child at more ease. This is also a nice time to invite the child to explore the drawing or play materials provided in the office.

It is important to identify what school and grade the child attends and whether it is a regular or a modified educational program. It is not infrequent that clinical concerns involve issues at school, so it may be that this information is more reasonably obtained when the clinical concerns are being discussed (see School History section to follow).

At the beginning of the first appointment, you should meet with the whole family (or all those family members who attend the first meeting) and talk as a family group in the presence of the child while the child is invited to play with the toys and games put out for the child. It is important during this time to ensure that the discussion is sensitive to and respectful of the child, with any harshly negative or critical comments and other forms of disparaging remarks about the child reserved for a separate interview where the child is not present. A parent should be helped to provide the history and developmental information in as positive or neutral a way as possible with respect to any issues or concerns. If the developmental history is extensive, arrange to meet separately with the parents to obtain this information. It will be more informative, and you and the parents can more easily focus on the critical issues of development without the child present.

When the interview involves an older child, the child can be invited to speak more actively about his concerns, and the dialogue between the child and the parents and other family members can be instructive. Observe whom the child sits closest to—whether the mother or the father—and observe any potential alliances between the child and other family members. Does the parent compare the child to a sibling? Observe the content as well as the nature of the dialogue between the child and parents: whether a parent appears cold, harsh, or critical toward the child, or on the contrary, is the parent infantilizing?

Case Example 4

One mother of an 8½-year-old boy was so worried about her son's ability to take care of himself that she continued to wipe his bottom for him. This boy had problems with independence and lacked the confidence that he could perform age-appropriate tasks himself. The mother was helped to step back, allowing her son to take appropriate responsibility for his own bodily functions.

The History of Presenting Problems

Gather as much information as possible about the presenting problems. When did the problem start? Did it start abruptly after a precipitating event, or has the problem been chronic but worsening? What makes the problem worse? Better? What is the impact of the problem on the child? On the family? This approach will often encompass issues of where (e.g., classroom versus playground versus home) and with whom (e.g., with Mom but not with Dad) the problems are worse or better. It will also often invite information about past and current therapies (e.g., psychotherapy, pharmacotherapy, educational programs) and recent changes in the child's life (e.g., change in family constellation, death of a family member, change of school, loss of friends, bullying). If the family can identify a period in time when the child was symptom free or showed evidence of minimal symptomatology, it may be possible to identify circumstances in the child's life that inform the assessment with respect to appropriate strategies of intervention;

for example, "She was doing alright until Suzie was born," or "He was doing okay before he started the advanced class at school."

When you obtain the history of the presenting problems, inquire about any previous psychiatric history and any previous assessments. Obtain permission to request copies of any previous psychiatric or psychological reports. Previous assessments will help guide the current assessment by revealing what gaps exist in understanding the child's psychiatric problems.

When you get the history from the parents about the child's problems, do not take the information at face value. This is especially true if the parents offer you conclusions about their child, such as "He never listens," "She hears what she wants to hear," "She is stubborn," "He is lazy," etc. Ask for examples with specific details, and draw your own conclusions. For instance, a parent may complain that Johnny never listens to them. On further inquiry, it appears that the parent is complaining that Johnny does not come when called. However, from Johnny's perspective, he had been watching his favorite television program, and there is 5 or 10 minutes to go before the denouement in which he will discover if the good guy survives and if the bad guy is captured, and he pleads to wait the extra 5 or 10 minutes to the end of his show. A detailed inquiry of this kind helps to put into perspective the nature of the parents' complaint and their relationship with their child.

This approach is especially important in situations when parents are angry with their child and convey a sense of blaming him. In these circumstances, the assessment requires skillful interviewing. The challenge arises in situations in which the parents may believe that a particular problem exists because of the child (i.e., what the child is *doing*), whereas the child will feel aggrieved, unsupported, and picked on or neglected (i.e., what the child feels is done *to* her). Our challenge is to find the appropriate balance in which the parents feel that they are supported, that their perspective is understood, and that they are receiving appropriate empathic understanding for their concerns, while at the same time the parents are helped to understand the child's perspective and the issues at hand over which they have some control and influence. A critical therapeutic strategy is to help the parents reduce their own sense of guilt and blame and move toward a more concrete problem-focused approach.

The Clinical Picture

Explore in detail the symptoms and clinical picture. Has the child's academic performance fallen? Has she withdrawn from her friends? Has the child started to have frequent stomachaches and miss many days of school? Is she depressed and tearful, or angry and irritable? All of these changes in a child can prompt clinical concern. It is not always straightforward to differentiate the principal difficulty from difficulties arising secondarily. It is essential to be aware of all aspects of the current dysfunction of the child, whether or not the temporal sequence can be disentangled. For example, it may not be possible to tease apart whether symptoms of depression and anxiety in a 12-year-old girl preceded or followed the onset of her fibromyalgia and her school refusal. Her family history included first-degree relatives with both depression and somatic complaints. Because the girl identified her fibromyalgia (fatigue, painful joints, and muscles) as the main impediment to school attendance, the treatment plan focused on pharmacological treatment of the pain and a graded approach to school reentry. Ongoing evaluation of depression and anxiety showed that these symptoms improved as pain decreased and normal activities were resumed. If depression had not remitted with treatment of the fibromyalgia, it would have been necessary to address and treat this symptom as a primary clinical problem.

A not uncommon parental complaint is that a child is difficult to manage at home. Here again, clarify whether this is of recent onset or longer duration. For example, the parents might complain that they have difficulty with their youngster because he doesn't listen to them. Although this had been a chronic problem, there has been a recent exacerbation. On further inquiry, you learn that one parent has recently taken on a new job (or alternatively, there has been a change in that parent's workload or work hours), so that the parent is less accessible and under more stress when at home and dealing with the child. Thus, the exacerbation in the behavioral problem is the result of a combination of the parent being less available to respond patiently and appropriately to the developmental needs of the child, and the child's behavior worsening in reaction to the felt change in the parent's availability and responsiveness.

Case Example 5

Anxiety at School and Changed Emotional Climate at Home. Jay is an 11-year-old girl who was referred because of concerns about anxiety symptoms. Jay had recently started at ABC School and reported that she was having difficulty following along in class. She would sit in class but could not understand what the teacher was explaining. In each class, Jay became progressively more and more worried as she found she could not understand, and finally she would begin to cry. Jay also developed stomachaches, was frequently tearful, and one time drew a picture of a weeping girl saying that she just couldn't go on.

During the interview, Jay revealed that she had always had trouble with change. She remembered particularly the trouble she had when she started kindergarten. Jay denied

symptoms of panic disorder. Furthermore, there did not appear to be any anticipatory anxiety. She said in the mornings she was too tired to think much about school. She simply got up and went. She reported, however, that she felt she didn't have enough time with her mom. Her mom was working, and she didn't see her as much as she used to.

Jay's father had recently had surgery and was not working since becoming ill. Jay's mother continued to work, but had longer days and appeared to be under some stress. Jay's mother expressed concern, even annoyance, that Jay might expect help with her homework after a long day at work. The parents were concerned about Jay's self-esteem, noting that she seemed to be critical of herself and did not show her usual confidence. Jay's father suggested that his wife was too critical and expected too much of Jay.

Comment. Several issues converge to create this picture of an anxious child. She has a long history of difficulty with change. She has started a new school. She has difficulty with the oral instructions and would need to have her hearing, auditory memory, and comprehension tested to assess her difficulty in following the teacher's instructions. There has been a two-fold change at home. Her father had surgery and is no longer working, and her mother has increased her work hours and is less available to Jay. Furthermore, father's perception is that mother is too critical of Jay. All of these elements converge to contribute to Jay's anxieties.

Impact on the Family

To fully appreciate the child's difficulties and the potential need for treatment, explore the impact on the family. Do the child's problems put the family in disarray, create tension in the family, or exacerbate conflict between parents? For example, severe separation anxiety in a 12-year-old essentially prevented the parents from going out alone because the child was in such distress and created such turmoil when the parents tried to leave. Another example is a child who had pica (i.e., eating of non-nutritive substances) and required constant supervision such that the family activities revolved around supervision duties. Families may be reluctant to reveal the amount of disruption the child's difficulties have caused because they love the child and do not want to appear selfish or bitter. They may have fears that the clinician will blame them for causing or perpetuating the child's problems, or they may have been adapting to the difficulty for so long that they are now unaware of the changes in their lives due to their child's struggles. Exploring the impact of the child's problem on the family is also an opportunity to compliment the family members on what they are doing well.

Key Point:

Many parents are relieved and appreciative when a professional acknowledges the energy and resourcefulness they have shown in coping with their child's problems.

Developmental History

The developmental history is often a useful introduction to exploring the past psychiatric history as well as an important part of the child psychiatric history in its own right. However, you *need not* obtain a complete developmental history in every case. The developmental history is usually more salient with younger children (i.e., under 7 years of age). Referral for clinical concerns in this age group more commonly involve developmental issues whose bearing on the clinical problems need to be understood.

With the child of 7 years of age or older who is being referred for an assessment for the first time, relevant developmental issues will commonly have revealed themselves before the end of the first grade of school. This is not to suggest that developmental issues are not relevant in this age group, just that given a limited amount of time with the family and child, a more focused assessment on current issues will usually be more fruitful.

A few key questions regarding developmental history will usually dictate whether a more complete history is required. For instance, if the parent reveals that the child was slow to speak or slow to achieve certain milestones, or there was evidence of fetal distress at delivery, then a more detailed inquiry is appropriate. If there is any doubt about the developmental status of the child, ask for more detail until you have satisfied yourself regarding the child's developmental progress.

It is best to obtain the complete developmental history from the parent(s) when the child is not in the room. Parents differ in their degree of caution about saying certain things in front of the child. The parents may omit certain information if they think it might affect the child negatively (e.g., the child was slow to talk, had poor motor skills, or was previously assessed for autism). In addition, be alert for the parents who may present too much information in front of the child. If you have concerns about the parents continuing a topic with the child in the room, you can remind the parents that there will be an opportunity to speak alone with you and that this topic might be better reserved for that time.

Begin taking the developmental history with questions about the pregnancy and birth. Ask whether the pregnancy was planned or unexpected. Were there any complications during the pregnancy or delivery? If the answer is yes, a more detailed inquiry is needed. Was the pregnancy full-term? Was the baby healthy at birth? Did mother and baby leave the hospital together? Was the child breast or bottle fed?

Developmental milestones are a common and easy way to roughly establish the individual child's developmental trajectory. Developmental problems may relate to delays in walking, delays in learning to speak, or other developmental problems. If the answers to the screening questions regarding the history of developmental milestones are negative, you need not explore the child's development in detail, except as it appears relevant to the child's clinical picture. For example, it is appropriate to inquire in some detail about the language development of a child with a history of learning difficulties.

The details of the pregnancy, delivery, and development may have been uneventful; however, important issues may nonetheless emerge. A mother may have regret and feel guilty that she was not able to breast-feed her baby and tends to overcompensate by infantilizing her child. A father who was unable to attend the birth of the child due to a business trip out of town may still feel he has less of a parenting role than the mother.

Ask about the child's temperament. Did the child quickly settle into a routine of eating, sleeping, and diaper changes? Or was the child fussy and colicky? Was the child adventurous and curious as a toddler? Or quiet and more reserved? Does the child persist at tasks? Or does she quickly lose interest and move to a new activity? How does the child respond to being told "no"? Does/did the child have temper tantrums? Is she independent? Or does she cling to the parent? Inquire about the child's reactions to separations, such as when left with babysitters or other adult caretakers.

The child's developmental history often serves as a lead-in to questions regarding psychological or behavioral problems. Were there any difficulties with toilet training? Does the child wet the bed at night? Were there any problems associated with feeding the child? Are the parents aware of any problems with the sleeping routine? Does the child have nightmares? What was the child's reaction to the birth of a new sibling? Important points of developmental transitions concern separation from the parents. How did the child manage school entry?

Inquire about the child's social skills and his social circle. Are there any social problems with peers either in the form of feeling rejected, neglected, or bullied? Does the child have an appropriate peer group? How many friends does the child have? Does the child have a best friend? Have you seen your child playing with his friends? What does the child do with his friends?

For example, in obtaining a history from the parents of a 4-year-old boy who appeared to have autistic disorder, the parents were quick to tell me that the boy had friends who played with him regularly. If true, this would challenge the initial diagnosis of autistic disorder. On further inquiry, it emerged that with his friends he played house and that he played the role of the baby, a role that could be played by a toy doll! From this report of the child's play, it is not possible to know whether the child is able to engage in developmentally appropriate reciprocal social interactions. Whereas without this detail we would perhaps eliminate the presumptive diagnosis of autism, simply knowing that the child played the role of a baby allows the diagnosis of autism to remain plausible.

Be sure to identify the child's strengths. It is important to balance the time in the interview asking about topics the child will perceive as areas of "weakness" or even "badness" with time asking and talking about the child's strengths. Strengths may be in the academic sphere, the social sphere, or the athletic sphere; the child may be musical, artistic, or mathematically inclined. These strengths provide a scaffold on which interventions can be based. A child's developing sense of confidence and self-esteem can be bolstered around these areas of strength. Hobbies can both develop areas of strength and be an expression of the child's areas of perceived strength. They provide opportunities to develop peer relationships and a potential avenue for the child to disengage from areas of conflict.

Key Point:

Whatever evidence for strength is present provides a scaffold on which interventions can be based. Helping a child develop a sense of confidence and self-esteem can be built around these areas of strength.

Past Medical History

Ask about any previous surgical procedures, chronic medical conditions, hospitalizations, or head injuries. Are the child's immunizations up to date? Does the child have any allergies? Does he take any medications? This information must be reviewed and incorporated into the formulation of the child's difficulties and the treatment plan.

School History

The child's history at school is a critical area of inquiry. When asking the child's age, inquire about the current grade and school. Find out whether the child is in a regular school program or whether it's modified in some way. Determine whether there is any concern with regard to any academic or learning difficulties. Does the concern arise from the school? If so, what is the nature of the concern? Are the parents concerned about issues at school? Are both parents, or only one? Is the child concerned?

A good way to begin is simply to ask the parent whether the child is working at grade level and if there have been any concerns with regard to academic progress. When such concerns exist, a more comprehensive assessment of the child's learning ability and behavior is required. If there are previous educational assessments or psychological testing, it is important to evaluate their validity and accuracy. With the parents' consent, the school psychologist or educational consultant can be contacted to help clarify the nature of the child's learning abilities and academic difficulties.

Learning difficulties can arise because of specific learning disabilities, or they can arise secondary to psychiatric or behavioral disorders. Inquire about symptoms of ADHD, depression, and anxiety, for example. These clinical symptoms are associated with decreased concentration, which could interfere with the child's ability to learn and progress academically. There may be other behavioral or emotional problems that interfere with the child's ability to learn, and these, too, should be ruled out.

It is important to ask how many schools the child has attended including the current school, how long the child was at each one, and the reason for each change of school. A change of school often is a traumatic event for a child and can precipitate emotional and behavioral difficulties. Adjusting to a new school, new class, new teacher, and a new peer group can be more challenging and anxiety provoking than adults commonly appreciate. Difficulty with adjustment to a new school may result in school refusal or develop into a school phobia. Be sure to be sensitive to the child's perspective when asking about school difficulties. In obtaining the school history, ask whether there have been behavioral difficulties and whether the child has had detentions, suspensions, expulsions, or been truant from school. To the extent that these have been present, you should detail the time frame and the reasons for these occurrences. Ask whether there is any history of bullying of the child or of other children by the child. Parents may be able to comment on the nature of the child's peer relationships at school. It is important to talk to the child about her school experience and experience in the playground, asking how the child gets along with other children and whether other children pick on her. Ask what the child does to cope with the teasing or bullying.

Key Point:

A change of school can be traumatic for a child, may precipitate emotional and behavioral problems, and can lead to school phobia.

Ask the parent, *"How is your child getting along at school? How is he progressing academically? Are you aware of any learning or behavior problems at school? Does your child get homework, and are there any problems with homework? Does your child show any persistent resistance or reluctance about going to school?"* Suzie was reluctant to go to school in the mornings. Her parents fought with her daily to get her to school, often forcibly putting her in a taxi or making her get into the family car to be brought to school. Suzie could not say why she did not want to go to school, but following a complete assessment she was found to be learning disabled and experienced school as an assault on her self-esteem. She was subsequently referred to a specialized school program at which her learning disabilities were recognized, and she no longer resisted attending class.

Key Point:

Conflicts regarding homework and school attendance are common among children with behavioral and/or learning problems.

Reports and Results

Obtain all the relevant reports and results including psychoeducational test reports from other agencies and the school. The psychoeducational reports are especially relevant when there are concerns regarding the child's learning and academic progress. The Wechsler Intelligence Achievement Test[8] and the Wechsler Intelligence Scale for Children[9] are common test instruments used by psychologists to assess a school-aged child's academic achievement and intelligence. This information can tell you whether the child is functioning at the appropriate grade level and whether his intelligence is within the normal range. If psychiatric rating scales such as the Achenbach Child Behavior Checklist[10] or the Teacher's Report Form[11] have been filled out, obtain these as well. These will provide a useful background of the child's behavior at a previous point in time as rated by the parents or teacher.

When there are questions or concerns about the child's behavior and progress at school, obtain the parents' permission to speak directly with the child's teacher. A 10-minute phone conversation with the teacher can be especially revealing and adds an important perspective on the nature of the child's difficulties.

Risk-Taking Behaviors

Risk-taking behaviors need to be evaluated for all children. The risky activities may be the main source of clinical concern and thus the reason for assessment (e.g., a 10-year-old boy setting fires). Risk-taking behavior may be an indication of the severity of a disorder or the child's attempt to cope with a disorder or difficulty (e.g., a depressed and

hopeless 12-year-old girl starts using ecstasy to feel connected to peers). It is important to clarify whether there are any legal issues, outstanding charges, concerns regarding the use or abuse of illicit drugs, or concerns about unsafe sexual activities. It is unusual to encounter prepubescent children with charges; however, this can occur and before beginning the assessment this should clarified. If there are outstanding charges, determine for whom the assessment is being conducted (i.e., whether it is court ordered); the family should be fully informed as to the nature and purpose of the assessment.

Parents should be asked whether they have any concerns about their child using drugs or being involved in inappropriate and/or unsafe sexual activity or whether the child has any past or current legal charges. Be certain to revisit these topics when speaking to the child alone. Many children will not divulge such information in front of their parents for obvious reasons. It is very helpful to have the parents' perspective before speaking to the child. The parents may report concern about the child using drugs, but when you speak to the child alone, she may deny drug use. Here, as in other parts of the assessment, it can be very informative to explore conflicting perspectives.

Self-Harm and Suicidality

The concern that a child will hurt herself or someone else is a common urgent clinical issue. The safety of the child is an essential part of *every* assessment. Children may have thoughts of harming themselves or others as a response to acute or ongoing stressors and clinical difficulties. They may have thoughts or acts of self-harm (e.g., hitting, cutting, burning), thoughts of suicide, suicidal plans, or suicidal intents. Although it is always a concern when a child voices or enacts a desire to hurt herself or someone else, there is a clinical spectrum of suicidality/homicidality in children just as there is in adults, and it is important to distinguish among the thoughts, plans, and intents of self-harm. The older the child, the more realistic her understanding of death and the more capable she is of forming and carrying out a plan. Younger or impulsive children may act without a clear understanding of the consequences (e.g., running out into traffic). Quiet, reserved children may not voice the depth of their hopelessness. It is important to ask parents about the child's potential for self-harm by asking whether the child has ever seemed sad or melancholy, whether the child speaks about the topic of death and dying, or whether the child has ever directly voiced that he wanted to die or harm himself. Ask whether the child has ever made an attempt to harm himself or someone else. If the answer to any of these questions is "yes," find out more. What has the child said? Does anyone else in the family say the same things? What has the child done? What were the circumstances of the talk/behavior? Was it after the child was reprimanded or did not get his own way? How did the parents respond to the child's words or actions? Does the child know anyone who has attempted or completed suicide? If so, this increases the risk that the child may make an attempt.

It is essential to ask questions about self-harm of the child without the parent present. Children do not easily offer information regarding their internal states, and direct questions typically provoke denials. Sometimes, you can prepare a child to discuss issues of self-harm by asking whether he ever gets sad feelings, or mad feelings, and if so what does he do with them. This may allow him to tell you more about his thoughts and intentions. Often, themes of sadness and melancholy will emerge through his drawings and provide a natural opening to ask about thoughts or behaviors of self-harm. If the child endorses thoughts of self-harm or suicide, these issues must be explored further (with the child and with the parents).

Child Abuse

Child abuse is another issue that should be addressed in every assessment of a child. It is important to listen to the description of relationships in the family and to observe how the family members interact in the office. It may be appropriate to ask whether a child has a temper, and if so, how the parent responds. These questions can often be raised when asking about the child's temperament: *"How does your child respond to being told 'no'? Does the child misbehave? What do you do when he misbehaves? How is he disciplined? Who is the one to most often discipline the child? Do arguments ever get physical?"* How do the parents handle disputes with each other? Does either parent have a temper?

Parents can be asked directly whether they have ever had concerns about the child being physically or sexually abused. As in the issues of risk-taking behaviors and self-harm issues, be certain that the child is also asked these questions without the parents present. The child can be asked directly about physical and sexual abuse: *"Do you ever get punishments at home? Do Mom and Dad ever get upset with you? What happens when they get upset? Do you know what makes them upset?"* This can lead to further questions about the nature and extent of discipline practices in the home. *"Has anyone ever touched you in parts of your body that you didn't want them to? Has anyone ever touched you in ways that made you feel uncomfortable? Has anyone ever touched your private parts?"*

If the child or parent(s) disclose information about child physical or sexual abuse, you are legally responsible to report the suspected abuse to the child protection services or Children's Aid Society. You do not have to have proof of abuse, only information leading to suspicion of abuse. It is the responsibility of the children's protection agency to investigate the matter further. It may or may not be advisable to tell the family that you are making the report to the children's protection services. In cases in which a child has disclosed abuse, there might be negative repercussions to the child at home if the family were to be informed that the report was going to be made. In other situations, physical abuse may arise from severe discipline thought to be appropriate to the parents' own upbringing or culture. In these situations, you can tell the family that the children's protection services can provide support to them in their child-disciplining methods and advise them that you are obliged to report the incident.

Providing a safe and friendly setting will sometimes lead to the spontaneous disclosure of abuse. For example, a 7-year-old boy was referred for assessment because while on the school bus he was found to have a knife with which he said he was intending to stab another boy. During the course of the assessment, while the youngster was playing with some wooden blocks, he casually revealed that even though his father would punch him and hit him, he would still give him lots of money if he won the lottery. In circumstances such as these, reporting to the local child protection services or Children's Aid Society is mandatory.

Family Psychiatric History

In conducting the assessment of the child, it is essential to gather information from the parents about a range of subjects that may not seem directly related to the child. You need to inquire about the parents' approach to parenting, the nature of their marital relationship, their understanding of the child's problems, and their own personal history.

Most parents are comfortable providing the details necessary to conduct the assessment, including details regarding their own personal history. However, sometimes parents may object, either overtly or in other more subtle ways. Some parents may feel that questions regarding their own personal history are intrusive and do not belong as part of the assessment of the child. Sometimes parents may feel that the inquiry into their own personal history suggests that they have a problem or that they *are* the problem. Approach this area tactfully and in a way that the parent understands its purpose and does not feel blamed or even attacked (see Family That Is Hostile to the Psychiatric Assessment section to follow).

One way to begin so as to minimize the discomfort of the parents is to start with a neutral line of inquiry. Begin with the child's developmental history, and then proceed to explore the range of the child's symptoms, including areas of strength and adaptation. It is then appropriate to inquire about the impact the child's problems have had on the family and on the parents. For example, discussing the child's learning problems may lead a parent to say that he, too, had problems in school, and his hope is that he can preempt similar problems for his child. Sometimes it is best to simply tell the parents that in order to understand the nature of the child's concerns it is often helpful to understand more about the parents themselves. If the inquiry into the parents' own histories is gentle and nonjudgmental, the parents are typically happy to share the information. It is important to frame the questions and the comments in such a way that the parents do not feel blamed for the child's problems. If the child's difficulties possibly have a heritable component, it may, in fact, help the parents to know this so that they can better understand and empathize with their child.

Help the parents explore their own experiences of being parented; this can lead to greater understanding of their feelings and reactions to their child. For example, a father who had a very lonely adolescence himself recognized how painful it was for him to watch his son not be able to make or keep many friends. Recognizing their own past histories can help parents make adaptations that are more helpful to the child's difficulties. It is not necessary and would be counterproductive to conduct a full psychiatric history of each parent. Instead, the approach should be to identify any past psychiatric history and any current psychological, marital, or psychiatric problems the parents may have that seem relevant to the child's problems.

You will need to get some background information on the parental relationship. If there are two biological parents, determine whether they are living together and/or married. Ask how long they have been together and whether there are other children in the family, starting with the oldest to youngest. Inquire about any medical, behavioral, or developmental problems in the other children and whether there is any medical history in regard to either of the parents. Ask whether anyone else in the family has ever had any problems similar to those of the identified patient. Ask whether either parent has ever had similar problems when they were children. In this context, it is appropriate to ask whether there have been any psychological or psychiatric problems in either parent or whether any other family members have received treatment for such problems. If the answer is yes, obtain details on the nature of the problems, the diagnosis if any, and the nature of any treatments. If the parents provide a diagnosis for themselves or a family member, obtain details on the nature of the symptoms to be certain that the diagnosis offered is consistent with the symptom picture presented. Sometimes, the family will be concerned that their child has the same problems as or will grow up to be just like a close relative who is perceived to be psychologically deviant or otherwise "never amounted to anything." Ask about such ghosts in the family

tree. For example, *"Who in the family is Johnny most like?"* or *"Is Johnny like anyone else in the family?"* This will help you focus on their true concerns.

Key Point:

Ask about ghosts in the family tree. Sometimes parents are afraid that their child will grow up to become like a mentally ill or delinquent family member.

In assessing the nature of the child's problems, it is essential to determine to what extent the family psychiatric history may have contributed to the onset or maintenance of the child's identified problems. For example, a parent with a history of alcoholism or substance abuse may create a tense and conflict-ridden home environment in which the child feels psychologically traumatized or otherwise blamed. Ultimately, the child may see the parent as a role model for the use of alcohol and other substances and feel permission to engage in similar risk-taking behaviors.

Case Example 6

Worried and Dysthymic. Amy had come to see me because a school worker was concerned about a story and drawing Amy had come up with. Her mother felt that Amy was having trouble at school, and the school workers seemed to think that Amy might have an attention deficit disorder.

Amy told me about the story that she had written in school. The story was about a girl who was sent away to a foster home and some kids who had been taken away by a bird. One of the kids taken by the bird was killed; then her mother died, and the bird let the kids go. She told me about some of her worries about her own mom, about how she worried that her mom would die. She remembered seeing her mother doing drugs, watching her mother inject herself, and said she felt sad about that, but also felt like shouting. She wouldn't shout, however, because she knew that she wasn't supposed to talk like that to grown-ups, and she was afraid that she might get grounded.

Amy said that she didn't tell anybody about those feelings, but she had those worries a lot. She acknowledged thinking about those things at school and that it made it hard to concentrate. She worried that her mom would die; she also worried about her friends and referred to one friend, Valerie, whose mother wouldn't let her play with her because of Amy's mom.

Amy also told me that she thought that she was bad because she did bad things, for example, not cleaning up her room, forgetting to turn off the television, or forgetting to take her lunch. When these things happened, her parents yelled at her. This made her feel bad.

Comment. In this example, Amy has difficulty concentrating in school, worried that something would happen to her mother and that she would be removed from her parental home. Furthermore, she believes she is bad and is unable to share or express her worries, concerns, or upsets. For common and ordinary happenings, such as forgetting her lunch, she is left feeling that she is bad. Although this girl may have an attention deficit disorder, to properly assist her there clearly are a large number of concerning issues that will need to be addressed.

INTERVIEWING CHILDREN

By now we have observed the child and family together, we have obtained the history of the presenting problems, and we have reviewed the relevant family history and child's development. The challenge now is to understand the child's perspective and child's mental state. In this section, we describe the approach to interviewing the child and illustrate some of the issues with clinical vignettes. We use the mental status to help organize the information from and about the child.

Observing Children: The Pediatric Mental Status Exam

How do we find out about the mental state of a child? Observation is a critical part of the mental status exam for adults and children alike; however, the younger the child, the more we rely on observation as the *sole* tool for examining mental state.

There is much information that can be obtained from even a very brief amount of time spent with a child. Observation of the child begins from the time of the first phone call made to the family home. There are occasions when the child can be heard in the background (e.g., being angry, demanding, or happy, or arguing with a sibling). Even from just hearing a child, you imagine the child in a certain way. Sometimes our imaginings of the child contrast strikingly with the child who later presents at the assessment. The child is usually first *seen* in the waiting room with the family while waiting for the first assessment. In the waiting room, you may observe an extremely shy child who was heard being very boisterous in the background when you were talking to the parent on the phone, or you may see the same boisterousness in the waiting room as you imagined from the phone call. Here again, much can be gleaned from a brief visual encounter in the waiting room.

Get a first general impression of the child with the family. Observe whether the child is close to the parent or playing independently across the room. Her play may be active

or quiet. Some aspect of the child or an aspect of how the child relates to the environment and/or parents may catch our attention. The child may appear very melancholy or extremely outgoing. She may appear delicate or somewhat awkward or clumsy. Whatever the first impression and the initial reaction, it is important to follow up with further observations and questions during the assessment. Also, watch for changes in the child as the assessment progresses, as different topics are raised for discussion, as different toys are used, and as different thematic material emerges in the child's play.

When observing children, it is helpful to organize the information under the following headings adapted from Greenspan and Greenspan[12]: (1) physical and cognitive development, (2) mood, (3) human relationship capacity, (4) affects and anxiety, (5) thematic development, and (6) subjective reactions.[7]

Each category also represents a line of development. Thus, as children get older, they gain gross and fine motor control; they develop a wider repertoire of moods and affects; they develop richer affects; they grow in their capacity for human relationships; and they are able to develop more complex play themes that reveal age-appropriate anxieties and developmental challenges. The ability to determine the age-appropriateness of children's skills and thoughts grows with the degree of experience working with children. Tables of developmental milestones can be very helpful to the beginning clinician.

Physical and Cognitive Development

As in each of the six categories, observation of the child's physical and cognitive development begins at the first meeting in the waiting room and continues throughout the assessment interview. Note the child's height, weight, and general health. Observe his posture and gait as he walks and moves. Some children may walk with a fluid athletic motion; others may have a stiff or awkward gait. Children will often move around the room or move between playing and being close to the parent. This tells you the child's general activity level as well as the child's balance and gross motor abilities.

Case Example 7

A 9-year-old boy was thought to be particularly oppositional and defiant because he would refuse to go to the playground during recess. Observing this boy's gross motor movements and gait, it became evident that he was poorly coordinated and feared falling and hurting himself during play. Furthermore, he had been the subject of teasing by his classmates because of his awkwardness at common childhood activities such as running, jumping, and playing ball games. He became exceedingly sensitive to being humiliated. When his coordination problems were

recognized and alternative arrangements made, his oppositional behavior decreased, and his anxiety about recess
diminished.

Observe the child's fine motor skills as she manipulates
blocks or Lego pieces as she plays. Note how the child
holds a pencil or crayon. What kind of movements does the
child use to draw? Are they large sweeping movements of
the whole arm or finely controlled movements of the hand
and fingers?

A child who does not respond to your words or gestures
may have a difficulty with hearing or language comprehension or may be preoccupied or anxious. You will need to
form an impression of the child's level of cognitive development, whether at an age-appropriate level or below; if
below an age-appropriate level, is there evidence suggesting possible mental handicap? Assess the child's use of
expressive language and language comprehension.
Children may demonstrate a particular sensitivity to one or
more sensory modalities. For example, a child may be easily startled by loud noises (e.g., blocks banging on the table
as they fall) or may show great interest in textures (e.g.,
repeatedly stroking a toy horse's mane).

Case Example 8

Thought Disorder or Severe Problems in Language
Comprehension. An 8½-year-old boy with severe language comprehension difficulties was referred for assessment because of his parents' concerns regarding his
anxiety. The child had seen a dentist a few days earlier and
was now scheduled for a follow-up dental appointment. An
interview with this youngster went as follows:

"What do you suppose you would like to do today?"

"I don't know."

"What things do you like to do?"

There is a long pause. "I don't know what things I like to
do."

"Do you like to watch television . . . do you like to play
with toys?"

Another long pause. "Well, I like to do a lot of things."

The child is then invited to play with some of the figures
and toys on the tabletop as he and the doctor sit on the floor
together.

"We'll put some of these things on the floor so you can
play with them if you like. Would you like to do that?"

"Yup."

"You have some animals and people too."

The child is moving blocks and various toys around.

"There are lots of people over there, aren't there?"

The child identifies two small figures saying, "This is
Dr. Y. He has bits of hair kind of like he's bald" (referring to
a hairless plastic figure of a boy). The child then identifies
this as a game called Family Matters.

"Okay, who else is in the game Family Matters?"

He begins to whisper, "Is maybe you can have some
time. I am having appointment. I am a dentist appointment
'cause I have a cavity. I have to get filled in by my head
'cause they're going to take some x-rays so I'm going to
have to use that now 'cause we never cured this before."

"Okay, alright."

"Cause my humor is kind of silly for me."

The child begins to mumble, and is invited to repeat
what he said.

"Taking a dentist appointment."

"You're taking a dentist appointment?"

"Yeah. He has a little cavity. I'm going to take it from him
'cause it's stuck there. He sure doesn't like it but he knows
there is too far and so he was losing a lot of hair so he needs
a new way. So I'm having this appointment, um, I'll mention what that's thing on the air. It's going to be up to my
hair so they're going to take it 'cause it's already sucked in.
I've never heard that before so I'm taking an operation test.
Well, they're going to put me to sleep with some magic pill
and then I have to do is really put me to sleep and take out
and there will be a hole and they're going to take it out and
put a radio in and it'll lose all its energy and then they'll
chop his head."

Comment. It's evident in this short vignette that this
youngster had an appointment with a dentist and was told
that he had a cavity that would need to be filled, and that to
do the procedure he would likely have an anesthetic so
that the procedure would be painless. It also appears that
this boy was confused and frightened by the procedure,
did not understand what was going to happen, and had the
idea that they were going to make a hole somewhere in his
head or mouth and put a radio in it. He clearly did not
understand what was going to happen to him and was
exceedingly frightened. Furthermore, as his conversation
continued uninterrupted, it became progressively more
disorganized and fantastical. His ideas were barely coherent, and he shifted between the first and third person so it
was hard to know about whom he was speaking. Without
knowing the context, this boy could be considered to have
a thought disorder and could be labeled psychotic. This
would be a great disservice since his problems have to do
with poor comprehension, not distortions in the perception of reality.

What is important in this context is to recognize that children can acquire and develop these fanciful and fantastical
ideas, and it does not mean that they are psychotic or otherwise lying or malingering. You need to understand the context and the possibility that there is difficulty with
comprehension. It is apparent in this example that this
child's misunderstanding of the nature of the dental
appointment has increased his anxiety. He worries that
they will chop off his head!

Mood

A child's mood is surmised by piecing together aspects of the child's facial expression, behavior, the content of play, and the feeling evoked in you as the interviewer.

Case Example 9

A 7-year-old boy came for an assessment. He sat between his parents and glared at me any time I mentioned "the problem" (encopresis). He physically covered his mother's mouth with his own hand so she could not say anything to me either. He later growled from under a chair and threatened to throw his snack (a tomato) at me. Over several sessions, he developed play themes of violence and aggression. This boy's mood was angry (and perhaps frightened).

Capacity for Human Relatedness

Observe the child's connectedness with the parent or family while in the waiting room, then observe how the child's relatedness evolves through the course of the interview. In the waiting room, note how far the child is from the parent. The child may be sitting on the parent's lap or engaged in activities at a distance from the parent. The child may be playing alone or playing cooperatively with other children. See whether it is parallel play (alongside but not with another child) or cooperative play. He might be playing alone yet be in close proximity to other children. For example, he might be coloring at a table with one or two other children and sharing crayons. Alternately, a child may be taking pieces from a shared Lego pile but is still disconnected from the other children playing with Legos. Or perhaps the child has isolated himself and is sitting alone in a far corner of the room reading.

How does the child greet you? Is he aloof and disinterested or warm and friendly? The speed of the connectedness and the quality and depth of connectedness should be noted. A child may introduce himself to you in the waiting room and then take your hand and say, "Let's go!" yet the relatedness may feel shallow. A child may be very hesitant in the first part of the interview, saying little and keeping a distance, but then warm up and range closer in physical space to you as the interview continues. The resulting connectedness may feel less in degree but deeper and richer than with the first child. Notice also if the child initiates relatedness. A child may see drawing materials on the table and may, even if he does not verbalize the request, communicate to you by looks and gestures a desire to draw. If you then nod assent and the child starts drawing, the child has then completed a circle of gestural communication, which he initiated. On the other hand, a child may not initiate and also may not respond to your verbal or gestural invitation to draw.

Your sense of personal relatedness to the child forms part of your assessment of the child. Is the child likeable, off-putting, or distant and hard to connect to? Your sense of relatedness to the child is derived from the child's physical proximity to you; the speed, quality, and depth of his connectedness to you; his ability to read and send signals (gestural or verbal); and his desire and ability to reciprocate relatedness. This information will help you understand the child and the issues that his parents and others may bring to your attention.

Case Example 10

Bobby, an 8-year-old boy referred for assessment, was diagnosed with ADHD and possible mild developmental delay. Bobby had difficulty making and keeping friends. He described how he wanted to tell his friends all about his favorite cartoon character or action movie, only to have his friends cover their ears and shout, "Be quiet!" In the play portion of the assessment interview, Bobby was in constant motion, moving from activity to activity around the room. He did not engage with the toys; rather, he fidgeted with them as he regaled me with a barrage of detail about the latest cartoon action movie. He was animated in his story telling and demonstrated the different voices of the various characters. Even so, as his commentary continued I realized that I could not follow the sense of his play or of his narrative. I became aware of my own sense of disengagement from Bobby; the more he talked and did, the harder it was for me to sense a meaningful relatedness to him.

Affects and Anxiety

Regardless of children's moods or overall emotional tone, they will display a range of affects during the interview. Of course, the affects displayed will contribute to your understanding of the child's mood. The child may have a wide range of affects, or the affect may be restricted or even flat. Different affects will emerge as different topics are discussed in the interview. The child may display sadness or anger when the area of difficulty is discussed or pride or pleasure when areas of strength are discussed. Different affects will also emerge as the child develops themes through playing and drawing. It is important to note the affect associated with a particular play theme and, in particular, the points of transition of affect.

Case Example 11

A 4-year-old boy who had been witness to and victim of physical domestic violence was engaged in imaginative play in which doll figures were being destroyed by an "evil overlord" and by large-scale natural disaster. He displayed anger and aggression during the disaster and fight, but he became very intensely solemn as he buried the dead figures. Shortly after the "burial," he jumped on the table and energetically sang, "I'm the king of the castle and you're the dirty rascal!"

Comment. The intensity and depth of this boy's affect was considerable. His switch from sadness burying the dead to energy and defiance being king was a flight from intense negative emotion and the anxiety it raised in him. It also speaks to this child's experience of being a victim and his struggle with feelings of both helplessness and aggression.

Thematic Development

The assessment of children requires a "playful ear." The interviewer needs to be attentive to the child's activities, affects, relatedness, and the sequencing of these through the play session interview. The child's playing, drawing, and talking, including silence and inactivity, are clues to themes and thematic development. What drama is the child playing out for you? Does the story plot progress, or is it fragmented? What is the child trying to convey about his ideas, feelings, and attitudes? Can this be found in the metaphor of the child's play? Here is a brief vignette to illustrate some of these ideas.

Case Example 12

Obtaining the Child's Perspective Through the Use of Play. Samantha is a 5-year-old who was brought for an assessment. Approximately a year ago, Samantha began having bad days during which she would begin crying and hiding under tables, would appear very upset, and would not respond to her teachers. Mother reported that the difficulties with Samantha began a couple of months after she began attending a new day care center. The difficulties seem to have increased over time.

Samantha presented as an attractive, blond-haired girl, who appeared about her stated age of 5 years. She played comfortably with the toys in the presence of her mother and father and was able to separate from her parents without incident. She soon settled into playing happily with the toys. She was an articulate youngster, who freely expressed her feelings and ideas and did this through the metaphor of little plastic figures of dogs that she had brought with her. She identified a particular dog as a boxer dog with angry feelings. The mother dog would take care of the situation by placing the boxer dog in its cage and in this way would contain him. Samantha told me that the dog had to face his feelings and face its bad days. She indicated that the dog would become angry because it had gotten grounded and referred to a potential conflict between the boxer dog and one of the cat puppets. Although the specific reference was uncertain, it appeared to be an allusion to a conflict with her younger sister, and she conveyed the notion that the dog would get punished or reprimanded even though it did not do anything.

In response to my question about magic wishes, she answered that she would become a horse—a stallion—and would knock people off her back. She became quite animated in doing this and showed me how she would throw them off her back by arching her back and jumping in the air. She showed some evidence of angry affect and conveyed a sense of tension, and she stated the need to confront problems, although at the same time she conveyed the sense of a lack of sufficient support or emotional resources to be able to do so.

Comment. The use of play material provides the opportunity for a child to express herself via the metaphor. In this particular example, although the child would likely be unable to answer direct questions about the nature of her problems or difficulties, through this play it becomes evident that she recognizes that she may have misbehaved and was reprimanded by being placed "in a cage." At the same time, however, she expresses the magical wish to be free of the people who are "on her back." She was quite excited and animated as she demonstrated this.

The inference in this assessment is that this child is speaking to perceived conflict and stress in the day care environment. Although you might be tempted to suggest that one needed to be firmer with her, it is evident that she feels that people have been treating her with a degree of firmness already, and instead she may need more support, guidance, and perhaps psychological space. In the course of the assessment, you would make note of other situations that may contribute to the child's difficulties, but in this instance, the balance of the assessment was essentially unremarkable.

Subjective Reactions

Children evoke strong feelings in us. When you first meet a child, you may have a strong sense of warmth and closeness, or you may get a sense of distance and aloofness. Your feelings are compiled from your observations of the child's physical presence, facial expression, emotional responsiveness, physical closeness, and ability to provide gestural cues and respond to the ones you provide. These feelings also inform each aspect of your observation of the child. How you feel about the child influences your assessment of the child's level of emotional maturity, mood and affect, capacity for relatedness, and play themes.

The feelings the child evokes in you are an essential tool in the psychiatric assessment of children. It is important not to dismiss your reactions as just a natural response to "a cute and cuddly child" or "an obstinate child." You should permit yourself to wonder what the child is doing to evoke such feelings in you. Be prepared to examine how the feelings the child evokes in you contribute to your overall understanding of the child. What is it about the child that makes you feel the way you do? Compare the feelings parents convey about their child with those the child has evoked in you. This can be instructive in deciding what treatment to recommend. (For an example of these issues, see the Step-Parent Family section to follow.)

Talking with Children

In most instances, your first contact with the child will be in the family context with parents present. This allows the child to meet you and have some sense of how you interact with him and his family. Once alone with the child, you can repeat or confirm some of the initial discussion of the introductory session; for example, *"Johnny, do you know why you came here today with your mom and dad?"* The child may say, *"Because I get into fights at school."* This then provides an opportunity to talk with Johnny about those fights. A useful tactic in talking with children where there is a concern that they might feel blamed is to adopt their point of view. For example, *"I wonder, does it feel like the other kids are picking on you or blaming you?"* This may then lead to a more complete discussion of Johnny's feelings that in fact he feels this way, blamed and picked on, and he is only defending himself or fighting back. After an exchange along these lines, it is then appropriate to ask Johnny whether he can tell you what he does or what he did that seemed to get him into some trouble. From there you can explore his relationships with other children—are there some kids with whom he plays and kids that he likes? What kinds of games do they play? You could pursue this line of inquiry to invite discussion about dreams or wishes. For example, a child might express retaliatory fantasies toward his detractors or dreams that he had that are often quite transparent. This provides a more complete insight into the nature of the child's thinking and the issues that need to be addressed.

Key Point:

When talking with children who may feel blamed or accused, it is often useful to adopt their point of view; that is, that they are the ones feeling victimized.

Oftentimes, it is precisely this deeper understanding of the child's perspective that is helpful in working with the parents so they appreciate and understand their child's point of view. A not uncommon dynamic that arises is one in which the parents see the child as bad, provocative, or disruptive, and they fail to appreciate what the child is experiencing and why the child is reacting in the way that he does. By your helping the parents to understand the feelings and state of mind of the child, the parents are able to be more empathetic to the child and respond more sensitively to the

child, and in that way shift the interaction from a battling, blaming perspective to a more helpful understanding and collaborative one.

In another situation, the attempt to engage the child, either in play or discussion, is met with the child moving from one activity to another, from one object to another, and wandering about aimlessly. Furthermore, the child appears to be unable to engage in any sustained activity that requires some degree of concentration. As well, attempts to engage in some conversation or dialogue will be met with simple one-word answers or "I don't know." Although the clinical interview does not usually lend itself to making the diagnosis of ADHD, this behavior raises a high index of suspicion. Confirmatory information from the child's school and further discussion with the parents can help establish such a diagnosis. Usually, the symptoms will have been present at least since the child began school and will continue unless treated. The more recent onset of such symptomatology raises a suspicion that there may be an alternative diagnosis.

Case Example 13

Attention Deficit Hyperactivity Disorder and Oppositional Defiant Disorder. Mrs. P came for an assessment with her son, Donald, who is 6 years of age. Mother and son were seen together. As the interview progressed, Donald, who presented as a pleasant-looking, blond-haired, solidly built youngster, began to openly challenge and provoke his mother. He tried to climb on the chairs to reach something that was clearly out of his reach; he threw paper and toys on the floor, and he began to pound on the windowpane and throw pillows on the floor. During this time, his mother tried to redirect him, curtail him, tell him to stop, and give him a time-out. In response, he threatened her, cursed at her, swung at her, and raced around the room away from her. He was clearly out of control, upset, and challenging. Donald tried to pretend that he was Spiderman, for instance, and his mother interjected, telling him that he was not Spiderman, to which he replied angrily that he was and tried to climb one of the cabinets as though to demonstrate his Spiderman powers. Mrs. P noted that Donald does behave this way from time to time, although he was more provocative today than he would normally be at home.

Mrs. P says that Donald is prone to get into fights with other children. He gets warning notices about his behavior on the school bus, and she cannot leave him alone with other children because he will get into fights with them. She reports that if he doesn't get his own way, he is prone to have a temper tantrum. For example, if they were quarreling over the television and he didn't get to watch the program that he wanted, he might carry on for 15 minutes to half an hour, kicking, screaming, throwing things, and cursing. She says this might occur three times a week.

Available history confirms behavioral, attentional, and learning problems in the school environment. Donald also shows delays in speech and language development. It is not known to what extent he may also have a learning disability, but with the history of speech, language, and behavior problems, there should be a high index of suspicion for a learning disability.

Comment. This is a child with serious behavior problems. He would qualify for a diagnosis of ADHD and oppositional defiant disorder. Further information and psychoeducational testing would be needed to determine the presence of a concurrent learning disability.

Normally, we pace the interview and the approach to the child depending on the nature of the child's difficulties and temperament. A child who is anxious and/or depressed will typically require a more gentle, graduated approach than a child with a history of externalizing symptomatology, such as aggressive or disruptive behavior. The child may require or insist that a parent remain in the room and be unwilling to be interviewed alone. If this is the case, his wish should be respected. It is often helpful to begin the initial approach to the child by focusing on some issue, activity, or event known to be of interest to the child. This is a good way to begin. Say, for example, *"I understand that you are a hockey fan,"* or *"I understand that you like the television program XYZ."*

Key Point:
_____

It is often helpful to begin the initial approach to the child by focusing on some issue, activity, or event known to be of interest to the child.

This can often lead to important and useful information. For example, one 11-year-old boy, who had been brought in for an assessment because of concerns about emerging psychosis or schizophrenia, had been watching the television program *X-Files*. This program involves a fictional story about supernatural events. Watching this program unsupervised, without clarification, this boy was allowed to believe that the supernatural events were in fact real, further blurring the boundaries between fantasy and reality. You could ask the child whether he believes that events such as those seen in a fanciful television program are real or are just pretend. This helps clarify what the child understands about what is and is not real.

The use of play material provides a vehicle through which one can engage the child in casual conversation while playing with or alongside the youngster. Sometimes, it is sufficient simply to sit quietly on the floor beside the child while she is playing. A helpful strategy in establishing

rapport with a child is to sit beside the child and assist her by passing her play materials while she builds a tower of blocks, for instance.

Key Point:
_____

The use of play material provides a vehicle through which one can engage the child in casual conversation while playing with or alongside her.

In the initial encounters with the child, particularly during the individual interview, the child should be informed that the information that is discussed is private, just between the child and you, although if there are any concerns with regard to personal safety, these would have to be shared with the parent. Information of a more general nature can be shared with the parent, and you can often share this information with the parent in the presence of the child. Sometimes it is useful to arrange a family meeting in which you can help the child express her point of view to the parents.

In interviewing a child, it is necessary to be flexible and patient. A younger child will enjoy play materials such as blocks, cars, dolls, human figures, and representations of the home. An older child can take advantage of paper, pencil, and crayons to color or draw. A game introduced by Winnicott called *Squiggles* is an easy, nonthreatening way to engage a somewhat hesitant or otherwise shy youngster.[13] The game is played simply by drawing a squiggle and inviting the child to make the squiggle into a picture and then to describe what it is he has drawn. This game goes back and forth, with players taking turns making their own squiggle. The child will reveal thoughts and feelings by the pictures he creates and the stories he develops around them. This provides another medium through which the child can express his point of view. Alternatively, ask the child to draw a picture of a person or of his family. Invite the child to tell you about the picture and what the people in the picture are doing. The child also uses play materials as a vehicle to express his ideas, concerns, and attitudes.

Once you are able to engage the child in conversation, it is best to conduct the interview as though it were a conversation, moving from one content area to another in as smoothly flowing a pattern as possible. Begin by discussing areas in which you know the child is interested, and then move to more neutral topics. In the course of the discussion, opportunities will present themselves to inquire about potential areas of conflict or concern (e.g., start by talking about video games [interest], which leads to discussion of bringing a "Gameboy" to school [more neutral], which leads to talking about a fight with another child and getting suspended from school [reason for referral]). Return to neutral topics or topics of interest/strength to settle the child if he becomes upset and also to draw the interview to a close. (Be cautious not to patronize the child, however.)

As previously mentioned, it can be revealing to ask the child about "three wishes." For example, *"If you had magical powers, what would you want to do with them?"* or *"If you had magical powers, what three things would you wish for?"* Inviting children to talk about their dreams or nightmares is also often useful. Children frequently describe dreams that are transparent, reflecting the state of their anxieties or concerns.

Difficult Patient Scenarios

The Silent Child

There are many situations in which the child will be silent. It is useful to know ahead of time whether the child is talkative or if you are dealing with a child who is known to be electively or selectively mute. Likewise, it is useful to gain some information from the parents ahead of time on the child's attitude toward the assessment and what the parents can tell you about the nature of the child's reaction to strangers.

If during the initial encounter the child is silent, do not press the child or otherwise try to make the child speak when she is reluctant to do so. Observing the child with the family and other family members, observing the child's play, inviting the child to use the play materials to act out a personal life situation or to draw pictures reflecting scenes of her life can often be quite revealing. When you approach the child gently and patiently, creating an atmosphere in which the child feels safe, often the child will gradually begin to speak and share her thoughts, feelings, and ideas. This may take more than one session, and you will need to be prepared for that.

In the event that you are dealing with a child known to be electively mute, it is unlikely the child will speak to you in the course of your initial assessment. For successful consultation, however, it is not essential that the child speak to you. Much information can be obtained from the parents, other collateral sources, and observation of the child's play and the child's interactions with other people.

The Angry Child

A child who presents angrily should be given the opportunity to express this anger and, to the extent possible, the reasons for the anger. Adopt an attitude of empathic understanding, allowing the child to express his anger as long as no one is injured or hurt.

Commonly, the child who is angry will feel justified in his anger. A helpful strategy is to convey to the child that you recognize that he may feel victimized and that from his perspective his anger may seem justified. Of course, it is important not to justify the child's anger but to help find appropriate outlets and appropriate ways of dealing with it. The child should be given opportunities to express and otherwise explain what it is he is angry about and how one might begin to address this anger. Not uncommonly, there will be issues in the child's current family situation or past history in which the child will have felt victimized or traumatized.

Case Example 14

A 10-year-old boy, Sean, says he hates a former friend Peter.

"It sounds like you have mad feelings about Peter."

"Yup, he lost my baseball bat."

"I guess that bat was pretty important to you."

"Yup."

"Was there anything special about it?"

Here Sean tells you that he got it from his dad, who has now moved away. The bat is one of his remaining ties to his father.

Comment. In this example, the loss of the bat has important symbolic meaning for Sean. Here you also gain a more complete understanding of Sean, the reason he was angry, and some leads on issues that may be relevant treatment foci.

> **Key Point:**
>
> ---
>
> One way to help a child talk about his anger is to help him distance it by identifying it as "mad feelings," for instance. By labeling them in this way it is easier to refer to them, and the child will not think you are saying he is angry—just that he has mad feelings.

The Step-Parent Family

The step-parent family is a particularly challenging family constellation. A not uncommon presentation occurs with complaints that the child does not listen, does not obey, and is considered to be provocative or challenging. Be alert to comments saying things like the child is manipulative or stubborn, or "deliberately does things to provoke or upset us." This family constellation can be particularly troublesome when the child's biological mother is uncertain of her parenting skills, has low self-esteem, and is dependent on the child's step-father. A considered danger is that the mother will side with the step-father in identifying the child as the problem or the provocateur.

Case Example 15

Harry was brought in for an assessment because of concerns regarding his behavior. He was described as difficult to manage with frequent temper tantrums, and he had destroyed property. Information from the mother differed

20

Assessment of Adolescents

PIER BRYDEN AND MARK SANFORD

INTRODUCTION

Braver physicians than we are quake in their boots when confronted by an apparently mute, surly adolescent dressed like a character from a film or music video too hip for us to know about and whose parents insist that their child is at acute risk and needs immediate intervention.

But do not fear. You have the skills and the ability to breach all but the most entrenched defenses, and as you do you are likely to find a grateful, intimidated adolescent who is willing to accept help, albeit on his own terms. In our experience, the majority of adolescents who come for consultation would die rather than acknowledge they want to be in our offices, but they demonstrate relief as the interview progresses if it's done in a competent manner that promotes trust.

In this chapter, we will discuss the purposes of your interview with an adolescent (Box 20-1); point out special considerations specific to interviewing adolescents, outline different stages of the interview, explore the use of semi-structured and structured interviews and rating scales, identify some common adolescent disorders, talk about how to approach difficult-to-interview adolescents, provide do's and don'ts for professional behavior, and finally, pull it all together in a discussion of formulation and a general approach to management of adolescent patients. We will use the interview from the Case Example to demonstrate concretely some of the pertinent issues.

We will also present how we interview—not the only or correct way, but the approach we have developed over years of cumulative clinical experience with adolescents. You will find an approach to interviewing and relationship-building with adolescents and their families that works for you and fits with your personal style. We hope only to provide you with some ideas and to provoke some thought about potential pitfalls that you are likely to encounter in your work with this population.

We also hope that you can benefit from the innumerable mistakes and faux pas we have made in accumulating our clinical experience. No doubt you will make your own—it's an inevitable aspect of our work—but we expect that you and your patients may be spared some of our more embarrassing errors after reading our chapter.

Given the clinical focus of this book and the guidelines around psychiatric interviewing you have already read in earlier chapters, we will skip over general aspects of psychiatric interviewing to focus on the specifics of interviewing and working with adolescents.

PURPOSE OF THE ASSESSMENT

There's no point denying that in providing psychiatric care to an adolescent population, you will have your work cut out for you. Adolescents don't usually refer themselves for psychiatric assessment; referrals tend to be made on their behalf by adults in their lives. The adolescent will be a more or less willing participant; in our experience, often less willing. Your initial job is therefore multidimensional: to ascertain who is concerned about the child, to identify which behaviors are a source of concern, to get a sense of the context for the concerns, and, as much as possible, to get the adolescent on board with assessment of the concerns and your proposed approach to dealing with them.

As with younger children, your focus in the assessment of the adolescent remains developmental. Your goal is to obtain descriptions of the adolescent's current functioning in a variety of different domains and to assess his level of functioning relative to that expected for the adolescent's age and stage of development.

Box 20-1. Goals of the Assessment Interview with an Adolescent

Build rapport with adolescent and family
Socialize adolescent patient to patient role
Delineate symptoms and signs of psychiatric disorder
Assess level of high-risk behaviors
Elucidate the history of the development of these symptoms, signs, and behaviors (e.g., onset, course and duration, intensity, context)
Assess for impairments in social functioning
Obtain developmental history to place detected disturbances in a developmental context
Determine presence of background risk/protective factors
Diagnose and formulate
Develop management plan
Conclude with adolescent and family having a better understanding of the nature of the referring problem and open to further assessment and treatment if indicated

---

As with any patient, but perhaps even more with an embarrassed adolescent who is a reluctant participant, your assessment should focus not only on the adolescent's difficulties and symptoms, but also on her strengths, talents, and areas of superior adaptation.

Finally, it's important to remember that to fulfill the comprehensive developmental assessment that is essential in this population, you will need additional informants such as parents, an approach that is less used in adult psychiatry. You may want to obtain information from other adults in addition to parents, for example, teachers, other health care professionals, coaches, probation officers, and other important adult figures in the adolescent's life. You will also want to explore sibling and family relationships, and this will often entail interviewing whole families together.

Case Example

Sanjay is a 16-year-old boy who has been sent to you for a psychiatric assessment for depression by his family doctor. Before you have a chance to invite the family into your office, Sanjay's parents begin to tell you in the waiting room that they are extremely worried about his heavy drug use. Sanjay sits glumly, not looking up as his parents talk to you.

SPECIAL CONSIDERATIONS WITH AN ADOLESCENT POPULATION

Let's look at what's different about adolescent patients like Sanjay.

High Velocity

Adolescence is a time of developmental high velocity. Consider that in the course of approximately 6 years of adolescence, the child moves from almost complete dependence on her parents for shelter, food, clothing, activities, transportation, health care, etc., to self-sufficiency. Concurrently, the child's parents must negotiate the shift from near-complete control of their child's day-to-day life to accepting the young adult's need to make her own decisions on issues both large and small.

Hostility

As we have said, adolescent patients do not always come for psychiatric assessment willingly and may be hostile to the whole process. Much can be accomplished by an acknowledgment of any valid reasons for such hostility. For instance, we encounter situations in which the adolescent has been misled by desperate parents as to the nature and purpose of their assessment, only to be told in the waiting room that they are in fact meeting with a psychiatrist. This issue will require open discussion with the adolescent if the interviewer is to stand a chance of getting his active participation in the assessment.

Most adolescents referred to a psychiatrist are referred because of a perceived developmental failure (e.g., academic, social, emotional or behavioral), hardly something they want to discuss with a stranger. In addition, adolescents are likely to be acutely aware of the stigma and shame that are unfortunately associated with seeing a psychiatrist. Given the difficulty many adults have dealing with this issue, it is hardly surprising that an age group characterized by heightened anxiety about identity issues and increased susceptibility to peer pressure as the gateway to social acceptance should perceive a psychiatric referral as potential social suicide. Other adolescents are concerned about a loss of control over their lives or of being labeled or criticized. Acknowledging these barriers to assessment will often help the adolescent to open up to you despite the anxiety of the situation.

Adultism

One of our colleagues addresses in her therapeutic work adolescents' expectation of "adultism" at the hands of adult authority figures,[1] an idea originally developed by Flasher.[1] Some aspects of adultism as practiced by adults when communicating with adolescents are talking down/over, brushing aside, pulling rank, changing rules, making them wait, forgetting to ask, and stifling them with adult worries. Some of the impacts of adultism on adolescents are feeling silenced and invisible; feeling under suspicion; feeling incompetent, intimidated, not consulted, and underestimated; and having their feelings not acknowledged.

As a result of these experiences with adult authority figures in their lives, adolescent patients may expect you to discount their experience or perspective, to listen to their parents rather than to them, and to impose judgments. These expectations interfere with a comprehensive assessment and development of a therapeutic alliance, and therefore you need to counter them actively in your approach to the adolescent patient.

Where's the Doctor?

It's informative here to look at what adolescents want from health care professionals. Ginsburg et al.,[3] in a survey of adolescents on factors affecting decisions to seek health care, found that adolescents prefer health care professionals who are honest, knowledgeable, experienced, and—presumably in the case of family doctors and pediatricians—who wash their hands in the teens' presence. They want physicians who treat patients equally, emphasize confidentiality, and relate well to teens. In addition, Wilkes[4] identified that adolescents want factual information rather than authoritative instruction on what to do, and they identified motivational interviewing as a positive strategy that provides adolescents with feedback on risks while promoting a sense of responsibility for their health.

The take-home message from these findings is that adolescents like their doctors to be doctors—not friends, not cool older siblings, not parents. They prefer doctors who are knowledgeable, professional, and trustworthy. We'll come back to what constitutes trustworthiness in a physician for your adolescent patients later; it is an important topic.

What does it mean to behave like a doctor? It means don't tell Sanjay you share his taste in music. Actually, it's probably fine if you do, but we are emphasizing here that it is best to avoid a common trap for professionals working with this population, that of trying to address the relationship's power imbalances by over-identifying with the adolescent.

There are a number of problems associated with trying too hard to break down the power differential between yourself and your patient by trying to place yourself in an adolescent world, however well-intentioned your goal. Developmentally, adolescents require adults in their lives to take on authoritative roles at times. It is misleading and erodes your patient's trust if you switch from someone who discusses a shared interest in body art to a person who tells the patient that she will not be allowed to leave your office or the emergency room because of safety concerns. It may help to remember that to the adolescent you represent both your profession and the mental health system, and if she feels betrayed by you, that sense of betrayal will color her view of other mental health professionals going forward.

Another point here is that you don't need to know up front about adolescent popular and recreational culture to help your patients. A more useful approach to the power imbalance in your relationship is acknowledging where you have power and expertise, and then balancing that by asking your patients to educate you where they have knowledge: their personal experiences and their adolescent culture. There are few things an adolescent will enjoy more than explaining to you why you are hopelessly out of it.

It Ain't What it Used To Be...

Have you used an Internet chat room? What about instant messaging? Did your recreational drug use as an adolescent include marijuana with THC concentrations of 3.5%, ecstasy, or crystal methamphetamine? Did you ever have a thousand people turn up to a party because of a cell phone invitation? Were there guns in your school? Were you worried about terrorist attacks? Global warming? Not getting into university because there were twice as many applicants as in previous years? Did you want to get into medicine and were not sure you could afford it because annual tuition fees cost the same as a small car?

Although all of us who survive adolescence may have similar developmental experiences, the context of adolescence for our patients has changed dramatically in the past decade as a result of technological, social, economic, and global change. One author has referred to adolescence in North America as a culture-bound syndrome, a reminder to clinicians to approach their adolescent patients from a stance of wanting to be informed and educated about their patients' cultures in the broadest sense of the term.[5]

Any attempt to stay abreast of adolescent culture, which is by definition restless and shifting, is likely doomed and would require you to spend your continuing medical education (CME) time reading music magazines, staying up until the wee hours watching fashion and music television programs, and frequenting adolescent chat rooms. Don't do it. It's undignified and developmentally inappropriate. It is better for your patients if you use your precious CME time keeping up to date with the ever-expanding research base in this field.

STAGES OF YOUR INTERVIEW

The interview of an adolescent should follow a general pattern (Table 20-1). In this section, we will discuss its various stages.

Stage I

Stage I involves meeting the adolescent and family, making introductions, explaining to the adolescent the format of the interview, finding out reasons for referral, establishing confidentiality, and building rapport. Your initial contact sets the tone for the assessment.

The adolescent and family will be vigilant at the outset of the session as to how you are going to approach them, and this will affect the whole assessment process and perhaps the treatment stage as well. You will need to be friendly and direct but also to be in charge of the assessment process, spending time explaining to the family what is going to happen.

Let's use the Case Example to walk you through how to meet Sanjay's need for privacy and a competent psychiatric assessment, his parents' need for information and reassurance, and your need to complete a safe, informative, and accurate assessment.

Don't get too hung up on introductions or worry too much about using first names versus your title. We introduce ourselves as Pier Bryden and Mark Sanford. Adolescents still expect adult authority figures to use titles and invariably address us as "doctor." On the rare occasions where an adolescent uses our first names, it can be an interesting insight into that adolescent's relationships with adults or use of bravura as a coping mechanism in anxiety-producing interactions with adults.

Remember that Sanjay is looking depressed and hostile. His parents are regaling the waiting room with their concerns about their son in their desperation to enlist your help. Your first job is to assert your comfort and willingness to structure a situation that is fast becoming uncomfortable for everyone in the room. Suggest that everyone may be more comfortable discussing the issues in private, and make a point of asking Sanjay whether he wishes to be interviewed alone first, or with his parents.

Let them know early on that there will be lots of time for you to obtain the required information. Adolescents and their worried parents cannot be rushed. You may have in mind a 50-minute oral exam format as an appropriate

Table 20-1. Stages of the Interview with an Adolescent

Stage	Components	Approaches
Stage I	Introductions, rapport-building, orientation to the assessment and confidentiality rules	Attend to obstacles to adolescent participation. Take time with adolescent. Carefully explain the interview process. Use direct straightforward communication. Don't "play" at being an adolescent. Don't neglect adolescent interests and nonproblematic areas of the adolescent's life.
Stage II	Generating a problem list and obtaining patient/family account of the history of the presenting problem	Use open-ended questions, and encourage description in the patient's own words. (*"Can you help me understand more about that? What else has been troubling you?"*) Avoid premature closure of the problem list.
Stage III	Detailed exploration of problems, systematic interrogation, and background history	Use a closed questioning style. Press for detailed descriptions of mental experience, behaviors, and context. Cover all important areas, including those avoided/difficult for adolescents to discuss (e.g., emotions, suicide, drugs, sexuality, traumatic experience, eating behaviors).
Stage IV	Mental status	Use specific questioning in areas not covered in course of history-taking. Cover psychotic experience, anxiety-depression, mania, and suicidal ideation if not covered earlier in interview. Get patient to describe experience in own words wherever possible.
Stage V	Standardized assessments	Use these for supplementary information relevant to diagnosis and to obtain baseline symptom severity. Do not neglect to review them.
Stage VI (see also Box 20-3)	Feedback of working diagnosis and formulation, treatment planning, and closure	Discuss differential diagnosis in terms of pros and cons of leading candidate diagnoses. Don't forget to provide feedback in reference to what are normal adolescent problems. Don't feel forced into making a firm diagnosis if it is very unclear. If you are reasonably confident regarding the diagnosis, say so—but remember to go soft with major mental illness diagnoses. Discuss likely course with no treatment and the range of treatments available.

time frame for the interview, but Sanjay and his parents likely do not.

Let's assume Sanjay gives the universal unhelpful adolescent response, "I don't care." You have a choice. Our tendency would be to respond by meeting with Sanjay first, demonstrating that he is your patient and that you are most interested in his perspective on things. If you do this, it will be important to reassure his parents that there will be an opportunity for them to meet with you alone and with you and Sanjay.

If it's clear that Sanjay would rather be getting dental surgery than meeting with you, say so. *"Sanjay, I get the strong impression it wasn't your idea to come here today. Whose idea was it?"* Not only have you given Sanjay the opportunity to express his feelings about being in your office, you will likely get information about the referral process.

"What are your parents and your doctor so worried about?" Again, you will get Sanjay's interpretation, as well as his views on his parents' focus of anxiety.

"Do you share their worry?" Here is a chance to assess Sanjay's insight and motivation to seek assistance.

In this instance, Sanjay denies that he is using drugs heavily, but he does express concern about his mood and his declining school performance. This is your opportunity to start building a treatment alliance, albeit with a different goal in mind from Sanjay's parents.

"Let's put the drug question aside for the moment [it's clear that you are not ignoring this important issue] *and focus on your mood and school work. Many of the adolescents I see have similar concerns."*

By the time you get back to the topic of drugs—which you will—you will have had a chance to talk with Sanjay about areas that are less threatening for him. You may also have an opportunity to reintroduce his parents' concerns, but from a perspective more in tune with his own. *"I'd like to know more about your drug use. It's often both a cause and a result of depressed mood in the adolescents I see."*

In situations where your patient is initially more forthcoming than Sanjay, it is usually helpful to ask the adolescent what the problems or symptoms she is describing mean to her (i.e., what is the salience of the symptoms to the adolescent herself). This will allow her to raise anxieties about the referral process that can be the focus of education and encouragement: "Well, I don't know whether I am depressed or not. Sometimes I think I am just exaggerating these feelings in my mind. I haven't had anything really bad happen to me. Sometimes, I feel I am just being a wimp." To which you might respond, *"No I don't think so. It's not normal to cry yourself to sleep each night and then to have to drag yourself out of bed mornings, and to get nothing done in class, day after day. You weren't like that last year. This sounds like depression, and it is a common myth that only people that have suffered horrendous circumstances get depressed. I think it was wise of you and your family to seek help for this."*

Trust Versus Secrecy

We feel confidentiality merits its own section in this discussion of the interview because it can be such a difficult and complex issue in this population. We know that adolescents like health care providers whom they trust and who assure them of confidentiality. Knowing this, you as a caregiver may feel pressure to win over the adolescent at all costs and may find yourself trapped in a promise of confidentiality that is likely to cause harm to your patient, potentially alienate his parents, and render you unable to help.

A relationship built on trust differs from one built on promises of absolute confidentiality or secrecy. It is a breach of your role as a physician for you to collude with an adolescent who is putting himself at significant risk. Therefore, at this stage of the interview, you must lay the groundwork for your and other professionals' future relationship with the adolescent. Trust is built here by your conveying honestly what you can keep to yourself and what the limits are to confidentiality. Your goal is not to trap the adolescent into disclosing something that he will later regret disclosing; rather, it is to start to build a therapeutic alliance based on trust, in which the adolescent knows that you will be taking a developmentally appropriate role as a health care provider. He will be allowed to make his own mistakes in areas where the consequences are not irrevocable, but you will intervene where his actions may cause him or another person significant harm. Remember that important developmental tasks in this age group are the mastery of impulse control and the appropriate calculation of risk. Your job may be that of both a role model and a tutor in these areas, as someone who helps the adolescent understand how to protect himself from harm in the course of his development.

An adolescent who knows from first contact what information you will or will not keep confidential has the choice of how much to reveal in the course of the interview. You may not get as much at your first meeting, but you are more likely to build and maintain a solid therapeutic alliance that will facilitate contacts with future caregivers as well as with yourself. Difficult gray areas include drug use and self-harm that is not suicidal in intent, and we will return to these later.

Here's how one of us (PB) frames the confidentiality issue for adolescents:

"Sanjay, I wanted to let you know about how confidentiality works here and what its limits are. What you tell me today is private between the two of us, unless you disclose something that poses a significant health risk to you or to a child under the age of 16. Since you and I may not agree on

what constitutes a significant health risk, I suggest that if you are wondering about something you want to tell me, before answering you should check whether it's something I will need to pass on."

Stage II

The next stage of the interview involves exploration of the presenting problem using open-ended questions to generate a problem list. Our discussion includes how to move beyond the one-word answer.

With an adolescent, you will need to have a flexible approach to asking questions. At this stage, it is best to use the open-ended question, which gives you a sense of the adolescent's concerns, together with her ability to articulate them in an effective manner. Her approach to answering such questions will throw light on her intellectual abilities, her willingness to cooperate with you in answering questions, her self-confidence, and her ability to attend and to concentrate—all essential aspects of the mental status examination.

But it is also possible that you'll find yourself with a near-silent, monosyllabic adolescent, in which case you will need to take on a much more active role than you may be used to. Start with the process. First make sure the adolescent is clear about the goal of the interview, and then label the difficulty both of you are having, and ask what it's about. *"Is it difficult talking about this stuff with someone you don't know? Are you so angry with your parents for bringing you that you can't bear to talk? Are you a shy person?"* Whether you get an answer you can work with or not, you may well have to begin with some sort of monologue to set your patient at ease. Sometimes, entire interviews with adolescents consist of asking whether what we're saying makes sense for the adolescent, along the lines of *"Many of the adolescents I see tell me that. . . . Is that true for you?"* Use information obtained from the referral source here, as often adolescents will comment on the accuracy of that information (or lack thereof). Often, a good tactic is to ask what the adolescent has told others about the problem. *"What did you say to her that made her so worried about you?"* This approach can bypass the difficulty that some adolescents have in talking directly to someone about their problem. Once comfortable with you, the adolescent will usually be able to be more open and direct. These interviews with the quiet adolescent are not particularly easy; they tend to feel more like a workout. But by the end of the interview, you can surprise yourself by how much information you've obtained by means of nods, shakes of the head, and yes or no answers.

In general, it is useful to take note of the language that the adolescent uses to describe her thoughts and feelings and where possible to use the adolescent's own language, but also to clarify what the adolescent means when using a particular term. *"You mentioned that school has been bugging you a lot lately. What else has been bugging you? When you say you feel bugged, can you describe in other words what that feels like, so I am clear what you mean?"*

Similarly, with your patient's parents, you are better off starting by giving them an opportunity to express their concerns in their own way. Unless they are mental health professionals themselves (in which case, interviewing them merits a chapter on its own), they are not familiar with the DSM-IV-TR and are likely to feel misunderstood if you are too hasty to couch their concerns in the form of specific diagnostic entities.

Stage III

The third stage of the interview involves detailed exploration (hypothesis-driven) of problems, exploring symptoms, system interrogation, functional impairments, strengths, interests, aspirations, and key background such as past medical history, family history, developmental history, school experiences, high-risk behaviors, and traumatic experiences

These middle stages of the interview are guided by the clinical hypotheses that you will develop based on the unfolding history. To be most efficient, during this stage you will generally use direct questions to explore in detail the nature of problems elucidated, including behavioral descriptions, timing and circumstances of onset, course over time, aggravating and ameliorating circumstances, general background factors, and factors known to be specifically linked to a problem or disorder. For instance, if you suspect Sanjay is depressed, this section of the interview will consist of a review of depressive symptoms (with descriptions of disturbances of mood), a review of anxiety symptoms, exploration of the temporal relationship between onset of drug use and depressive symptoms, and inquiry into adverse life events such as humiliating social experiences. For example, *"What was happening in your life when you first began to feel sad in this way? When did you begin drinking every night alone? What were your reasons for drinking like this?"*

The interview should go beyond describing the presence or absence of certain symptoms (which could be obtained from a standardized interview or self-report questionnaire) to enable you to understand—as far as possible from self-disclosure—the context for symptoms, as well as the relationships among different symptoms and between symptoms and life experience. The first step in any differential diagnosis process is to establish whether the patient's experience is outside the range of normal experience. This depends on both a quantitative evaluation of each symptom (*"How often? How severe? How persistent?"*) and on qualitative evaluation (*"When and where does that happen? Why do you feel that way?"*).

For instance, in Sanjay's case, it may be relevant to tease out whether his irritable withdrawal from his parents is confined to the day of the assessment, is a general feature of their relationship, describes all of his relationships with adults, or describes all of his relationships. Beyond that, is this a feature of his relationships all the time, over the whole of his life, or just since he was "ditched" by his girlfriend? Early in the interview, we caution against premature closure of the problem list. But in this middle stage, it is important to focus in order to rule in or out the most likely diagnoses, taking note of unanswered questions that will be the subject of future inquiry with the patient and other informants. You might ask collaborative sources, *"Was Sanjay always an irritable child? When did he begin to withdraw from the family? What do you think was going on at that time? Was anyone else feeling low or depressed around then?"*

You will see that there is an inexhaustible supply of questions, and it can be difficult to choose the right ones. As experienced interviewers, we sometimes fail to ask the key questions early in the assessment process. To minimize this, we suggest that you develop a set of general questions that you will ask in most if not all situations. Supplementary questions will arise from your ongoing formulation of the case, your knowledge of the important developmental influences on psychopathology, and what you are learning of the unique individual experience of the adolescent. For instance, you should always inquire about victimization experiences, police involvements, family conflict and violence, psychotic symptoms, drug use, and eating behaviors because these are often areas that adolescents will fail to report or where they may be evasive. (*"Sanjay, have you ever been in trouble with the police? If the police knew what you were doing, would you be in trouble? Have you ever been teased by others? Have you ever been hurt physically by another person? What about being intimidated by someone?"*) Because peer/older sibling/parent drug use is known to be a strong determinant of adolescent drug use, in this scenario you would want to know about the drug use and attitudes of Sanjay's peers/siblings/parents. You might ask, *"Do your friends use drugs as well? Do you have any friends who don't use cannabis or other drugs? What does your older brother think about your using drugs? Do your parents smoke/drink alcohol/use cannabis or other drugs? How much?"*

In Sanjay's specific case, you might find that there is a peculiar aspect to his drug use or situation that warrants further investigation. Let's say that his father is employed in the narcotics squad of the local police force, and Sanjay is particularly disparaging when mentioning this. You would want to assess whether this fact has any bearing on his drug use: *"What is your dad's attitude to drugs? Can you talk with him about these things? What does he do when you come home stoned? What did your parents do when your mom discovered your marijuana stash in the liquor cabinet? What was your reaction to that? What is it like having a dad in that line of business?"*

With these questions, you are beginning to explore meaning attached to Sanjay's behavior as well as the family context. Often you will be surprised by what you find, but don't fall into the trap of believing that all behavior is meaningful, or that it always represents an expression of family conflict. Behaviors are often multi-determined, and it is also important to recognize that symptomatic adolescents will induce behavioral changes in other family members and that normally well-functioning parents will sometimes lose their composure in face of adolescent provocations. Similarly, don't be too anxious to explain everything in terms of a single empirical or theoretical model (always an approximation of what is happening in the individual case), or as a result of psychiatric disorder. Adolescents will be reassured by developing a better understanding of symptoms/behaviors, even if this entails labeling of an experience as outside the range of normal, but they will revolt against all-encompassing generalizations about themselves and their family.

It is often surprising to listen to adolescents provide a long list of their parents' shortcomings, only to leap immediately to their defense if they perceive the interviewer is blaming them for their problems. As with children, it is important to anticipate loyalty conflicts in adolescents that will inevitably arise in the interview situation. Questions directed to adolescents about parental illnesses, substance abuse, discipline, and parenting practices will provoke ambivalent responses in the adolescent, and it will often be necessary to acknowledge this: *"I can see that it is upsetting for you to talk about your mom's drinking. Is it difficult to discuss these things with a stranger?"* Ideally, the adolescent should come to see the doctor as an advocate for him but also for other family members.

As this stage of the interview proceeds, you will be able to build a list of diagnostic possibilities and place them in order of likelihood. For instance, Sanjay may report the full range of depressive symptoms, but he may report them as only occurring at home, where he is pressured by an overbearing parent who does not accept that he has a learning disorder, although this has been documented through psychological assessment. The parent spends hours standing over him as he works—or doesn't—at his homework. He uses drugs to get to sleep at night because he is so stressed at the end of these sessions, and he worries constantly about school, his future life, and whether his friends will tease him about his appearance. Given this story, major depression appears less likely than a generalized anxiety disorder or adjustment disorder, and stress in family relationships now appears to be a major causal factor that will need to be addressed in treatment.

The key message we would like to convey is that there are multiple goals to each interview. The interviewer must get a good description of the adolescent's mental and behavioral disturbances by questioning the adolescent and others (e.g., parents) and through observation. This is central to the diagnostic process, the ruling in and out of the various diagnostic possibilities. The interviewer must also explore whether known causes for any disorders are present. This information may support a particular diagnosis but is most important in understanding the adolescent and his disorder and may lead to specific interventions. Finally, it is important to understand the unique characteristics of the adolescent, his unique life experience, and his own interpretation of those experiences. This will inform you as to how to approach the adolescent about diagnosis as well as the priority he places on treatment, and may affect the types of treatment offered. Do not expect to be able to achieve this kind of understanding in a one-shot consultation interview that would likely focus on one goal, often determining symptoms and signs of disorder.

This is the stage of the interview where "medicalizing" the interview is helpful. Adolescents have generally had the experience of being asked intrusive, health-related questions by their family doctor, pediatrician, or school nurse. Allying yourself with these other authority figures may potentially accentuate the relationship's power imbalance, but it will also help your patient with any shame she has in talking about difficult and at times intimate subjects.

In line with this medical approach, we approach difficult areas by couching our questions in terms of risk behaviors or other factors known to cause or relate to psychiatric problems. Here's an example: *"Sanjay, you may not know this, but depression in your age group has been associated by researchers with difficult or unwanted sexual experiences. Can you tell me about any sexual experiences you've had, either wanted or unwanted? Depression has also been linked with questions about sexual orientation. Have you experienced attractions to members of your own sex? It's a fairly common experience for people your age to have and to wonder about."*

When talking to adolescents about sex, always specify what you consider to be sexual experiences. Adolescents often tell us that they are not sexually active only for us to find out later that they have experienced mutual masturbation, oral sex, even anal sex without labeling it as sex because it wasn't considered sexual intercourse. This is not unreasonable, perhaps, given that some prominent politicians have expressed similar perspectives!

It can help the conversation along to normalize aspects of adolescent sexual development without implying that your patient is developmentally delayed if he hasn't had the experiences you are asking about. *"Sanjay, some adolescents your age are pairing off in romantic relationships. Is that happening with your friends? Is it something you're interested in yet?"*

Exploring risk behaviors and risk factors is also a way to introduce questions about school and social life. Framing questions in this way emphasizes you are not asking in order to label or judge the adolescent, but to explore possible medical symptoms. *"Mood disorders* [or anxiety disorders, alcohol and substance use disorders, eating disorders, etc.] *in people your age may be associated with changes in academic performance or in relationships with family and friends. Have you noticed any changes?"*

Other questions about school and social life might include: *"Are you someone who prefers to spend time alone or with other people?" "Is your school clique-y? What are some of the cliques? Where would you say you fit?" "Are you a one-on-one person, or do you prefer large groups?" "What aspects of school do you prefer—its academic or social life? Where do you fit academically? Are you an average, below-average, or above-average student? Are you planning on post-secondary education?"*

Remember to ask about changes in these areas, and focus on transition times (such as from grades 5 to 6 and 8 to 9) that tend to stress children and adolescents who are struggling developmentally. You may have noticed that we sometimes introduce potentially shaming topics using language that implies volition on the part of the patient. It's much easier for an adolescent to tell you that she doesn't choose to participate in her school's social life than that she's a social outcast; that she chooses not to spend her time on her math homework but instead on her guitar playing, rather than that she is flunking most of her subjects; that she has decided to get some work experience rather than that she will be working in a fast-food restaurant next year because her marks weren't good enough for the community college program she wanted. You will get a more accurate picture later as the adolescent comes to trust that you are not judging her, but at this point it does no harm to let your patient save face and tell you her troubles at her own pace.

Here are our approaches to other important questions to ask of an adolescent patient:

- *"Sanjay, how many of your friends are using alcohol and drugs regularly? What are they using? What have you tried? What do you like most? What effect does it have on you?"*
- *"How much does it take to get you drunk/high? How often do you drink/smoke/snort? With whom and where do you drink, etc.?"*
- *"Do you tend to be more or less affected by the drugs than your friends? Have any of your friends ever expressed worry about your alcohol or drug use?"*

- *"Have you ever had an unwanted sexual experience while drunk or high?"*
- *"Have you ever gotten into trouble with the police while drunk or high?"*
- *"Do you ever drive, or have you driven with someone, while intoxicated?"*

Notice how we are seeding psychoeducational points in our questions about drug and alcohol intake that we can return to in our feedback to Sanjay on high-risk behaviors.

If it appears that Sanjay is drinking or using drugs heavily, it is important to find out how he is funding these behaviors because often the need to pay for drugs and alcohol may lead to further high-risk activities such as stealing, dealing, and exchanging sex for money or drugs. As already noted, it is also important to find out more about drinking and drug use in the home. *"Who in your family drinks? Who uses street drugs? Are you concerned about their use?"*

Even if the adolescent expresses no concern about parental or sibling drinking or drug use, ask about quantities and frequency, as lack of concern does not necessarily mean there isn't a problem. Interestingly, even those adolescents who are indulging in high-risk drinking or drug use are censorious regarding parents' habits, dislike seeing their parents in an intoxicated state, and will often try to separate themselves physically and psychologically from them. In this circumstance, some of the adolescent's problem behaviors may serve the purpose of establishing a negative identification with the parent.

Other important areas in the adolescent history include screening questions for eating disorders, criminal activity, self-harm, and trauma. Given the existing research on the dangers of providing teenagers with information about behaviors aimed at achieving weight loss, if you ask about purging, use of diet pills, or excessive exercise, balance these questions with psychoeducation about the relative ineffectiveness of these as weight-loss aids, together with information about their dangerousness.

When asking about a history of criminal involvement, make sure you phrase your questions in such a way that it is clear to the adolescent that you are asking about criminal behaviors, not labeling him as a criminal. *"Some adolescents we see end up in trouble with the law because of bad judgments or choices they've made. Have you had any charges against you? Warnings? What about your friends?"* *"If the police knew what you were doing, would you be in trouble?"*

Self-harm is increasingly prevalent among adolescents in North America, ranging from body piercing and tattooing that may be compulsive and masochistic to cutting and burning arms, feet, abdomen and thighs, and even genitalia. It is important for clinicians working with adolescents to approach the topic of these behaviors with sophistication, recognizing that there are a variety of possible causes and different levels of severity of self-harm. Body piercing and tattooing for most adolescents is a form of self-expression or group identification; only for a minority will it represent a form of psychopathology. Parents, too, may need to learn that not all self-harm is suicidal in intent, nor is it always attention seeking and therefore to be disregarded. You as a clinician are wise to ask about these behaviors calmly but with concern, conveying that while you are not likely to overreact to any disclosures, you take these behaviors seriously and perceive them as requiring attention. *"Some of the adolescents we see respond to strong emotions that seem overwhelming by hurting themselves. They might burn themselves, bang their heads, or cut their skin. For some adolescents, frequent body piercing and tattooing may be a form of self-harm. Have you ever used these types of behaviors as a way of coping with out-of-control feelings?"*

The disclosure of self-harm to parents is a controversial area for mental health professionals working with adolescents. Some disclose it or encourage the patient to disclose with the limit that if the adolescent is unable to do so, the professional will after a certain period of time. Others don't disclose it if they perceive the behavior to be relatively low risk. We can't give you a right answer but can share our biases with you. One of us (PB) had the experience early in her practice of meeting a young girl who was scratching her arms superficially with razors. At the initial assessment, PB agreed not to tell the girl's parents about the self-harm, since she felt it did not constitute a significant risk. A few days after the assessment, the girl rolled up her sleeve so that her mother could not avoid seeing recent scratches and told her mother that she had told the psychiatrist who had told her that she did not need to tell her mother. PB received an outraged phone call from the girl's mother informing her that she would be seeking further psychiatric consultation elsewhere. In retrospect, it is clear that the girl wanted her mother to be aware of her self-harm and may indeed have disclosed to PB in the hopes that she would pass on the information.

We both endorse giving the adolescent control of how and when (within a limited time frame) to tell her parents about current or recent self-harm, while letting her know that if she cannot, we will. We are transparent to the adolescent about our rationale: the injuries may cause permanent scarring, infection, or unpredictable trauma to a vein or artery; and parents are likely to be more worried and upset if they find out about such behaviors in an uncontrolled way. The majority of adolescents we see accept these parameters as common sense.

Stage IV

Stage IV of the interview deals with mental status features not already covered in detailed exploration and through observations.

Even with a laconic adolescent, there may be a myriad of clues to diagnosis in your nonverbal mental status exam (Box 20-2). Ask about clothes, jewelry, tattoos and piercings, and head gear. Again, you don't have to know about gang insignia to ask whether a head scarf or a ring has special significance. If sleeves are rolled up, look for scarring or signs of intravenous drug use. If clothes are unusually layered or baggy on a thin female, consider a potential eating disorder. If Sanjay is fidgety and sweaty, is he hyperactive, anxious, or in potential withdrawal? If he's relaxed and smiling, is it appropriate, or is he high?

How an adolescent answers your questions will help you to judge whether his reported academic performance is affected by his symptoms. Characterize his vocabulary, fluency, and syntax; note whether you share a first language or if he is responding in what is a second or third language for him. Notice his use of expletives. Even now, it's unusual for most adolescents to swear repetitively in front of a strange adult without some sort of apology or acknowledgment.

As with other age groups, body language may be useful in conveying nonverbal reluctance or anxiety in an ostensibly amicable interview. PB remembers interviewing a well-groomed, courteous young woman in a school uniform accompanied by her parents. The girl stated repeatedly that she had no difficulty with being assessed, but she spent the entire interview poking hard at the chair arm with a hair slide. She disclosed in a subsequent interview that she had recently discovered that her father was having an affair and that she was furious with him for dragging her to see a psychiatrist when she felt his infidelity was the source of her change in mood and academic and social functioning, as well as their family conflicts.

Hygiene is an interesting issue. Most parents will try to coerce their adolescent into cleaning up for the doctor. If parents fail and your patient turns up with greasy, uncombed hair and filthy clothes, is this is a statement to you, to his parents, or is it indicative of grave impairment of his ability to function day to day?

We have given up on trying to evaluate whether clothing and makeup are age-inappropriate, given the downward expansion of corporate marketing of sexualized clothing aimed at preteens. Further on in an interview or relationship, you may get useful information from asking your patient about how her style represents her social affiliations, interests, etc.

Thought content and perceptions are essential aspects of the adolescent's mental status, which you may have an easier time getting at by asking about favorite music groups or films. Many adolescents can recite entire lyrics of loved songs that express a world view or perspective that feels identical to their own. It's important to explore in detail for psychotic thought content and perceptual abnormalities; this is the age group in which the major psychotic disorders first appear. Psychotic symptoms that occur in conjunction with drug use cannot be attributed definitively to substance abuse; it may be that the substance use is a form of self-medication. Adolescents will frequently conceal psychotic symptoms such as hallucinations and delusions because the stigma of mental illness is especially strong during this developmental stage, and psychosis is likely to be terrifying to the adolescent. It will often take sensitive questioning to unearth these experiences. It is important to listen closely for suggestions of psychosis and introduce questions consistent with exploring these themes. For instance, a very isolated adolescent may report "rumors" circulating at school. The interviewer can comment, *"Rumors often circulate at school, and it's very tough if that's going on. What do you think the rumors are about? Who do you think is spreading them around?"* or *"Have you worried at all that these students mean to hurt you? How would they go about that?"* or *"How sure are you that*

Box 20-2. Special Considerations in Mental Status Exam with Adolescents

APPEARANCE

Clothing, insignia, tattoos may have gang significance or indicate other important identity issues

RAPPORT/DEMEANOR

Often very influenced by context of medical assessment
Pay close attention to nonverbal behaviors
Watch for different demeanor in presence of parents

MOOD

Mood state also greatly affected by interview context
Depressed mood state often experienced as ego-syntonic by adolescents
Irritable behavior may represent different underlying mood states
Many unwilling to report anxiety symptoms
Explore for concealed suicidal ideas and behaviors

THINKING/PERCEPTION

Adolescent persecutory ideas often involve family, may appear normative
Often reluctant to reveal psychotic experiences
May be difficult to disentangle effects of hallucinogenic drugs

INSIGHT/JUDGMENT

Can't always take initial adolescent denial/minimization as sign of poor insight as it may be a manifestation of reluctance to acknowledge a need for help *this is what's going on?"* Another aspect making assessment difficult is that family members are often the subject of an adolescent patient's delusions, and it can be difficult to separate delusional concerns from the usual adolescent-family relationship concerns. Take the following, for example: "My sister is a real a pain. She is always trying to get my parents' attention away from me," versus "If my sister wasn't there, I would have lots of friends. She spoils all my chances for meeting people, she wants me to fail and kill myself so she can have my parents to herself. Yes, she is only 8 years old, but she has always had it in for me." Questions that are rooted in an adolescent's actual experience are superior in eliciting psychotic symptoms than the usual standardized questions such as, *"Have you ever heard voices or sounds that others couldn't hear?"* However, frequently there will be no indication to undertake this subtle questioning, and the more direct approach will be in order. We would suggest a preliminary remark such as, *"Sometimes when people's feelings are all jumbled like this, they have odd experiences like hearing voices. This can be quite scary as it feels like losing your grip on things. Has this ever happened to you?"*

Assessing emotion in adolescents is usually difficult because they may lack words to describe their feelings adequately. The adolescent may not be able to go much further than to say that she "doesn't feel good." Sad, depressed feelings and pessimistic ideas are frequently experienced (or communicated) as ego-syntonic: "That's just the way things are," or "I don't go because it's totally boring hanging out at those parties." In your interview, you will need to press the adolescent to try to find words to express how she feels, to describe what actions she wants to take when in a particular mood state (e.g., withdraw, cry, punch the wall), and to describe any mood changes. A parent's objective description of the adolescent's behavior can help round out the picture: "She just looks miserable, won't speak to us, and lies about in her room for days at a time."

Adolescent boys are loath to admit any anxiety. The question "Is there anything you are scared of?" will almost inevitably draw a negative response. It is useful to substitute the terms "nervous" or "stressed" and ask about situations that make him feel that way. Questions such as these include the following:

- *"Everybody gets nervous sometimes, perhaps before an exam or speaking in class. When do you feel like that?"*
- *"What does that feel like?"*
- *"Do you notice any changes in your body when that happens? Like feeling your heart racing, etc.?"*
- *"What other situations would get you feeling that way? Do you try to avoid those situations? What other situations will you stay away from because you feel uncomfortable?"*

Some will react with anger and irritability. Again, it will be useful to get a detailed description of behavior from a parent including signs of autonomic arousal, situations that always produce specific responses, and situations that are avoided. It may be that similar behaviors were noted earlier in development and were more readily acknowledged as anxiety responses or were associated with reassurance-seeking.

Suicidal and homicidal ideation must also be explored in detail. Adolescents are a high-risk group (15 to 25 per 100,000) for suicide. You should not rely on simple yes/no answers to questions about suicidal ideas and behavior. Watch carefully for hesitation in answering these questions because this often indicates that you should push a little further even if the adolescent has answered in the negative. Ask directly whether the patient would reliably report on this sort of behavior. We are no longer surprised by the number of adolescents who are willing to tell you, when challenged, that of course they wouldn't be stupid enough to tell you if they were feeling suicidal. Many adolescents (and parents, interestingly) think suicidal thoughts are normal in this age group, so it is important to reiterate to your patient that you take any such thoughts seriously. On the other hand, it's also helpful to reassure parents that not every adolescent who listens to Kurt Cobain or who has read his diaries is an acute suicide risk. Explore how often suicidal ideas are present, how pressing they are, details of specific content and circumstances, what the adolescent does in response to these thoughts, occurrence of any impulsive or planned suicidal behaviors, and—if these have occurred—what was done afterward. These questions tend to be more acceptable to adolescents when clearly linked to your assessment of their depressed mood and feelings of helplessness and hopelessness. *"Sanjay, many adolescents who feel the way you do have thoughts of harming themselves or ending their lives. Has that been true for you?"*

An adolescent's own account of her difficulties will usually offer clues to her insight, judgment, and motivation for change. It is unlikely, although possible, that parents are entirely mistaken about their child's functioning. Complete denial of difficulty on the part of the adolescent may connote anger at, and resistance to, the assessment but may also point to deeper problems with impulse control, self-awareness, empathy, or conscience.

Finally, how an adolescent relates to his or her parents during the interview is a goldmine of information. Does she comment on their contributions verbally or nonverbally, with overt contradiction or rolling of eyes? Does he sit close to one or both parents or strategically place himself as far away as possible? Does everyone look as though they come from the same family, or is the adolescent dressed in such a way as to distance herself from her parents' economic or sociocultural background?

Stage V: Supplementary Information

The clinical interview, which we have described in detail, remains the main tool available to us as psychiatrists assessing adolescents. It is important to recognize some of its problems. First and foremost, it relies on a minimally willing subject and a degree of self-awareness on the part of the subject. Unfortunately, most adolescents—and indeed most adults—are limited in their ability to describe their own experience. Therefore, it is necessary whenever possible to supplement the history with direct observations, something much easier to achieve in inpatient settings. A second problem is the lack of reliability of the clinical interview; different interviewers will obtain different stories, and adolescents will tell different stories at different times. As a result, it is helpful to get the perspective of different informants and to interview the adolescent on different occasions.

It is also useful to supplement the interview with standardized assessments. We do not use the available structured and semi-structured interviews in clinical practice except with adolescents who are participating in research protocols. They tend to be unwieldy, and interviewers must be trained for reliability. This is onerous and requires regular training sessions, not always feasible for a purely clinical service. The available interviews also lack the flexibility of the clinical interview for exploring background contextual factors, and, arguably most importantly, are boring and repetitive for the adolescent.

We do use a variety of standardized questionnaires. These have the advantage of being relatively quick to complete. We choose well-standardized instruments that provide excellent information regarding diagnosis and in determining the severity of symptoms. There are many available instruments, but we use the Child Behavior Checklist (parent-report, teacher-report , and adolescent self-report versions).[6] These are broad, well-standardized questionnaires that cover a wide range of psychopathology. We also use instruments targeted at specific symptoms (e.g., Children's Depression Inventory[7] or the Beck Depression Inventory,[8] Multidimensional Anxiety Scale–Child version,[9] Drug Abuse Screening Test,[10] the Eating Attitudes Test[11]).

It may seem obvious, but if you are using questionnaires to gather information, it is essential to look at the results, including any written comments. Adolescents and parents will often use these forms to communicate specific concerns and expect that you will be reading them (why else would you give them?). One of us (no initials given because of residual shame) has had the unfortunate experience of having to call back some days later a patient who disclosed acute suicidal ideation on a questionnaire that she had not disclosed in the clinical interview. We would like to save you and your patients from a similar risk.

You will also need to know how to interpret scale scores to obtain the most information from them. This means that you will need to know how to interpret a z-score and t-score, to be aware of clinical cutoffs, etc. If you have not been taught these basic statistics, we suggest you consult your service psychologist, who should be able to help with a quick tutorial.

Stage VI: Closing the Interview

During the final stage of the interview, you will give feedback about differential diagnosis and formulation, have a discussion of the adolescent's view of these formulations and what treatments work, negotiate around further investigations and management, and discuss what is to be shared with parents (Box 20-3).

The optimal outcome for the first assessment is to arrive at the preferred diagnosis and to outline a treatment plan, which can be discussed with the adolescent and/or family. Given sufficient interview time, it is usually possible to achieve this, although usually there will be unanswered

---

Box 20-3. Feedback Regarding Diagnosis and Management

Prepare the adolescent as to what feedback will be given to the parents.

Explain the diagnostic process, including the idea that the diagnosis may be in error, the idea that the diagnosis may change with time, and the purpose of arriving at a preferred diagnosis (emphasizing how it can guide treatment).

If the diagnosis is uncertain, say so.

If the diagnosis is relatively certain, discuss the main possibilities and the pros and cons of your preferred diagnosis.

Proceed gently in sharing the diagnosis of stigmatizing disorders.

Don't lecture; keep this stage of interview as interactive as possible.

Ask the adolescent (and the parents) for their opinions.

Provide a brief preliminary formulation that covers possible causes.

Don't forget to discuss adolescent/family strengths and weaknesses and protective factors.

Discuss first what the likely outcome of the disorder will be without treatment (natural history of disorder).

Discuss the pros and cons of treatment and the level of evidence supporting different treatments.

Ask about adolescent (and parent) treatment preferences.

Don't rush the adolescent into deciding on a specific treatment.

Give time for further assessment and later discussion.

If there is an urgent or dangerous situation, be prepared with adequate security support, discuss your concerns frankly, and act to ensure immediate safety of the adolescent.

questions and other diagnoses that will need to be ruled in or out at subsequent interviews. Sometimes, the differential diagnosis is long even at the end of the first interview. In this situation, it is best to summarize what you have learned so far, to acknowledge that you are unsure about how best to describe or diagnose the problem, and to outline the next steps in your investigations together, recruiting the adolescent to explore some aspect of the history or to monitor symptoms.

A chief goal of each interview is to reach an understanding on the part of the interviewer as to the nature of the problem and the mental and social functioning of the patient. It is equally important that the adolescent herself develop a better understanding of her problems, or her disorder if she has one. This is often achieved throughout the interview as the adolescent begins to articulate for the first time her experience, and in doing so, to make links with life events. Discussions toward the end of the interview will consolidate these insights and provide an opportunity for the clinician to make links and to educate about the features of specific disorders.

It is important that the interviewer not go beyond what she can state with some confidence; to do so risks being dogmatic or formulating prematurely. Too much education about a disorder early in the assessment process might suggest certain symptoms to the adolescent and lead to invalid symptom reports. It is important to assess the adolescent's preexisting knowledge of psychopathology, exposure to other clinicians, and likelihood that the report is being influenced by others' expectations. When you are in doubt about the validity of the report, probe for more descriptions of experience, avoid using the common broad language of symptoms (the meaning of which has become degraded through nonspecific usage, e.g., depression, paranoia, panic, mania, "on a high"), and obtain objective accounts from unbiased observers. It may be necessary to see the adolescent yourself several times before reaching a judgment about the presence or absence of specific symptoms, such as depressed mood.

This is not a chapter on formulation, but it is also important to attempt to arrive at a formulation of the patient's problems. That is, what are the remote and proximal causes of the disorder, and what are the factors that aggravate or ameliorate the disorder or interfere with treatment? It is helpful, with experience, to be able to develop an initial formulation as the interview progresses. Obviously, this is easier to do in less complicated cases when the adolescent is able to provide a full and convincing history. In the closing stage of the interview, it is appropriate to begin to discuss your formulation with the patient. Adolescents and their parents are, like most of us, exquisitely sensitive to the possibility of blame. The biopsychosocial formulation is a useful tool in helping

to convey that you do not perceive any single etiology to a disorder.

An example of a way to close the interview is as follows: *"Sanjay, I think we are in agreement that you have been quite depressed since the summer. I am thinking that your marijuana habit is fairly recent, and it is likely that you have been smoking up at night alone as a way of coping with this depression. What do you think? It hasn't helped that at the time you started to feel depressed, your father lost his job. Worrying about him seems to have been related to your depression getting worse. In fact, both of you have gotten more and more depressed together. Do you see any connection there? I agree it can be really stressful living with a depressed parent. There has been so much depression affecting your family that it seems likely that you may share a vulnerability to depression with your father. That doesn't mean you and your father are the same or that you will be affected in the same way, but it may mean that if you are in a stressful situation that you may be more likely to get depressed than someone who doesn't have any vulnerability. However, it is complicated; many factors may contribute to depression, and we don't fully understand how this happens."*

This kind of feedback should be interactive. A monologue by the interviewer that is too long will lose the adolescent. Further, there is much to be gained from eliciting the adolescent's responses to the feedback. Often the adolescent will weigh symptoms, stressors, and risk factors differently, and this will lead to a more accurate and useful formulation—one that can lay the groundwork for discussing treatment.

The last stage is to discuss further investigations and treatment: *"We do know that depression will usually lift on its own, but it can take a very long time for that to happen. There are treatments that can speed up recovery from depression, and some are even helpful to reduce the likelihood of its returning. How much do you know about depression and its treatment?"*

It is useful to discuss first whether you think treatment is necessary and what is likely to happen without treatment before discussing benefits and risks of specific treatments, whether they have been tested out in trials, etc. Asking the patient's treatment preferences indicates that there are treatment choices and that the adolescent will be central in making the final choices. It is helpful to discuss treatments in general terms and ask preferences, even when there is doubt about the diagnosis and preferred treatment. This will indicate to the adolescent that you are serious about finding some way to help him.

It may be obvious, but when you are unclear about what is wrong with the adolescent, don't worry about conveying this uncertainty to adolescents and their families. It is an opportunity to enlist them in further information gathering and observation, reinforcing the theme that they have expertise that is unavailable to you. Even if you are fairly certain of the diagnosis, particularly when it is of a serious and disabling illness such as schizophrenia or bipolar disorder, convey that a definitive diagnosis will take time and that further exploration will be necessary to confirm your diagnosis. This is accurate information and will allow your patient and his family to come to terms with the diagnosis at their own pace.

Probably the best advice to leave you with is to make sure to close without any major surprises for the adolescent. If Sanjay has disclosed serious drug use to you by the end of the interview, or if you are suspicious that he is using more than he is willing to disclose, you will need to assess whether this can be disclosed to the parent. Again, this is a difficult issue with respect to the limits to confidentiality. Generally, we would encourage the adolescent to disclose something of his drug use to the parents. If he refuses, we would generally not divulge the information directly. However, we would advise the adolescent that this is a major issue that might interfere with any useful treatment and that it will need to be revisited frequently. One of us (PB) also advises her patients that she will be discussing high-risk behaviors in general with parents: *"Sanjay, while I will not discuss the specifics of your drug and alcohol use with your parents without your permission, I will be letting your parents know that I am aware of their concerns, that drug and alcohol abuse may accompany depression in adolescents, and that I will continue to assess and monitor your use of substances as part of treatment as I would with any depressed adolescent in my care."*

The no-surprise approach is particularly important in a crisis or emergency room assessment. If you are thinking of hospitalizing an adolescent involuntarily, let him know that this is a possibility early in your interview—once you have a security guard or staff member available to assist you if the adolescent tries to leave. If you've had a "warm, fuzzy interview" in which the adolescent has opened up to you only to find out at the end that you also have a policing aspect to your role, he will feel justifiably manipulated.

We therefore talk with the adolescent about diagnostic possibilities and treatment options before meeting again, usually at the end of the assessment with him and his parents. This gives him an opportunity to voice any concerns or misgivings about what is to be said to parents. It also provides you with a sense as to what treatments the adolescent is willing to consider, rather than having to deal in the last 5 minutes of your interview with Sanjay informing his parents that he will have nothing to do with any of your suggestions. It won't look good if you end the interview at this point. If Sanjay or any child who needs help is refusing it, you will need to advise parents on how to proceed and what options are available to them in applying pressure on their child where appropriate.

If you are left with a diagnostic question mark such as drug use, be up front about how you intend to explore it further. Sanjay may be interested in getting help for depression but completely uninterested in talking about his drug use. Make your limits clear at the outset; it will save you much grief later. Let him know you are happy to treat his depression but cannot leave the drug question aside, given its importance in its own right and in terms of its likely effect on treatment response. Ask his permission to perform random drug screens, explaining that it will help both of you to avoid debates about his use, and that this is your standard practice in such situations. Stand firm. You may lose him in the short term, but you have conveyed that you are neither a pushover nor a fool, at the same time conveying a nonjudgmental, concerned stance.

CONCLUSION

We hope we have conveyed some of the complexities and challenges of interviewing adolescents, as well as its rewards. Adolescents are a patient population who underutilize the health care system despite high rates of morbidity and mortality, some of which stem from developmentally normal experimentation with high-risk behaviors. This is also a common age for the onset of a variety of psychiatric disorders, some of which will persist into adulthood. Psychiatrists with comfort and expertise working with this age group may play a crucial role in intervening in specific instances in time to prevent tragedies such as suicide and accidental deaths that remain too prevalent among these patients.

And, on a lighter note, we have both found working with adolescents humbling, sometimes exasperating, never boring, and frequently enjoyable. We recommend it highly.

REFERENCES

1. Jasper K: Personal correspondence.
2. Flasher J: Adultism. *Adolescence* 13(51):517–523, 1978.
3. Ginsburg KR, Menapace AS, Slap GB: Factors affecting the decision to seek health care: the voice of adolescents, *Pediatrics* 100:922–930, 1997.
4. Wilkes M: A primary care approach to adolescent health care, *West J Med* 172:177–182, 2000.
5. Hill R, Fortenberry JD: Adolescence as a culture-bound syndrome, *Soc Sci Med* 35(1):73–80, 1992.

6. Achenbach T: *Child Behavior Checklist for Ages 4–18,* Burlington, VT, 1991, University of Vermont.

7. Kovacs M: *The Children's Depression Inventory (CDI),* North Tonawanda, NY, 1982, Multi-Health Systems.

8. Beck AT, Steer RA, Brown GK: *Beck Depression Inventory: second edition (BDI-II) manual,* San Antonio, TX, 1996, The Psychological Corporation, Harcourt Brace & Co.

9. March JS: *The Multidimensional Anxiety Scale for Children (MASC),* North Tonawanda, NY, 1997, Multi-Health Systems.

10. Martino S, Grilo CM, Fehon DC: Development of the drug abuse screening test for adolescents (DAST-A), *Addict Behav* 25:57–70, 2000.

11. Garner DM, Olmstead MP, Bohr Y, Garfinkel PE: The eating attitudes test: psychometric features and clinical correlates. *Psychol Med* 12:871–878, 1982.

21

Assessment of Older Adults

KENNETH I. SHULMAN AND IVAN L. SILVER

INTRODUCTION

Geriatric psychiatry has been referred to as "general psychiatry—only more so." A psychiatrist working with geriatric patients must be extremely versatile and have a wide range of knowledge and skills applicable to the assessment of mental and behavioral disorders of old age. Hence, this chapter will focus on the "added value" necessary for adequate assessment of an older adult building on the issues relevant to a mixed-age adult population.[1] These special considerations include the following: (1) flexibility of place and mode of assessment; (2) the ability to integrate and synthesize a lifelong history of many years; (3) knowledge and assessment of medical comorbidity (especially neurological disorders) as well as an assessment of drug sensitivity and drug interactions; (4) incorporation of the informant/caregiver role; and (5) assessment of cognitive status, including capacity assessments.

Throughout this chapter, we have highlighted clinical tips for clinicians. These are based primarily on our clinical experience, which we happily share with the reader.

PLACE AND MODE OF ASSESSMENT

One of the fundamental differences in assessing older adults is that the traditional place of assessment in the doctor's office, be it in the community or in a hospital setting, is often not an optimal or even practical place. Indeed, a psychiatrist, mental health clinician, or multidisciplinary psychiatric service must have the flexibility, where appropriate or necessary, to assess persons in their own residential settings—be they houses, apartments, or institutional facilities.

Especially if dementia, cognitive impairment, or extreme frailty is a consideration, the patient's own setting is the preferred location for the psychiatric assessment. This is not just optimal, but a necessity at times. In some cases, seeing persons in their own settings helps to determine important environmental factors that may affect their care and management.

Because of the complex and often multifaceted nature of psychiatric disorders in older adults, it may very well be desirable to conduct the assessment with at least one other health care professional to deal with other psychosocial and practical issues related to independent activities of daily living. Where the resources are available, the psychiatric assessment of an older adult is optimally done by a multidisciplinary team based in a general hospital setting, where access to medical consultation and investigation is readily accomplished, given the common medical comorbidity associated with psychiatric disorders. The traditional method of a psychiatrist operating in an office outside of an institutional setting, with little access to other health care professionals or investigative resources, is not only impractical but represents poor quality of care for this population; it should be actively discouraged by a health care service.

Not uncommonly, the psychiatric assessment will call for laboratory investigations, especially hematology; electrolytes; thyroid, hepatic, and renal function; and vitamin B_{12} and folate. The need to rule out systemic medical conditions such as hypothyroidism and vitamin deficiencies means that ready access to laboratory services is important. Sending elderly and frail patients to private laboratories in the community is impractical and may place a significant burden on both the patient and the family. Secondly, neuroimaging is a frequent component of assessment to rule out cerebrovascular pathology, dementia, or other space-occupying lesions when a differential diagnosis of depression or dementia is an issue. Hence, access to computed tomography (CT), single-photon emission CT, and magnetic resonance imaging scans is an important component of the assessment of many older adults and needs to be available as appropriate.

Furthermore, we take the position that all psychiatric assessments of older people should be preceded by a screening assessment by a primary care physician who is responsible for making the referral. This ensures that a medical screening has taken place, including a careful review of medications that can significantly affect mental status.

ROLE OF THE CAREGIVER/INFORMANT

The involvement and contribution of an informant/caregiver are vital to the adequate psychiatric assessment of an older adult. Without an objective informant, in a large number of cases the psychiatrist or the psychiatric team will not have adequate information to establish an accurate diagnosis, formulation, or management plan. Thus, we take the position that all psychiatric assessments of older people should include the involvement of an informant or caregiver who lives with the patient or has a good knowledge of the patient's daily functioning.[2,3] Too often, we find ourselves limited in assessing an older person without full information from another informant and, indeed, with an inaccurate perception of the issues or the patient's level of function.

Clinical Tip

When a caregiver indicates that there is something wrong, this is almost always the case. We qualify the caregiver's assessment of changes or concerns when he offers his own explanation for the cause of the changes. For example, caregivers will frequently misinterpret motivational deficit and cognitive impairment as a sign of "depression."

Unfortunately, the historical psychiatric culture has traditionally excluded families from being active participants in both the assessment and ongoing management of major mental disorders. This culture has evolved in part because of legitimate concerns about confidentiality and the primacy of the doctor-patient relationship. In our experience, you can still sensibly maintain appropriate confidentiality as well as a positive therapeutic alliance without excluding families or stonewalling them from having access to information or even communicating concerns, as has often being reported to us by family members. Caregivers and families should be equal partners in the therapeutic alliance. In the care of older adults, the well-being and quality of life of those around them are as much a part of the clinical equation as that of the patient. In dealing with older adults and their families, you must modify the traditional "doctor-patient relationship" to include the "doctor-*family* relationship." This is especially true when the patient is incapable or extremely frail.

A general principle would be to try to see the patient first and give her the sense that her concerns are being valued, especially if there is any element of suspiciousness or paranoid beliefs directed at the family or caregivers. However, where cognitive impairment is the primary concern, there is little value in spending a great deal of time attempting to take a history and learning facts from such a person. In circumstances like that, when it is obvious that you are dealing with a significant cognitive concern, you may want to interview the family member or caregiver first and obtain an external perspective before bringing in the patient, where the focus is primarily on mental status and cognitive assessment. Flexibility is always the important principle in assessment, and clinicians need to both obtain as much information as possible before the assessment and use their intuition in determining how to go about the assessment of older adults. Seeing such a patient and her family members or caregivers together is generally not conducive to the orderly determination of history or mental status. Seeing persons together is designed for two purposes. The first is to determine the nature of their interaction and to have an opportunity to observe such interaction in the office or home setting. The second reason to see people together is to give the same feedback and the same message to both patient and family to minimize miscommunication and misunderstanding. Generally, we recommend that the patient and the family member/caregiver be assessed separately, but that feedback be given together when possible. Sometimes, having the caregiver present during the cognitive assessment can be helpful to highlight the degree and significance of cognitive impairment when caregivers are unaware or in denial.

MENTAL STATUS EXAMINATION

The mental status examination of the older adult is not fundamentally different than the mental status examination of mixed-age adults. Hence, the examination in the form of a semi-structured interview takes place throughout the history-taking process. Indeed, mental status begins from the moment one observes the patient walk into the room and continues in a flexible fashion throughout the course of the assessment.

The special aspect of mental status that distinguishes an older adult from a younger adult has to do with the need to do a careful cognitive assessment in all cases.[4] No matter how intact an older adult appears, our experience is that if we neglect to do a formal cognitive screen during the initial consultation/assessment, we always regret this and often find ourselves having missed significant cognitive impairment because of the superficial appearance of intact cognitive function. This is the case in many persons experiencing the onset of dementia. They maintain their social graces and may have been functioning at a previously high level or held a position of high esteem. You might feel reluctant to address formal cognitive screening for fear of embarrassing the person. This is almost always a mistake, and some form of formal cognitive assessment is essential in every case involving older adults. (A discussion of the techniques of cognitive screening will follow.)

Cognitive screening can start at the very beginning of the interview, without offending the patient and potentially threatening the kind of therapeutic alliance that is necessary to elicit adequate information for the purposes of diagnosis. Hence, we recommend that the initiation of the interview take place as follows: Carefully observe the patient's appearance and behavior from the outset. Does the patient seem bemused or bewildered on entry into the room? Is there evidence of disinhibition or socially inappropriate behavior? Is the patient's dress appropriate and coordinated?

Clinical Tip

"THE AGE AND DATE OF BIRTH" COGNITIVE SCREEN

Early in the interview, when taking basic demographic information such as name, place of residence, marital, occupational, or retirement status, one can easily insert two questions that function as an effective cognitive screen: *"How old are you? What is your date of birth?"* In the context of demographic inquiry, these are innocuous questions that do not threaten the patient, but they often will reveal problems in cognition when there is difficulty recalling age, or when the age and date of birth are not congruent.

As in younger adults, the initiation of the interview with an older adult should use questions that are as open-ended as possible, after demographic information and age and date of birth are determined. The open-ended questions provide two important outcomes. First, they allow the examiner to tap into important ideational, psychological, and emotional material that emerges spontaneously from patients who are troubled. Secondly, the open-ended questions and lack of structure will help to reveal any evidence of speech disturbance, such as dysphasia or thought disor-

der, which may occur in major psychiatric disorders. If the patient is talkative, it is well worthwhile to invest 1 or 2 minutes to allow the patient free reign while carefully observing for content and process.

Clinical Tip

THE "WHITE ROOTS" SIGN

Grooming is often a clue as to level of functioning and the presence of cognitive impairment. However, for older women who are in the habit of dyeing their hair, there is a special opportunity. We have often been able to diagnose a major depression by simply observing the white roots of a woman who has been in the habit of dyeing her hair. A major depression affects motivation, initiative, and in severe cases, will actually affect an older woman's long-established pattern of attending the hair salon on a regular basis. Knowing that hair grows roughly at the rate of half an inch a month will reveal that a 2-inch band of white root suggests a 4-month major depression. Of course, this clinical tip needs to be corroborated by history and the rest of the mental status examination. Nonetheless, suspicion about a major depression based on this type of observation can be helpful and can direct the examiner to the more critical questions necessary to establish a diagnosis of major depression versus dementia.

We hasten to add that this same clinical tip may apply increasingly to older men who develop the same pattern of maintaining a youthful appearance.

DIFFERENTIAL DIAGNOSIS OF PSYCHOTIC SYMPTOMS IN THE "3DS"

Regarding mental status examinations in which psychotic symptoms in the form of delusions or hallucinations are present, we provide in Table 21-1 a useful method of differential diagnosis on the basis of the quality of those symptoms. The differential diagnosis of the "3Ds"—dementia, delirium, and depression—is the most common diagnostic challenge in older adults. Delusions in dementia tend to be compensatory in nature; that is, they compensate for memory and cognitive deficits. They are typically of a rather vacuous, mundane, and banal quality and when present, are

Table 21-1. Differential Diagnosis Psychotic Symptoms

	Dementia	Delirium	Depression
Delusions	Compensatory	Nightmarish	Nihilistic
Hallucinations	Variable	Visual	Auditory
Quality	Vacuous/banal	Frightening, bizarre	Self-deprecatory

often characterized by suspiciousness or frank paranoid ideas usually related to stealing.

Clinical Tip

Any older adult who presents for the first time with stealing delusions (usually involving a daughter-in-law) is suffering from a dementia until proven otherwise.

Clinical Tip

The delusions of delirium have an entirely different quality and resemble the experience of a nightmare, tending to be frightening and bizarre in nature. This phenomenon, coupled with visual hallucinations, and acute onset are almost always pathognomonic of delirium.

The delusions and hallucinations of major depression with psychotic features are characterized by the term *nihilistic,* originating from the Latin word *nihil* (meaning "nothing"). Depressive delusions are typically self-deprecatory in nature and characterized by a sense of nothingness, both in self-worth and value. Hence, delusions of poverty, worthlessness, and hopelessness, all with a nihilistic quality, characterize psychotic depression. Somatic delusions related to gastrointestinal functioning are also common in older adults suffering from major depression with psychotic features (e.g., the belief that one is riddled with cancer). Hallucinations, when present in psychotic depression, are of an auditory rather than visual nature and tend to convey the same self-deprecatory and accusatory tone of the delusional material. Typically, these are voices hurling insults and condemnations and demeaning the patient.

HISTORY-TAKING

Given the many years to review in a history, it is important that you not be overwhelmed by too many details and that you develop the capacity to filter relevant from irrelevant material. Otherwise, a history of 80 or 90 years could potentially overwhelm you and even discourage you from becoming involved in the assessment of the older adult. Consequently, focusing on major events and patterns of behavior is vital if you are to assess an older adult in a timely and clear manner.

Understanding the early development of an 85-year-old person does not require detailed attention to the age at which that person first began talking or walking or developed bladder and bowel control. Rather, you need to know whether there was more or less a normal developmental course and whether there were major disruptions to development in the form of early trauma or losses, such as the death of a parent or divorce. Patterns of adjustment to school, social relationships, intimate relationships, occupation, retirement, bereavement, and disability need to be incorporated in a fashion that gives you a concise synthesis rather than a detailed and over-inclusive history. All too often, a sexual history may be omitted because of embarrassment related to asking the relevant questions. Changes in sexual function and activity can provide helpful cues about the emergence of mood and degenerative brain disorders.

You need to pay particular attention to the medical history, again highlighting major illnesses, operations, and any previous history of head injury. Moreover, a detailed description of current or recent drugs used, especially when there have been recent changes, is vital to the assessment of the older adult.

The age at onset of symptoms is also a very important variable in assessing not just the clinical course but also the role of familial or genetic vulnerability. Early-onset symptoms tend to be more genetically determined and reveal a constitutional vulnerability that is more severe than a late age of onset of mental disorder, where medical and neurobiological factors (especially drugs) may play a more important role and, therefore, may have implications for investigation and further assessment.

3Ds REVISITED

Table 21-2 identifies the way in which history-taking can help to differentiate the 3Ds: dementia, delirium, and depression. First, the onset of the history of present illness is in itself most revealing. Typically, dementing illnesses have an insidious, chronic course prior to the time of assessment. This is often in the order of years' or at least 6 months' duration, as opposed to the onset of a delirium, which in most cases is acute. In delirium, changes in mental state—be they cognitive or psychotic in nature—are in the order of 24 to 48 hours in duration before coming to clinical attention. Finally, major depression has an onset of symptoms that are subacute, in the order of weeks to months. Thus, simply knowing the timeline of the presenting symptoms can go a long way to help to differentiate the 3Ds from one another.

The longitudinal course of the illness is also helpful in differential diagnosis. Dementias, by their nature, are degenerative conditions, and a progressive cognitive decline over a long period of time would be confirmatory of

Table 21-2. Differentiating the 3Ds in the Assessment of an Older Adult

	Dementia	Delirium	Depression
Onset	Insidious	Acute	Subacute
Course	Progressive	Increased mortality	Recovery/recurrence
Medical status	Variable	Acute illness drug toxicity	Rule out medical illness
Family history	10% familial dementia	Negative	Mood disorder, substance abuse

have a familial incidence, but only in about 10% of cases, and these tend to be early-onset Alzheimer cases.

Clinical Tip

If the presenting picture is that of a depressive condition, a strong family history of dementia should raise suspicions that the depression may be the forerunner of an eventual dementing illness.

---

this syndrome. The course of delirium is very different. Many delirious patients do make a full recovery; however, there is a very high mortality associated with delirious episodes, particularly those that occur in the hospital setting. Recent evidence also suggests that there is a higher incidence of progressive irreversible dementia following delirium compared with age-matched control subjects.

The clinical course of depression is usually characterized, as it is in younger adults, by recovery and recurrence, with periods of relatively good functioning in between. However, you must also be prepared to deal with chronic unremitting depression in older adults.

A medical history is also helpful in differential diagnosis. In dementia, the medical status is extremely variable, including severely ill, frail, bed-ridden persons as well as those who are perfectly healthy, robust, and independent from a physical perspective. With delirium, on the other hand, an acute systemic illness has overwhelmed the central nervous system, and it behooves you as a clinician to refer any patient suffering from delirium to a medical practitioner. However, careful attention to drug toxicity is an important aspect of the assessment of delirium. Psychotropic agents, particularly those with anticholinergic properties, are often implicated. Finally, in major depression, inquiry about medical illness is also an important component of the assessment. Typically, a major depression is not necessarily associated with an underlying systemic illness. However, a refractory depression raises the index of suspicion and should lead you to increased efforts to rule out an underlying systemic medical illness, especially carcinoma.

Even in older adults, family history is especially helpful in the diagnosis of a mood disorder. Like mood disorders in younger adults, major depression still carries with it a significant familial or genetic vulnerability. Although this is less so in the late-onset depressions of older adults, you still need to make a careful inquiry into the family history of mood disorder or substance abuse. On the other hand, dementias also

COGNITIVE ASSESSMENT

Before beginning a discussion of the cognitive assessment, it is important to highlight the fact that cognitive screening alone is never diagnostic. There is no cognitive screening measure that is an "Alzheimer test." Consequently, the cognitive assessment must always be integrated with the history and investigations to establish a diagnosis. Nonetheless, the cognitive assessment is a vital part of the overall assessment of *all* older adults, given the prevalence of dementia and other neuropsychiatric conditions. These include focal lesions due to cerebrovascular disease, toxicity associated with many drugs, and even cognitive impairment that is associated with major depressive illness, which tends to be primarily of an attentional and motivational nature. Cognitive assessment can also determine whether the impairment is diffuse or focal, and whether it involves only amnestic functions or simply frontal/executive functions. Finally, the severity of impairment is also determined by formal cognitive assessment, and this is particularly important in monitoring change over time, as current neuroimaging and laboratory investigations are not able to monitor or assess cognition.

Because dementia is such a prevalent and important aspect of the psychiatric assessment of older adults, its early detection is important for a number of reasons. The first is to provide an explanation for the patient and his family for changes in intellectual functioning, behavior, or other aspects of mental status. Second, the early detection and diagnosis of dementia allow for planning financial affairs and other aspects of a patient's life while he is still legally capable of doing so. Third, the establishment of a diagnosis of dementia alerts clinicians and families to the increased risks for delirium, particularly in relation to driving. Finally, from a clinical perspective, the development of medications known as cognitive enhancers in recent years makes the diagnosis of dementia and the initiation of a clinical trial important in affecting the clinical course of the illness.

Two of the major obstacles to effective cognitive screening are the discomfort felt by the clinician posing the questions and the actual potential of the questions to offend patients by virtue of their threatening or embarrassing qualities. Consequently, the entrée or segue into the formal cognitive assessment is an important clinical skill that calls for a sensitive approach to the patient.

Clinical Tip

BEGINNING THE FORMAL COGNITIVE ASSESSMENT

Our recommendation is to seize on any point in the interview in which the patient spontaneously refers to memory impairment or subjective concerns about cognition. This is a good opportunity to follow up with the patient's own concern: *"In light of the concerns that you seem to have about your memory, perhaps I could follow that up with some questions that may allow me to determine how your memory is today."*

Otherwise, at a certain point you can simply move into the cognitive assessment by telling the patient that it is important for you to assess "concentration and memory." By adding the word *concentration,* it tends to diffuse the angst around the testing of memory. Avoid the use of words like *test* and replace them with terms like *assessment.*

MINI-MENTAL STATE EXAMINATION, OR "THE FOLSTEIN"

Although imperfect and featuring the deficiencies described below, the mini-mental status examination (MMSE) has emerged as the most widely used cognitive screening instrument in the world.[5] It has become the lingua franca of cognitive assessment. Consequently, when you want to communicate in short-hand the cognitive status or severity of cognitive impairment, you often do this simply by relating the score of the MMSE out of a maximum of 30. A mild cognitive impairment score ranges from 20 to 30, moderate impairment from 10 to 20, and severe impairment less than 10. The MMSE is heavily weighted toward tests of orientation, short-term memory, and language, with only one visuospatial test (the intersecting pentagons). MMSE headings include orientation, registration, attention and calculation, recall, and language. The MMSE does have a number of limitations, not the least of which is the amount of time required for administration. It takes usually about 10 minutes to administer, which consumes a significant amount of assessment time. Nonetheless, because of its widespread use, popularity, and communication value, we recommend that all psychiatric assessments of older adults include an MMSE.

You should be cognizant that education and language are significant factors that influence the score on the MMSE. There is a clear effect of extreme age, education, and language on the MMSE score. The average 90-year-old will do worse than the average 80-year-old on the MMSE, and this must be factored into the interpretation of scores. Those with education levels less than 6 years will also be affected and may reveal false-positive scores. Conversely, highly educated and intelligent persons may score 29 or 30 on the MMSE and yet suffer from a clinically significant dementia as elicited by history from caregivers and family members. The MMSE also has limited sensitivity to change.

Clinical Tip

Perhaps the most glaring deficit of the MMSE is the fact that it does not test frontal lobe or executive functions. Consequently, the cognitive assessment of the older adult, in addition to the MMSE, must include specific frontal lobe and executive testing.

Clinical Tip

CHECK FOR TONGUE IN CHEEK

A little-known complication of the Mini-Mental State Examination relates to the significant public health problem of orthopedic injuries resulting from the MMSE. Marshal Folstein, the originator of the MMSE, seems to be unaware of the potential impact of the "three-stage command." The direction to "take a piece of paper in your hand, fold it in half, and place it on the floor" reveals the potential for aggravation of back problems that could result from this apparently innocuous instruction (Figure 21-1).

Notwithstanding the widespread use of the MMSE, it is worthwhile thinking about the qualities of an ideal cognitive screening test. We would suggest the following properties that should be sought as more screening tests appear in the literature: (1) it should be quick, well tolerated, and easy to administer and score; (2) it should be relatively independent of culture, language, and education; and (3) it should possess appropriate psychometric properties, including inter-rater reliability, test-retest reliability, a good balance of sensitivity and specificity, and a high level of predictive validity. One such popular screen is the clock drawing test.[6] In this test, a pre-drawn circle (approximately 10 cm in diameter) is placed before the patient with the following instruction: "This is a clock face. Please fill in the numbers and then set the time to 10 past 11."

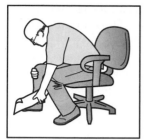

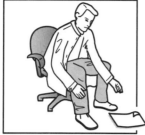

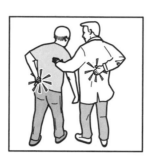

FIGURE 21-1 *Possible injuries incurred during the MMSE. (Reprinted with permission from Shulman K, Feinstein A:* Quick cognitive screening for clinicians, *New York, 2003, John Wiley & Sons.)*

Clinical Tip

CLOCK-DRAWING TEST INSTRUCTIONS

This verbatim instruction is necessary to avoid the word *hands*. Using the word *hands* may give the patient a clue when abstract ability is impaired and may mask such impairment. Clock-drawing is a useful cognitive screen because it casts a very wide net in terms of the cognitive functions necessary to complete the task. These brain functions include comprehension, abstract thinking, planning, visual memory, visuospatial ability, motivation, and concentration. It also includes an important frontal lobe function, the ability to inhibit the stimulus to point the hand to the number 10 when given the instruction "10 past 11."

Clock scoring has always been a problematic issue because of the complexity of evaluating the multiple components of a clock. As research has progressed, it seems apparent that the simpler the scoring system the better. A recent four-point scoring system recommends that 0 be applied to an intact clock, 1 to mild impairment, 2 to moderate impairment, and 3 to severe impairment (Figure 21-2).

A very brief screen that combines the clock-drawing test with a three-word recall test is known as the Mini-Cog.[7] It demonstrates good psychometric properties in screening for dementia by use of an algorithm (Figure 21-3).

Qualitative errors can also be assessed in the clock-drawing test by observing for perseverative responses, where numbers are repeated, and poor planning, which results in numbers being poorly spaced around the circle. Concrete and conceptual deficits are also easily elicited by the clock-drawing test. Like all mental status examinations, the clock-drawing test represents an opportunity to monitor change over time with a simple visual document.

ASSESSMENT OF FRONTAL LOBE/EXECUTIVE IMPAIRMENT

The frontal lobes oversee a number of important functions that include concentration and attention, verbal fluency, and abstract ability, as well as insight and judgment. The clock-drawing test does allow for the elicitation of

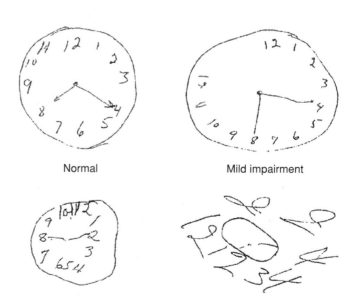

Normal   Mild impairment

Moderate impairment   Severe impairment

FIGURE 21-2 *Consortium to Establish a Registry for Alzheimer's Disease (CERAD) scoring for clock-drawing test. (Reprinted with permission from Shulman K, Feinstein A:* Quick cognitive screening for clinicians, *New York, 2003, John Wiley & Sons.)*

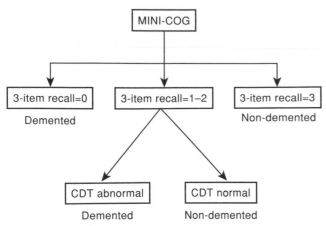

FIGURE 21-3 *Mini-Cog screening tool for dementia. (Reprinted with permission from Shulman K, Feinstein A:* Quick cognitive screening for clinicians, *New York, 2003, John Wiley & Sons.)*

frontal lobe/executive impairment through its wide cognitive net. However, other more specific tests are also appropriate and easily incorporated into a cognitive screen. In particular, word fluency has proved to be a valid and reliable method. We use a *phonemic* prime such as the letter *F* with the instruction: *"List as many words as you can that begin with the letter* F *in the next minute."* (A native English speaker with high school education should be able to generate approximately 14 words.)

Clinical Tip

Patients with frontal lobe/executive impairment characterized by disinhibition will often blurt out a common swear word beginning with *F* as the first reaction to such a direction. We hasten to add that this is not a diagnostic symptom because many false positives are found within the general population.

The second component of word fluency includes a *semantic* prime: *"Name as many four-legged animals as you can in the next minute."* As a general rule, patients with Alzheimer's disease with mainly parietal/temporal impairment will have more difficulty with the semantic prime, whereas patients with primarily frontal lobe/executive dysfunction may have more difficulty with the phonemic prime. (Similar to *F* words, an average of 14 words is expected.)

Perseveration is often assessed by tasks that require shifts of mental set. This can be tested by the alternate sequence diagram of three multiple loops and asking the patient to copy such loops and then continue the pattern across the page. Patients with perseverative responses add extra loops to the three that are recorded. You can also have the patient copy a line of alternating triangles and rectan-

gles. Another alternate sequence test includes the "go-no-go" sequence. In this test, the examiner taps twice and asks the patient to tap once, then asks the patient to tap twice when the examiner taps once. Using random tapping of one or two taps allows the determination of whether the patient can adjust and switch sets accordingly, or if the patient lapses into a perseverative response by mimicking the number of taps the examiner makes.

Abstract ability is best tested by questioning similarities such as, *"How are an orange and apple alike?" "What is similar about a bus and an airplane?" "What is similar about a table and a chair?" "What is similar about a sculpture and a painting?"*

A variant of the clock-drawing test is designed to detect frontal lobe/executive impairment specifically. This is known as the CLOX test.[8] It involves a first component (CLOX 1) in which the patient is asked to draw a free-hand clock in response to a command. If the patient is unable to do this or cannot do it accurately, he is then asked to copy a drawing of a completed clock (CLOX 2). In the case where CLOX 1 is impaired but CLOX 2 is intact—that is, the copying ability is retained—there is evidence to suggest that this is a specific measure of frontal lobe/executive impairment (Figure 21-4).

A variation on the cognitive tests described previously can be completed in a timely fashion and can provide valuable information for the assessor of older adults.

CAPACITY ASSESSMENTS

Although it is beyond the scope of this chapter to go into medicolegal detail, psychiatric assessments of older adults often involve capacity assessments. This may apply to such basic issues such as the capacity to consent to treatment, the capacity to consent to long-term care, or the capacity to give instructions for power of attorney for property or personal care. It may also include more complex capacities such as financial and driving capacity. In all of these assessments, the general cognitive screen is relevant insofar as it gives a general indication of the global functioning of an older adult. However, all capacities are task specific and are governed by the following principles: (1) understanding of relevant facts; and (2) appreciation of the consequences of taking or not taking a specific action. In older adults, however, these types of assessments are very common and, in addition to the cognitive screen and the specific questions that are relevant to each task, one must always include related and valuable information from key informants and caregivers. Careful documentation should be made of cognitive status, responses to specific questions, and the detailed probing of rationale for decisions, with the aim to demonstrate the ability to appreciate

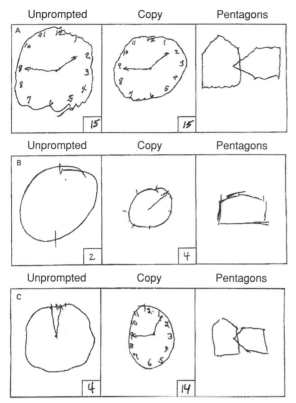

FIGURE 21-4 *CLOX test in Patients A, B, and C. (Reprinted with permission from Shulman K, Feinstein A:* Quick cognitive screening for clinicians, *New York, 2003, John Wiley & Sons.)*

consequences. This will provide for the best capacity assessment and will protect the patient from challenges to her competency.

Consider the following three clinical cases.

Case Example 1

Refractory Headaches. An 80-year-old single retired librarian presented with refractory headaches and secondary depressive symptoms. She had a history of narcotic analgesic use for the persistent headaches but without significant benefit. Relevant background history revealed that her mother had also suffered from late-onset headaches but eventually progressed to an advanced dementia and was placed in a nursing home for the last few years of her life.

The mental status examination on initial assessment revealed evidence of agitation, depressive symptomatology, and a predominant preoccupation with complaints of unremitting and intractable headaches. Despite the apparent intact cognitive presentation and no cognitive concerns expressed by the patient or her husband, an MMSE and clock-drawing test were conducted. The MMSE score on

initial assessment was 28/30, and the clock-drawing test was perfectly intact.

The patient was treated aggressively for her major depression, but, despite a wide range of pharmacological treatments and electroconvulsive therapy, it remained treatment-refractory, as did the complaints of headaches. Interestingly, while complaining bitterly of headache, the patient did not present as objectively distressed.

Detailed neuropsychological testing shortly after her initial assessment was inconclusive, although there was evidence of subtle cognitive dysfunction at that time. Her full-scale IQ was still in the average range, and the results of the dementia rating scale, one of the standardized neuropsychological instruments, were also within normal limits. However, it was of interest that she scored in the low-average range on executive tasks.

Fortunately, the standardized cognitive screening instruments provided a baseline for subsequent comparison. Figure 21-5 reveals the progression of her clock-drawing ability to the point that 3 years after the initial assessment in which she drew a perfectly normal clock, she was demonstrating severe impairment including right/left reversal and an inability to complete the task. At the same time, her MMSE score deteriorated over time from the initial score of 28/30 to 16/30 less than 3 years after the initial assessment.

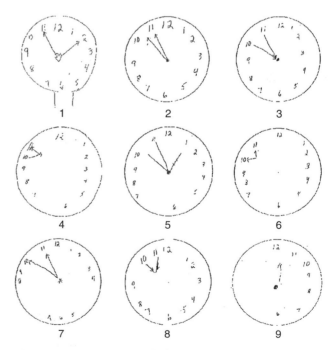

FIGURE 21-5 *Consecutive clocks drawn over a period of 3 years that show progression and fluctuation in cognition as part of a slowly developing dementia. (Reprinted with permission from Shulman K, Feinstein A:* Quick cognitive screening for clinicians, *New York, 2003, John Wiley & Sons.)*

During this time, despite the persistent headaches and depression, it was evident that the patient was developing a progressive and irreversible dementia that was proving to be identical to that of her mother.

Comment. This case once again highlights the fundamental importance of performing a cognitive screen in *all* older adults presenting for psychiatric assessment. Although initially there were no concerns about the patient's cognitive function, and indeed her screening tests were within normal limits, the family history was suggestive of a vulnerability to dementia. The ability to repeat the same standard cognitive screens elicited the clinical pattern of declining cognitive function and with time indicated more clearly the true underlying nature of this condition.

Case Example 2

Drug Toxicity. An 82-year-old retired salesman suffered a stroke causing a right-sided hemiplegia and was admitted to a rehabilitation hospital. In the immediate post-stroke period, he was observed to be emotionally labile, and his physicians treated him with the tricyclic antidepressant amitriptyline in doses that increased to 150 mg daily (recall the role of anticholinergic properties in delirium). He was maintained on this regimen at the time of the requested psychiatric consultation because of persistent lability and mood symptomatology.

At the time of initial assessment, this man showed evidence of gross cognitive impairment and marked disorientation. His MMSE score was 10/30 on initial assessment. His clock-drawing test (Figure 21-6) also showed evidence of gross disorganization, poor planning, and concrete thinking.

A provisional diagnosis of toxic delirium was made based on clinical presentation in the context of the relatively high doses of a tricyclic antidepressant. The amitriptyline was immediately discontinued, and the patient was followed up 2 and 5 weeks later. As seen in Figure 21-6, his clock-draw-

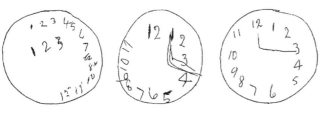

| Day one | Two weeks later | Five weeks later |

FIGURE 21-6 *Improvement to clock-drawing test after toxic delirium subsides. (Reprinted with permission from Shulman K, Feinstein A:* Quick cognitive screening for clinicians, *New York, 2003, John Wiley & Sons.)*

---

ing showed progressive improvement with better spacing, a return of symbolic representation of time by hands, and eventually a virtually normal-looking clock when he was asked to denote 3 o'clock. His MMSE score concomitantly improved from 10/30 to 22/30. He was left with mild cognitive impairment.

Comment. This case highlights the very common clinical problem of medications causing central nervous system toxicity or delirium. In this case, the *anticholinergic* effect of the antidepressant was primarily responsible. Once again, cognitive screening served to monitor change in cognitive status and helped to confirm the initial diagnosis of toxic delirium as the evidence mounted that his cognition and clinical condition were improving with the elimination of the toxic substance.

Case Example 3

Importance of the Doctor-Family Relationship and the Role of Caregivers. A 74-year-old retired truck driver was referred for assessment by a neurologist who had been treating his wife for a particularly aggressive form of Alzheimer's disease. Her behavior and severe impairment made it very difficult for him to manage his wife at home, and he sought help from the local social service agencies. Despite several attempts at providing in-house support and eventual admissions to hospital, this gentleman continued to have difficulty accepting the dramatic change in his wife's clinical condition. The disruption in their long-standing and happy marital relationship was extremely painful for him. This loss was a great stressor for him, and over time he became increasingly despondent, irritable, and angry at the formal caregivers and physicians who became involved at various points in the care of his wife's dementia. Indeed, he became so emotionally unstable and frustrated by his situation that he became verbally aggressive and was sometimes perceived as threatening toward the formal caregivers. This, in turn, resulted in a reaction from the health care agencies involved with him, and he was eventually charged by the police with threatening behavior and had to appear in court.

Fortunately, the judge was able to recognize the extent of emotional distress in the husband, and he was referred for psychiatric assessment. This, in turn, revealed a strong family history of mood disorder and suicide in his father and paternal grandfather. One of his sons was also showing evidence of significant depressive symptoms affecting his education. On clinical examination, the caregiver/patient did indeed present with marked irritability, hopelessness, and fleeting suicidal ideation. He readily acknowledged a change in his mental state and its influence on his ability to cope as well as his behavior toward the formal caregivers who were involved with his wife and him.

Treatment with antidepressants over a period of a few weeks and modified cognitive behavioral therapy resulted in a dramatic change in his mood state. He was much more realistic and was able to put into perspective the events that had transpired in the past year, including the dramatic change in his wife and his need to regroup and adjust to the reality of his wife's situation.

Comment. This is a classic example of the necessity of addressing the identified patient and the caregiver as an inextricable dyad. In this case, the irritability and anger that manifested themselves in association with his wife's progressive dementia were a reflection of a developing major depression, which in turn was related to the familial/genetic vulnerability that was elicited by history during the formal psychiatric assessment. Irritability and anger may very well be the predominant symptoms of a depressive illness at any age.

SUMMARY

The assessment of older adults need not be a daunting or overwhelming challenge for clinicians. A clear systematic approach to history-taking and mental status examination will commonly allow for an accurate provisional diagnosis. Special expertise in cognitive assessment is necessary, as is the retention of basic medical knowledge with particular attention to the role of medications. Even with these clinical skills, you must function in a health care system that is adequate and flexible enough to address the complex and multifaceted needs of older adults and their caregivers.

REFERENCES

1. Silver I, Herrmann N: History and mental status examination. In Sadavoy J, Jarvik L, Grossberg G, Meyers B, editors: *Comprehensive textbook of geriatric psychiatry*, ed 3, New York, 2004, WW Norton, pp 253–280.
2. Jorm AF, Jacomb PA: The Informant Questionnaire on Cognitive Decline in the Elderly (IQCODE): sociodemographic correlates, reliability, validity and some norms, *Psychol Med* 19:1015–1022, 1989.
3. Mackinnon A, Mulligan R: Combining cognitive testing and informant report to increase accuracy in screening for dementia, *Am J Psychiatry* 155:1529–1535, 1998.
4. Shulman K, Feinstein A: *Quick cognitive screening for clinicians*, New York, 2003, John Wiley & Sons.
5. Folstein MF, Folstein SE, McHugh PR: Mini-Mental State: a practical method for grading the cognitive state of patients for the clinician, *J Psychiatr Res* 12:189–198, 1975.
6. Shulman KI: Clock-drawing: is it the ideal cognitive screening test? *Int J Geriatr Psychiatry* 15:548 561, 2000.
7. Borson S, Scanlan J, Brush M, et al: The Mini-Cog: a cognitive "vital signs" measure for dementia screening in multi-lingual elderly, *Int J Ger Psychiatry* 15:1021–1027, 2000.
8. Royall DR, Cordes JA, Polk M: CLOX: an executive clock drawing task, *J Neurol Neurosurg Psychiatry* 64:588–594, 1998.

22

Family Assessment

Gabor I. Keitner, Christine E. Ryan, and Nathan B. Epstein

INTRODUCTION

Family members can be a valuable resource in obtaining detailed information about the patient and his family life and in providing different perspectives on the presenting problems, range of symptoms, and the patient's course of illness. Understanding the patient's family functioning may provide important information on how the family can help or hinder the patient's recovery from an illness episode or manage a chronic illness.

For example, research has shown several areas in which the family may influence the patient: helping with medication and treatment compliance, keeping track of medication side effects and prodromal and residual symptoms, providing social support and encouragement, sharing responsibilities, and lessening patient anxieties. Families can help patients remain positive, can help them deal with illness conditions, and can facilitate/encourage communication between providers. Conversely, families might hinder a patient's progress by directly or indirectly putting pressure on the patient to get better and "pull himself together," particularly if the patient's illness causes a financial burden by a lengthy hospital stay or time away from work. Resentment toward the patient may surface as family members pinch-hit for the ill member. Critical, hostile, or overinvolved family members can influence hospitalization or relapse rates for patients with a number of psychiatric illnesses. Fear and anxiety on the part of a family member may exacerbate the patient's unease, and this may lead to the patient's deciding to stop taking the medication. Finally, the quality of the marital and sexual relationship may affect, and be affected by, the patient's illness.[1,2]

Assessing the family's functioning can help to inform treatment options. Conducting an in-depth assessment of the family can be viewed as a checklist of the family's functioning, similar to how you obtain a mental status checklist for a patient before recommending treatment. Like a mental status checklist, a comprehensive family assessment should be focused and systematic. The comprehensive assessment of a family as presented here is based on the McMaster approach to evaluating and treating families and derives from the McMaster Model of Family Functioning (MMFF),[3] one of the most developed and validated family treatment approaches in the field. The assessment is one component of working with and understanding families. The family assessment provides an in-depth, systematic evaluation on six fundamental aspects of family life: problem solving, communication, roles, affective responsiveness, affective involvement, and behavior control. Although this list is not exhaustive, it includes basic areas of family life that affect a family's functioning. To get comfortable with this assessment, you should become acquainted with other aspects of the McMaster approach to working with families.[4,5]

Briefly, *problem solving* is a gauge of the family's ability to work out difficulties to a level that maintains effective family functioning. *Communication* refers to how a family exchanges information. *Roles* include the repetitive patterns by which individual family members fulfill family functions. *Affective responsiveness* is defined as the ability to respond to stimuli with a range of feelings, and *affective involvement* is a measure of the degree to which family members show interest in and value the activities of other family members. *Behavior control* is the pattern a family adopts in handling three types of situations: those that are physically dangerous, those meeting psychobiological needs and drives, and those involving socializing behavior within and outside the family.

To evaluate families (including the patient) on all these dimensions without overburdening either you or the family, you need to be focused, clear about what questions to ask (and why), and able to keep the interview moving at a comfortable pace. By using a framework such as the McMaster approach, you will be able to engage all family members and obtain complete information about the family's functioning. Following established guidelines has added benefits, especially for an inexperienced clinician or a seasoned therapist who is learning to incorporate a family assessment into her overall evaluation.

BEFORE THE FAMILY ARRIVES

Patient Issues

To optimize an understanding of the patient's issues, you will gather information from the referral source, which may include documentation from a medical chart or a brief discussion with a referring clinician. At a minimum, you will need to know the reason for the referral and the purpose of the family assessment. Although the method of assessing the family will not change if the goal is to provide a consultation or a second opinion, you will need to be clear with the patient and family members concerning the nature of the meeting because a comprehensive, thorough family assessment often is used to initiate the treatment process and will be used to inform any treatment recommendations for the patient and/or family.[6]

Information on the patient's medical and psychiatric illness, currently used medications, family history of medical or psychiatric illness, and presence of psychosocial stressors provides important data for you to know. Although these areas will be covered in the family assessment interview, pertinent knowledge obtained before the family interview can alert you to particular areas of concern, complex issues, or apparent difficulties within the family.

Family Issues

Approaching family members to invite them in for a family assessment may differ depending on the clinical setting. In general, it is easier to get families to come in for a comprehensive family assessment meeting when a patient is hospitalized, versus obtaining an appointment for those patients who are attending an outpatient clinic. The severity and seeming urgency of an inpatient hospitalization tend to mobilize families sufficiently to overcome whatever

ambivalence or resistance they have to being seen. It seems to be easier for a family to put off making the effort to coordinate schedules to come to a family meeting if the identified patient is not in a serious crisis. Nonetheless, arranging for family meetings in either setting can take place if certain principles are kept in mind.

It is important for you to explain to the patient and the family that the purpose of the assessment is to understand the overall system in which the patient is embedded. All members of the system affect and are affected by the system. No individual can be understood without an understanding of the system in which he is embedded. The assessment is used to gain a better understanding of how everybody sees the problem at hand, to gather information to allow for a more comprehensive treatment plan, to provide an opportunity for all members involved in trying to cope with the situation to ask questions of you, and to solicit the help of all involved in setting up a meaningful treatment plan. It is important to get across the message that the aim of the meeting is not to try to find a source of blame for the patient's problems. Many family members have had unpleasant experiences with therapists who, in their attempts to try to arrive at an understandable "cause" for the patient's illness, have too readily identified some dynamic issue in the family as that cause. There has been an unfortunate tendency in the family therapy field to confuse correlation with causality. In addition, it is often unclear whether dysfunctional family patterns that are apparent on evaluation are the antecedents or the consequences of a patient's clinical presentation.

Key Point:

Don't blame the family for the patient's problems. One of the most valuable results of a family evaluation is obtaining the perspectives of many family members. Rather than assigning blame, the assessment is useful for pinpointing areas of family dysfunction that may be amenable to change.

It is helpful for you to explain to the patient and family members that a family assessment is a standard part of your treatment approach and that the family is not being singled out because of an assumption about their particular family difficulties. It may also be worth noting that understanding the social environment of the patient usually helps to determine the most helpful treatment course. Without understanding all the relevant circumstances surrounding the patient and family that a family assessment provides, suboptimal treatment may result.

You should keep in mind that patients often assume that family members are not interested, willing, or able to come to a family meeting. This may reflect their misperceptions about their families' investment and motivation in their care and/or patients' ambivalence about having family members attend; it may also represent mood-congruent cognitive distortions. Do not take this at face value! In such cases, it is often helpful for you to contact the family members directly (with the patient's permission) to extend the invitation to the family members directly. More often than not, the patient's assumptions about lack of caring by family members is erroneous and reflects her own ambivalence about reaching out to significant others for help.

As a rule, it is useful to have as many family members and significant others in the patient's social field to come for an initial assessment as possible. In addition to the most immediate family members living with the patient, it is often helpful to meet with others who are significantly involved in the patient's life. These could involve extended family members, good friends, employers, mental health care providers, and spiritual counselors. The goal of the initial family assessment is to obtain a clear understanding of the range of problems and strengths within the family and the extent of resources that are available to deal with the problems. You and the patient invite all those deemed appropriate to meet this goal, and this may involve 2 to 10 persons, at least, at the first session. Subsequent assessments or therapy sessions can be reduced to various subgroups, but initial assessment sessions are more productive in clarifying the problems at hand if they are more inclusive.

> **Key Point:**
>
> Meet with as many family members as possible. One reason to be more inclusive is that you do not know in advance who will be the most helpful in understanding what the family problems are.

To manage the range and number of people who may be present at such an evaluation, it is important that you have a clear idea of the goals of the assessment. As outlined in greater detail below, the primary goal of such an assessment is to obtain a clear perspective of how the various family members view their problems that in their mind relates to the patient's presentation of symptoms. One of your major tasks in the assessment process is to ensure that *all* parties have an appropriate opportunity to present their view of the problems. The challenge is to provide such an opportunity to all family members without allowing any of them to dominate the discussion. For example, you can stop the person when you have a clear sense of what she is saying and summarize her point. Then, ask for her feedback on its correctness, and move on to the next question (or the next family member). It is important for you to have as few preconceived notions of what goes on in the family as possible. Beginning therapists tend to identify with their

patients' view of reality, which often is at odds with the view of many others. Sometimes, inexperienced therapists jump on the first problem presented and spend too much time on it without finding out about other family problems. The goal of the family assessment is to broaden such perspectives to reflect more accurately the world that the patient lives in and to help patient and family members to arrive at a consensus.

> **Key Point:**
>
> Don't identify with the patient's perspective. Your role is to understand the whole system. Often, you will learn new information from family members that modifies what the patient has initially reported. In fact, one of the reasons to obtain a family assessment is to learn other perspectives from those close to the patient.

The age range of family members invited to the initial family assessment ranges widely. There is no age at which a family member should be excluded from such a meeting. The presence of infants and young children adds to the assessments of families, both in terms of what children present with their own perspectives and in terms of observing the behaviors of these children, as well as the ways in which family members deal with them. Some patients become very protective about the notion that their young children might be adversely affected by the revelation of potential problems in the family environment and try to exclude children from attending these meetings. In fact, the opposite is often the case. It is rare that children in conflicted families are not aware of such conflicts. The lack of resolution of such conflicts creates a greater burden for children than the opportunity for resolution of such conflicts presented by family meetings. Children are often reassured by the reality of seeing their family problems being managed in a professional environment.

CONDUCTING THE FAMILY ASSESSMENT

You have three main goals when conducting a family assessment. First, you orient the family to the interview process and establish an open and collaborative relationship with the family and any additional guests. Second, you and family members (and guests) identify all current problems in the family, including the problem that precipitated the meeting. Third, you identify the family dynamic patterns that seem to be related to the family's functioning. You should keep in mind that dynamic patterns may be causal or correlational. Specific issues that you describe are presented to the family so that they can verify the accuracy of the information, accept the formulation of the problem, or amend it as needed.

The amount of time taken to assess the family, as well as the number of assessment sessions, will vary according to your level of experience and the nature of the family's problems. Although therapists are expected to take longer when first learning to conduct a family assessment, they soon become familiar with the process, and the interview becomes a natural part of their assessment. A useful analogy of the family assessment (i.e., family checklist) is a mental status checklist. Although a thorough assessment may initially seem time consuming, it will ultimately result in a careful delineation of family issues and highlight both family strengths and family deficits.

Basic information of the family assessment is obtained from family member reporting. Use observation of behavior throughout the family interview session to form impressions of the family's functioning. During the session, identify and clarify any contradictions between stated information and observed behavior, and between contradictory information taken from different family members. Remain respectful of family members when trying to reconcile differing perspectives on an issue. Offer an impression based on the information received, and elicit corrections or agreement from all family members before proceeding to the next topic in the assessment.

The family interview consists of four identifiable components: orientation, data gathering, problem description, and problem clarification.

Orientation

In the first step of the family interview, you will ask each family member why he thinks he is in the family session, what he thinks will happen during the session, what he hopes will come out of it. It is important to ask these questions of every person who is in the session. The family soon learns that every member will get a chance to talk and that each person's opinion will be considered. Furthermore, it becomes clear that family members may have different yet valid perspectives on the same topic of concern. Finally, family members learn to listen to what others are saying.

After all persons have responded, summarize the ideas put forth by the family members, and then provide your own ideas about why the family is there. In the summary, note facts about the family in general, state what you hope to achieve in the assessment session, and identify what you plan to do in the session. Before proceeding, explain the rationale for seeing the entire family. You can take this opportunity to explain that the way a family functions has an influence on a person's behavior, and that how a person behaves can affect the way a family functions. Serious events that affect one family member will affect the family

and the way it operates. For these reasons, it is important that you understand the family. To understand the family, you should go on to explain, you will be asking questions of each family member on a variety of issues—but all will be related to the way they function as a family. From time to time, summarize what you have learned and ask for input and corrections from family members. At any point, individual family members can ask questions of you. If there are no questions at this point, you can ask if it is alright to proceed with the assessment. Do not continue unless all persons have agreed.

Data Gathering

In this step of the family interview, data are gathered about the presenting problem, the family's overall functioning, additional investigations (if needed), and other problems.

During the data-gathering step, you will ask family members what *they* think are the problems in the family. This helps to get them focused on the issues, gives them an outlet to express their feelings, and creates an atmosphere for listening and discussing. In this section, we pose several questions to ask the family. The questions are meant as suggestions for understanding the family system and not as a list in which every question needs to be asked.

Presenting Problem(s)

You begin by asking the family to describe the problem that brought them to seek help. You should spend enough time in gathering the data so that you have an accurate picture of the nature and history of the problem. This includes exploring the factual details of the problem, the affective components, historical perspective, precipitating events, who is mainly involved in the problem, and how.

An example of a presenting problem is the following: John's teacher calls to discuss problems he is having at school. The call, what the teacher said, the mother's observation of John's withdrawal and increased disobedience are factual details. The mother's reaction of frustration, the father's anger at John and his wife for not disciplining him, and John's feeling of guilt are affective components. Information that the problem began 6 months ago, seemed to improve for a while, and then worsened are historical components; the father's change in jobs is a precipitating event; and John's entering adolescence is a developmental issue.

When the family describes the presenting problem, you would use the appropriate dimensions of the McMaster approach to frame the issues. In the presenting problem noted above, you would explore how the family attempted to solve the difficulty (problem solving), how they talked with each other about it (communication), and what behavioral issues were involved (behavior control). Other issues may arise when you explore the presenting problem. For example, the mother may feel that the father does not support her efforts in disciplining any of the children; the father may feel no understanding about his work situation; the son may notice the conflict between his parents, feel neglected, and act out.

You would then summarize your understanding of the problem as presented by the family, ask for corrections from each person, and make sure everyone is in agreement about the problem(s): John has become more difficult to manage in the past 6 months; the mother does not feel support from the father; the father is frustrated about his job change and lack of understanding from his wife, contributing to his overall sense of failure. Both parents are not able to solve the problems and have difficulty in talking to each other, increasing the tension between them and making them both unhappy. These problems did not seem to exist before the father's job change, suggesting that may be the major stressor.

Overall Family Functioning

Once an assessment of the presenting problem is completed, you move to the next step, assessing the family's functioning. First, you should let the family know that you will change the focus to ask questions about how they generally operate as a family.

You will assess the family on the six dimensions of the MMFF: problem solving, communication, roles, affective responsiveness, affective involvement, and behavior control. The assessment focuses on delineating family strengths and weaknesses in each area. The important point in this step is to evaluate aspects of the family's overall functioning and avoid formulating conclusions based only on data obtained from the presenting problem, which is more likely to be negative. As you go through each dimension, you explain what you are doing (*"Now, I would like to discuss how you deal with problems in general," ". . . how you talk with each other," ". . . some of your feelings," ". . . rules you have in the family,"*) and help the family discuss each area in an open, direct manner. After each family dimension is discussed, give the family an understanding of their strengths and shortcomings before moving on the next area of family functioning. In each case, emphasize family strengths and ask whether your impression is accurate.

Problem Solving

To explore problem solving, ask the family to identify a few problems that have occurred in the last couple of weeks and discuss problems that were solved and problems they had difficulty with. Ask each person about her reactions to the problems, when she was upset, and attempts made to resolve the problem. The following questions are a guide for understanding how the family negotiates the six steps of problem solving.

1. Problem identification: *"When the problem arose, what did you think was going on? Did you think anything else was involved? Did you all see the problem in the same way? Who first noticed the problem?"*

2. Communication to appropriate resource: *"When you first noticed the problem, whom did you tell? When did you tell? Did others notice the problem but not say anything? What stopped you from saying something?"*

3. Consider alternatives: *"What did you think of doing about the problem? Who thought of the plan? Did other people have ideas? Did you share your ideas?"*

4. Decision and action: *"How did you decide what to do? Who decided?"*

5. Monitor the action: *"When you decided on the action, did you follow through? Who did what? Do you usually check to see that things get done? Who usually checks?"*

6. Evaluate the process: *"How did you do with that problem? Do you usually discuss what you did as a family?"*

Finally, you should ask a few summary questions, such as, *"Is this the way you usually handle problems? What is different? In general, what do you think makes it hard for you to handle problems as a family?"* When exploring problem solving, it is important to understand how the family deals with instrumental as well as affective issues surrounding the problem. Instrumental issues refer to day-to-day practical issues such as making a decision about a purchase, fixing something that is broken, and arranging transportation to after-school activities. Affective issues deal with emotions. Once you have an understanding of the family's problem-solving abilities, you can move on to another area of family functioning. The fewer number of unresolved problems in the family and the more steps taken in the problem-solving process, the healthier is the family's functioning. If family members differ widely in how they tend to resolve their problems, you should determine which areas cause the most difficulty. As the family accomplishes fewer problem-solving steps and denies or mislabels the problem, they move toward the unhealthy end of the spectrum. Research indicates that families that are most disturbed consistently deny or mislabel problems and have long-standing unresolved problems, and the problems create conflict and dissension in the family.

Communication

To assess communication within the family, you will observe communication patterns during the assessment process and stimulate discussion among family members to produce observable behavior. You should explore the nature and the extent of communication in the family along two continua—clarity-masked and direct-indirect—to evaluate the family's functioning in this area. *Clarity* refers to information being transmitted in a relevant, clear, concise, and consistent manner. *Masked* communication may be vague, indirect, muddied, or unclear. *Directness* refers to the verbal (or nonverbal) message being given to the intended receiver. Communication may be *indirect* when the message is given to an inappropriate person or directed to no one in particular.

Questions to examine the nature and extent of communication might include the following: *"Do people in this family talk with each other? Who does most of the talking?"* For each person the therapist asks, *"With whom do you talk? How often? Do you feel free to say things?"* Other questions probe the clarity and directness of communication.

1. Clarity/masked continuum: *"What is she telling you? How did John let you know that? Do you feel that you can get your ideas across to others in the family?"*

2. Direct/indirect continuum: *"How do you let your dad know how you are feeling? Do you talk to your brother directly? To whom do you talk?"*

When you assess the family's overall functioning, you should give more weight to the parents' (rather than the children's) communication pattern. If the level of communication is low and if a greater number of family members display low levels of communication, then the family's level of communication is considered poor. Healthy families communicate clearly and directly in instrumental and affective areas of communication. Families move toward the unhealthy end of the spectrum when the communication is less clear and direct and when affective communication is distorted. Communication of families at the very disturbed end of the dimension is consistently masked and indirect in both instrumental and affective areas.

Roles

To assess a family's role functioning, you will consider two types of functions (i.e., necessary and other) and two areas of functioning (i.e., instrumental and affective). *Necessary* role functions that are *instrumental* include provision of resources, whereas *affective* role functions are nurturance, support, and adult sexual gratification. Other role functions may include social or cultural, such as maintaining relationships with extended family and friends. Life skills development and systems maintenance compose both instrumental and affective areas of functioning. The following lists examples of questions used in these areas.

1. Provision of resources: *"Who brings in the money? Are there separate bank accounts? Who gets the groceries and prepares meals? Is it always the same person? Do you have a car? How do you get to work, school, and other activities?"*

2. Nurturance and support: *"To whom do you go when you need someone to talk to? Is it helpful?"* If there are small children, you should ask which parent usually comforts the child. How do the parents divide their availability to the children?

3. Adult sexual gratification: You should ask these questions when the parents are alone or when the children are extremely young. Older children can be asked to leave the session for a short time so that you and their parents can discuss a few adult issues, or the questions can be asked at the end of the session after excusing the children from the room. Before the children leave the room, you should assure them that they will not be discussed and no plans will be made unless they are present. Single parents are also asked how they meet their sexual needs. *"How do you feel about the affectionate and sexual aspects of your relationship? Are you satisfied with all aspects of your sexual life? Do you feel that you satisfy your partner? Can you easily say `no' to your partner?"*

4. Life skills development: *"Who usually sees what's happening with the children's education? Who helps with homework? How do you handle stages that the children go through? Who's responsible for teaching manners? Sex education? Adults go through stages also . . . who is involved in discussions about job changes? How do you help each other develop?"*

5. Systems maintenance: *"Who is involved in major decision-making? Who keeps track of the health of the family? Who handles the monthly bills? Who cleans the house? How do you handle repairs to the house? The car? Who disciplines the children?"*

Two other types of questions include role allocation and role accountability.

6. Allocation: *"How do you decide who does the jobs? Do you talk about it? Do any of you feel overburdened about your jobs? Would you like the decision about jobs to be handled differently?"*

7. Accountability: *"How do you check that a job gets done? What happens if a job isn't done?"*

To assess the family's role functioning, you must consider whether the necessary functions are being fulfilled, whether family members are satisfied with the way responsibilities are shared, whether there is consensus regarding the allocation of roles, and whether the roles are appropriately assigned to family members. Also, you should determine whether there is collaboration in fulfilling the role functions, a process in the family to make sure the jobs are completed, and flexibility within the system to reassign roles as needed. A healthy family fulfills all necessary role functions, cooperates, ensures functions are fulfilled, and has some flexibility to shift role functions if necessary. Role functioning moves toward the unhealthy end of the spectrum as the family shows less and less effectiveness in accomplishing basic functions. At the most disturbed end of the spectrum, one or more basic functions are not fulfilled, and there are major problems with allocation and accountability.

Affective Responsiveness

To assess the affective responsiveness of the family, you will consider the pattern of the family's responses to affective stimuli. This dimension refers to feelings that the person experiences and focuses on the person as the locus of response. Ask each family member about his experiences (and examples) of feelings of two kinds of emotions: welfare emotions (e.g., love, affection, tenderness, support, joy, happiness) and emergency emotions (e.g., anger, depression, sadness, hurt, fear, tension, rage, hate). When assessing each, check whether the person feels he over- or under-responds in each area of emotion. Other family members may confirm or adjust the perceptions of a person's emotional response.

Some questions that will elicit information on emotional response include the following: "*What was your response to . . .? How did you feel? Do the rest of you feel like that? Do you ever sense that you don't feel emotions that you should or that others do? Are you a family that responds with a lot of feelings? Some feelings more than others? Do you feel that you under-respond? Are there feelings that you experience more intensely than you think reasonable in a particular situation?*"

Assess whether the family's affective response is appropriate in intensity and duration for a particular situation. Since there is such a large range of possible emotional responses and a variety of stimuli, you must take into account the total scope of responsiveness. At the healthy end of the spectrum, families are capable of a full range of responses with appropriate intensity and emotion. Families can be at a healthy level even if they occasionally respond with inappropriate affect or include a family member who cannot respond emotionally to the full range of affect. Families are rated at the disturbed end of the spectrum if they are extremely constricted in the range of emotions and/or are consistently inappropriate in quality or quantity of emotional response.

Affective Involvement

Next you will explore the affective involvement of the family and rate it on six identified styles: absence of involvement, involvement devoid of feelings, narcissistic involvement, empathic involvement, overinvolvement, and symbiotic involvement. You should be interested in whether family members show an appropriate amount of interest and concern for each other, the nature of their involvement, how much they give of themselves, and how they are supportive of each other.

Questions may include the following: "*Who cares about what is important to you? What activities or interests are important to you? How does the rest of the family respond to these? Are they interested? Too interested? Do you feel that others in the family don't care or notice what happens to you?*" For parent-child dyads, questions may include: "*Do you feel people in the family are overprotective or overinvolved in your life? How do you handle it? How do you get them to stop?*" For parents: "*How do you relate to each of the children? Do you listen? Do you feel that your relationship with your child is close enough?*"

You can assess different styles of affective involvement along a continuum. Families at the healthy end of the spectrum show empathic involvement and are characterized by a positive interest in each other without intruding. In descending order of effectiveness, other styles are overinvolved families, narcissistically involved families, and families devoid of feelings. The least effective and most disturbed type of involvement includes families at either pole; that is, those with lack of involvement or a symbiotic involvement.

Behavior Control

To obtain an assessment of behavior control, investigate the rules adopted by the family to handle behavior in three specific areas: physically dangerous situations, meeting psychobiological needs (e.g., eating, drinking, sleeping, sex), and socializing behavior between family members and with people outside the family. Four styles that can be conceptualized as determining standards for rules and for the range of acceptable behavior are as follows: rigid, flexible, laissez-faire, and chaotic. You can use the following set of questions to help elicit the rules for each family.

Begin by commenting that all families have rules and ways to handle behavior in certain situations, and it is helpful to know how this family's rules work. Then you can ask, "*Do you have rules for table manners, going to bed, drinking (alcohol), and bathing? Are they consistent in each area, or do they vary? Are the rules the same for everyone? Do you expect everyone in the family to eat together? How do you handle dangerous situations? Can you give an example of a dangerous situation and how you would handle it?*"

clinical relevance of demographic variables. It will leave you, at least, with an appreciation of what you need to be aware of before beginning the interview. At best, it will inspire curiosity and further reading on the issues only briefly addressed here. You will be exposed to a variety of approaches and suggestions about how to use these approaches flexibly and adaptively. Depression cannot be dismissed as a nebulous entity. With thoughtfulness and familiarity, the illness, its signs, and its symptoms can be easily grasped.

The Different Faces of Depression: What Does "Depressed" Mean?

The term *melancholia* was first used around 400 BC by Hippocrates to describe a state similar to what is now known as a major depressive episode. About 30 AD, August Cornelius Celsus described melancholia as a depression caused by black bile. In the 12th century, Moses Maimonides claimed melancholia was, in fact, a discrete disease entity. Emil Kraepelin, a 19th-century psychiatrist, played a significant role in bringing the term *depression* into common usage to replace the diagnostically nonspecific term *melancholia* (the term is now used to denote a specific subtype of depression, described later).

In its broadest use (Figure 23-1), depression is an emotion (e.g., sad/low/gloomy mood) that can be considered within the range of normal experience by virtually everyone (except that painfully optimistic 5% of individuals).

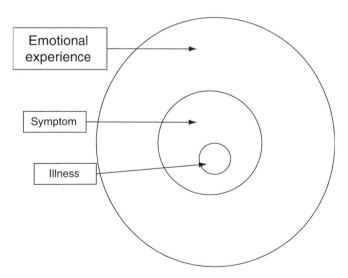

FIGURE 23-1 *Over-simplification of the many uses of the word "depression."*

This emotion is often experienced when things don't go our way: a parent or spouse doesn't show enough love, we get a poor grade on an academic test, or a job interview is unsuccessful. Less frequently, the term *depression* is used to describe a symptom of a medical illness (e.g., post-stroke or as part of anemia) or a symptom of several psychiatric illnesses (e.g., anxiety disorders, schizophrenia).

So, you wonder astutely, what is the difference between the ubiquitous emotional experience and the symptom? As a symptom, depressed mood is persistent and consistent. That is, it recurs for a number of days, and for a significant portion of those days. The anemic or anxious *or* depressed patient can feel sad for most of the day for the better part of 2 weeks. So, you again wonder astutely, what is the difference between the symptom and the illness? In its most restricted sense, depression refers to an illness that is characterized by depressed mood *along with* other symptoms. The anxious patient may well experience depressed mood, but does she lack the ability to enjoy good things when they happen? Does she constantly evaluate herself negatively? Does she think about killing herself? (If the answer to these questions is affirmative, of course, comorbid psychiatric diagnoses must be considered). The more restricted definition of depression as an illness will be referred to as Major Depression in this chapter.

So this constellation of symptoms can be clustered together in a meaningful and valid way, and can be reliably examined by different individuals and nonetheless likely be identified as the same illness. But what of individual differences, such as those that were alluded to in the cardiac comparison? The truth is that how an individual experiences major depression may be as idiosyncratic as a how people experience headaches. Some are triggered; others are not. Some vary with the time of day, with the season, or with the menstrual cycle. At times, depression seems predictable, and at other times it comes out of nowhere. Its onset can be sudden or insidious. It has the capacity to affect a number of different domains, in various combinations. It is often a chronic, recurrent illness. For some, all episodes are alike; for others there are marked differences in symptom constellations.

Key Points: Bright Metaphor

The onset of depression can take a variety of paths. Think of depression as a person's internal light turning off. For some people this happens suddenly, as when a lightbulb burns out, with no apparent warning. For others, the onset of depression is like a light being turned down with a dimmer; they can't say exactly when the process started, but they know it's been progressing steadily. For others still, the onset of depression is like a fluorescent bulb going out; their depressive

Key Points: Bright Metaphor—cont'd

symptoms sputter and cough before alleviating temporarily, only to sputter and cough again before finally persisting. The latter two presentations can delay the patient's presentation to a physician. With the dimmer scenario, the patient often thinks the process will halt on its own, or even reverse itself. He may begin to believe that depression is part of his makeup, of his personality. With the fluorescent scenario, the ominous flickering is often ignored until the bulb stops working entirely. In many cases, depressive symptoms and associated disability predate the onset of full-fledged major depression.

Subtypes of Depression: Melancholic, Atypical, Catatonic, Postpartum, Seasonal, and Others

There have been many different subtypes of major depression described over the decades. Few have withstood scientific scrutiny, and only four remain in the *Diagnostic and Statistical Manual of Mental Disorders*, Fourth Edition, Text Revision (DSM-IV-TR). Table 23-1 identifies the various subtypes and the important features of each. The first group are those that still remain in the DSM system. However, in clinical practice you will hear references made to a wider range of subtypes, so it is wise to familiarize yourself with as many as possible.

Table 23-1. Depression Subtypes

Subtype	Features
Melancholic	See DSM-IV for specific criteria. Bottom line? SEVERE depression

Atypical	Two uses of this term:
	  1. Atypical symptoms: increased weight, increased sleep
	  2. Atypical depression:
	    a) Reactive mood
	    b) Two or more of following:
	      i. Weight gain
	      ii. Hypersomnia
	      iii. Leaden paralysis
	      iv. Rejection sensitivity

Catatonic	Rare; can be considered a psychiatric emergency as patients are frequently unable to eat, drink, or communicate
Postpartum	Speaks for itself; within 4 weeks of childbirth officially
Seasonal	• Onset/remission at characteristic times of year • Seasonal episodes substantially outnumber nonseasonal episodes • Atypical symptoms (increased weight and sleep) predominate
Psychotic	• Psychosis exclusively in context of major depressive episodes • Significant treatment implications (i.e., need for antipsychotics)
Anxious	Three potential definitions: • Depression comorbid with anxiety disorder • Depression with anxiety as predominant mood • Anxious symptoms in absence of an anxiety disorder plus depressive symptoms in absence of a mood disorder; but combination results in dysfunction
Agitated (versus Retarded)	This distinction is not currently in vogue, because: • Many depressions involve combinations of both types of symptoms • No apparent impact on prognosis or therapeutic intervention Some researchers assert that a significant proportion of agitated depressions are in fact mixed episodes, indicative of an underlying risk for bipolar disorder.
Endogenous (versus Reactive or Precipitated)	Also not in common contemporary use, due to lack of differences in symptoms or outcome; is the relationship between depression and life events "chicken or egg"? (see discussion in Life Events section to follow)
Minor (versus Major)	Minor has fewer symptoms, less impairment than Major, but responds to the same treatments
Chronic (versus Acute)	Rule of thumb: • Acute up to 6 months • Subacute 6 to 24 months • Chronic more than 2 years The longer the duration, the worse the prognosis
Premenstrual	Symptoms generally occur 1 week prior to menses, and resolve within 1 to 2 days of menses At least five symptoms required for diagnosis: • In general, same symptoms as in major depression, in addition to: (1) Bloating and other physical premenstrual symptoms; (2) Irritability; (3) Lability
Bipolar (versus Unipolar)	Depressive symptoms tend to be atypical; important to examine carefully for history of a manic, hypomanic, or mixed episode

*Doctor: Have you ever had 2 weeks or more when you felt **sad** or **blue** almost all day, almost every day?*

Part 2 of the SSQD addresses alternative descriptors for depressed mood, and should be included if the response to Part 1 is negative:

*Doctor: Have you ever had 2 weeks or more when you felt **low**, **gloomy**, **down in the dumps** almost all day, almost every day?*

If the response to Parts 1 and 2 are both negative, SSQD Part 3 should be used to screen for anhedonia:

*Doctor: Have you ever had 2 weeks or more when you **lost interest** in things almost all day, almost every day?*

Notice the three crucial components of each of these questions:

1. Primary symptom of depression (depressed mood or anhedonia) is addressed.

2. Minimum duration of symptoms is addressed (at least 2 weeks).

3. Persistence ("almost all day") and consistency ("almost every day") of the symptoms are addressed.

The truth is that there is no such entity as the SSQD; we've just introduced it here to demonstrate clearly the importance of being inclusive when screening for major depression. The same approach can be utilized when assessing for current major depression by simply changing the tense. For example:

Doctor: For the past 2 weeks have you been feeling low, gloomy, down in the dumps almost all day, almost every day?

Good work. You've taken our advice seriously, screened carefully—in a *sophisticated* fashion—for depression, and you now have preliminary evidence of a possible episode of major depression. You should now proceed to a full evaluation of the depressive episode.

Anchoring the Episode

By and large, major depression is an episodic illness. People with major depression may have multiple episodes, some of which meet full diagnostic criteria and others of which do not. Your first task is to identify an episode that is most likely to yield a positive diagnosis. So, how do you choose an episode? This is an exquisite art that takes years of experience with dozens of complex clinical cases, and masterful mentoring by dexterous diagnosticians to achieve aptitude. Alternatively, you could ignore the asinine alliteration in the previous sentence and just ask about the *worst* episode! The logic here is that if the patient's *most* depressed period does not constitute an episode of major depression, then it is highly unlikely that any of his other periods of depressed mood will either. Having said that, there are other episodes that you can target in your interview. Sometimes patients have difficulty recalling depressive symptoms that occurred in past depressive episodes, so that if the worst episode was more than a few months ago, they may not have accurate access to full recollection of their specific symptoms. Alternatively, some very severe episodes may not achieve full symptomatic criteria. Therefore, you may want to ask about the first, most recent, longest, or best-recalled episodes (see Table 23-5).

So, you've identified a "candidate" episode for further questioning. The next important step is to identify a catch phrase or *key words* of sorts that represent the time period of interest that you can use to introduce your enquiry about symptoms. For example, typical catch phrases include "during that 6 months last summer . . .", "over the past several weeks . . .," "during that month after you lost your job . . .," "in that 18-month period in the late 1990s," etc. It is important to introduce your enquiry about *each and every* symptom with some acknowledgment of the time period addressed in the catch phrase. Once you've established with the patient that you are inquiring about the

Table 23-5. Anchoring Episodes of Depression

Episode for Anchoring	Advantage(s)	Disadvantage(s)
Worst	High yield for a major depressive episode	If episode occurred in the distant past, specifics might be incompletely recalled
First	Usually unaffected by confounding variables such as medications or residual symptoms of previous episodes	May be of low severity and is the most historically remote
Most Recent	Usually the easiest to recall in its entirety	May be confounded by residual symptoms and/or side effects to medications
Best Recalled	Self-evident	May not achieve symptomatic criteria
Longest	Increased probability of sufficient symptoms for diagnosis, and of recall	May be symptomatic fluctuation, resulting in difficulties anchoring a clearly delineated time period

specific time period, you can go on to introduce your subsequent questions with simply "During that time . . . ," "During the period we've been talking about . . . ," "When that happened . . . ," or "At that time. . . ." We suggest that you return to the specific catch phrase with every question (or every few questions if you are convinced the patient understands the pattern) to ensure that patient remains constantly anchored with respect to the episode.

This issue of anchoring the episode and identifying a catch phrase is critical in the diagnosis of major depression—or any recurrent mental illness, for that matter. Although it may seem laborious at first, try answering this question in your own mind: "Think of a time when you felt worried." Our bet is that if you think about this for 10 seconds, you'll come up with more than one occasion. If you then had to answer the question, "Did you have muscle tension?", how would the interviewer know which occasion you were describing? Or even if you were relating the muscle tension to a specific time when you were also anxious? Suffice it to say that this is a significant issue in psychiatric interviewing, such that *if you take one message from this entire chapter this is quite possibly the most important. 75% of your final exam mark for this section will be based on your understanding of this issue. (Joking, of course—just wanted to produce anxiety and muscle tension in you to prove a point.)*

Current Symptoms

When asking about the symptoms of depression, you can use a number of strategies to organize your questions so that you ensure that each diagnostic symptom is reviewed. Common acronyms include "Sad Facies" and "Sige Caps," although you may find that a more personal mnemonic is easier to remember (Table 23-6). Another way to approach each of the nine DSM-IV-TR symptoms is to organize them by topics. The advantage of this approach is that the transitions from question to question are likely to seem more logical to the patient and easier for you to remember.

In-Depth Guide to Asking Questions About the Symptoms of Major Depression

Rule number one in asking about depression is NOT to ask questions about more than one symptom at a time. If you ask someone, "Have you ever had 2 weeks of feeling sad, poor concentration, low energy, and crying all the time?" and the patient says, "Yes," what is he saying "yes" to? And worse, if he says, "No," have you really screened out all these symptoms at once? Asking questions this way is like using the same swab on three successive children in a family practice to test for strep throat! OK, so it's not quite as bad, but you get the point. Having said this, it is quite permissible to use several words to describe one symptom: that is, when asking about depressed mood, it is advisable to use several words like *down, low, blue,* as you will see in a few sections of this chapter.

Rule number two: you must establish that the symptom is distinctly different, in terms of quality, frequency, and/or severity, from what he may have experienced premorbidly or just prior to the episode of interest. Although someone may have felt guilty from time to time before becoming depressed (a lifetime absence of guilt would be of some concern!), it may be that now he experiences guilt virtually every day (increased frequency). Although someone may have had chronic difficulty getting off to sleep before, now he is having trouble with early morning wakening (increased severity). And although he might have had

Table 23-6. Mneumonics for Depression Symptoms

Sad Facies	Sige Caps	Depression
Sleep	**S**leep	**D**epressed mood
Appetite	**I**nterest	**E**nergy
Depressed mood	**G**uilt	**P**sychomotor changes
Fatigue (low energy)	**E**nergy	**R**educed concentration in decision-making
Agitation (or retardation)	**C**oncentration	**E**steem decreased, **E**xcessive guilt
Concentration	**A**ppetite/weight	**S**leep changes
Interest (or anhedonia)	**P**sychomotor	**S**uicidal ideation
Esteem decreased, **E**xcessive guilt	**S**uicide	**I**nterest decreased
Suicidal ideation		**O***
	N.B: Depressed Mood noticeably missing from this mnemonic	**N**utritional changes (appetite and weight)

*"O" stands for **o**ther related syndromes and is a reminder to consider "manic, panic, organic." That is, be vigilant in screening for organic causes of depression (medical conditions, medications, substances), underlying bipolar illness, and comorbid anxiety disorders.

thoughts of death before, now these thoughts have more of an imperative to act on them (change in quality). So check out these important types of changes when assessing current symptomatology.

With these rules firmly ensconced in your brain, the following paragraphs should give you sufficient arrows in your quiver to make sure you hit the mark and diagnose or rule out major depression.

Depressed Mood
Mood

Elsewhere in this chapter the importance of flexible questioning for the symptom of depression has been mentioned. Less than half of patients can identify "depressed" or "sad" as the principal feeling state of their major depression. It bears repeating: asking if someone feels or has felt sad, low, blue, gloomy, down in the dumps, etc., increases the yield of positive diagnosis threefold! Are there other words that might reflect someone's feeling of depression? What about "miserable"? Unfortunately, this is too nonspecific. As is "awful." These are very generic descriptions of having difficulty. So pick words that have the right mood tone to them. In addition, 5% of people have great difficulty putting any words to their emotional state; these people are said to have *alexithymia* (*a* = unable, *lex* = using words, *thymia* = mood). It is particularly important to try to use as many appropriate descriptors for these people as possible, but often these people are more likely to endorse irritability or the anhedonia item (see following material).

Irritability

Often the only manifestation of depressed mood is irritability. Nobody has really defined the irritability of depression with any precision, and this is a problem considering that irritability is a cardinal feature of the polar opposite of depression, namely *mania*. Table 23-7 may help to sort out, in many cases, whether the irritability may be part of a mania or part of a depression, but it is just a rough guide.

Typically, the following question is used to screen for irritability:

"Over the past few weeks have you been irritable with people, getting into lots of arguments, or having outbursts of anger?"

As will become clear, this question, by itself will pick up the irritability of both mania and depression, and so it may be helpful to keep Table 23-7 in mind.

Crying, Tearfulness

This is often simply observed by you or by family members, but sometimes the only "evidence" you have is the patient's own report. Many people describe "crying jags" or "outbursts." The quality of this symptom is that it is almost uncontrollable; it occurs with any valence of emotion, positive or negative, and it often prevents them from socializing, watching the TV, or having conversations with people. To be so out of control in a public way is devastating for many people with depression. Interestingly, it is one of the first symptoms to improve when someone is treated for depression. But that is beyond the scope of this chapter. Because it is so often observed, it is not commonly asked about. Nonetheless, it is recommended that you record whether this symptom is present, as it may help understand many aspects of people's behavior when they are depressed and because it is a helpful early sign of response.

Table 23-7. Irritability in Depression and Mania

Feature	Major depression	Mania
To whom the irritability is directed	Irritability is much more likely to be expressed toward loved ones and people who live in close proximity.	Expressed with less selectivity. Therefore, coworkers, strangers, other drivers, etc. receive the wrath of the irritability, although simply as a virtue of time spent together, family is more likely to receive the brunt.
Triggered or not	There is often a "hook to hang the hat" of irritability on. The "infraction" may be small or insignificant, but there is usually a trigger for the irritable outburst.	The irritability is expressed virtually spontaneously. Some patients talk about walking on their own and feeling rage, and yelling, when there is no particular precipitant.
Remorseful?	People with depression most often feel awful about how they are acting and hate the fact that they are irritable.	People experiencing a mania are usually remorseful only once the episode is over. During the episode, they do not recognize their behavior as irritable or feel justified in behaving that way.
Associated behavior	The irritability of depression is often associated with distress and expression of other negative emotions such as tearfulness and anguish.	The irritability of mania is often associated with rage and aggression, either verbal or physical.

Energy

Many people mistake "low energy" for "low interest" or even "poor concentration." For example:

Dr. W: Have you had trouble with your energy in the past 2 months while you've been feeling blue?

Patient: Yes! It's just so hard to get out of the house.

What does this mean—has it been hard because she is too exhausted or doesn't have the motivation, or are too anxious? If you ask this kind of question, you must probe further and not accept the nonspecific answer.

Dr. W: Do you mean it's been hard to get out because you are too tired to move?

Patient: Yes! I just don't have the energy to do the things I used to want to do.

Are you sure now that this patient has endorsed the energy item? Even though she has responded with a resounding "yes!", don't be sure.

Dr. W: Do you mean that you are just too physically tired, that your muscles feel weak or exhausted?

Patient: No, not really. I just don't feel like I want to go and do things anymore.

One way to reduce the number of clarifying questions is to ask, "Over the past 2 months have you been more physically tired or exhausted than before/usual?" If the answer is no, then add, "Have you been more physically fatigued than you would expect after doing even small amounts of activity, such as walking a few blocks or going out shopping?" If the answers are "No" to both, it is unlikely this person has this symptom of depression, because this items specifically refers to the physical aspects of fatigue, and not the cognitive or hedonic aspects of concentration or motivation.

Psychomotor Agitation and Retardation

Not to overwhelm you, but this item is actually four symptoms in one! The four symptoms are:

1. Psychic agitation—feeling "wired," "revved up," "on edge," or "very tense inside." It refers to the internal experience of being agitated.

2. Motoric agitation—this refers to pacing, fidgeting, wringing hands, or motor restlessness. It is the objective or motor manifestation of agitation.

3. Psychic retardation—feeling "slowed down," "slowed thinking," "slowed emotional responsiveness," or "having few thoughts." This is the internal experience of slowed mentation or slowed processing of emotional information.

4. Motoric retardation—this would be seen as significantly reduced movements, slowed walking, slowed reaction time, immobility, or staring for extended periods.

Although many people talk about "psychomotor slowing" or "psychomotor agitation," these four symptoms may occur in any combination and may change over time or from day to day in major depression. For example, the classic state of "psychomotor retardation" is catatonia. Catatonia is, in fact, characterized more often than not by motoric retardation in the context of profound and overwhelming psychic agitation. For this reason (i.e., the profound psychic agitation), the treatment of catatonia is usually sedation! Many patients tell us that they are fidgety and restless (motoric agitation) but at the same time have almost no thoughts, or feel their emotions are "on delay." Some people report that some days they feel clumsy and have slowed reaction times while at the same time they feel "wired" and "like I'm crawling out of my skin." Still others report being physically slowed down and yet are wringing their hands and picking at their skin! So rather than just looking for the pure states in which there is a perfect match of psychic and motoric states, with no cross-contamination with the polar opposite state (this is actually very rare in our experience), it is much simpler to inquire, sequentially, about each of the four symptoms previously described and then sit back, in wonder, at the remarkable combinations and permutations of psychic and motoric retardation and agitation that present themselves. The DSM-IV-TR excludes psychic agitation or psychic retardation alone from its definition of this symptom complex. In practice, however, a positive response on any of the four symptoms in this complex, with concomitant dysfunction, should suggest that the criterion is endorsed. Whether you go by the DSM-IV-TR or not, to ensure a complete grasp of your patient's mental state, it important to evaluate and monitor the progress of each symptom in this complex.

Concentration, Indecisiveness

Sample question: *"Over the past 3 weeks, while you have been feeling low, have you had difficulty concentrating?"*

This is relatively straightforward; the majority of people will give you a clear and helpful answer. However, many people will look at you with uncertainty, because "concentration" may have several meanings to them, or may be a concept they have not associated with their current state. Whether someone answers yes or no or has a quizzical look, it is always important to get some example of the problem concentrating before you accept that this criterion is met. As mentioned, concentration is often confused with for other symptoms.

Patient: Yes! I just can't read a book now.

Dr. T: Is that because you don't have any desire to read, or are you having difficulty concentrating on the words you are reading?

Patient: (quizzical look)

Dr. T: Do you find that you get to the end of the paragraph and can't recall what the beginning of the paragraph was about? Do you find that you go over and over sentences and words and still can't follow the plot or story?

In fact, there are several ways of getting at poor concentration using common activities. It is important to first establish that people do routinely participate in these activities!

1. *"Can you sit through an entire movie, or do you lose track of the story line?"*
2. *"When you read the paper, can you finish an article or do you lose the train of the article?"*
3. *"Can you follow a conversation, or do you get lost after awhile?"*

The shorter the activity that someone has difficulty concentrating on, the more severe is the symptom.

Decisiveness can also be part of this symptom grouping. Some people may have a personality style that includes difficulty making decisions, but this symptom often is expressed in the "little decision," such as, what to wear, what to do on the weekend, what to do with spare time, what to cook, what to eat, what to say in social settings. A sample question might be the following:

Dr. I: "Over the past 6 months, have you had difficulty making decisions, even small decisions, like what to wear or where to go when you have some time?"

This grouping, poor concentration and difficulty with decisions, can be very disabling and is associated with significant dysfunction, because these cognitive functions are required in virtually all activities.

Although it is not a symptom included in the DSM-IV-TR criteria for major depression, the vast majority of people with depression also complain of impaired memory and/or attention. Unfortunately, many conditions are also associated with impaired memory. Nonetheless, it is still reasonable to inquire about memory and attention, and if these are impaired, this information can be used in clinical practice to support the diagnosis of major depression.

Feelings of Worthlessness or Excessive or Inappropriate Guilt (not merely self-reproach or guilt about being sick)

Many people do not know that, next to suicidal ideation, this is the most unpleasant and unwanted symptom of major depression. It is also sometimes difficult to evaluate. Why? Because many people with depression exhibit guilt trait as well as guilt state. In other words, many people with major depression have persistent feelings of guilt even when not in an episode of the illness, and these feelings may intensify when they are acutely depressed.

"During the past 5 weeks, when you have been feeling down-in-the-dumps, have you felt more guilty than usual, guilty about things you have nothing to do with or over which you have no control?"
Or
"Over the past 5 weeks, have you been feeling down on yourself?"
Or
"Over the past 5 weeks, have you lost confidence in yourself?"

Sometimes we ask all of these questions, because they all reflect slightly different aspects of worthlessness or guilt. Familiarize yourself with these types of options, and you will be able to identify this criterion in more than 85% of people with depression.

A more advanced issue arises when you realize that guilt is ubiquitous! Many people with a chronic illness of any type, medical or psychiatric, experience guilt that is related to their loss or change in role function at home or at work, etc., and is not a specific symptom of the illness. They feel they are letting down their family, their coworkers, and their friends, because they are not able to complete the tasks that would be assigned to them, and that this adds burden to others. Recent studies have identified several key statements that people with depression endorse that distinguish the nature of their guilt from that of people with a chronic illness. The sorts of statements include those listed in Box 23-1.

You can turn these statements into questions if you are faced with the need to distinguish the guilt associated with chronic disability from the guilt associated with major depression. In fact, it is very common that people with medical illnesses also develop or have preexisting major depression, and in these circumstances the distinction is even more important. In fact, we find that:

"Do you feel like you are a bad person?" and *"Have you been feeling a strong sense of regret?"* are simple and very helpful in making the distinction. Don't forget—guilt may reach delusional intensity with people believing they are

---

Box 23-1. Statements of Guilt and Shame Endorsed by People with Major Depression that Distinguish Them from People with Chronic Medical Illness

"If I could live my life over again, there are a lot of things I would do differently."
"I often have a strong sense of regret."
"I would give anything if, somehow, I could go back and rectify some things I have recently done wrong."
"I want to sink into the floor and disappear."
"I feel like I am a bad person."

truly to blame for things that they have no responsibility for, or feeling profound self-loathing over events that are trivial, or believing they are truly "bad to the core," even when they are upstanding members of their community or believing that they are being punished by some higher power for their sins, even when they have done nothing particularly wrong or bad. Although this kind of delusional guilt is relatively uncommon in the community at large, it may be seen in patients with severe depression who present to the emergency room or on inpatient mental health units.

Increased or Decreased Sleep

Decreased sleep may be at the beginning of the night (initial insomnia or troubling getting to sleep), and/or the middle of the night (middle insomnia or trouble staying asleep/waking frequently), and/or at the usual waking time (terminal insomnia or waking early than anticipated). Increased sleep is usually manifest by waking much later than expected, and/or earlier bedtime, and/or increased napping. Most depressed people, whether they have insomnia or hypersomnia, awake unrefreshed and feel they could or should sleep more or better, although there is no specific criterion on the DSM-IV-TR for this symptom or complaint.

Sample questions:

Initial insomnia: *"During the past few years, when you have been feeling gloomy, have you had trouble getting to sleep?"*

Middle insomnia: *"During the past few years, have you been able to stay asleep? Do you wake frequently during the night?"*

Terminal insomnia: *"During the past few years, do you find you wake up much earlier than you would expect to or than you would like to and can't get back to sleep?"*

Hypersomnia: *"During the past few years, how many hours, including nighttime sleep and naps, have you been sleeping, in general? How many hours did you used to sleep before you started to feel gloomy?"*

Or

"Do you find that you are sleeping much longer than normal . . . whether that means sleeping longer during the night or taking naps during the day so that the total hours of sleep is longer than before you became depressed?"

Increased sleep and increased appetite are often called the "atypical" features of major depression. The word "atypical" is used to imply that this constellation is unusual and not the way most people with depression present. However, most epidemiological studies now demonstrate that up to 40% of people with major depression do have the "atypical" profile. In some studies, this profile outnumbers the "typical" profile. So, although the word no longer really reflects the statistical evidence, it has stuck.

One more note: here's a question for you—on average, how many hours a night have you slept in the past month? It's a complicated question and often difficult to answer. Do you include weekends? What about those couple of late nights studying/partying/watching *Sex in the City* reruns? Remember that recollection of sleep quality and times is notoriously inaccurate, so try to find corroborating information if at all possible.

Suicidal Ideation and Thoughts of Death (not just fear of dying)

Questioning regarding suicidal ideation is probably the most daunting of all symptoms for students and staff alike. You need to practice your questioning and make sure you are confident about what you would like to ask and how to respond. If you give the subtle message to the patient that thinking about or planning suicide is socially unacceptable or frightening to you, you may get a spuriously negative response. For example,

Dr. L: Have you ever . . . some people when they are really, really depressed start to think . . . you aren't thinking about killing yourself, are you?

This question demonstrates a discomfort with the subject and, because it is framed in the negative, is almost asking the person to say no. Probably every teacher will give you slightly different advice on how to deal with these questions. Some suggest gently introducing the subject area before asking specifically about suicide. For example, "Sometimes people with depression start to think about their own life and wonder if life is worth living." Others recommend heading straight into the topic and dealing with it up front and in a nonjudgmental, matter-of-fact way—for example, "Have you been thinking about killing yourself?" There is no absolutely correct way; however, the question must be asked, whether you "ease into" it or not. There are four separate questions or issues that are all related to suicidal ideation and should be asked:

1. *"Do you think life is worth living?"* This ascertains a general sense of a person's will to live or hopelessness.
2. *"Have you been thinking about harming yourself or have you harmed yourself?"* Many people wish to harm themselves but have no desire to die. The wish to harm themselves may be part of major depression or, not infrequently, part of another illness or personality disorder.
3. *"Have you been thinking about death?"* Many people with major depression become preoccupied with death as a concept, even their own death, but may not be thinking about taking their own life.
4. *"Have you had thoughts about taking your own life or about wanting to die?"* Taking one's life assumes an active process, whereas wanting to die may reflect more passive suicidal ideation.

Case Example 2

Scott: A Tale of Two Viewpoints. The abbreviated version of events is this: after helping cover the very vicious Chechen war in 1995 for the Canadian Broadcasting Corporation, I returned to our base in Moscow. Julia and I were living there while I worked as the bureau's producer. It was a demanding job that involved long hours, high stress, and frequent travel to hard places. Nothing, however, was quite as intense as Chechnya.

We'd spent much of our time in the war zone documenting the horrors that had taken place, atrocities that did not seem to differentiate between military and civilian targets. We also spent a lot of time running: diving into muddy ditches as Russian fighter jets swooped low, hiding in basements as cluster bombs exploded nearby, and scrambling for protection behind the nearest solid wall when mortars began to thud. And increasingly, at night, I spent time soothing, or rather, numbing, what I'd seen with alcohol.

Although I wasn't even aware of it, I had been through a very traumatic experience. And that trauma, on my return to Moscow, would manifest itself. What started with a feeling of being energized on having emerged intact from Chechnya would accelerate in the weeks and months to come. Neither Julia nor I knew what hypomania was, but I was in the throes of it. It would eventually lead to the loss of my position, a full-blown psychosis in China, and a rather memorable involuntary hospitalization in a crumbling asylum on the outskirts of Hong Kong.

The experience was, by turns, exhilarating, mystical, and ultimately terrifying. It was also appallingly expensive, and I blew pretty much every dime we had with a mania-fueled plan to export antique Chinese furniture. (It seems I was ahead of the curve; several stores in Toronto now sell precisely the goods I was snapping up.)

We'd love to tell you the full story, but neither the space nor the focus of this chapter permit. We do, however, heartily encourage you to read *The Last Taboo: A Survival Guide to Mental Health Care in Canada*.[1] You'll find the full version there—along with the answer to one of the most pressing questions of the 21st century: "What ever happened to the furniture?"

What we can offer in this section is a sense of what our own initial experience with psychiatrists was like. Because there was very limited contact with psychiatrists in Hong Kong (although the psychiatric ward nurses were friendly), we'll leave out that part and start this journey in Canada. It begins on the very day we returned to the country, shortly after getting off a jet in Saskatoon.

Doctor #1 was a dour man, seemingly incapable of even a brief smile. I met him after being taken for an examination at a local hospital soon after arriving from Hong Kong.

His cursory examination, in an emergency ward waiting room, consisted of his asking me a few questions about what had happened. I told him I was a Buddhist and an entrepreneur (both of which seemed quite true at the time), and that we'd bought a whack of furniture.

"And you don't think there's anything wrong with you?" he asked sternly.

"No," I replied. "I'm feeling better than I've ever felt in my life."

He looked at me with an odd expression that appeared to be either disdain or disgust. "Then we've got a problem," he said curtly. He then walked out the door and closed it with an abruptness that closely reflected his overall demeanor. Even my father, who'd been in the room during the encounter and personally knew this physician, thought he'd acted like a jerk.

It may well be that this physician felt some empathy, but he did not impart one iota of concern over my well-being. I left the hospital hoping I would never see him again. I didn't.

Doctor #2 was a staff psychiatrist at the University Hospital in Saskatoon, where—to please my family—I agreed to go for another assessment only a day or two after the experience with the first doctor. This psychiatrist smiled when he met me, laughed at some of my better jokes, and appeared genuinely interested in the "transformation" that I explained had taken place while abroad. (Despite the Haldol I'd been taking since my hospitalization in Hong Kong, I was still high as a kite at this point.)

Rather than treating me like a problem, this doctor seemed genuinely interested in finding solutions. My lasting impression is that he was incredibly patient with me, pointing out that some of my recent behavior just didn't jive with what the rest of my life had been like. Being manic, of course, I had an answer for everything. He'd listen to those answers, but would point out inconsistencies for which I had no explanation.

The still-buzzing mania had left me quite agitated, unable to sit still for very long, and certainly unable to shut up. At one point, he pointed this out and said it's quite common for someone with mania to have those symptoms. I believe I then tried my best to sit still (to demonstrate that I was, indeed, well) but simply couldn't do it.

Using this kind of empathetic logic, it wasn't long before, on some level, I started to think there might just be something to what he was saying. It was enough for me to consent to another meeting along with Julia and other members of my family.

Julia. The gathering Scott refers to was the one and only family meeting ever held during his treatment and recovery. I remember it well. There we all sat, in a semicircle facing a psychiatrist in a large office at the University Hospital:

Scott and his sisters, his mother, stepmother, and father, and me. The psychiatrist drew a neat sine-wave pattern of mood fluctuations on a chalkboard. He talked about mood cycles and mood stabilizers—entirely new terminology to us—and about the highs and lows that lay ahead. I remember lapping up his every word, his every scribbling, while Scott, still manic, barely listened. I remember the intense desire to learn every detail of this disorder whose name I'd only recently heard for the first time.

The psychiatrist, as I recall, was the only calm person in the room; the rest of us were frazzled, confused, overwhelmed, and exhausted. I had barely begun to make sense of everything that had happened to us, having just returned from Hong Kong where I'd spent 3 weeks chasing after my increasingly erratic and unrecognizable spouse. I was the only one who'd been with Scott through the building mania and subsequent psychosis. His parents and siblings, meanwhile, had been on the receiving end of many disturbing late-night phone calls across continents.

Like many family members, I knew almost nothing about mental disorder, and even less about Scott's particular diagnosis. (I think I'd vaguely heard the term "manic-depression" before, but I had no idea what it actually was and had never, to my knowledge, met anyone who'd been diagnosed with it.) What I needed most urgently was information—plain, easy to understand information. I appreciated the doctor's forthright manner, his patience in answering our questions, and his sense of humor in dealing with Scott's buoyant mood. At one point, Scott decided he'd had enough of this meeting, and he walked out; the doctor seemed neither surprised nor perturbed and pressed on without Scott. His calmness helped calm us, too.

There was another purpose to the meeting beyond education. Although Scott was taking the medications prescribed in Hong Kong, he still did not believe there was anything wrong with him. The mania was slowly subsiding, but now he was talking about going off the pills and returning to Toronto. Scott did not, however, meet the criteria for involuntary committal. (It's a scenario I've since heard from countless frustrated family members.)

The psychiatrist believed that Scott needed to be admitted to hospital and had called us all together to discuss how best to convince him to do so voluntarily. It was the one time, in the 9 years since Scott's diagnosis, that a doctor has offered to involve the family in the treatment plan. And it came at a critical turning point. Had Scott stopped taking his medication, his condition would have undoubtedly worsened. He would likely have been hospitalized involuntarily a second time. After the trauma of his initial hospitalization, his trust in the system might have been broken for good. With the whole family's involvement, we were able to avoid those dire circumstances.

At the psychiatrist's suggestion, we presented a united front, gently encouraging Scott to give the hospital a try. The important thing, we were told, was that we all work together. And it worked. Scott later told me that although he still didn't believe he was ill, he was swayed by the unanimity of our persistence. It's a good example of how medical professionals can include the family to the benefit of everyone involved.

As deftly as this particular psychiatrist handled the situation, he got a few other things wrong. He told us, for example, that Scott would need to be on mood stabilizers for the rest of his life; that even with medication he would continue to experience highs and lows beyond the "normal range"; that if Scott ever stopped taking his medications, he was pretty much guaranteed of a rapid relapse. All this, of course, is straight out of the textbooks. Still, all of the above turned out, in our case, to be incorrect.

After a couple of years of stability and a return to work, Scott did decide to try life without medication. He made the decision in consultation with his new psychiatrist, and with me. Remembering the Saskatoon doctor's warnings, I was dead set against it, terrified of a relapse—another explosive mania or intransigent depression. But Scott persisted despite my concerns; he felt it was important to at least try. (As a professional writer, he also felt that the mood stabilizers suppressed his creativity.)

For the past 6 years, Scott has remained both medication and relapse free. He's been able to work full-time at a high-pressure job, endure the deaths of four close family members, write two books, buy a house, and maintain a loving relationship with me. In other words, he's been able to live a healthy and productive life, with care and attention to lifestyle but without the use of medications.

I raise this not to be dismissive of psychiatric drugs, which are essential to many people's ongoing mental health. No doubt, Scott's circumstances are unusual; by any textbook's standards, the odds were stacked against him being where he is today.

But I do believe our story raises a few crucial points: there are exceptions to every rule in psychiatry as in all other endeavors; there is still much we do not understand of the why's and how's of mental illness; and, above all, each one of us truly is unique. These are points worth remembering with every new patient you treat.

GETTING DIAGNOSED

"Ah, Clara! No one knows the suffering, the sickness, the despair, except those so crushed."

—Composer Robert Schumann in a letter to his wife, 1838

Consider, for a moment, what it's like to be on the receiving end of a diagnosis. Although this field often makes analogies between physical and mental illness, getting tagged with a DSM-IV-TR label is quite different from hearing the doctor say, "You've got the flu." The patient is not merely being told he's ill, he's being told he's mentally ill. And each person—including you—brings to the clinician's office his own preconceptions about what it actually means to be mentally ill.

You've likely seen research suggesting that only a small minority of people with a diagnosable mental disorder seek help (some data suggest about one in four). The rest suffer in silence, often for years—especially men. "Men tend to suffer in silence. And they tend to self-treat using other means. And obviously the most popular means in the adult male population, unfortunately, is alcohol," Bill Ashdown, president of the Mood Disorders Society of Canada, told us.[1]

Stigma, along with lack of information and education needed to make healthy choices, is a big part of the reason why. Who wants to admit to a mental health problem in a world that often fears, shuns, and despises the mentally ill? As we wrote,[1] "Who dares admit to being crazy, nuts, or loony?" People have told us they feared being locked up for life, having their children taken away from them, losing their jobs, and more.

In the face of so many myths and misconceptions, it's remarkable that anyone ever does come forward. It takes real courage to reach out for help and to admit you might need it. Some persons will confide first with a family member, close friend, or perhaps even a minister or spiritual advisor. Others might phone a crisis line, or tell their family physician they're in need of help. Still others may have help imposed on them because of conflicts with work or the law, or through an involuntary admission. In some cases, the first contact with the formal mental health system is after a suicide attempt.

Regardless of the circumstances, the diagnosis, or particular symptoms, the first impression you as the clinician create—how comfortable you make the person feel and how supportive, hopeful, and encouraging your manner is—will make a tremendous difference in the faith each person places in you and her willingness to accept the help you offer. Those first few minutes are absolutely crucial.

"They have to have a sense, hopefully from the first moment they make contact with that psychiatrist—whether it's over a telephone or in the waiting room—that 'I think this might work. I kind of like this person,'" says Dr. Michael Myers, former president of the Canadian Psychiatric Association. "He or she seems sensitive, they seem kind, they seem polite, they're making me comfortable and, most importantly, they're listening."

As part of our research for *The Last Taboo*,[1] we asked Dr. Myers how he goes about making that first crucial assessment of a new patient. His Vancouver psychiatric practice is devoted exclusively to treating physicians, medical students, and their families, earning him the nickname "the doctor's doctor." Because his approach is so thorough and firmly rooted in the biopsychosocial model, we quoted him at length in our book, and will do so again here:

> If I'm assessing a new physician in my practice and, say, I think he or she has major depression, what I want to do is take a very good genetic, family history to find out if there've been any family members with a history of mood disorder. I need to know his general medical health to make sure there aren't physical factors contributing to his symptoms: thyroid disease or other endocrine problems. I want to know about any medications or street drugs that he might be taking, and any previous depressions. I also want to know, of course, about his alcohol use. So a lot of that stuff is all in the area of biological psychiatry. . . .
>
> But then I want to have a very detailed developmental history on him. I want to know if his parents split up, for instance, when he was a child or adolescent. Whether or not he might have been abused, whether or not he might have had a learning disability. Whether or not he might have had some catastrophic event that might have put him off-course for a while. So all of the psychological factors that might have contributed to his self-esteem, his personality development, things like that. . . .
>
> Now the sociocultural part is whether or not he's, say, a member of an ethnic minority. . . . Did he grow up in poverty? . . . Religious persecution? Gay bashing? Things like that. . . . It's the last part, the psychosocial part, that helps a lot in setting up your psychotherapy plan. So even if I conclude that this guy needs to go on an anti-depressant, that's fine, I'll monitor his mood. But I want to also get at any of the other stuff that's in his background.

This is the kind of comprehensive assessment you would no doubt want if you were sitting in a doctor's office or hospital room feeling frightened and confused about the state of your mental health. Unfortunately, we've heard from many people who said they received far less—people who told us psychiatrists had them in and out the door in a matter of minutes, and treated them not as living, breathing human beings but as a cluster of biochemical symptoms.

We're not about to delve into any lengthy debates about nature versus nurture. But we'll briefly summarize what we've learned over the years. It is both simple and complex. And it is this: many patients, regardless of symptoms, will arrive at your door because something very real—and often unpleasant—has happened in their lives. There will be others for whom mental illness apparently drifted in of its own neurophysiological accord, with no apparent core issue other than a genetic susceptibility. And there will be a third category—likely the largest—for whom their current distress appears to be a blend of the above.

Whatever the cause, all three of these groups—indeed, anyone who sets foot in your office or emergency department—generally share a few things in common: They are in pain. They are seeking relief from their suffering. And in nearly all cases, they are looking to you for far more than a prescription; they are looking for understanding, empathy, and a message of hope.

COMMON REACTIONS

You will have many tools available for making a diagnosis, but remember that patients and their families will have few at their disposal for *receiving* one. You might be surprised at how much the responses can vary. Being handed a diagnosis has different implications for different people. For some, finally having their affliction identified and named can bring tremendous relief. It can point the way toward treatment, management of symptoms, and hope. For others, hearing that they have a mental illness can trigger anger, denial, sadness, self-loathing, and just about everything in between.

In Scott's case, the initial diagnosis from the psychiatrist in Saskatoon didn't mean much because he was so high. But when the mania finally quelled, a well-meaning social worker sat him down and spoke the following words: "You have bipolar affective disorder. You will have this illness the rest of your life. You will have to avoid stress, not drink or use drugs, and stay on medication."

She said Scott would be disabled for some time, then she offered this optimistic note for the future: "It's unlikely you'll ever work in journalism again."

The overall message was that Scott's life, as he knew it, was over. What was even harder to digest was the message that this was something over which Scott had absolutely no control (with the exception of adhering to medication). The die had been cast. It was like being punched.

Not surprisingly, Scott's response was one of shock. And shock is one of six different reactions that we've heard of from users of mental health services (Box 24-1). There may well be more, but these are certainly the most common.

Box 24-1. Common Reactions to Diagnosis

Relief
Shock/panic
Denial
Anger
Confusion
Guilt

How a person responds to a diagnosis will to a certain extent be "soft-wired," based on her understanding of mental illness, conceptions or misconceptions, experience, and interaction with others with mental illness (including her own family members), dealings with mental health service providers, and a host of other experiential factors to which you may not (yet) be privy.

As well, the stage, severity, and type of the illness will also play a role. A hypomanic patient, for example, might well dismiss your opinion and want to leave. (He does, after all, have better things to do—like make money and have sex.)

We know of cases where the lack of insight was so profound that the patient was able to convince the clinician that he was, in fact, well. (Julia believes that in the early stages of his hypomania, Scott could have convinced all but the most seasoned of psychiatrists that he was perfectly fine.)

There will also be people, as you will shortly discover, who believe (in some cases, legitimately) that they do not have a mental illness and that the symptoms with which they present are simply a normal human response to trauma. They will reject (in some cases, legitimately) any talk of "lack of insight" or "denial." And, despite the fact they may be in desperate pain and need of help, they might simply be offended by talk of "illness" and walk straight out your door.

Rather than parse the entire DSM-IV-TR, let's have a broad look at the possible reactions to getting diagnosed, and helpful ways in which you might respond.

Relief

A patient might react with an expression of relief: "Thank goodness we've figured out what's wrong. I've been struggling with this for ages. But it all makes sense now." A potential response from the doctor might be to say, *"Well, now that we know what's been going on, we can work on a plan to get you feeling better."*

Denial

Another reaction might be one of denial: "I'm not crazy. It's my family that's sick," or "You don't understand me," or "I just think differently than other people—there's nothing wrong with that." Appropriate responses from the clinician might include the following: *"I'm not suggesting you're crazy,"* or *"I hear what you're saying"*—anything to indicate that you have, indeed, been listening to the person's concerns. *"But I think you'd agree, based on what you've told me, that something's troubling you. All I'm interested in is helping you get back to your usual self."*

Anger

Patients might react to a diagnosis with anger: "Screw you and your diagnosis of borderline personality disorder. I was sexually abused as a child, and I'm offended you would suggest my response to trauma is an "illness." How dare you!" A clinician might respond to this by saying, *"I know from what you've told me that there are legitimate reasons for your pain—and I'm not in any way trying to minimize that. Nor am I saying you have to accept my opinion on this. We're just trying to explore some possibilities at this stage."*

Confusion/Fear

Alternatively, the patient being diagnosed might react with feelings of confusion. For example, "What does this mean? I don't understand what you're saying. Does this mean I'll have to be locked up for life?" A potential response might be: *"It's okay to be a little confused about this—many people are. But there's no need to be frightened. Determining what the problem is will help us get you feeling better. And don't worry, we are not going to lock you up. The only circumstances where you might be hospitalized against your will are if you feel so bad that we're worried you might hurt yourself or someone else and you aren't prepared to get help. We are going to help you get better."*

Panic

Another possible reaction is panic: "I can't be mentally ill! I have a job, I have a family. I have a reputation! What will people think of me?" To this, a clinician might respond as follows: *"Lots of people with jobs and families have been diagnosed with a mental disorder and are able to live normal lives. You don't have to tell anyone until you're ready—and you certainly don't have to worry that I'll share this with anyone."*

Guilt

Lastly, a patient receiving a diagnosis might react by feeling guilty: "It's all my fault. If I was a stronger person, this wouldn't be happening to me. I have nothing to complain about—I shouldn't even be here. I should be able to get out of this rut on my own." A possible response to this might be, *"If you broke your leg, you wouldn't be trying to fix it yourself. And you wouldn't be blaming yourself either. Try to remember that this is not your fault. You haven't done anything wrong. There are things you can do to help yourself. But we can help you as well."*

Responding to Reactions

The theme, you'll no doubt have noticed, is one of optimism and empathy. Show the person across from you that you are not only listening to her concerns but also can help to address them.

As you'll have seen above, it's helpful to relate the behaviors and feelings the person is experiencing to recognized symptoms of disorder. For example: *"You've been spending lots of money and have come up with an unusual array of business schemes lately. You've also told me that you haven't been sleeping much. Would you agree with this? The behavior that you've described is typical for something we call bipolar affective disorder. I think it's possible that's what you've got, though I'll have to know more about you before we can be sure. It's treatable, and with the right medication and therapy, we hope to have you back on track before too long."*

As mentioned, patients will have their own preconceptions of mental disorder. And in an age where celebrity confessions about depression or eating disorders have become common, we've noticed people are sometimes more comfortable with these more "popular" disorders. Disorders involving psychosis seem far more frightening. Yet even with schizophrenia, which many would argue has the worst public image of the lot, there are more positive ways to frame the diagnosis. For example: *"The voices you've been hearing and the paranoia you're feeling are consistent with schizophrenia. I don't know what you know about this disorder, but there have been tremendous advances in treatment in recent years. It might take a little while to find the treatment that works best for you, but once we do, we should be able to get those symptoms under control."*

It's worth noting that a label cannot always be cast in stone. Many people have complained to us of having had an incorrect diagnosis—even multiple incorrect diagnoses over many years—something that doesn't instill much confidence regarding practitioners. One study by the Canadian Mental Health Association's British Columbia division found that nearly half of people surveyed had been incorrectly diagnosed at least once. So a willingness to reconsider is important.

It's also important, especially in this growing age of biological psychiatry, to remind ourselves that distress does not always equal disorder. Sometimes a decision not to diagnose is the best assessment of all.

GOOD DOCS, BAD DOCS

"I think it's really important for the consumer/patient to demand a lot from their physicians and to challenge their physicians to provide them with the kind of service that they need to have. I think that traditionally the process has been a different way, and I'm not in favour of that."

—Dr. Stan Kutcher, former Head of the Department of Psychiatry at Dalhousie University[1]

One of the trickiest things about psychiatry, it seems to us, and what separates it from many other areas of medicine, is that so many of your patients will take so many different paths to recovery. There is no one prescribed course of action that applies to all because recovery is such an individual process.

Likewise, there is no one definition of what makes for a "good" clinician. Patients' opinions of what they like in a mental health professional will vary widely. Flexibility and an open mind are extremely important for all of these reasons.

That said, we can offer some of the common points that keep cropping up—a few refrains we heard over and over again when we asked what people liked or didn't like. But before we summarize a few key points, we would like to raise one overarching theme that can be summed up in a single word: empathy.

We could go on at great length about the importance of empathy, but it might start sounding touchy-feely. Someone who has written eloquently on this topic, however, is Dr. Richard B. Goldbloom—the father of the editor of this very book. "Empathy alone is certainly no substitute for scientific knowledge, nor for first-class clinical skills or diagnosis and treatment," he wrote several years ago.[2] "However, empathy also should not be regarded as some form of 'warm and fuzzy' bedside manner that features a gentle touch and a velvet voice. Empathy is the expression of true insight into how patients and families feel and an appreciation of the difficulties they face."

If you've got a highlighter handy, it's worth underlining the previous paragraph. These are wise words, and timeless in their truth.

Remember, empathy does not mean "I feel your pain." It does, however, indicate you're making an effort to understand it. And that means a great deal to a patient.

MORE THAN JUST PILLS

There is one recurring message that we have heard from those we've met in our research. We have heard it said with anger, frustration, sadness, and despair. And we have heard it often. As one woman told us, "I'm a person! I'm much more than biochemicals."

We do not doubt, for a millisecond, the importance of targeted and precise psychiatric medications. There are countless millions who owe their day-to-day functioning, and even their lives, to accurate diagnosis and a therapeutic regimen that includes medication. We've interviewed scores of people for whom the right drugs have brought respite, relief, stability, and even sanity.

And yet, as the field continues its remarkable advances in the world of biological psychiatry, we believe a good clinician must try to avoid a common trap in this field: viewing a human being solely as a cluster of symptoms in need of a prescription.

It's easy to forget, with the great strides that have been made in recent years, that there is still much we do not understand about mental illness. Yes, we can describe the origins of mental disorder as "biopsychosocial," but what does that really mean in terms of how a human being—your patient—has developed and experienced that disorder? It can be temptingly easy to put the focus on the "bio" and pay lip service to the "psychosocial." Pills seem faster, tidier, and more "scientific."

"It's not like you just add them all together," Dr. John Strauss, Professor Emeritus at Yale, told us a few years back. "We don't really understand, I think, how the *bio*, the *psycho*, and the *social* interact."

Many, many patients have told us they're turned off by the "take-your-pills-and-see-you-later" approach. And many—even most, based on our research—will need more than pills to recover. This passage from a woman who appeared in our second book[3] sums it up very eloquently: "I am not against medication. What I am opposed to is this: a biological mindset that prescribes without listening, the practice of declaring the human condition a disease. Sometimes the heart of sickness is a festering story. That story needs to be told, and it needs to be heard."

The woman who wrote that passage spent 7 months in a psychiatric hospital where doctors prescribed an array of medications to no effect. What ultimately helped her, and what has kept her out of hospital ever since in spite of a bleak prognosis, was intensive therapy with a doctor she trusted. "I used to think he saved my life," she wrote. "Now I know he did more than that; he taught me how to save my own."

Enough said.

OTHER COMMON CONCERNS

In interviews and correspondence with people across the country who have seen a psychiatrist, some common refrains quickly emerge. We offer these not as indictment but as information from which you can learn.

Not Listening

The idea that the clinician did not listen to the patient is by far the most common complaint we heard. The doctor slots the patient in for 15 minutes, asks a few questions by rote, barely glances up from his notepad, and then scribbles down a prescription. The doctor does not seem to want to hear how the patient is feeling (beyond a narrow range of symptoms) or to consider what the patient thinks might have prompted those feelings. The patient feels like it's over before she even sat down.

Presenting Only One Treatment Option

Since mental disorder often leads to feelings of helplessness and loss of control, people need to feel that they have some say in their treatment plan. Presenting a range of alternatives, including self-help groups or options like cognitive behavioral therapy, also helps build trust; the person doesn't feel like he is being told what to do. (Besides, as we said before, recovery often takes more than a prescription.)

Failing to Secure Informed Consent

In the complaint that the clinician failed to secure informed consent, the key word is *informed*. Far too many people have told us that they were handed a prescription with little or no information provided about benefits and risks, including side effects. Not only is this bad practice, it also can turn people off of medication for good. And it can destroy that crucial element of trust; the patient is left to wonder whether the doctor tried to "pull one over on him" by failing to warn him about the potential downsides of taking a particular drug.

Lack of Information and Encouragement

Another common complaint is that the doctor sends a patient out the door without any resources. People consistently told us they wanted information to help them make sense of this confusing new world, to help them overcome their fears surrounding a diagnosis, and to realize that they are not alone. Yet they have no time or energy to devote to finding this information, especially early on when the disorder is consuming their lives. To understand and to accept a diagnosis, people (including family members) need to be told where to find helpful books, Websites, and support groups.

Pathologizing of Emotions

The doctor assumes that the emotions surrounding the trauma and chaos caused by mental disorder are symptoms of illness rather than natural reactions to it. Because a person has been diagnosed as "mentally ill," you may assume that his insight is poor and that feelings of hopelessness, fear, anger, etc. are a part of the illness rather than a fairly

normal response to it. We refer you back to the William Anthony exercise above.

Dismissing Alternative Therapies

Patients often complain that the doctor sees no role for alternative therapies beyond the regimen or therapeutic approach prescribed. This occur despite the growing body of evidence that some people benefit from non-mainstream approaches, whether that be St. John's wort, prayer, self-help groups, and more. We've heard that people find the "My way or the highway" approach to be egocentric and ultimately harmful to the therapeutic relationship. We encourage you not to reject or deny the patient permission to explore other beneficial (or even benign) treatment options, providing they're not contraindicated. Although people are looking for your expertise and your best recommendation, they also want to know the full range of options and want to do some exploring for themselves.

Overmedication

Sometimes the doctor prescribes medications at levels that result in intolerable side effects for the patient, or she prescribes a staggering kaleidoscope of drugs in the hope that eventually the right combination will alleviate symptoms (or stop the patient from complaining). We've heard from top clinical pharmacologists that "there are some horrendous doses out there." We encourage you to prescribe only what is necessary to alleviate the symptoms, and to listen when patients say they think they might be taking too high a dose. We've heard far too many times from people who complained about intolerable side effects only to have their physicians say they'd simply have to put up with them. Other people tell us that the sexual dysfunction caused by some psychotropic medications causes great distress, but that their doctors somehow don't seem to understand or even ask about this embarrassing but real experience.

Lack of Goal-Setting

The complaint that doctors fail to set goals has come to us from people on both sides of the couch or desk. Some patients have plodded along with psychiatrists (and some psychiatrists have plodded along with patients) for years without ever assessing whether the process is working and whether goals are being met. We'd strongly encourage you, as you embark on a therapeutic relationship, to discuss what the patient would like to achieve and what her goals are. Perhaps you'd like to clarify your own expectations, whether it's the required notice for a cancellation, medication adherence, commitment to psychotherapy, etc. We'd also encourage you and your patient to agree on a time frame after which you'll both assess whether you feel the goals are, in fact, being met.

So, those are some of the things that can go wrong. And we're going to examine a few of them in a case study of Clara, who is now 47 years old and thriving as a family physician.

Case Example 3

Clara had a strong family history of bipolar disorder. She had her first episode of depression at the age of 13 years. She suspects both a genetic link and family dysfunction (due to untreated mental illness in her mother) contributed to her own vulnerability. As a first-year university student, she was troubled enough by her mood to visit a psychiatrist. During that first visit, the psychiatrist assessed her symptoms as "normal, age-appropriate angst" and sent her away.

During her second year of university, still struggling, she again sought help. This time, she began to see a psychologist regularly for psychotherapy only. Her depression did not lift, and Clara, a top student who now found herself unable to cope, dropped out of university. Despite the fact that she clearly met all criteria for major depressive disorder, no referral for pharmacological consultation with a psychiatrist was offered. She would not return to school for a decade. "I feel as if I wasted a lot of years," she told us.

In her 30s, Clara returned to university to study medicine. But the depression kept recurring. She again consulted a psychiatrist and was finally prescribed antidepressants. This would resolve the depression but also gave her insomnia. Inevitably, she'd go off the medication, and the depression would return. This cycle was repeated several times over. Every time she started a new course of medication, her mood would lift and she would experience bursts of energy that seemed, on the surface, to indicate that she was "recovering." What was actually happening was that she was having periods of hypomania. "I wasn't floridly manic, just hypomanic, so it kept getting missed," she says. "I would just look like this very competent kind of person in their office . . . But the insomnia should have tipped them off."

"I really wish the diagnosis had been made (earlier) because my life just kept getting worse and worse over the 7 years I was on antidepressants. I was functioning at a far lower level than I was when I started them. I felt such profound despair that I wanted to die, basically."

The psychotherapy, which also lasted 7 years, wasn't helping much either. Clara believes, in retrospect, that her psychiatrist should have better assessed whether the treatment was resulting in any sort of net benefit. But goals were never discussed with this psychiatrist.

"What I really think was remiss was for this fellow not to have asked himself objectively to evaluate: was progress occurring? And second of all, to have done this with me as

well. It's just criminal to keep somebody who's suffering in that state when a treatment clearly isn't effective," she says.

Four years ago, Clara finally switched doctors and was diagnosed with bipolar disorder—something her mother had as well. But Clara (who had been told by all her previous shrinks that she was not bipolar) was terrified of that label. It conjured up demons from her own chaotic upbringing. And the psychiatrist, she says, was not empathetic.

"There was not one iota of empathy for the total terror I had. He made it a lot harder for me because when I started to be defensive about it and to offer counter-arguments to the diagnosis, his response was to say: 'I think that's just psychological. You don't want to be bipolar because your mother's bipolar.' Well, that's right! But he took a very adversarial role and it was horrible. And it would have been so nice to have had some empathy."

It would also have been nice, says Clara, if her psychiatrist had addressed her concerns over potential side effects, especially the more severe ones, however rare. "When I asked him about adverse effects, he just said, 'Well, I know you can get a rash.'" This dismissive approach continued when Clara did begin taking medication. "Every time I complained of side effects, he would dismiss my claims and essentially argue that I was in a power struggle with him. Every single time."

Clara eventually connected with a psychologist whose approach worked for her. "She was always positive, never critical of me. And as she says, her approach was to work with people's strengths." Clara supplemented that psychotherapy by seeing a new psychiatrist on an as-needed basis for medication adjustments. Both professionals, she says, treated her with empathy and respect.

In the early days of adjusting to her new diagnosis, Clara also took tremendous comfort from a self-help book that included positive narratives from people with bipolar disorder. "That helped me so much because these were people who were able to convey a sense of self-esteem and self-respect despite the fact that they had this diagnosis. And that was so important to me."

One of the things that most helped her to recover, however, was decidedly nonmedical. She rediscovered her love for playing the cello—an artistic outlet that she'd dropped at age 15. "My whole energy returned when I went back to playing the cello. I had a purpose and energy," she says. Playing chamber music, she developed a social network—something that she had longed for during her years of illness.

On a follow-up interview 1 year later, Clara had stopped psychotherapy. But her personal growth had clearly continued. "I've found a strong spiritual life involving regular meditation practice has enabled me to go past this need," she said. "The gift of a supportive spiritual community has made this possible. Ultimately, I think this practice has provided me with much more than anything in the domain of psychology or medicine, although a mood stabilizer is a precondition for enjoying this strength."

Clara also says her psychologist played an important role in her personal evolution from psychotherapy to spirituality simply by "recognizing and encouraging my spiritual interest." She also says, "It's nice to know there's a trustworthy professional to go back to if I need psychotherapy (in future)."

There is much this physician/patient has learned during her long journey: the importance of informed consent, of social connections, and of spiritual and artistic outlets in conjunction with psychotherapy and medications.

"My life is together now," she says, "but it's too bad that it didn't happen earlier."

THE GOOD STUFF

When we asked people what they did like about their psychiatrists, what kept them coming back and helped them in recovering. The responses were remarkably similar:

- He listened to me.
- He was honest with me.
- He offered hope.
- He empathized with what I was enduring.

Notice that none of these statements has anything to do with correct diagnosis or even treatment (which presumably is a given in the patient's mind). Rather, they are all along the lines of "people skills." As you have no doubt read in other textbooks, the element of trust is never more important than in a mental health professional's office. We would like you to really think about that for a moment, by trying to put yourself in your patient's shoes. Recognize that for some patients, your office may be the only place on earth they feel safe. It is your obligation to honor that trust. And when you do so, the rewards can be astounding.

Our book *Beyond Crazy*[3] is a collection of personal stories by and about people who have had contact with the mental health system, either as patients or family members. The roughly 40 people we profiled in the book spoke to us with honesty and clear-eyed reflection. All of them had recovered—they had moved beyond their diagnosis— and all of them had thought hard about what they'd been through.

Here's just one example. In Halifax, Nova Scotia, we met with a former nurse and health care administrator who first found herself on a psychiatric ward at the age of 47. Her rapidly cycling bipolar disorder was difficult to treat; she lost a high-paying job, a large home, and much of her self-esteem and went through many combinations of medica-

tions before finally finding the one that worked. The pain on her face as she described these years of struggle was painful to witness. But then we asked about the psychiatrist who had stuck with her throughout, and in an instant the woman's face lit up.

"She is phenomenal," we were told. Her explanation of what that word meant is every bit as illuminating:

"She's smart without pushing that at you. She's a fantastic listener. She keeps giving you hope; she's able to tell you when you're going through a certain thing what it will be like: 'Just hang in, hang tough, and it's going to get better.' There has not been one thing she's ever told me that hasn't proven to be the case. . . . She really knows you as a person and when you go there, if you're talking about your meds, or talking about something in the past, or a person in your life, she never has to refer to a paper. She just knows everything about you; she remembers it. It's like you are a person. . . . I could not believe there would be a light at the end of the tunnel, and she kept encouraging me and telling me about other patients who felt the same way, and [saying] it will happen."

This one quote, describing this one psychiatrist, encapsulates all of the "good doctor" qualities noted above.

On a personal note, I (Scott) can relate to a lot of what she says. When I returned to Toronto after being hospitalized in Hong Kong, I was eventually referred to a psychiatrist who had a good reputation dealing with bipolar affective disorder. I was taking a heavy dose of Haldol, shuffling instead of walking, and in a suicidal depression.

The depression, some might argue, was biochemical in nature. The truth was, I felt like dying because there was truly very little then left to live for. My career was in ruins; my reputation was toast, and I'd spent every dime we had. I was collecting disability that barely met the bills. Oh yes, and I had some $25,000 worth of antique Chinese furniture to try to sell.

The medications, too, were really hell. Despite the fact the psychosis was long gone, I had been kept on that heavy dose of Haldol. I could barely think, barely move. I didn't even know (because no one had told me) whether the physical symptoms I was experiencing were due to the meds or caused by the mental illness itself. It took herculean effort simply to get out of bed.

And so, doped to the gills and wanting to die, I was desperately hoping that this psychiatrist would be able to help. I drove (and probably shouldn't have) to the hospital where he practiced and waited outside his office. And waited. And waited.

The doctor was very late—which sent a signal to me that I wasn't very important—and was dismissively apologetic when he did finally arrive. He took a minimal, cursory history of what happened and prescribed medication. He said I'd be off work for months to come.

To his credit, the doctor did say he treated plenty of successful people with this disorder. The passing comment did offer some hope that things might improve. What was missing, however, was a sense that he was committed to helping me get well. To him, it seemed, I was simply another case. I left disappointed, drove home, and went back to bed.

Another appointment was made with a psychologist through an employee assistance program. I remember needing, desperately, someone to understand how this episode had completely shattered my life, how catastrophic it all was. The psychologist said he'd been through a rough time once, too. He explained how, in a hockey game, an errant puck had shattered his teeth and he'd had to have dentures made. He looked, expectantly, as if we should be bonding for life over this shared tragedy.

I remember telling him there was a big difference between a career-ending episode of mental illness and a set of false teeth. And there was, of course. Again, I left the office of a professional feeling disheartened.

Finally, some months later, we managed to make an appointment with another psychiatrist with a reputation as a bipolar specialist. The depression at this stage was so bleak there was a complete and utter absence of hope that things could possibly ever improve one iota. Together, Julia and I attended the appointment.

I explained, and we explained, everything that had happened. The psychiatrist took notes, listened intently. She also had, in her body language, attentiveness and eye contact, something I hadn't found during all the previous appointments. It was empathy.

"Can you help me?" I asked at the end of the appointment. I remember the quiet, hopeful desperation with which I asked the most important question of the session.

"Yes," she said with caring but professional confidence. And with that single word, for the first time since the whole nightmare began, I felt a glimmer of hope.

FAMILIES

We cannot emphasize enough that psychiatrists ignore family members at their peril. Good or bad, supportive or not, spouses, parents, and other close family members are going to play a major role in your patient's recovery. Why not use that to everyone's advantage? To do so, you'll need to do the following:

1. Find a way to include a family member in the treatment plan
2. Encourage that family member to find supports of her own

Unfortunately, neither of these appears to be common practice. One Canadian survey asked more than a thousand family members to describe their experiences with the mental health system; the responses were a litany of frustrations and unmet needs. Family members noted that patients are seen by mental health professionals for as little as a few minutes per week, while families live with them the rest of the time.

It was a very common sentiment. Too often, psychiatrists seem not to want to receive the kinds of information family members are uniquely equipped to provide—information that can make a real difference in a person's recovery.

Conversely, family members also feel short-changed on the receiving end of the information loop. "It seemed logical to me that an informed partner is essential in the overall recovery," one man wrote.[3] (His wife struggled for years with treatment-resistant bipolar disorder.) "After all, we spend far more time with the patient than doctors do. Yet I was often considered a nuisance for asking questions, and . . . was simply left out of the information loop."

Our situation was fairly common: Scott's mental health got worse before it got better, and that took a huge toll on both of us. In fact, research shows that family members can themselves become ill, both physically and mentally, because of the enormity of stress. Day after day, they ride the roller coaster with their unwell family member. Too often, the disorder becomes all consuming; family members, especially those living with an unwell person, forget to look after themselves. While their loved one consults with doctors, therapists, and other professionals, family members are too easily left entirely alone.

Which is pretty much what happened to me (Julia). Over the years, no doctor ever told me that I could or would make a difference in Scott's recovery. No doctor ever said I mattered in any way whatsoever. I simply was not on the radar screen. And yet we both agree that my role was an important one. It's that way for every caring family member (as the research confirms). If I had left Scott because I didn't get the supports I needed, it would have taken him longer to recover. It would have cost the health care system more money. And it would have cost Scott in much more profound ways.

A good clinician recognizes all of the above and works to keep the family support system strong while his patient struggles towards recovery. In at least one instance, I was, at my insistence, able to have an impact on Scott's psychiatric treatment. My involvement was never solicited, but in this case I felt driven to offer it. Although Scott was seeing his psychiatrist in Toronto regularly, his depression was not lifting. He was taking various dosages of several medications and on disability leave from work. The depression immobilized him; it got so bad that at times he could not even lift a fork to eat. He was also experiencing a lot of suicidal ideation—something that terrified me, even though he had promised his psychiatrist that he would never act on it.

I became so concerned that, with Scott's permission, I phoned the psychiatrist, describing in detail just how severe his symptoms had become. The psychiatrist did not offer any comment at the time; it was a one-way conversation. But she clearly listened. At the next appointment, she recommended Scott be hospitalized again. It was the last hospitalization to date—one neither of us relished. But it did seem to help.

Many family members report that if they do offer their observations, they're treated as if they are meddling, too pushy, or overly involved. No doubt there are cases in which family members can be part of the problem. Not every family is functional. But we have heard from many, many family members who have only their loved one's best interests at heart and would do anything to help, and who bemoan the fact that their role has been minimized or ignored.

There are obvious legal and ethical implications regarding confidentiality. But what we've heard from both patients and family members is that clinicians too often don't even ask whether a patient would like a member or members of his family involved.

We ask you to think hard about your own approach to dealing with family members and your willingness both to include them and to acknowledge that this inclusion can be an important part of your patient's treatment plan.

PLEASE, HAVE A SEAT

We don't have a clue what you're taught, if anything, about how to set up your office. But, based on personal experience and what we've been told by others, we'll try to offer a few tips.

Of course, since it's the place where you'll be spending many hours every day, you'll want it to be comfortable for you. But a driving concern should really be, how comfortable is this for the patient? (One psychiatrist we know had his walls dominated by large works of art, some of which were truly disturbing. It may well suit his personal tastes, but it's not a particularly welcoming venue for patients!)

Personal practices and tastes vary, but our sense is that a mental health professional's office should include comfortable furniture that puts the patient at ease. Where possible, we've been told by patients that they appreciate having a choice of where to sit down, whether in chair or on a couch. (And we don't necessarily mean lying on a couch like the Freudian New Yorker cartoons. Just sitting on a comfy couch can put some people at ease.)

What is less preferred, but still common, is a rigid seating arrangement where there are simply two chairs in the clinician's office, directly facing each other. There's no choice whatsoever. When you're feeling powerless, as most people are as they set foot in this kind of office, even having the option of selecting a seat that makes you feel comfortable is important.

Lighting can also make a difference. Adjustable lighting from floor lamps or adjustable ceiling spots can make your office more conducive to a trusting conversation. Fluorescent ceiling lighting tends to have an institutional, clinical feel.

One psychiatrist we know of has a couple of different chairs and a very soft couch. She keeps a plate with small polished stones on a low table in front of the couch. She even has a candle on that table. She tells us some patients instinctively pick up a stone and hold it in their hands while they speak. Some have asked her what the candle is for. She tells them, simply, "Some people are more comfortable speaking by candlelight." Many, she's found, ask if they could try that.

We're not suggesting that you stock your office with incense and lava lamps. But a choice of seating options, relaxing and inoffensive artwork, a few plants, and some options for lighting can help put your patient at ease.

PLEASE, HAVE A BED

Hospitalization is, of course, a necessary option for some patients at certain points in their illness. And it can be a frightening prospect for some—especially those who have had previous, negative experiences on inpatient wards. It can also be frightening for those who have never been hospitalized but who have many preconceptions about what the "loony bin" will be like.

In cases where hospitalization is required, we believe patients appreciate being told what to expect during their stay. It's worth explaining, for example, that the ward will not allow "sharps," and that any razors, scissors, etc. will likely have to be handed over on admission. It can be quite a surprise to a patient unaware of the practice to have to surrender such items when walking through a hospital door. Similarly, your patients will appreciate being told if there are night checks on their ward. It's a bit disconcerting to the uninitiated to have a nurse shine a flashlight in your eyes at 2:00 in the morning.

Encourage your patients to take comfortable clothes, some reading material, and anything else that might make them comfortable during their stay. But perhaps the most important thing you can do during a patient's hospital stay is the following: make a professional visit.

Remember, being on a psychiatric ward is unlike a stay in other hospital wards. Friends, and even family, often don't want to visit the place. People rarely send flowers or cards. Other patients in varying degrees of distress may make it an unpleasant experience. Your patient may be assessed by an unfamiliar staff psychiatrist, social worker, occupational therapist, etc. It can be a very isolating experience. So in cases where you have a long-term therapeutic relationship with the patient, we'd urge you, when realistically possible, to make a professional visit to check up on your patient.

We would also urge you, except in cases where hospitalization is required by mental health legislation considerations, to explore whether other alternatives might be more appropriate. There are a growing number of "safe houses" for people in crisis, and they have a good track record. Such safe houses generally are comfortable, short-stay respites with on-site support. They are frequently built in renovated homes and house relatively small numbers of clients. They are often based on nonmedical models, meaning the emphasis is on supportive listening and practical advice to help someone through a period of crisis.

Unfortunately, psychiatrists sometimes confuse *nonmedical* with *anti-psychiatry*. Most safe houses that we're aware of actually welcome support from the medical model and encourage clients with psychiatrists to maintain their contact and to keep taking medications during their visit.

Ultimately, whether your patients belong in a hospital or a safe house (or simply back at home) will depend on the severity of their symptoms, whether they pose a danger to themselves or others, and what your own clinical instincts tell you. We would urge you, however, to consider alternatives such as safe houses when the nature of distress seems to be more of an episodic crisis rather a clinical deterioration.

We'd also encourage you, where appropriate, to discuss these options with your patient. The cases that follow illustrate what the experience of hospitalization can be like.

THE UNSPOKEN DIAGNOSIS: STIGMA

"We are all differently organized; and that I feel acutely is no more my fault (though it is my misfortune) than that another feels not, is his. We did not make ourselves, and if the elements of unhappiness abound more in the nature of one man more than other, he is but the more entitled to our pity and our forebearance."

—Lord Byron, 1813

Stigma is the single biggest reason why we, the authors, do what we do—why we share our own personal stories and why we've written two books and given dozens of speeches across the country. Stigma is not a figment of a patient's imagination. It is real; it is pervasive (although, we hope, gradually declining), and it will have a profound effect on many of the people you treat.

Being perceived as a lesser human being plays with your mind. It impedes recovery and can have a dramatic impact on a person's day-to-day living. Here's just one quote from a World Psychiatric Association report[1]: "Stigma can become the main cause for social isolation, inability to find work, alcohol and drug abuse, homelessness, and excessive institutionalization, all of which decrease the chance for recovery."

We could cite many, many studies on this subject, but let us offer here just a few comments from the people who've lived with stigma first-hand: "We knew we had a stigma attached to us," said a high school teacher who'd spent time in a psychiatric hospital. "We knew the visions people would get on the 'outside' if we told them we were in a psychiatric hospital. . . . But deep down inside, you are still you. It may be lost for a while, but you are there."

Ian Chovil recalls hanging around with a group of other young men who shared his diagnosis of schizophrenia. They also shared something else: a desire to connect with the world beyond their illness. "So we'd see a group of women. And we'd think, well, what are we going to say? 'Hi, I have schizophrenia and I'm on disability.' I mean, there was no way you could approach or talk to anybody. You feel like a real loser, no one would ever want to talk to you."

Clearly, stigma can have an impact on virtually every aspect of a person's life: from work to love life and beyond. One survey, conducted by the Canadian Mental Health Association, Ontario Division, asked people who worked in the mental health field for their opinions on how stigma affects social and family life. Based on their personal experience and those of their clients, the respondents said stigma impaired the following:

- Social and family relationships (84%)
- Employment (78%)
- Housing (48%)
- Inclusion in the community (22%)
- Self-esteem (20%)

As a document published by the World Federation for Mental Health[5] points out, misconceptions still abound. "Those with mental illnesses, some would say, are getting what they deserve as a result of their own personal inadequacies," it states. "They are perceived, for example, as lacking the motivational resolve to overcome their problems, as lazy, as self-indulgent in their emotions; they simply have given in to stress and failed to pull themselves up by their bootstraps as would a person of stronger character."[4]

In truth, many of the people with mental disorder that we've met are among the strongest people we know. You'd have to be, given the misconceptions that abound. Public understanding of mental illness, though growing, is still poor. Many wrongly associate a diagnosis of mental disorder with violence, developmental delays, or laziness.

One person experiencing the stigma of mental illness described her situation as follows: "My name is Catherine and I am from Montreal. In 1994 I had a big psychosis and was hospitalized for 6 weeks. Though my breakdown did not occur at work, I was very open and told my coworkers what happened to me. Since then they do not treat me the same way. First of all, they believe that I am not capable of handling stress, so they believe that I am not capable of handling certain tasks. Also, I have overheard one of my coworkers tell a new employee that I had gone wacko. I work part-time now, and people think that I am just lazy and that I go home early to watch soap operas. I find myself in the situation that I must find myself another job where nobody knows my past, so that I can be treated like a normal human being again."[1]

To be treated like a normal human being. It's all that anyone wants. And when mental health professionals—who are themselves stigmatized to a certain extent within the medical community—unknowingly use language that stigmatizes their patients, it can make things worse. We cringe, and so do others, when we hear them refer to people as "a schizophrenic," or "an anorexic." Use of such labels as nouns tends to define the person as the illness.

This is more than mere political correctness. Having a mental illness can be terribly isolating because society looks at the label instead of the person. When we reduce people to these labels (as opposed to "John, with a diagnosis of schizophrenia"), we dehumanize them.

We'd also encourage you to *ask* your patients or clients, once you've established a therapeutic relationship, if stigma is a concern for them. If they say it is, ask how it has affected their lives. You'd be surprised at the myriad of ways stigma can impair one's opportunities, and ultimately, one's self-perception. You may not be able to fix society's attitudes, but you can acknowledge and empathize with the very real pain those attitudes cause.

We'll close this segment with an ugly but true incident that illustrates just how widespread stigma can be. It happened, quietly, on the manicured grounds of a major psychiatric hospital in Toronto in 1997. There, just a few meters from a busy sidewalk, was a simple sign. It was supposed to read: "Dogs must be kept on a leash." Except someone had crossed out the first word and replaced it with something else. It now read, "Nuts must be kept on a leash."

That sign remained for 8 months, until someone sprayed black paint over the offending word.

Now, imagine a slightly different scenario. Picture a similar sign on the grounds of a synagogue. If the word "dogs" had been replaced by "Jews," people would have been out-

raged. The police likely would have been called. The act would have been described, accurately, as a hate crime. And, rest assured, the sign would have been replaced immediately. Instead, for 8 long months, that sign at the hospital remained unaltered. It would have been impossible for staff to miss it. It would have been impossible for patients to miss it. I would have been impossible for the public to miss it. And yet no one did a thing.

We'd encourage you to do your part. And the mere recognition that stigma plays a role in the lives of your patients is an important first step.

RECOVERY

As we reach the conclusion of this chapter, we're faced with the realization that there is still much more we'd like to say. So much that you could almost build a book around the topic. Except we don't *want* to write another book about mental health, at least not now. And that, believe it or not, is significant. It's significant because I (Scott) don't want mental illness to play a prominent role in my life anymore. Nor, rest assured, does Julia.

We know that when mental illness strikes, it can take over nearly every facet of a person's life. His personal relationships, professional aspirations, and even his financial situation can sometimes be rattled to their very core. The illness becomes the all-consuming beast, the thing around which everything else in life starts to revolve. (And this is true for family members as well.) Will the medications work? When will I get back to work? What will people think of me? Will I be mad forever? Will I ever enjoy life again?

We know of many people who obsess on these issues—not because of any obsessional thought disorder, but because mental illness *is* a catastrophe. Or it certainly has the potential to become one.

When I finally became symptom free, I still didn't feel "better." I felt like a manic depressive, with all the flaws, frailties, and uncertainty that go with that package. I felt that way for a long time and tried to find some meaning in the experience through the books listed in the Recommended Readings list.

Most important, though, is that I had unknowingly and unwillingly *adopted* the role of patient—a role of diminished expectations and unpredictability that we'd been told at every turn our lives would now consist of, all the way through from that initial diagnosis with the social worker in Saskatoon.

Julia, bless her, never lost faith, nor did family members and a small but loyal circle of friends. But many in the mental health system, unfortunately, repeatedly gave me the message that my life was forever altered and that things would never again be "normal"—with one important exception: the psychiatrist who told me she would help me.

That psychiatrist spent a great deal of time trying to explore the impact that single, rollicking mania had on our lives. She listened to me vent about the treatment I'd received from my employer and my despair at how friends had turned away. She tried different medications when the side effects of one became intolerable and had give-and-take discussions about my desire to explore alternative methods of therapy. She was also willing to accept that psychiatry, despite the current biological revolution, does not yet have all the answers. In short, she respected me as a person. And in doing so, she fostered in me a sense of hope that a life beyond simply being a psychiatric patient was achievable. And it was a life worth living.

In 1993, Dr. William Anthony wrote an eloquent paper about recovery.[5] In it, he stated that "a common denominator in recovery is the presence of people who believe in and stand by the person in need of recovery." His reasoning for this, based on decades of interviews with people who had recovered, was as follows: "Seemingly universal in the recovery concept is the notion that critical to one's recovery is a person or persons in whom one can trust to 'be there' in times of need."

The manner in which you choose to "be there" will ultimately define the kind of clinician you become. We hope, and trust, you'll choose with a blend of wisdom, professionalism, and compassion.

Do that, and your patients will do more than thank you. Eventually, they'll get on with living again.

REFERENCES

1. Simmie S, Nunes J: *The last taboo: a survival guide to mental health care in Canada,* Toronto, 2001, McClelland & Stewart.
2. Goldbloom RB: *Pediatric clinical skills,* ed 3, Philadelphia, 2003, WB Saunders.
3. Simmie S, Nunes J: *Beyond crazy: journeys through mental illness,* Toronto, 2002, McClelland & Stewart.
4. Wahl OF: *The stigma of mental illness,* 1999. World Federation for Mental Health Website: http://www. wfmh.org/stigma.htm
5. Anthony WA: Recovery from mental illness: the guiding vision of the mental health service system in the 1990s. *Psychosoc Rehabil J* 16(4):11–23, 1993. Retrieved from http://www.bu.edu/cpr/catalog/articles/1993/anthony1993c.pdf

RECOMMENDED READINGS

Capponi P: *Upstairs in the crazy house,* Toronto, 1992, Viking.
Goodwin DW, Guze SB: *Psychiatric diagnosis,* Oxford, 1996, Oxford University Press.
Pert CB: *Molecules of emotion,* New York, 1999, Touchstone.
Redfield Jamison K: *An unquiet mind,* New York, 1995, Alfred A. Knopf.
Solomon A: *The noonday demon: an atlas of depression,* New York, 2003, Simon & Schuster.
Styron W: *Darkness visible,* New York, 1992, Vintage Books.

Index